Orbital Apex and Periorbital Skull Base Diseases

Tak Lap POON • Calvin MAK
Hunter Kwok Lai YUEN
Editors

Orbital Apex and Periorbital Skull Base Diseases

Springer

Editors
Tak Lap POON
Department of Neurosurgery
Queen Elizabeth Hospital
Hong Kong, China

Calvin MAK
Department of Neurosurgery
Queen Elizabeth Hospital
Hong Kong, China

Hunter Kwok Lai YUEN
Ophthalmology and Visual Sciences
Hong Kong Eye Hospital
Hong Kong, China

ISBN 978-981-99-2988-7 ISBN 978-981-99-2989-4 (eBook)
https://doi.org/10.1007/978-981-99-2989-4

This Springer imprint is published by the registered company Springer Nature Singapore Pte Ltd.
The registered company address is: 152 Beach Road, #21-01/04 Gateway East, Singapore 189721, Singapore

Foreword

I am privileged to be given the opportunity to read all the chapters of this book *Orbital Apex and Periorbital Skull Base Diseases* and honoured to be asked to introduce the book. This truly multidisciplinary collection of manuscripts is in a concise and appropriately referenced textbook format. Authors come from specialists of the orbit and its neighbourhoods, i.e. ophthalmology, neurosurgery and otorhinolaryngology. The materials do not come from "copy-and-pasted" paragraphs of the published journal articles or textbooks. Each chapter is meticulously written, based on materials from their own clinical practice and teaching, through their subspecialty development, with passion for the region. Authors are congratulated for providing a readable textbook on the subject for clinicians making early diagnosis and appropriate treatment.

Neuro-medical Centre, HKU-Shenzhen Hospital
Shenzhen, Guangdong, China
The Chinese University of Hong Kong
Hong Kong SAR, China

Wai S. Poon

Contents

Part I Surgical Anatomy

1 **Optic Canal** ... 3
Tak Lap POON

2 **Anatomy of the Orbital Apex** ... 7
Shuk Wan Joyce Chow

3 **Superior Orbital Fissure and Inferior Orbital Fissure** ... 13
Atsushi Okano, Stefan Lieber, and Shunya Hanakita

4 **Cavernous Sinus and Internal Carotid Artery** ... 21
Ramez W. Kirollos

5 **Paranasal Sinuses** ... 33
Hung Wai Cho

Part II Diagnosis and Radiology

6 **History** ... 39
Sai Lok Chu

7 **Physical Examination** ... 43
Carmen K. M. Chan

8 **Principles of Imaging for Orbital Apex Pathologies** ... 51
Koel Wei Sum Ko and Wai Lun Poon

Part III Spectrum of Diseases

9 **Optic Nerve Neoplasm** ... 67
Noel C. Y. Chan

10 **Orbital Apex Vascular Disease** ... 85
Affan Permana Priyambodo and Zharifah Nafisah Fauziyyah

11 **Orbital Apex Infective Diseases** ... 97
Matthew C. W. Lam and Carmen K. M. Chan

12 **Orbital Apex Inflammatory and Infectious Diseases** ... 103
Yuk Fai Cheung

13 **Periorbital Skull Base Neoplasms** ... 115
Ehsan Dowlati, Max Fleisher, and Walter C. Jean

14 **Periorbital Bony Diseases** 131
Shuk Wan Joyce Chow

15 **Traumatic Optic Neuropathy** 143
Ka Hing Lok

Part IV 360 Degree of Surgical Approaches

16 **Choices of Approaches** 151
Stacey Lam and Hunter Kwok Lai YUEN

17 **Transcranial Approach to Optic Canal and Orbital Apex** 159
Tak Lap POON

18 **Transcranial Approach to Cavernous Sinus and Middle Cranial Fossa** 165
King Fai Kevin Cheng and Wai Man Lui

19 **Infratemporal Fossa and Orbital Apex** 175
Kentaro Watanabe

20 **Endoscopic Endonasal Approach to Optic Canal and Orbital Apex** 187
Karen Kar Wun Chan, Christine Chi Ying Lam, and Kelvin Kam Lung Chong

21 **Endoscopic Endonasal Approach to Cavernous Sinus and Middle Cranial Fossa** 195
Arianna Fava, Paolo di Russo, Thibault Passeri, Lorenzo Giammattei, and Sébastien Froelich

22 **Endoscopic Endonasal Approach to the Infratemporal Fossa** 211
Stefan Lieber and Sébastien Froelich

23 **Endoscopic Transorbital Approach to the Optic Canal and Orbital Apex** 223
Ben Ng, Hun Ho Park, and Calvin MAK

24 **Endoscopic Transorbital Approach for Orbital Apex Lesions** 229
Chiman Jeon and Doo-Sik Kong

25 **Endoscopic Transorbital Approach to Infratemporal Fossa** 233
Calvin MAK and Ben Ng

26 **Surgical Treatment for Traumatic Optic Neuropathy** 239
Yi Kui Zhang, Hunter Kwok Lai YUEN, and Wencan Wu

Part V Radiotherapy for Neoplasm

27 **External Radiotherapy for Orbital Apex Lesions: Principles and Practice** 249
Jeannie Chik, K. M. Cheung, Chi Ching Law, James Chow, Gavin Cheung, K. H. Au, C. W. Y. Kong, and K. H. Wong

28 **External Photon Radiotherapy for Benign Orbital Apex Lesions** 257
K. M. Cheung, Jeannie Chik, Christine Kong, and K. H. Wong

29 **External Photon Radiotherapy for Malignant Orbital Apex Lesions** 273
Jeannie Chik, K. M. Cheung, James Chow, Gavin Cheung, C. W. Y. Kong, and K. H. Wong

30 **Proton Therapy for Malignant Orbital Apex Lesions** 283
Chi Ching Law

About the Editors

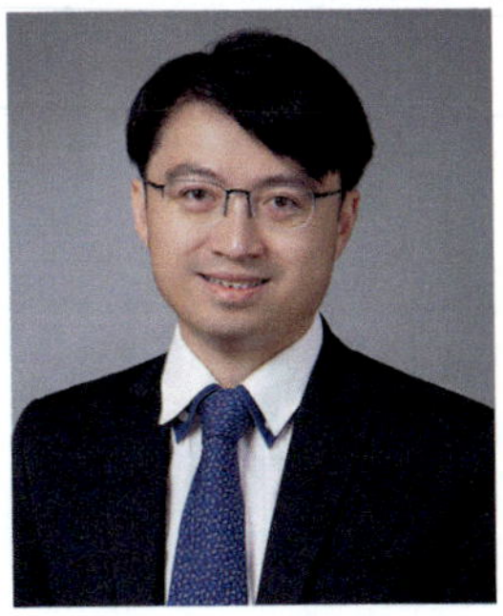

Calvin MAK is a consultant neurosurgeon at Queen Elizabeth Hospital in Hong Kong and is also appointed as Clinical Associate Professor (Honorary) of the Department of Surgery in the Chinese University of Hong Kong. He graduated from the University of Hong Kong and obtained his FRCSEd(SN) fellowship. His main clinical and research interests are endoscopic and complex skull base surgery. Dr. Mak performed the first endoscopic transorbital surgery for brain tumours in Hong Kong, and is course director for dissection courses on endoscopic transorbital surgery. He has been invited as faculty and instructor for various international skull base courses and meetings. Dr. Mak currently serves as Honorary Secretary of the Hong Kong Neurosurgical Society, first vice-president of the Hong Kong Neuro-oncology Society, executive board member of the Asian Congress of Neurological Surgeons, delegates to the Executive Committee of AASNS and WFNS, and council member of the China Greater Bay Area Neurosurgical Alliance. He is also a pioneer in smart hospital development and digital transformation of hospitals in Hong Kong. Dr. Mak was awarded the Ten Outstanding Young Persons in Hong Kong in 2022. He also received the Outstanding Team Award in 2021 and the Young Achiever Award in 2020 from the Hospital Authority of Hong Kong for his contributions and aspirations.

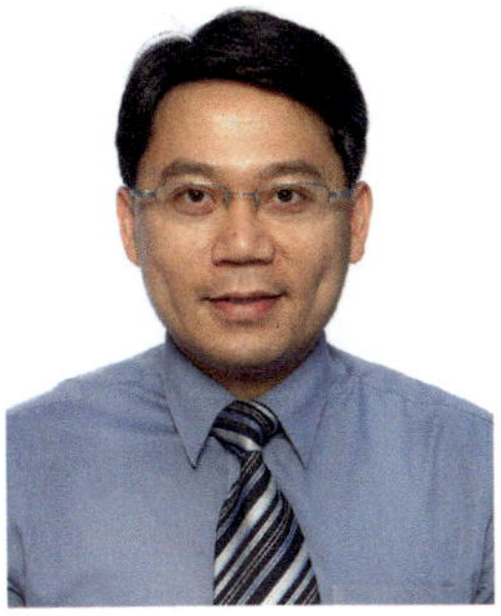

Hunter Kwok Lai YUEN is Hong Kong Eye Hospital Deputy Hospital Chief Executive, consultant ophthalmologist and head of Orbital and Oculoplastic Service. He is also the chairman of Ophthalmology Coordinating Committee of the Hospital Authority in Hong Kong.

Prof Yuen is the Clinical Professor (Hon) of the Department of Ophthalmology and Visual Sciences, the Chinese University of Hong Kong, and Honorary Professor of Department of Ophthalmology, Hong Kong University. He has published more than 110 peer-reviewed international publications and numerous book chapters.

Prof Yuen is the past president of Asia Pacific Society of Ophthalmic Plastic and Reconstructive Surgery (APSOPRS), vice-president of International Society of Dacryology and Dry Eye (ISDDE) and secretary general of Asia Pacific Society of Ocular Oncology and Pathology (APSOOP). He is a member of Orbital Society, fellow of Academy of Asia-Pacific Professors of Ophthalmology (AAPPO) and one of the Ten Young Outstanding Persons in Hong Kong in 2007. He was also awarded with the Asia Pacific Academy of Ophthalmology (APAO) Yasuo Tano Travel Grant, APAO Distinguished Service Award, APAO Achievement Award, APAO Outstanding Service in Prevention of Blindness Award and APAO Senior Achievement Award.

With his outstanding involvement and achievements in numerous NGOs and charity activities, Prof Yuen was awarded with the Hong Kong Volunteer Award in 2011. Prof Yuen was also invited as visiting Professor of Zhejiang University, China; Dalian Medical University, China; Shantou University Medical College, China; and King Khaled Eye Specialist Hospital (KKESH), Saudi Arabia. Prof Yuen was selected as 'Asia-Pacific Eye 100', one of the 100 most influential Ophthalmologists 2022 by the *Asia-Pacific Journal of Ophthalmology* (APJO).

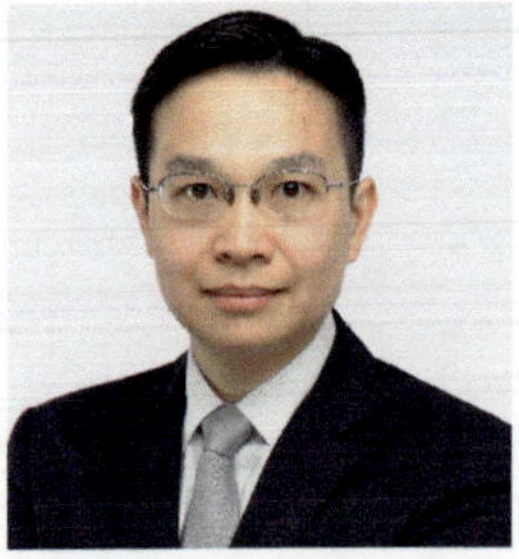

Tak Lap POON graduated from the medical school of the University of Hong Kong in 1998. In 2006, he stayed in London with Mr. William Harkness from the Great Ormond Street Hospital and Mr. Andrew McEvoy from the National Hospital for Neurology and Neurosurgery as his overseas training in the fields of epilepsy surgery and stereotactic and functional neurosurgery. Currently, Dr. Poon is the Deputy Chief of Service and Consultant Neurosurgeon of the Queen Elizabeth Hospital, Clinical Associate Professor (Honorary) of the Department of Surgery, Chinese University of Hong Kong, and coordinator of the neurosurgical services including stereotactic and functional neurosurgery, epilepsy surgery, movement disorder, stereotactic radiosurgery, and endovascular surgery. His interested sub-specialties in Neurosurgery include movement disorder surgery, epilepsy surgery, awake craniotomy, stereotactic and functional neurosurgery, stereotactic radiosurgery, and endovascular intervention. Besides, Dr. Poon is the current President of the Hong Kong Epilepsy Society, a council member of the Hong Kong Movement Disorder Society, a board member of the executive committee of the Asian-Australasian Society for Stereotactic and Functional Neurosurgery, and a council member of the Hong Kong Society of Interventional and Therapeutic NeuroRadiology.

Part I

Surgical Anatomy

Optic Canal

1

Tak Lap POON

Abstract

The optic canal is the connecting bridge between the orbital and intracranial compartments. The connections include bony structures, vasculatures, and nervous tissues. Pathologies around the orbital apex can also spread in or out from the orbital side to the intracranial side and vice versa. This chapter is intended to describe the relevant surgical anatomy and the anatomical and physiological variants.

Keywords

Optic canal · Orbital apex · Optic nerve · Hypophyseal artery · Ophthalmic artery

1.1 Introduction

The orbital apex is the area between the orbit and intracranial space. The human orbit communicated with the intracranial cavity via the middle cranial fossa through two major channels, namely, the optic canal and superior orbital fissure. The optic canal is a funnel-like tubal structure as part of the sphenoidal bone that extends from the optic foramen to the orbital apex. The optic canal transmits the optic nerve, meningeal sheaths, ophthalmic artery, and sympathetic nerve fibers [1].

1.2 Embryology

The formation of cartilaginous optic foramen happens in the third month of gestation. Ossification of foramen subsequently starts and completes between 12 and 17 weeks of gestation. When the fetus reaches the fifth month of development, the bony optic foramen will be transformed into a bony optic canal, and this transformation is closely attributed to the developmental process of the optic strut into the anterior-inferior and posterior-superior components.

The development of orbit in fetal status usually follows a linear growth. Previous research showed that the optic canal reaches the maximal growth when the length of the fetus approaches 400 mm. There is a gender difference with male fetuses usually having a larger diameter of orbit than that of female fetuses.

1.3 Bony Boundaries of Optic Canal

The optic canal with its intraorbital end (optic foramen) is bordered by the body of the sphenoidal bone medially, the superior root of the lesser wing superiorly, the optic strut inferolaterally, and the anterior clinoid process laterally (Fig. 1.1). There is no gender difference in optic canal shape and dimensions of the infraorbital foramen (IOF) and supraorbital foramen (SOF) [2]. On endoscopic view

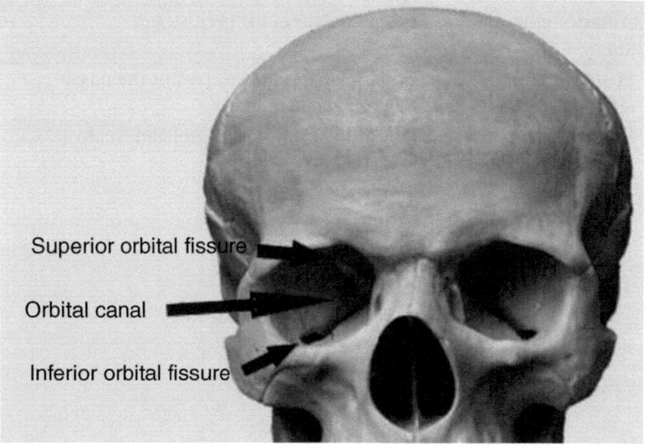

Fig. 1.1 Bony relationship of the optic canal

T. L. POON (✉)
Department of Neurosurgery, Queen Elizabeth Hospital, Hong Kong SAR, China
e-mail: ptl220@ha.org.hk

T. L. POON et al. (eds.), *Orbital Apex and Periorbital Skull Base Diseases*, https://doi.org/10.1007/978-981-99-2989-4_1

via transsphenoidal route, the optic protuberance, carotid protuberance, medial opticocarotid recess, and lateral opticocarotids are important bony landmarks related to the optic canal [3, 4].

1.4 Vasculature

There are two main arterial supplies to the optic nerve along the course from the intracranial to the intraorbital compartment. The hypophyseal artery mainly supplies the intracranial and intracanalicular parts of the optic nerve, while the ophthalmic artery supplies the rest of the optic nerve via the long ciliary artery and central retinal artery. The ophthalmic artery arises from the internal carotid artery in different positions. About 40% arise from the upper internal part of the carotid artery, 30% arise from the frontal internal part, 20% emerge from the upper central part, and 10% left at the end of the cavernous segment of the carotid artery [5]. The ophthalmic artery runs inferior to the optic nerve within the optic canal. One study showed that ~13% of the ophthalmic artery locates infero-medially to the optic nerve and, in about half of the cases, the artery moves infero-laterally along its course [6]. It is physically separated from the optic nerve by a dural barrier. Rarely, the ophthalmic artery enters the orbit through a separate bony canal.

Branches of the ophthalmic artery and the supplying anatomical structures are stated in Table 1.1.

Table 1.1 Branches of the ophthalmic artery and their supplying structures

Arterial branches	Supplying structures
Central retinal artery	Inner layer of retina
Long posterior ciliary artery	Iris through the circulus arteriosus major
Short posterior ciliary artery	Choroid, ciliary process
Lacrimal artery	Lacrimal gland, anterior portion of the eyeball and part of the eyelid
Anterior ethmoidal artery	Ethmoidal air cells, periosteum
Posterior ethmoidal artery	Ethmoidal air sinuses, part of the nasal mucosa and septum
Supraorbital artery	Part of the orbit, face, forehead, scalp

1.5 Nerves

The optic nerve is the only cranial nervous structure that is housed in the optic canal. It is the second cranial nerve with continuity of cranial meninges and serves as the transmission of vision signals from the retina to the visual cortex. The postganglionic sympathetic nerves arising from the carotid plexus run along with the optic nerve [7].

1.6 Cranial Aperture of the Optic Canal and Morphometry

The proximal end of the optic canal is called the cranial aperture of the optic canal (CAOC). It transmits the optic nerve, ophthalmic artery, and sympathetic fibers between the orbital cavity and middle cranial base. The morphometry and the shape had been studied widely to have a better understanding of this complex structure [8]. Ten et al. have studied the computed tomography images of 200 children to analyze the shape, location, and diameters of CAOC [9]. The followings are the measurements:

- Area: 17.53 ± 2.8 mm^2
- Width: 6.12 ± 0.84 mm
- Height: 4.35 ± 0.64 mm
- Angle of optic canal: $39.28 \pm 5.3°$ (axial plane) and $16.01 \pm 6.76°$ (sagittal plane)
  (The area, width, and height are measured in the coronal plane on the CT scan. The angle of the optic canal is measured in both axial and sagittal planes on the CT scan.)

It was observed in Ten et al.'s study that the height and the width of CAOC remain almost static after the prepubescent period, while the area will continue to evolve during the growth period of time. The shape of CAOC in the coronal plane was classified into four types (Fig. 1.2). The proportion of different types is teardrop 46.5%, triangular 39%, oval 11.8%, and round 2.8%. The shape is associated with surrounding important bony structures including the anterior clinoid process and optic strut.

Zhang et al. have studied on the computerized tomography (CT) the optic canals of 335 adult patients. The mean

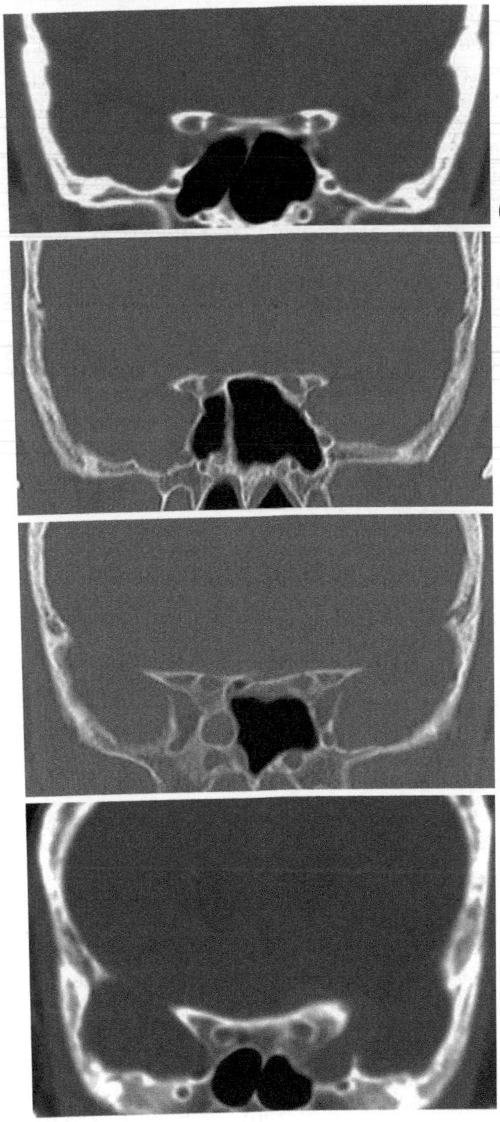

Fig. 1.2 Types of cranial aperture of the optic canal (CAOC). (**a**) Teardrop shape, (**b**) Triangular shape, (**c**) Oval shape, (**d**) Round shape

canal length was 5.61 ± 2.22 mm. The right optic canal was larger than the left (the right side was 12.12 mm, while the left side was 11.55 mm) [10].

1.7 Physiologic Variants

Variants of optic canal include duplicated optical canal and keyhole anomaly. A duplicated optic canal is rarely found in ~0.6–3% of the population [11]. If duplication is present, the optic nerve usually courses through the higher canal. Keyhole anomaly occurs in ~1.6–2.6% of orbits, of which the optic canal has a grooved floor with a keyhole appearance [12]. Along with some duplicated optic canal cases, the origin of the ophthalmic artery is at the intracavernous part of the internal carotid artery. In these cases, the ophthalmic artery could pass through the superior orbital fissure instead of the optic canal [13].

1.8 Translaminar Pressure Difference (TLPD)

Since the optic canal is the narrowest point of the optic nerve subarachnoid space, it creates a watershed region for cerebrospinal fluid (CSF). The translaminar pressure difference (TLPD) is derived by the pressure gradient between the intraocular pressure (IOP) and the cerebrospinal fluid (CSF) pressure in the subarachnoid space surrounding the optic nerve. The concept of TLPD was first introduced in the twentieth century by Kasmir Noishevsky. The microscopic anatomy of the optic canal including the size, intracanalicular dural-pial adhesions, and the resultant patent subarachnoid space may alter the TLPD. Examples of ocular pathologies that involve TLPD are glaucoma, papilloedema, or space flight-associated neuro-ocular syndrome (SANS). Pircher et al. have retrospectively reviewed the CT images of the cranium and orbits in 56 cases with normal tension glaucoma (NTG) and 56 age- and gender-matched subjects without optic-related diseases. It was found that patients with NTG house a significantly smaller optic canal cross-sectional area with a mean area of 14.5 ± 3.5 mm^2 [14].

1.9 Additional Canal Connecting to the Orbit with the Cranial Cavity

Normally orbits are connected to the cranial cavity via the optic canal and the superior orbital fissure. In addition, there are other inconstant canals named orbitomeningeal foramen (Fig. 1.3). A review study of 1000 skulls and 50 CT images found that orbitomeningeal foramina were present in ~60% of skulls and ~54% of CT images. Usually two to five foramina were identified. The meningo-lacrimal and meningo-ophthalmic arteries and meningeal branches of the lacrimal and supraorbital arteries, together with some other minor small arteries, are vasculatures that passed through the foramina [15].

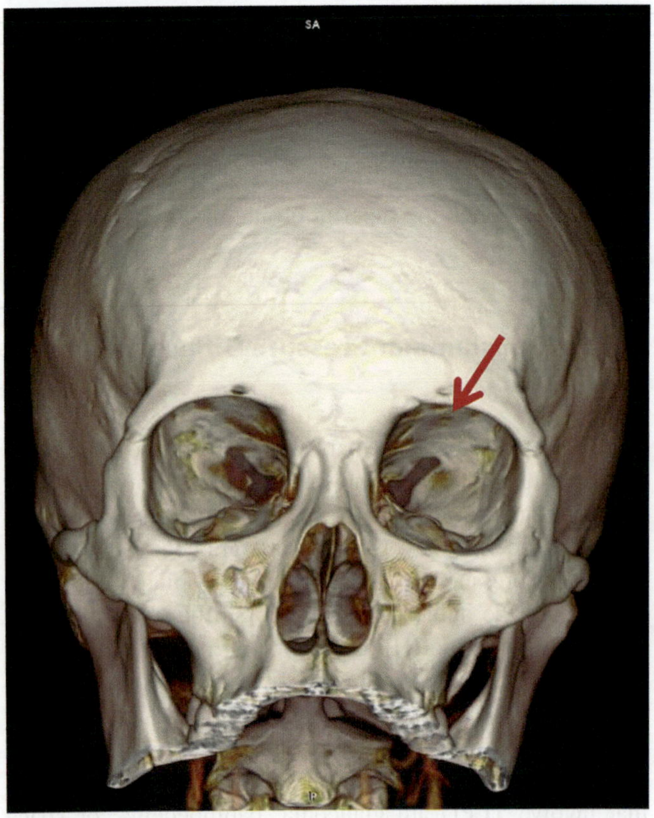

Fig. 1.3 The orbitomeningeal foramen in the left orbit CT scan (red arrow)

References

1. Maniscalco JF, Habai MB. Microanatomy of the optic canal. J Neurosurg. 1978;48:402–6.
2. Sinanoglu A, Orhan K, Kursun S, Inceoglu B, Oztas B. Evaluation of optic canal and surrounding structures using cone beam computed tomography: considerations for maxillofacial surgery. J Craniofac Surg. 2016;27:1327–30.
3. Hart CK, Theodosopoulos PV, Zimmer LA. Anatomy of the optic canal: a computed tomography study of endoscopic nerve decompression. Ann Otol Rhinol Laryngol. 2009;118(12):839–44.
4. Yilmazlar S, Saraydaroglu O, Korfali. Anatomical aspects in the transsphenoidal-transethmoidal approach to the optic canal: an anatomic-cadaveric study. J Craniomaxillofac Surg. 2012;40:198–205.
5. Ganiusmen O, Citak G, Samancioglu A, Korkmaz H, Binatli AO. Anatomic evaluation of the ophthalmic artery in optic canal compression: a cadaver study of 20 optic canals. Turk Neurosurg. 2017;27(1):31–6.
6. Zoli M, Manzoli L, Bonfatti R, Ruggeri A, Mariani GA, Bacci A, Sturiale C, Pasquini E, Billi AM, Frank G, Cocco L, Mazzatenta D. Endoscopic endonasal anatomy of the ophthalmic artery in the optic canal. Acta Neurochir. 2016;158:1343–50.
7. Govsa F, Erturk M, Kayalioglu G, Pinar Y, Ozer MA, Ozgur T. Neuro-arterial relations in the region of the optic canal. Surg Radiol Anat. 1999;21:329–35.
8. Kalthur S, Periyasamy R, Kumar S, Gupta C, D'Souza AS. A morphometric evaluation of the optic canal: comparative study between computerized tomographic study and direct anatomic study. Saudi J Med Med Sci. 2015;3(3):204–8.
9. Ten B, Beger O, Esen K, Adanir SS, Hamzaoglu EC, Cicek F, Taghipour P, Kara E, Vayisoglu Y, Talas DU. Anatomic features of the cranial aperture of the optic canal in children: a radiologic study. Surg Radiol Anat. 2021;43:187–99.
10. Zhang X, Lee Y, Olson D, Fleischman D. Evaluation of optic canal anatomy and symmetry using CT. BMJ Open Ophthalmol. 2019;4:e000302.
11. Bertelli E. Metoptic canal, duplication of the optic canal and Warwick's foramen in human orbits. Anat Sci Int. 2014;89:34–45.
12. Engin O, Adriaensen GFJPM, Hoefnagels FWA, Saeed P. A systemic review of the surgical anatomy of the orbital apex. Surg Radiol Anat. 2021;43:169–78.
13. Regoli M, Bertelli E. The revised anatomy of the canals connecting the orbit with the cranial cavity. Orbit. 2017;36(2):110–7.
14. Pircher A, Montali M, Berberat J, Remonda L, Killer HE. The optic canal: a bottleneck for cerebrospinal fluid dynamics in normal-tension glaucoma. Front Neurol. 2017;8(47):1–7.
15. Macchi V, Regoli M, Bracco S, Nicoletti C, Morra A, Porzionato A, De Caro R, Bertelli E. Clinical anatomy of the orbitomeningeal foramen: variational anatomy of the canals connecting the orbit with the cranial cavity. Radiol Anat. 2016;38:165–77.

2 Anatomy of the Orbital Apex

Shuk Wan Joyce Chow

Abstract

The orbital apex is a complex region in the orbit which contains important structures such as the optic nerve and ophthalmic artery. Although much research has been dedicated to the anatomy of this region, there has been a lack of consistency in the definition of the precise location of the orbital apex. In the modern era of microscopic and endoscopic surgery, where new approaches and methods are advocated for pathologies in the orbital apex, a detailed understanding is vital to avoid major complications in these patients.

Keywords

Orbital apex · Optic nerve · Ophthalmic artery · Superior orbital fissure · Inferior orbital fissure · Orbital surgical landmark

2.1 Introduction

The orbital apex is a complex yet important structure in the orbit. It houses the optic canal, superior orbital fissure, and inferior orbital fissure, which act as corridors for crucial nerves and arteries to travel from the brain to the globe. There has been voluminous research in the literature describing the anatomy of the apex. However, there has been a lack of consistency in defining the precise location of the orbital apex, which has led to confusion in conveying important surgical landmarks between surgeons. Danko and Haug [1] described the orbital apex as the distance from the infraorbital rim to the annulus of Zinn, measuring approximately 39.1 mm in length. Yilmazlar et al. [2] measured the distance between the orbital apex to the tubercular recess, which was between 11.22 and 11.47 mm. Martin et al. described the orbital apex (optic canal) to be about 7 mm posterior to the posterior ethmoidal canal in their paper on the "Rule of Seven" in the microsurgical anatomy of the orbit (Fig. 2.1) [3]. Other studies measured distances from the infraorbital rim to the lacrimal crest or lateral orbital rim [2, 4–13]. In daily practice, a common understanding of the orbital apex can be defined by the coronal plane of the posterior ethmoidal foramen and the optic canal [14]. Nevertheless, in-depth knowledge of surgical anatomy is crucial to avoid complications that may arise from surgical procedures in this critical area.

S. W. J. Chow (✉)
Department of Neurosurgery, Queen Elizabeth Hospital, Hong Kong SAR, China
e-mail: csw814@ha.org.hk

T. L. POON et al. (eds.), *Orbital Apex and Periorbital Skull Base Diseases*, https://doi.org/10.1007/978-981-99-2989-4_2

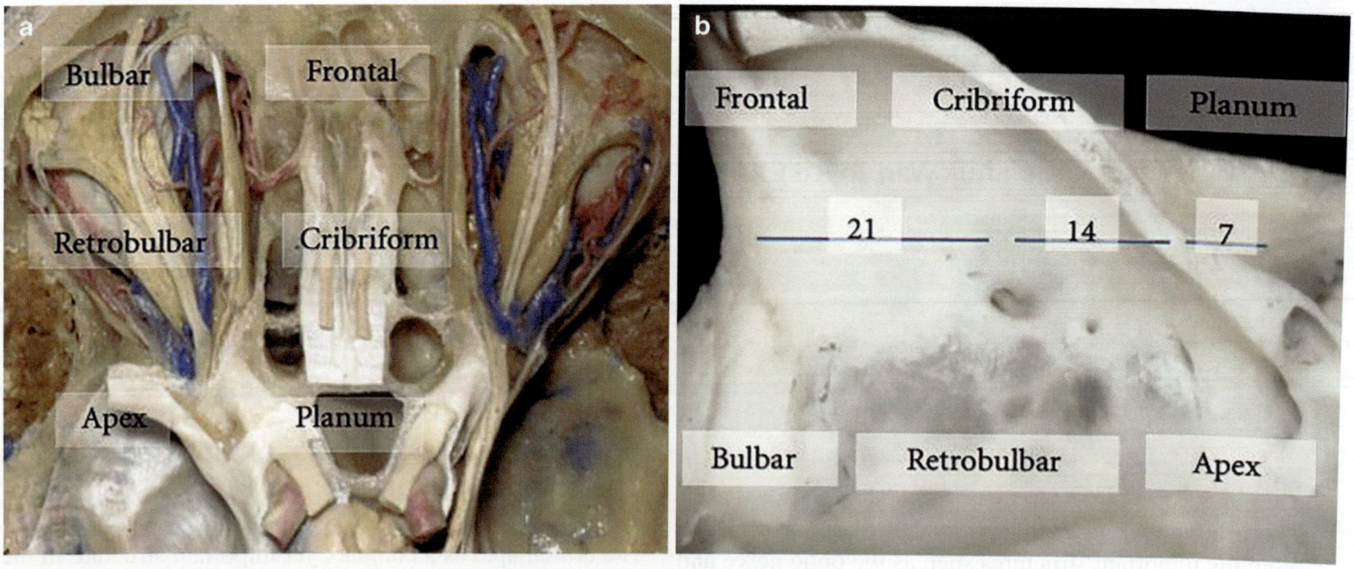

Fig. 2.1 (**a**) The orbital apex shown from a superior view posterior to the retrobulbar region. (**b**) It is about 7 mm posterior to the posterior ethmoidal canal according to the bony landmarks in the orbit. (Used with permission from [3])

2.2 Surgical Anatomy

2.2.1 Skeletal Anatomy of the Orbital Apex

The bony orbital apex is the narrowest part of the orbit, where all the nerves, arteries, and muscles of the orbit pass through this narrow space into the globe. The roof of the apex is formed by the lesser wing of the sphenoid bone, the lateral wall by the greater wing of the sphenoid, the medial wall by the ethmoidal sinus, and the floor is formed by the orbital plate of the palatine bones.

The optic canal (OC) is found within the orbital apex, measuring about 8–10 mm in length. It is bordered by the lesser wing of the sphenoid bone superiorly, the anterior clinoid process laterally, and the optic strut infero-laterally. The sphenoid sinus forms the medial wall of the optic canal. The optic strut separates the optic canal and the superior orbital fissure (Fig. 2.2). In 0.64–2.98% of orbits, there may be duplication of the OC, in which the lower canal usually contains the ophthalmic artery and the upper canal of the optic nerve [15–17].

The bony cleft between the orbital roof and the lateral wall is the superior orbital fissure (SOF). It is bounded by the greater wing, the lesser wing, and the body of the sphenoid bone (Fig. 2.2). Cadaveric dissections [13] have concluded important variations in the shape of the SOF. Reymond et al. identified two types of SOF in 100 human orbits, one with a significant narrowing near the midpoint, type a, and the other without, type b (Fig. 2.3). The size of the SOF did not differ much statistically, yet the distance of the optic nerve to the SOF is considerably shorter in type b which is of great clinical importance to the operating surgeon.

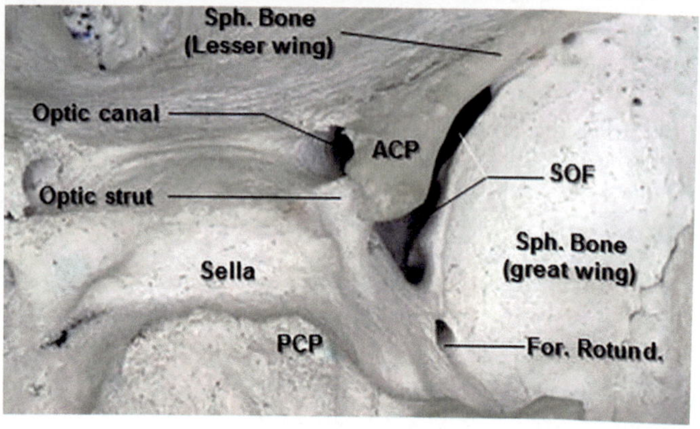

Fig. 2.2 A coronal view of the skull bone showing the orbital apex as the narrowest part of the orbit. It is bordered by the lesser wing of the sphenoid at the orbital roof, the greater wing of the sphenoid laterally, the ethmoid sinus medially, and the orbital plate of the palatine bone at the floor. The optic strut separates the optic canal and the superior orbital fissure. (Used with permission from [25])

The inferior orbital fissure (IOF) is located between the lateral wall and the floor of the orbit. The anterior margin is formed by the zygoma, and the medial side is the maxillary bone. The IOF is an important surgical landmark for both transcranial and transorbital approaches. The lateral part of the fissure contains mainly smooth muscle and fat tissues and is a point for bone cuts during orbitozygomatic approaches. Medially, the fissure communicates with the pterygopalatine fissure and connects to the nasal cavity.

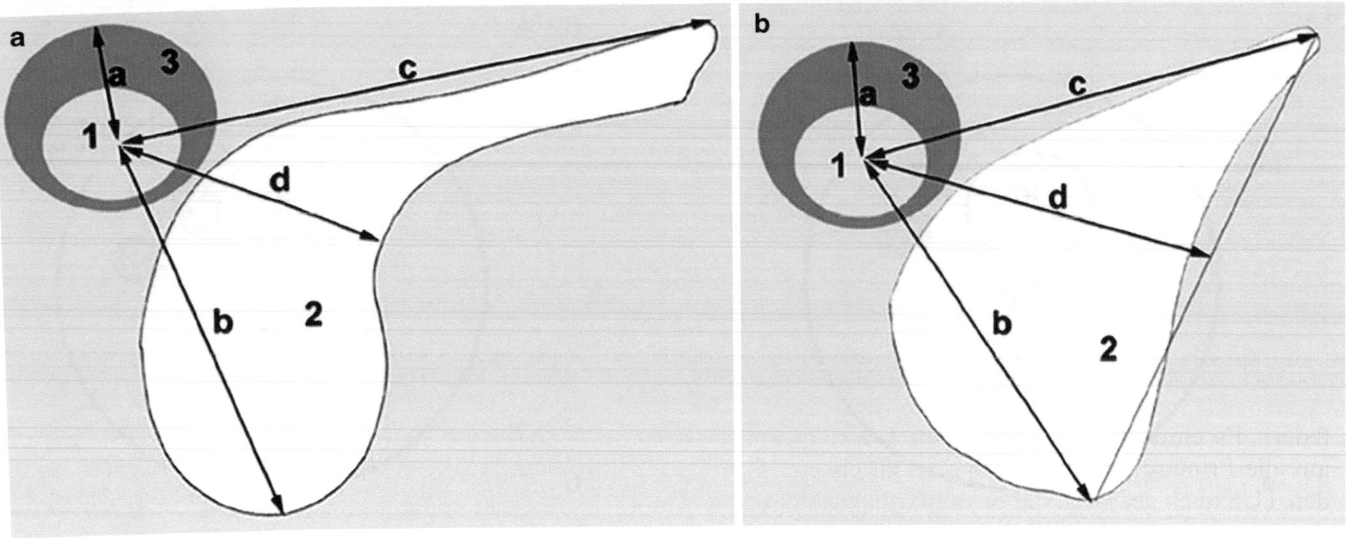

Fig. 2.3 Anatomical variations as described by Reymond et al. (**a**) Type a: significant narrowing near the midpoint. (**b**) Type b: no narrowing at the midpoint. (Used with permission from [13])

2.2.2 Soft Structures of the Orbital Apex

2.2.2.1 Optic Canal

The optic canal (OC) contains the optic nerve (ON), ophthalmic artery (OA), and the postganglionic sympathetic nerves from the internal carotid artery (ICA). The ophthalmic artery has an intra-orbital course that runs around the optic nerve. Arising from the internal carotid artery just medial to the anterior clinoid process, it enters the optic canal inferior and lateral to the optic nerve within the dural sheath. It then travels superior to the optic nerve 80–85% of the time from the lateral to the medial side and continues forward along the medial orbital wall under the superior oblique muscle [5, 6, 13, 18]. The central artery of the retina is a small but important branch that arises near the orbital apex [19–22]. It arises quite consistently from the ophthalmic artery at 10–15 mm posterior to the globe to penetrate the optic nerve and occupy a central distance to supply the retina.

Another variant of the ophthalmic artery is that it may enter through the SOF in 5–6% of cases [19, 22, 23]; hence, a thorough understanding of the anatomy is essential to avoid serious complications such as ischemic optic neuropathy.

2.2.2.2 Superior and Inferior Orbital Fissure

The superior orbital fissure can be divided into three separate compartments, i.e., lateral, central, and inferior, by the annulus of Zinn [24, 25]. The annulus of Zinn, referred as the "tendinem verum" in 1780, is a common annular tendon on which the four recti muscles insert.

The lateral component is the narrow part of the fissure and contains the trochlear nerve, frontal nerve, lacrimal nerve, and superior ophthalmic vein. The central part is the area enclosed by the annulus of Zinn, the oculomotor foramen, through which the ON and OA enter from the optic canal and the superior and inferior divisions of the oculomotor nerve, the abducens nerve, and the nasociliary nerve enter from the SOF. The inferior part is just below the tendinous ring and comprises mainly adipose tissue, but sometimes the inferior ophthalmic vein can be found. In Reymond's anatomical study, the arrangements of these nerves and vessels can differ into four types, with the greatest variation observed in the superior ophthalmic vein (Fig. 2.4). The inferior orbital fissure contains the infraorbital artery, infraorbital nerve, maxillary division of the trigeminal nerve, and zygomatic nerve.

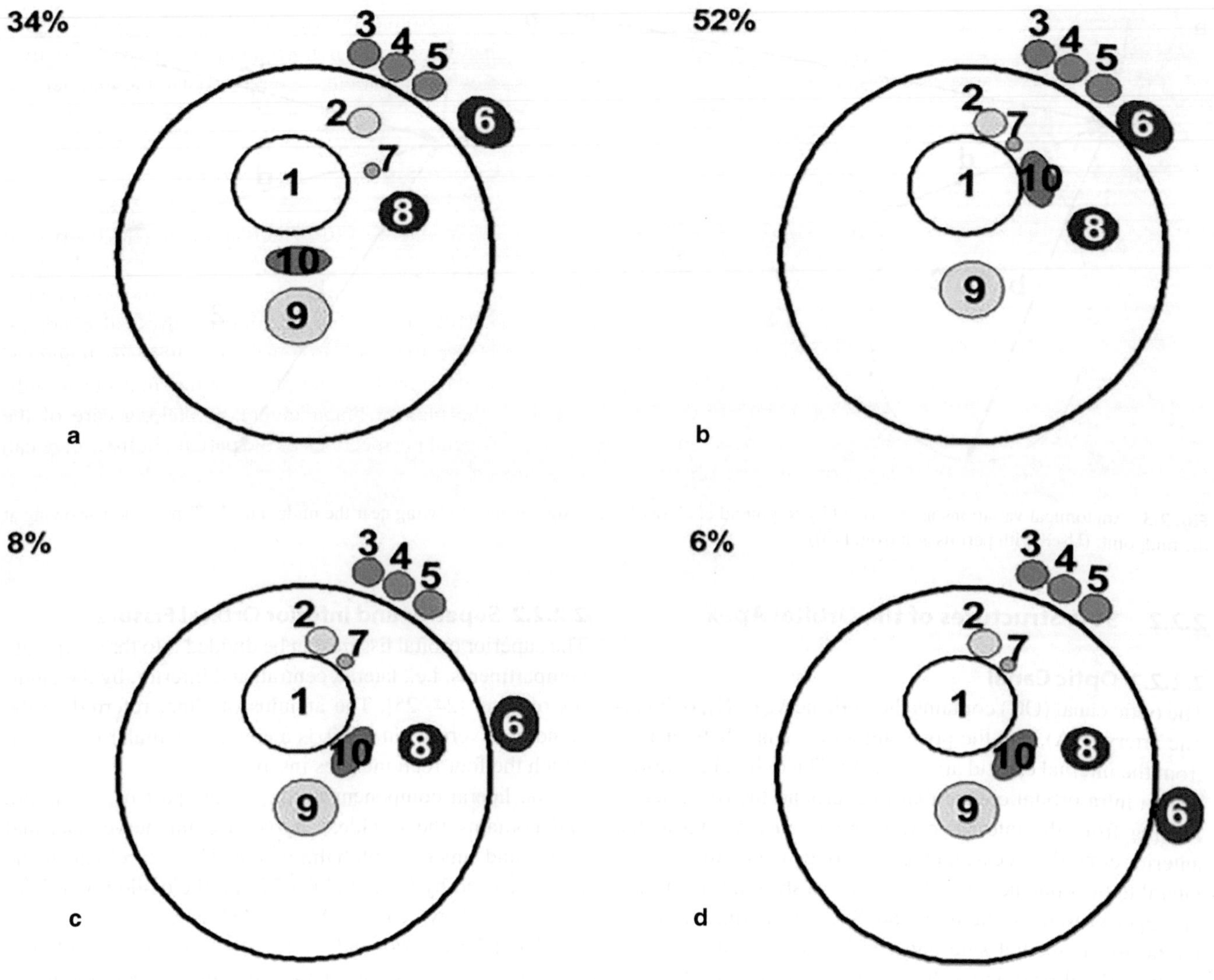

Fig. 2.4 Types of arrangement of nerves and vessels within the orbital apex. (**a**) Layout A. (**b**) Layout B. (**c**) Layout C. (**d**) Layout D. (1) Optic nerve, (2) superior branch of the oculomotor nerve, (3) trochlear nerve, (4) frontal nerve, (5) lacrimal nerve, (6) superior ophthalmic vein, (7) nasociliary nerve, (8) abducent nerve, (9) inferior branch of the oculomotor nerve, (10) ophthalmic artery. (Used with permission from [13])

References

1. Danko I, Haug RH. An experimental investigation of the safe distance for internal orbital dissection. J Oral Maxillofac Surg. 1998;56(6):749.
2. Yilmazlar S, Saraydaroglu O, Korfali E. Anatomical aspects in the transsphenoidal-transethmoidal approach to the optic canal: an anatomic-cadaveric study. J Cranio Maxillofacial Surg. 2012;40(7):e198.
3. Martins C, Costa e Silva IE, Campero A, Yasuda A, Aguiar LR, Tatagiba M, et al. Microsurgical anatomy of the orbit: the rule of seven. Anat Res Int. 2011;2011:1–14.
4. Renn WH, Rhoton AL. Microsurgical anatomy of the sellar region. J Neurosurg. 1975;43(3):288–98.
5. Piniara A, Georgalas C. Surgical anatomy of the orbit, including the intraconal space. Endosc Surg Orbit. 2021:18–27.
6. Engin, Adriaensen GFJPM, Hoefnagels FWA, Saeed P. A systematic review of the surgical anatomy of the orbital apex. Surg Radiol Anat. 2021;43(2):169–78. https://doi.org/10.1007/s00276-020-02573-w.
7. Ji Y, Qian Z, Dong Y, Zhou H, Fan X. Quantitative morphometry of the orbit in Chinese adults based on a three-dimensional reconstruction method. J Anat. 2010;217(5):501.
8. Kang HS, Han JJ, Oh HK, Kook MS, Jung S, Park HJ. Anatomical studies of the orbital cavity using three-dimensional computed tomography. J Craniofac Surg. 2016;27(6):1583–8.
9. Turvey TA, Golden BA. Orbital anatomy for the surgeon. Oral Maxillofac Surg Clin North Am. 2012;24:525.
10. Smerdon D. Anatomy of the eye and orbit. Curr Anaesth Crit Care. 2000;11(6):286.
11. Forrester J V., Dick AD, McMenamin PG, Roberts F, Pearlman E. Anatomy of the eye and orbit. Eye. 2016.
12. Sanchez-Diaz PC. Anatomy of the eye and orbit—the clinical essentials. Optom Vis Sci. 2018;95(7):627.
13. Reymond J, Kwiatkowski J, Wysocki J. Clinical anatomy of the superior orbital fissure and the orbital apex. J Cranio Maxillofacial Surg. 2008;36(6):346–53.

14. Aldea S, Brauge D, Gaillard S. How I do it: endoscopic endonasal approach for odontoid resection. Neurochirurgie. 2018;64(3):194–7. https://doi.org/10.1007/s00701-021-04900-5.
15. Patil GV, Kolagi S, Padmavathi G, Rairam GB. The duplication of the optic canals in human skulls. J Clin Diagn Res. 2011;5(3):536–7.
16. Bertelli E. Metoptic canal, duplication of the optic canal and Warwick's foramen in human orbits. Anat Sci Int. 2014;89(1):34.
17. Ghai R, Sinha P, Rajguru J, Jain S, Khare S, Singla M. Duplication of optic canal in human skulls. J Anat Soc India. 2012;61(1):33.
18. Scangas GA, Bleier BS, Dagi-glass LR. Anatomy of the orbit and paranasal sinuses. Endosc Surg Orbit. 2018;1:1–9.
19. Perrini P, Cardia A, Fraser K, Lanzino G. A microsurgical study of the anatomy and course of the ophthalmic artery and its possibly dangerous anastomoses. J Neurosurg. 2007;106(1):142.
20. Zoli M, Manzoli L, Bonfatti R, Ruggeri A, Mariani GA, Bacci A, et al. Endoscopic endonasal anatomy of the ophthalmic artery in the optic canal. Acta Neurochir. 2016;158(7):1343.
21. Huynh-Le P, Natori Y, Sasaki T. Surgical anatomy of the ophthalmic artery: its origin and proximal course. Neurosurgery. 2005;57(4 Suppl):ONS-236.
22. Michalinos A, Zogana S, Kotsiomitis E, Mazarakis A, Troupis T. Anatomy of the ophthalmic artery: a review concerning its modern surgical and clinical applications. Anat Res Int. 2015;2015:1.
23. Regoli M, Bertelli E. The revised anatomy of the canals connecting the orbit with the cranial cavity. Orbit. 2017;36:110.
24. Shi X, Han H, Zhao J, Zhou C. Microsurgical anatomy of the superior orbital fissure. Clin Anat. 2007;20(4):362.
25. Natori Y, Rhoton AL. Microsurgical anatomy of the superior orbital fissure. Neurosurgery. 1995;36(4):762.

Superior Orbital Fissure and Inferior Orbital Fissure

3

Atsushi Okano, Stefan Lieber, and Shunya Hanakita

Abstract

The microsurgical anatomy of the superior orbital fissure (SOF) and the inferior orbital fissure (IOF) is still important for tumors invading the orbit, cavernous sinus, optic canal, or middle fossa. Advances in endoscopic endonasal approaches have expanded their use for lesions at the orbital apex, SOF, and IOF. Thus, we illustrated the osteology of the orbit, the anatomy of SOF and IOF in craniotomy, and endoscopic endonasal surgery using dissected specimens. The anatomy of these areas should be well-understood when performing surgery for these lesions.

Keywords

Endoscopic endonasal surgery · Front-temporal craniotomy · Inferior orbital fissure · Orbital muscle of Müller · Superior orbital fissure

3.1 Osteology of the Orbit

The superior orbital fissure (SOF) connects the orbit to the middle cranial fossa. The cavernous sinus is located posterior to the SOF, and the orbital apex is located anteriorly to the SOF. The SOF is located between the greater and lesser wings and the body of the sphenoid bone (Fig. 3.1a). The annular tendon attaches to the superior, inferior, and medial aspects of the optic canal and the most medial aspect of the lateral margin of the SOF (Fig. 3.1b). The annular tendon subdivides the SOF into three separate compartments: a superolateral segment (11a), a central segment (11b), and an inferomedial segment (11c) [1]. The lateral margin of SOF, formed by the thin edge of the greater wing, is the sharpest and most defined border. The lower edge of SOF is separated from the foramen rotundum by the maxillary strut which is a bridge of bone [2] (Fig. 3.1c). The superior wall of SOF is formed by the lower surfaces of the lesser wing, the anterior clinoid process, and the adjacent part of the optic strut (Fig. 3.1d).

The inferior orbital fissure (IOF) is a narrow cleft with long anterior and posterior borders and narrow medial and lateral ends. It is bounded posteriorly by the greater wing of the sphenoid, laterally by the zygomatic bone, medially by the sphenoid body, and anteriorly by the maxilla and a short segment formed by the palatine bone (Fig. 3.1a). The IOF is divided into three compartments: a posteromedial segment (13a) that runs from the maxillary strut to the posterior border of the infraorbital groove, a middle segment (13b) that spans the width of the infraorbital groove, and an anterolateral segment (13c) that runs from the anterior border of the infraorbital groove to the most anterolateral aspect of the IOF (Fig. 3.1b). In the posteromedial portion of the IOF, the foramen rotundum, SOF, and pterygopalatine fossa communicate with the orbit and cavernous sinus. The middle segment of the IOF connects the infratemporal fossa and the anterolateral part of the IOF communicates with the orbit and the temporal fossa. The anterolateral part of the IOF is the part into which the two cuts of the one-piece orbitozygomatic (OZ) craniotomy extend (Fig. 3.1e, f).

The structures that pass through the posteromedial part of the IOF are small branches of the maxillary artery, tributaries of the inferior ophthalmic vein, and the infraorbital and zygomatic branches of the maxillary nerve (Fig. 3.2a). After passing shortly through the pterygopalatine fossa (PPF), the infraorbital nerve enters the orbit through the middle part of the IOF along the infraorbital groove and canal. The infraorbital nerve passes through the infraorbital foramen to reach the cheek (Fig. 3.2a). The zygomatic nerve arises from the maxillary nerve in the PPF, courses forward

A. Okano (✉) · S. Lieber
Department of Neurosurgery, Lariboisière Hospital, University of Paris Diderot, Paris, France
e-mail: okano-cib@umin.ac.jp

S. Hanakita
Department of Neurosurgery, Saitama Medical Center/University, Saitama, Japan

T. L. POON et al. (eds.), *Orbital Apex and Periorbital Skull Base Diseases*, https://doi.org/10.1007/978-981-99-2989-4_3

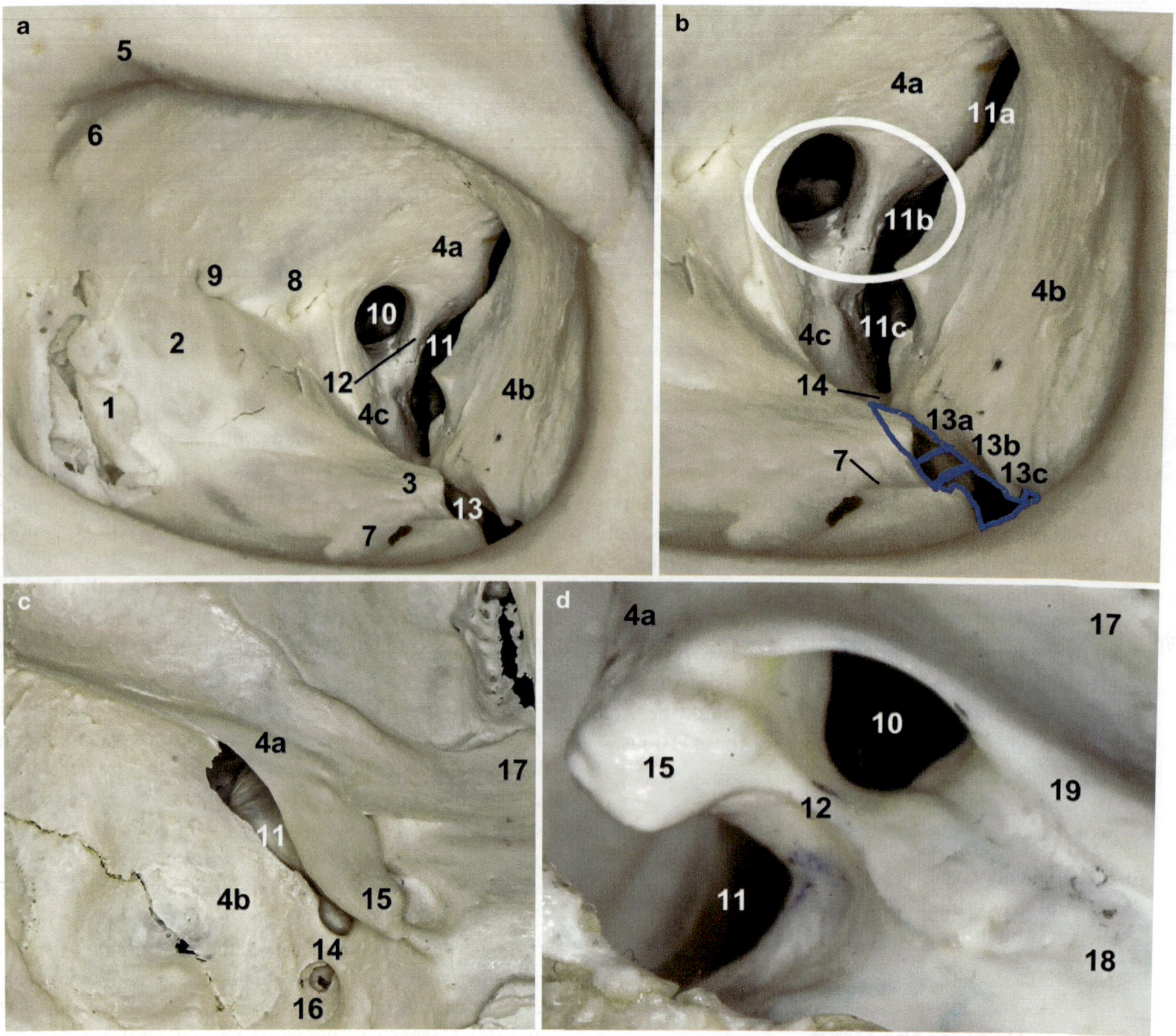

Fig. 3.1 Osteology of the orbit. (**a**) Oblique view of the left orbit oriented along the axis of the optic canal. (**b**) Enlarged view of the left orbit. The annular tendon (white ring) is attached to the optic canal and the most medial aspect of the lateral margin of the superior orbital fissure (SOF). The annular tendon subdivides the SOF into three separate compartments: a superolateral segment (11a), a central segment (11b), and an inferomedial segment (11c). The infraorbital fissure is divided into three compartments: a posteromedial segment (13a), from the maxillary strut to the posterior border of the infraorbital groove; a middle segment (13b), the width of the infraorbital groove [7]; and an anterolateral segment (13c), from the anterior border of the infraorbital groove to the most anterolateral aspect of the infraorbital fissure, (**c**) Osteology of the anterior and middle cranial fossae. (**d**) Osteology of the sellar region, oblique view oriented along the axis of a left optic canal. (**e**) The infraorbital fissure pointed from the intra orbit to the extra orbit. (**f**) The infraorbital fissure pointed in orbitozygomatic approach. 1, middle turbinate (the lacrimal bone is partially missing in this specimen); 2, ethmoid bone; 3, orbital process of the palatine bone; 4, sphenoid bone: 4a, lesser wing, 4b, greater wing, 4c, body; 5, supraorbital notch (or foramen); 6, trochlear fossa; 7, infraorbital groove; 8, posterior ethmoidal foramen; 9, anterior ethmoidal foramen; 10, optic canal; 11, SOF: 11a, superolateral segment, 11b, central segment, 11c, inferomedial segment; 12, optic strut; 13, IOF: 13a, posteromedial segment, 13b, middle segment, 13c, anterolateral segment; 14, maxillary strut; 15, anterior clinoid process; 16, foramen rotundum; 17, planum sphenoidale; 18, tuberculum sellae; 19, limbus sphenoidale

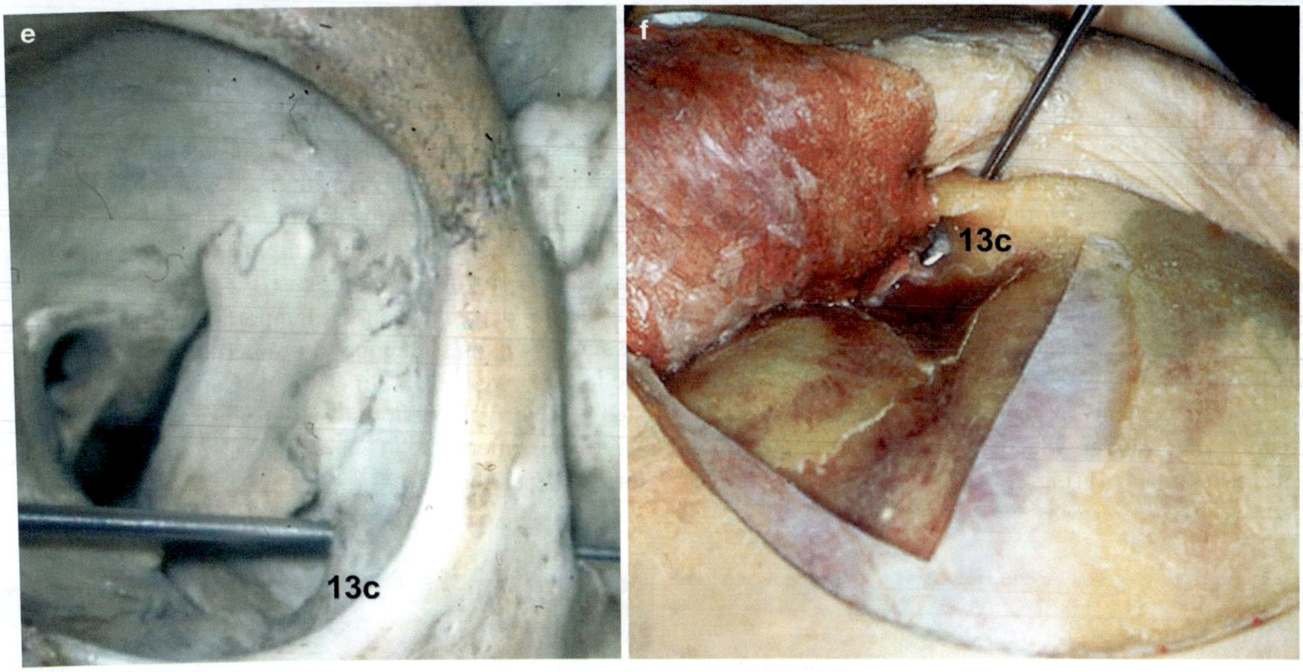

Fig. 3.1 (continued)

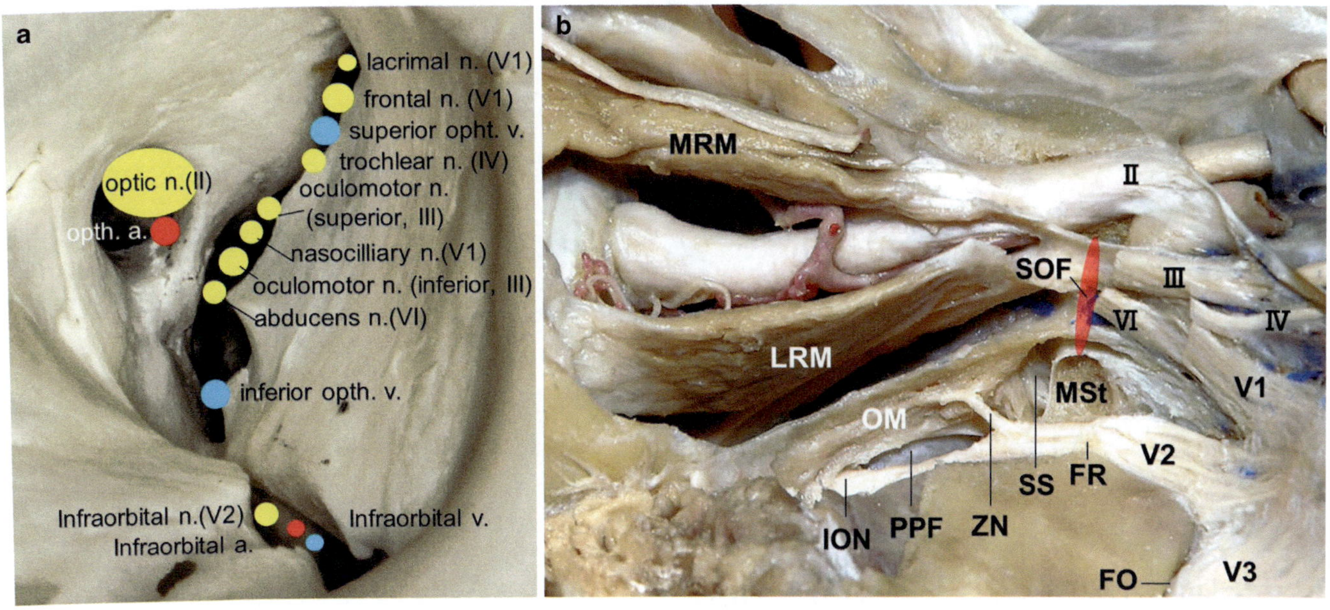

Fig. 3.2 (**a**) Compartments of a superior orbital fissure, an inferior orbital fissure, and an optic canal. The lacrimal nerve, the frontal nerve, the trochlear nerve, and the superior ophthalmic vein pass through a superolateral segment of the superior orbital fissure (SOF). The oculomotor nerve, the nasociliary nerve, the oculomotor nerve, and the abducens nerve pass through a central segment of SOF. The inferior ophthalmic vein passes through an inferomedial segment. The optic nerve and the ophthalmic artery pass through the optic canal. The infraorbital nerve, the infraorbital artery, and the infraorbital vein pass through a posteromedial segment of the infraorbital fissure. (**b**) Cadaveric dissection of the lateral sellar orbital junction. The orbital muscle of Müller (OM) extends posteriorly and medially to reach the superior orbital fissure (SOF) and the anterior confluence of the cavernous sinus. As the OM courses posteriorly, it lies above the maxillary strut (MS). In the posteromedial aspect of the inferior orbital fissure, the muscle lies between the orbit and pterygopalatine fossa, where it serves as the roof of the latter and contacts the maxillary nerve. The zygomatic nerve enters the OM, dividing it into two: a superior and an inferior bundle. *II*, optic nerve; *SOF*, superior orbital fissure; *III*, oculomotor nerve; *IV*, trochlear nerve; *V1*, ophthalmic branch of trigeminal nerve; *V2*, maxillary branch of the trigeminal nerve; *V3*, mandibular branch of trigeminal nerve; *VI*, abducens nerve; *ION*, infraorbital nerve; *MSt*, maxillary strut; *FO*, foramen ovale; *FR*, foramen rotundum; *SS*, sphenoid sinus; *MRM*, medial rectus muscle; *LRM*, lateral rectus muscle; *PPF*, pterygopalatine fossa; *OM*, orbital muscle of Müller; *ZN*, zygomatic nerve

and runs upward through the fissure and inside the periorbita of the lateral orbital wall, and gives rise to the zygomaticotemporal and zygomaticofacial nerves and sensory branches to the skin over the malar eminence and lateral orbital rim [3] (Fig. 3.2b). The orbital muscle of Müller forms a bridge over the IOF and separates the orbit from the pterygopalatine fossa, infratemporal fossa, and temporal fossa. The superior surface of Müller's muscle is associated with the orbital contents, especially the inferior rectus muscle, the inferior branch of the oculomotor nerve, and the inferior ophthalmic vein and its tributaries. The inferior surface of the muscle is associated with the pterygopalatine fossa and its contents, primarily the maxillary, zygomatic, and infraorbital nerves, which are all surrounded by adipose connective tissues [4] (Fig. 3.2b).

3.2 Surgical Anatomy of the SOF and the Inferior Orbital Fissure (IOF) in a Frontotemporal Craniotomy

The heads were fixed in a Mayfield head holder (Integra life science corporation, USA) with 5° of extension and 45° of rotation toward the opposite side. Frontotemporal craniotomy was performed [5, 6]. A slightly curved skin incision was started in front of the tragus (Fig. 3.3a). The temporal muscle was detached from the temporal bone using the interfascial dissection technique to protect the frontal branch of the facial nerve (Fig. 3.3b). The MacCarty keyhole was created to identify the periorbita and the dura of the frontal lobe (Fig. 3.3c), after which frontotemporal craniotomy was performed (Fig. 3.3d).

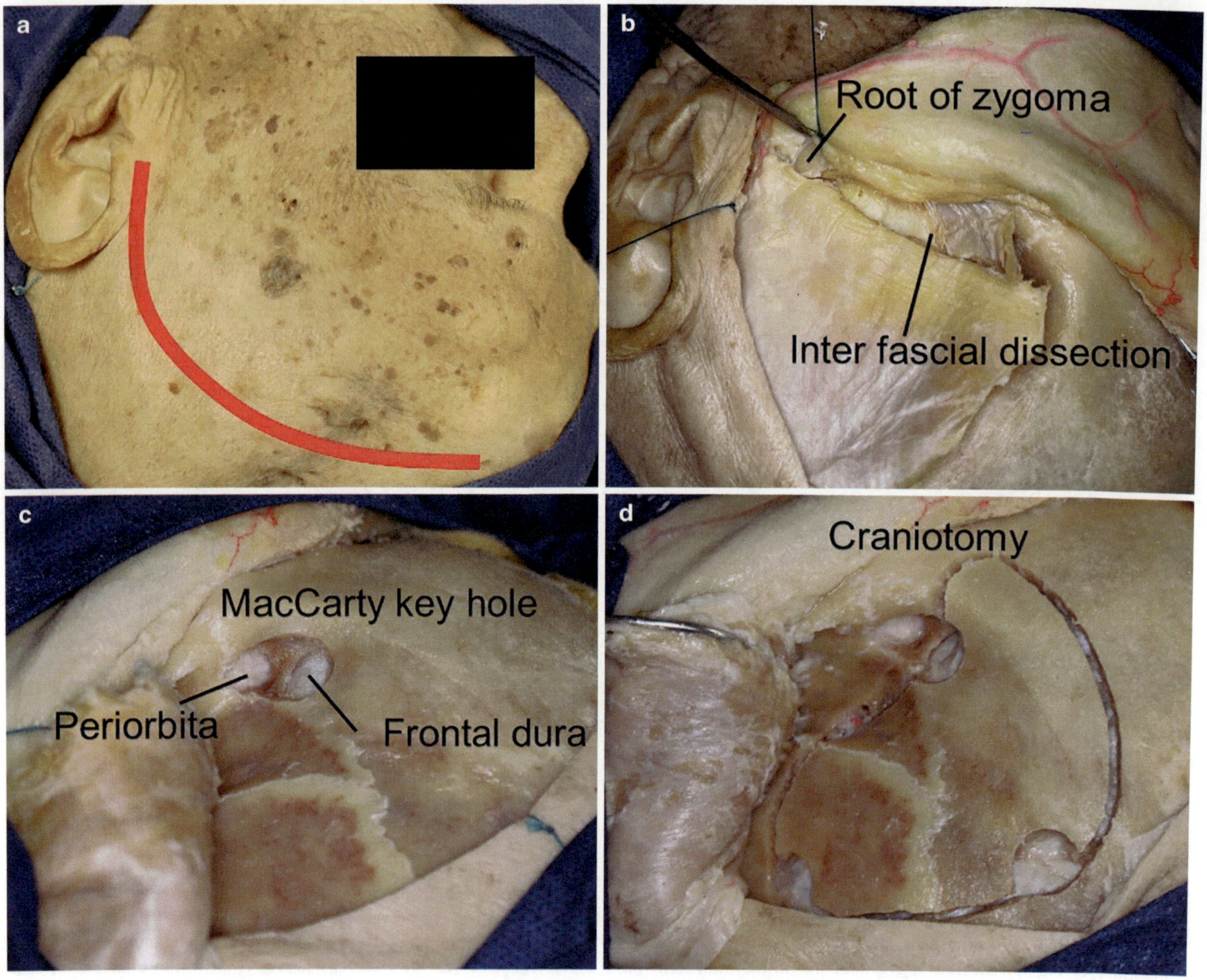

Fig. 3.3 Stepwise left frontotemporal craniotomy. (**a**) A slightly curved skin incision for the frontotemporal craniotomy starting in front of the tragus. (**b**) An interfascial dissection. The root of zygoma is well exposed. (**c**) Creating the MacCarty keyhole to identify the periorbita (PO) and the dura of the frontal lobe. (**d**) Frontotemporal craniotomy

The greater sphenoid wing, the lesser sphenoid wing, the temporal base floor, and the sphenoid ridge were fully drilled to be able to observe the temporal base more widely (Fig. 3.4a). Then, after pealing the lateral wall of the cavernous sinus, the ophthalmic nerve, the maxillary nerve, and the mandibular nerve could be seen. The ophthalmic nerve was going into the orbit passing through the superior orbital, the maxillary nerve to the pterygopalatine fossa through the foramen rotundum, and the mandibular nerve to the infratemporal fossa through the foramen ovale (Fig. 3.4b). After

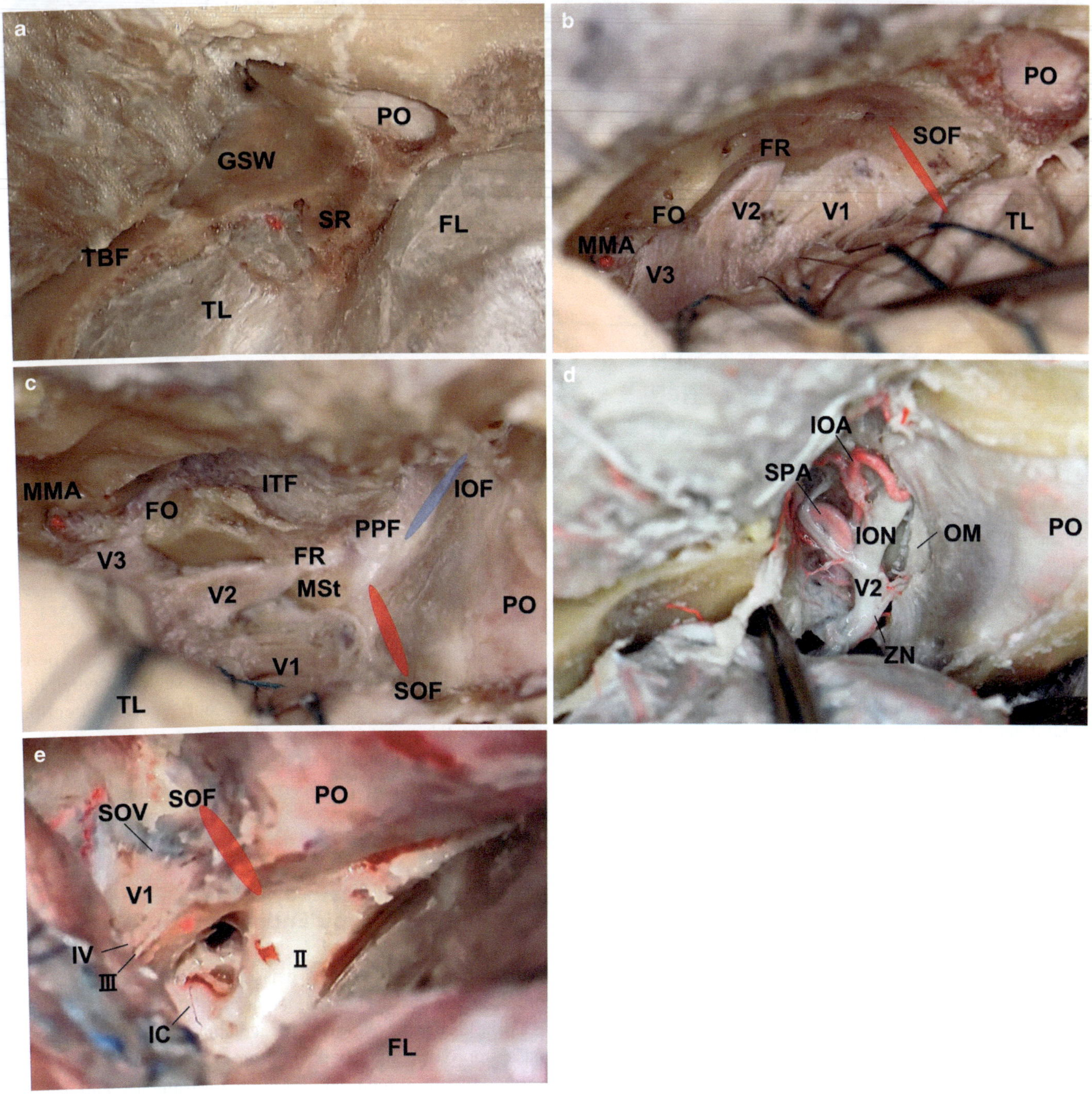

Fig. 3.4 Stepwise exposure of a superior orbital fissure (SOF) and an inferior orbital fissure. (**a**) After drilling through the greater sphenoid wing, the lesser sphenoid wing, and the temporal base floor. (**b**) After peeling the lateral wall of the cavernous sinus. The temporal base is widely exposed. (**c**) After opening the foramen rotundum and the foramen ovale. (**d**) After opening the pterygopalatine fossa (PPF) and removing the fat in the PPF. The inferior orbital nerve (ION), the sphenopalatine artery (SPA), and the infraorbital artery come into view. The orbital muscle of Müller (OM) indicates the level of the infraorbital fissure and separates the PPF from the orbit. (**e**) After the anterior clinoidectomy. The SOF is well exposed. *PO*, periorbita; *GSW*, greater wing of sphenoid bone; *TBF*, temporal base floor; *SR*, sphenoid ridge; *TL*, temporal robe; *FL*, frontal lobe; *SOF*, superior orbital fissure; *FR*, foramen rotundum; *FO*, foramen ovale; *V1*, ophthalmic branch of trigeminal nerve; *V2*, maxillary branch of the trigeminal nerve; *V3*, mandibular branch of trigeminal nerve; *MMA*, middle meningeal artery; *ITF*, infratemporal fossa; *IOF*, inferior orbital fissure; *PPF*, pterygopalatine fossa; *MSt*, maxillary strut; *OM*, orbital muscle of Müller; *ZN*, zygomatic nerve; *ION*, infraorbital nerve; *IOA*, infraorbital artery; *SPA*, sphenopalatine artery

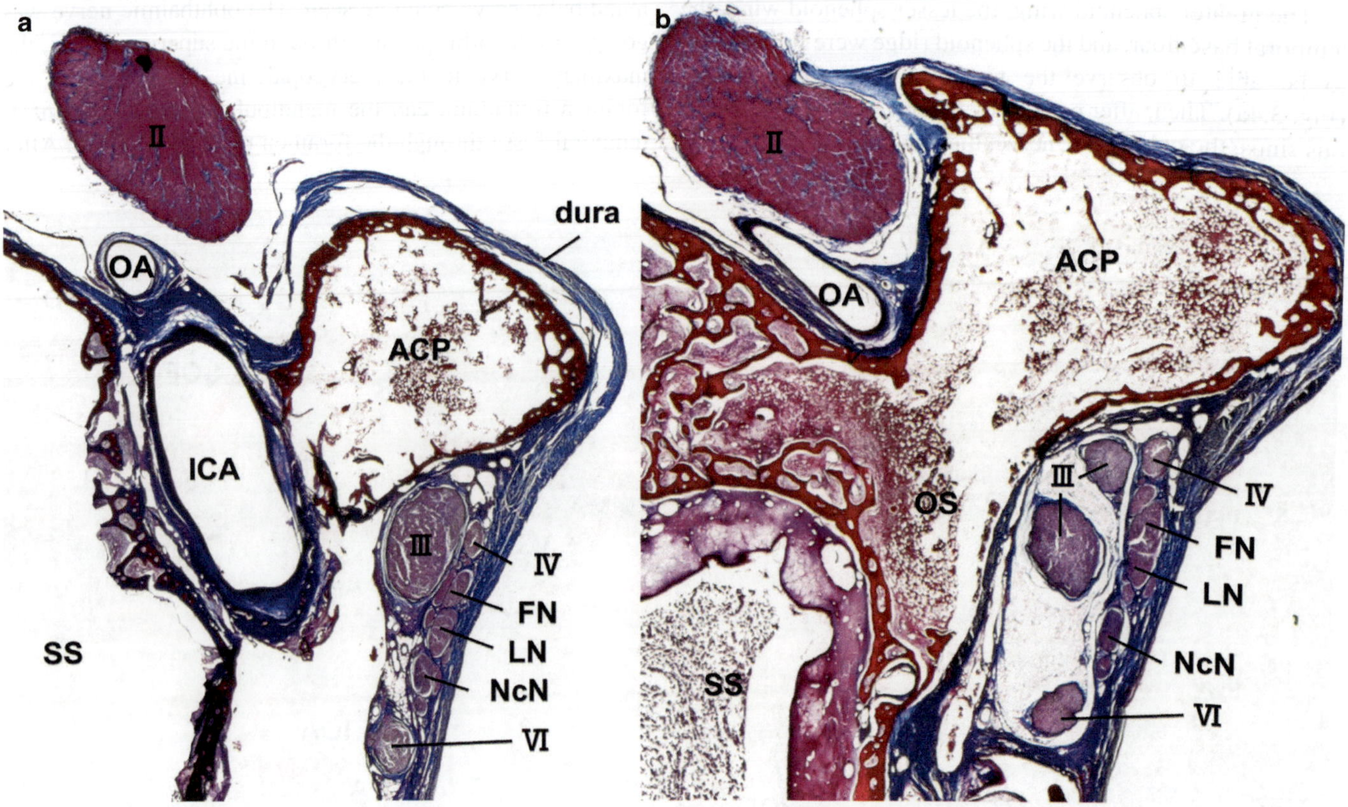

Fig. 3.5 Coronal histological sections of the left cavernous orbital region. (**a**) Section is at the level of clinoidal segment C5 of the Internal carotid artery. (**b**) The section is at the level of the optic strut. *II*, optic nerve; *OA*, ophthalmic artery; *ICA*, internal carotid artery; *ACP*, anterior clinoid process; *SS*, sphenoid sinus; *III*, oculomotor nerve; *IV*, trochlear nerve; *FN*, frontal nerve; *LN*, lacrimal nerve; *NcN*, nasociliary nerve; *VI*, abducens nerve; *OS*, optic strut

opening the foramen rotundum, the pterygopalatine fossa and the infraorbital fissure could be seen (Fig. 3.4c). After opening PPF and removing the fat in the PPF, the inferior orbital nerve, the sphenopalatine artery, and the infraorbital artery come into view. The orbital muscle of Müller indicates the level of the infraorbital fissure and separates the PPF from the orbit (Fig. 3.4d). Figure 3.4e shows the optic nerve, the SOF, the oculomotor nerve, the trochlear nerve, the ophthalmic nerve, and the internal carotid artery after drilling the anterior clinoid process. Extradural anterior clinoidectomy was performed using the detailed technique published [7]. The clinoid space is limited superiorly and laterally by the dura that covers the superior and lateral aspects of the anterior clinoid (Fig. 3.5a). Its medial aspect is formed by the optic nerve sheath. Just below the optic nerve sheath is the inferior root of the lesser sphenoid wing (optic strut), which extends from the base of the anterior clinoid process to the body of the sphenoid bone (Fig. 3.5b). The size and shape of the optic strut varied in our specimens, with a diameter ranging from 3 to 7 mm and section shapes extending from round to oval [7]. The clinoid segment of the internal carotid artery runs along the posterior margin of the optic strut and is covered by a thin periosteal membrane (Fig. 3.5). The inferior surface of the clinoid space is formed by a thin layer of periosteum that covers the oculomotor nerve such that when the anterior clinoid process is drilled out, special attention should be taken not to damage the oculomotor nerve, especially thermal damage besides mechanical damage. The trochlear and frontal nerves cross over the oculomotor nerve anteriorly.

3.3 Surgical Anatomy of the SOF and IOF in Endoscopic Endonasal Surgery

Endoscopic dissection was performed using the technique published by our group [8]. Each head was fixed in a Mayfield head holder and positioned for a standard endoscopic endnasal approach. Endoscopic end-nasal approaches were performed using standard endoscopic instruments and rigid 4-mm-diameter endoscopes that were 18 cm in length with 0° and 30° lenses (Karl Storz, Tuttlingen, Germany). Bone resection was performed with a high-speed drill (Midas Rex [Medtronic, Jacksonville, Florida, USA]), and intraoperative images were taken and stored with the Karl Storz Aida system (Karl Storz).

A middle turbinectomy was first performed to approach the orbital apex. Then, the uncinate process and the bulla ethmoidalis were subsequently removed, followed by a maxillary antrostomy. The junction between the lamina papyracea and the posterior wall of the maxillary sinus indicates the level of the IOF (Fig. 3.6a). The antrostomy was extended anteriorly to expose the proximal part of the infraorbital nerve on the roof of the maxillary sinus. Posterior ethmoidectomy and sphenoidotomy were then performed to expose the medial wall of the orbital apex. The nasal mucosa above the inferior turbinate was incised vertically and elevated to expose the orbital process of the vertical plate of the palatine bone and its ethmoidal crest. The sphenopalatine foramen and artery were then identified, and the sphenopalatine foramen was unroofed. Using Kerrison rongeurs or a diamond drill, the lamina papyracea and the superior part of the posterior wall of the maxillary sinus were gently removed to expose the periorbita, the medial margin of the IOF, and the pterygopalatine fossa (Fig. 3.6b). The palatine nerves running down into the palatine canal were identified. The bone that forms the medial margin of the IOF between the lamina papyracea and the posterior wall of the maxillary sinus is tightly adherent to the orbital muscle of Müller, which is made of smooth muscle fibers that span the IOF from one margin to the other. Detailed histological images of this area are shown in this manuscript (Fig. 3.6c, d). The zygomatic nerve arises from the maxillary nerve after the foramen rotundum. It crosses the IOF and runs upward along the lateral wall of the orbit (Fig. 3.6e). The function of the orbital muscle of Müller and the zygomatic nerve varied among the individuals and was not clearly understood. Hence, they could be sacrificed on necessity, and the removal of those structures allowed wide exposure of the greater wing of the sphenoid bone. When the bony structures surrounding the foramen rotundum (such as the maxillary strut and the superior margin of the pterygoid plate) were carefully removed, the infraorbital nerve was isolated and became retractable, which further facilitated the exposure of the greater wing of the sphenoid bone through the rostral space of the infraorbital nerve. Simultaneously, the supraorbital nerve was disclosed behind the foramen rotundum on the rostral side of the infraorbital nerve, with the greater palatine nerve on its caudal side. Then, with careful removal of the greater wing of the sphenoid bone, we could finally reach the anterior aspect of the temporal base dura mater (Fig. 3.6f).

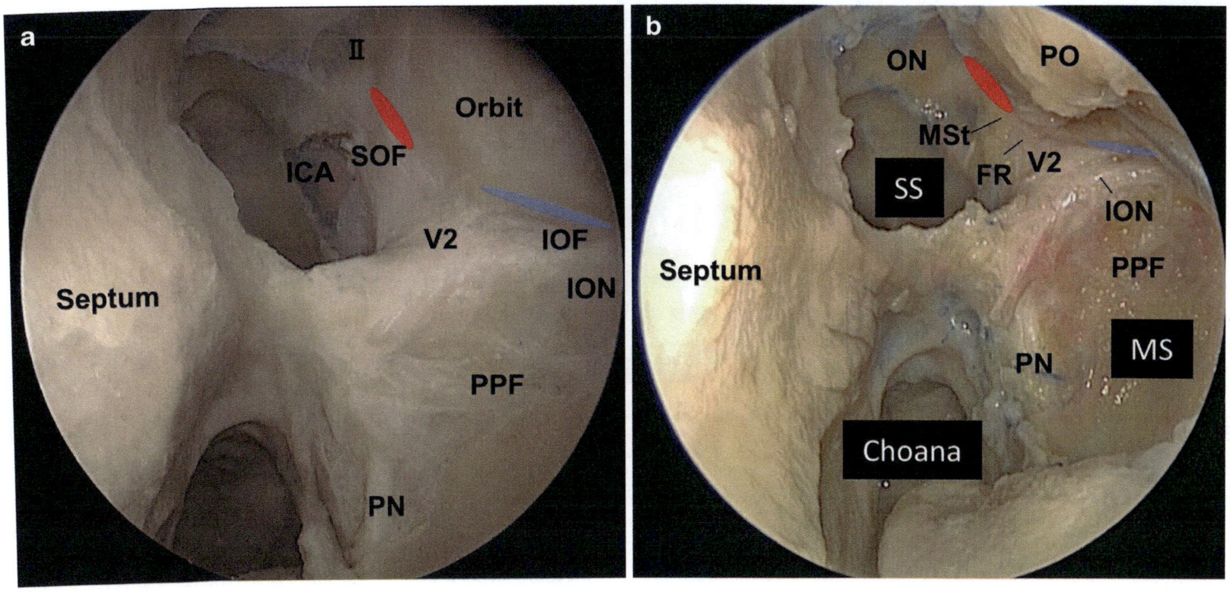

Fig. 3.6 Stepwise procedure of the endoscopic endonasal approach. (**a**) Endoscopic view (30° endoscope, left side). After exposing the vertical plate of the palatine bone. The orbital process, the roof of the sphenopalatine foramen, and the posterior wall of the maxillary sinus are removed. The medial wall of the superior orbital fissure (SOF) and the foramen rotundum is then progressively removed using a high-speed drill. (**b**) Endoscopic view (30° endoscope, left side). After antrostomy, the pterygopalatine fossa is widely opened. The medial wall of the SOF and foramen rotundum is removed. (**c, d**) Coronal histological sections of the left orbital apex region (**c**) and the left cavernous sinus and parasellar region (**d**). (**e, f**) Endoscopic view (30° endoscope, right side). Opening of the pterygopalatine fossa. *ICA*, internal carotid artery; *II*, optic nerve; *PN*, palatine nerve; *PPF*, pterygopalatine fossa; *SOF*, superior orbital fissure; *IOF*, infraorbital fissure; *V2*, maxillary branch of the trigeminal nerve; *ION*, infraorbital nerve; *PO*, periorbita; *MSt*, maxillary strut; *FR*, foramen rotundum; *PN*, palatine nerve; *SS*, sphenoid sinus; *MS*, maxillary sinus; *OA*, ophthalmic artery; *MRM*, medial rectus muscle; *IRM*, inferior rectus muscle; *LRM*, lateral rectus muscle; *III*, oculomotor nerve; *IV*, trochlear nerve; *V1*, ophthalmic branch of trigeminal nerve; *OM*, orbital muscle of Müller; *CS*, cavernous sinus; *ZN*, zygomatic nerve; *GWS*, greater wing of sphenoid bone; *MPM*, medial pterygoid muscle; *IOA*, infraorbital artery; *SPA*, sphenopalatine artery; *TD*, temporal dura; *PPG*, pterygopalatine ganglion; *IMax*, internal maxillary artery

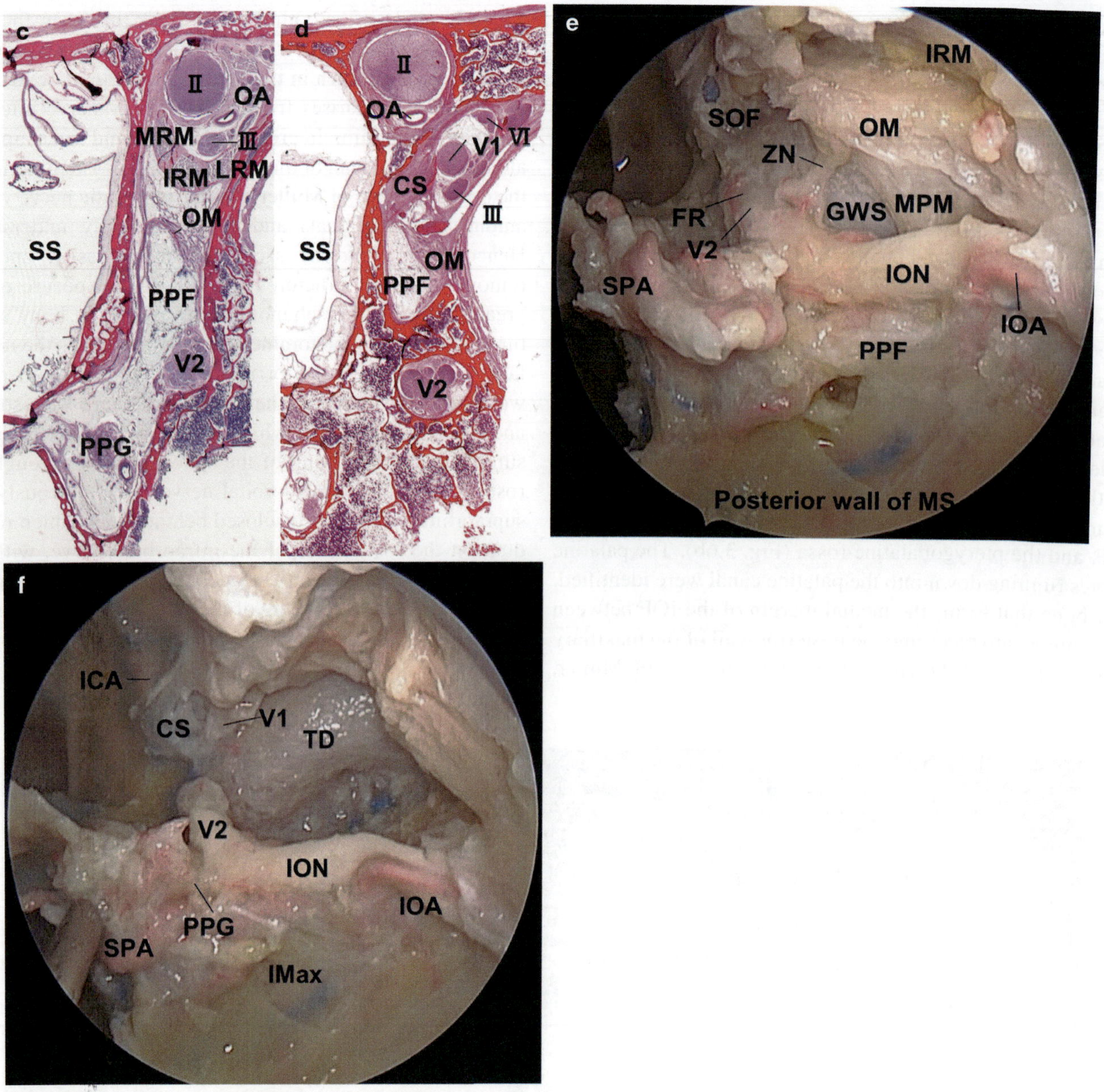

Fig. 3.6 (continued)

Competing Interest The authors declare no competing interests.

References

1. Lieber S, Fernandez-Miranda JC. Anatomy of the orbit. J Neurol Surg B Skull Base. 2020;81(4):319–32.
2. Natori Y, Rhoton AL Jr. Microsurgical anatomy of the superior orbital fissure. Neurosurgery. 1995;36(4):762–75.
3. Shimizu S, Tanriover N, Rhoton AL Jr, Yoshioka N, Fujii K. MacCarty keyhole and inferior orbital fissure in orbitozygomatic craniotomy. Neurosurgery. 2005;57(1 Suppl):152–9; discussion -9.
4. De Battista JC, Zimmer LA, Theodosopoulos PV, Froelich SC, Keller JT. Anatomy of the inferior orbital fissure: implications for endoscopic cranial base surgery. J Neurol Surg B Skull Base. 2012;73(2):132–8.
5. Froelich S, Aziz KA, Levine NB, Tew JM Jr, Keller JT, Theodosopoulos PV. Extension of the one-piece orbitozygomatic frontotemporal approach to the glenoid fossa: cadaveric study. Neurosurgery. 2008;62(5 Suppl 2):ONS312–6; discussion ONS6–7.
6. Oyama K, Watanabe K, Hanakita S, Champagne PO, Passeri T, Voormolen EH, et al. The orbitopterygoid corridor as a deep keyhole for endoscopic access to the paranasal sinuses and clivus. J Neurosurg. 2020;134(5):1480–9.
7. Froelich SC, Aziz KM, Levine NB, Theodosopoulos PV, van Loveren HR, Keller JT. Refinement of the extradural anterior clinoidectomy: surgical anatomy of the orbitotemporal periosteal fold. Neurosurgery. 2007;61(5 Suppl 2):179–85; discussion 85–6.
8. Hanakita S, Chang WC, Watanabe K, Ronconi D, Labidi M, Park HH, et al. Endoscopic endonasal approach to the anteromedial temporal fossa and mobilization of the lateral wall of the cavernous sinus through the inferior orbital fissure and V1–V2 corridor: an anatomic study and clinical considerations. World Neurosurg. 2018;116:e169–e78.

Cavernous Sinus and Internal Carotid Artery

4

Ramez W. Kirollos

Abstract

The anatomy of the cavernous sinus (CS) as an enclosed venous space with trabeculations surrounding the cavernous segment of the internal carotid artery (ICA) is described. This includes the anatomy of its dural boundaries and formation together with its relationships to surrounding structures. Details of its venous tributaries and connections and the associated cranial nerves are described. The anatomy of the ICA at the skull base is detailed in a useful anatomical orientation relevant to surgical procedures, and a correlation between intracranial and endonasal skull base anatomy is provided. The relevance of the surgical anatomy of the CS and ICA to the operative management of orbital lesions is discussed.

Keywords

Cavernous sinus · Internal carotid artery · Oculomotor nerve · Trochlear · Trigeminal nerve · Abducens nerve · Orbit · Superior orbital fissure

4.1 Anatomy of the Cavernous Sinus

4.1.1 Definition and Formation of the Cavernous Sinus

Each of the paired cavernous sinus (CS) is an enclosed venous space surrounding the "cavernous" segment of the internal carotid artery (ICA) and is limited by four dural walls. These are a roof superiorly; a medial and a lateral wall meeting inferiorly, giving it a triangular shape; and a posterior wall. The CS is narrow anteriorly and widens posteriorly [1, 2].

The dura covering the brain on forming the walls of the CS splits laterally and includes the cranial nerves within its two layers, whilst medially it forms its medial wall (Fig. 4.1). The wall of the CS on the middle fossa skull is formed by the periosteal layer.

The multiple venous tributaries form venous confluences end in venous spaces within the CS that are in the shape of a plexus or "caverns" separated by trabeculations allowing

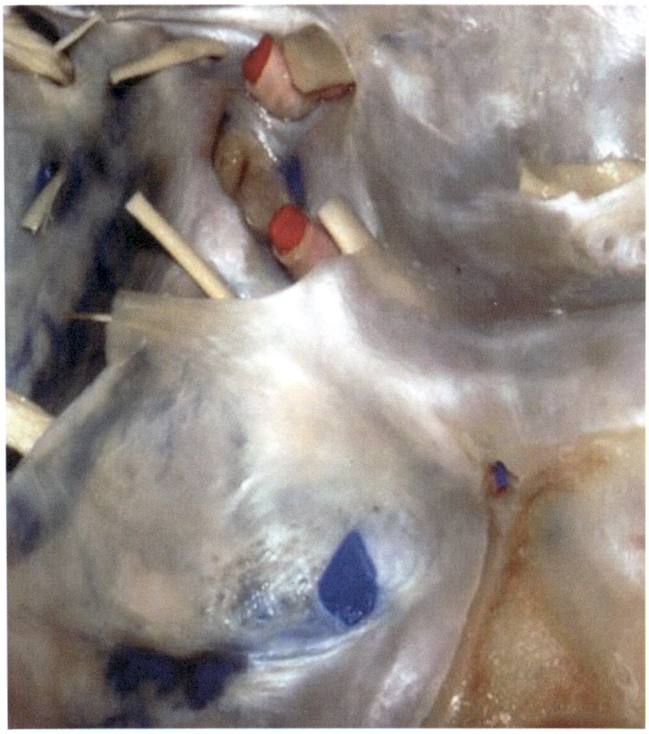

Fig. 4.1 The CS is located on either side of the body of the sphenoid bone and sella, extending from the SOF anteriorly to the level of the dorsum sellae posteriorly and lying over the petrous apex. The right CS is shown covered by the dura of the middle cranial fossa, forming the outer layer of the lateral wall of the CS and extending over the Gasserian ganglion in the Meckel's cave. The third nerve is seen entering the roof of the CS at the centre of the oculomotor triangle, the margins of which are formed by the interclinoid and the anterior and posterior petroclinoid dural folds

R. W. Kirollos (✉)
National Neuroscience Institute (NNI), Singapore, Singapore
Duke-NUS Medical School, Singapore, Singapore

T. L. POON et al. (eds.), *Orbital Apex and Periorbital Skull Base Diseases*, https://doi.org/10.1007/978-981-99-2989-4_4

varying degrees of separation or connections between the different caverns [2]. This is reflected potentially by the varying degrees of ease in controlling venous bleeding on surgical breach of the different compartments of the CS.

4.1.2 Location and Relationships of the CS

The CS is located in the parasellar area with the body of the sphenoid bone in the centre, harbouring the sella turcica and the sphenoid sinus. The anterior extent is the superior orbital fissure (SOF), and posteriorly they end at the level of the dorsum sellae and lie over the petrous apex [1–4].

The dural *roof* extends between the petrous apex and anterior and posterior clinoid processes forming the oculomotor triangle as the posterior part of the roof. The margins are formed by the interclinoid dural fold, between the clinoid processes, medially; the anterior petroclinoid fold, between the anterior clinoid process (ACP) and petrous apex, laterally; and the posterior petroclinoid fold—between the posterior clinoid process and the petrous apex—posteriorly (Figs. 4.1 and 4.2). The dura of the oculomotor triangle extends as the dura at the inferior margin of the ACP. The carotid-oculomotor membrane extends medially from the lower margin of the ACP to the optic strut at the medial extent of the proximal dural ring of the ICA. At the anterior extent of the roof, the clinoidal triangle, between the optic and oculomotor nerves, is covered by the ACP with the optic strut anteriorly separating the optic canal from the SOF (Fig. 4.2). The cavernous ICA emerges through this part of the roof.

The *lateral* CS wall is between the anterior petroclinoid fold starting at the roof superiorly to the level of the lower margin of the carotid sulcus on the sphenoid bone inferiorly. It is between the lateral end of the SOF anteriorly to the edge of the Meckel's cave posteriorly (Figs. 4.3, 4.4, and 4.5). The dura separating the CS from Meckel's cave lies just lateral to the posterior CS.

The *medial* CS dural wall extends from the medial edge of the SOF to the dorsum sellae posteriorly. It slopes from the roof at the interclinoid fold to the level of the carotid sulcus inferiorly to the join the lateral wall, giving the triangular shape of the CS in the coronal plane. As such the medial wall separates the CS from the lateral sella and lies lateral to the body of the sphenoid bone.

The relatively wide extent of the *posterior* wall of the CS is from the lateral dorsum sellae medially to the lateral edge of the Meckel's cave ostium laterally and from the petrosphenoid fold superiorly to the petroclival fissure inferiorly (Fig. 4.6).

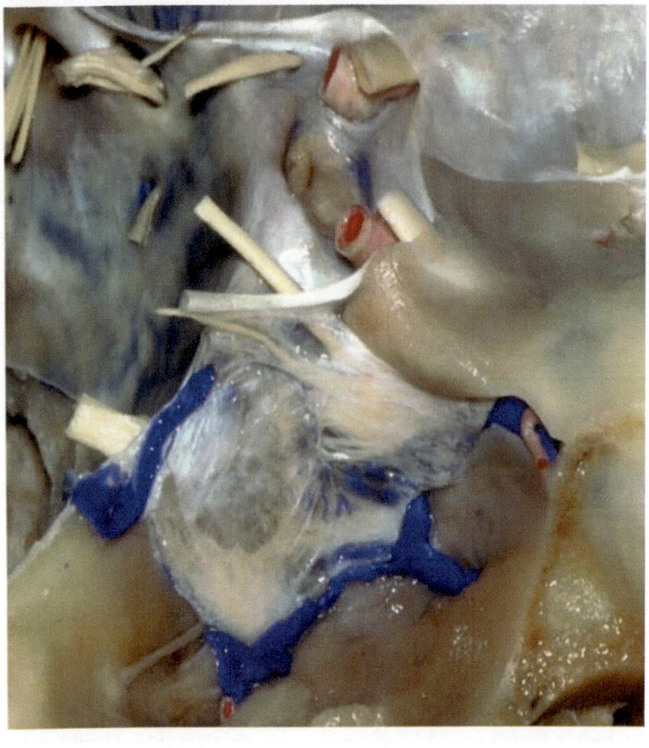

Fig. 4.2 The clinoidal triangle is between the optic and oculomotor nerves. The cavernous ICA is emerging through the carotid-oculomotor membrane at the anterior part of the roof of the CS and is covered by the ACP with the optic strut anteriorly separating the optic canal from the SOF. The outer dural layer of the lateral wall of the CS and Meckel's cave has been peeled off. The course of the third and fourth nerves in the lateral wall of the CS separated from its interior by the deep layer of the lateral wall is seen towards the SOF. The superior petrosal sinus is running at the superior edge of the petrous bone over the ostium of the Meckel's cave where the root of the fifth nerve is seen entering. The meningo-orbital arterial branch of the middle meningeal artery is noted to enter the orbit through the lateral aspect of the SOF

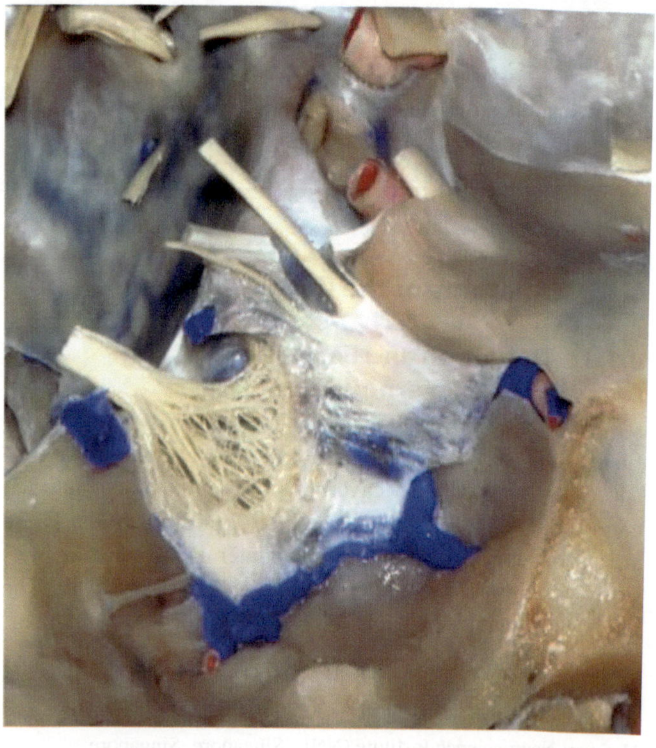

Fig. 4.3 The pericavernous venous plexus and extensions to the foramina ovale, rotundum, and spinosum are exposed. A dural wall between the posterior CS and Meckel's cave separates the CS from the Gasserian ganglion and V2 with V1 entering the lateral wall of the CS above its inferior limit and below the third and fourth nerves

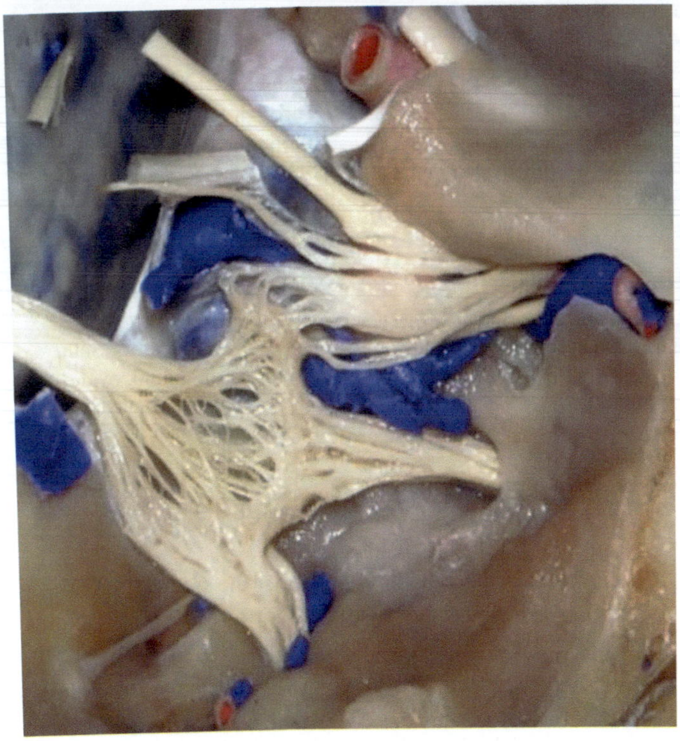

Fig. 4.4 The course of cranial nerves related to the lateral wall of CS (third, fourth, and V1) is fully exposed. The antero-inferior venous compartment of CS is joined by the SOV passing from the orbit through the SOF and inferior to the V1. A venous confluence is joining the superior petrosal and basilar venous sinuses to the supero-posterior venous compartments of CS

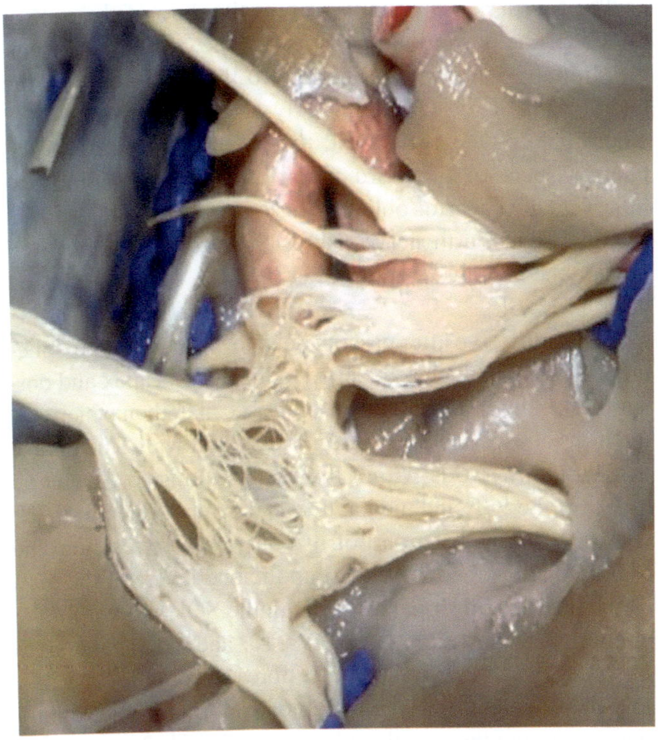

Fig. 4.5 The lateral aspect of the cavernous ICA segments is partially exposed. The sixth nerve is passing under Gruber's ligament into Dorello's canal in the vicinity of the basilar venous sinus. It is within the CS, and its course is medial to V1. On approaching the orbit, it joins the other cranial nerves travelling in the lateral wall of the CS to pass through the SOF. The clinoidal segment of the ICA is medial to the ACP

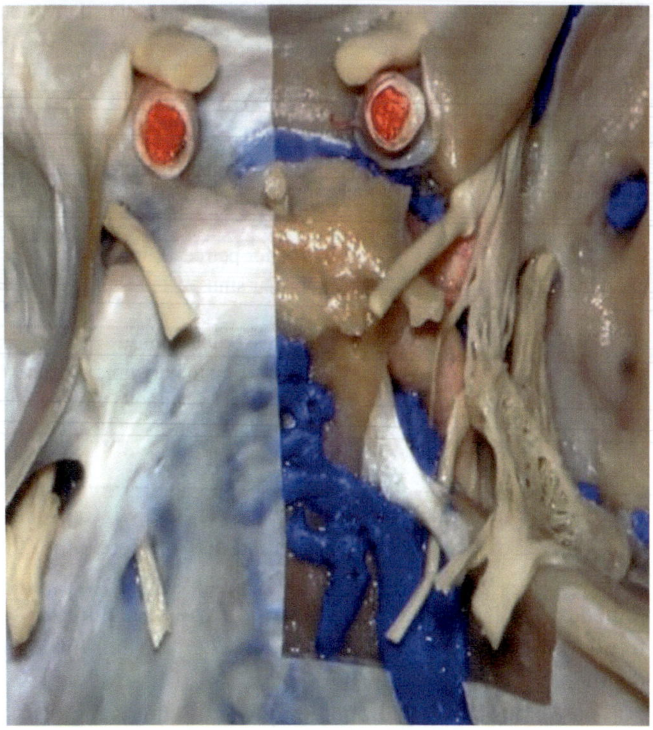

Fig. 4.6 The basilar venous plexus at the dorsum of the upper clivus and the inferior petrosal sinus are related to the sixth nerve as it enters Dorello's canal. This joins the posterosuperior venous compartment of the CS. The cavernous ICA separates on either side—between it and the CS medial and lateral walls—two of the venous compartments. The medial compartment is joined by the anterior intercavernous sinus and the narrow lateral venous compartments of CS. The emergence of ICA through the roof of the CS is posterior to the optic strut and medial to the ACP

4.1.3 Venous Connections and Extensions

The CS is connected circumferentially to the superior ophthalmic vein (SOV) and inferior ophthalmic vein (IOV), Sylvian and sphenoparietal sinus, superior petrosal, inferior petrosal, and basilar and intercavernous sinuses (anterior and posterior) from anterior in a clockwise fashion on the right and anticlockwise on the left. In addition, it has connections to the pterygoid plexus inferiorly (Table 4.1) [1, 2].

The venous plexus within the dural walls of the CS does have extensions connecting with other veins in adjacent regions. Although the CS venous spaces may extend into the SOF, the CS is in proximity but not directly straddling other foramina and fissures such as the foramen rotundum, ovale, or spinosum and the sphenoid emissary foramen. As such venous connections through these to other compartments may connect directly within the CS or via a pericavernous venous plexus (Fig. 4.3). Such extensions include those surrounding the V2 (maxillary) division of the trigeminal nerve that is not anatomically part of the CS and through the proximal dural ring around the clinoidal segment of the ICA and the ICA canal.

The SOV crosses from the medial aspect of the orbit above the optic nerve, passes between the superior and lateral recti, goes through the SOF outside the annulus of Zinn,

Table 4.1 The direction from which the CS is connected to the various tributaries, with their regions of drainage and course

Direction	Connection	Region	Course
Anterior	SOV	Orbit	Though SOF
	IOV		Through IOF
Lateral	Middle and inferior cerebral veins, Sphenoparietal sinus	Lateral cerebral hemisphere, anterior and middle cranial fossae	Along the superior margin of SOF
Posterior	Superior petrosal sinus	Posterior fossa	Along the superior ridge of the petrous bone
	Inferior petrosal sinus		Along petroclival fissure
Posteromedial	Basilar sinus	Contralateral CS	Posterior aspect of the upper clivus
	Intercavernous sinuses		Anterior and posterior Sella
Inferior	Connection to pterygoid plexus (via the pericavernous plexus)	Pterygopalatine and subtemporal fossae	Foramina rotundum, ovale, or spinosum and the sphenoid emissary foramen

and drains into the CS. It travels between the V1 (ophthalmic) and V2 divisions of the trigeminal nerve to reach the CS (Fig. 4.7). Prior to entry to the CS, frequently the SOV is joined by the IOV and drains via a single trunk. The IOV less frequently drains to the CS separately after passing through the inferior orbital fissure (IOF).

The venous drainage from the Sylvian fissure and parts of the middle and anterior cranial fossae drain through the sphenoparietal sinus which has a course along the sphenoid ridge and lateral margin of the SOF to reach the CS.

The large venous confluence at the posterior wall of the CS connects the convergence of the basilar and the superior and inferior petrosal sinuses. The basilar sinus at the posterior upper clivus and dorsum sellae communicates both CS as an intercavernous connection. This drains into the posterior CS, and the posterior CS dural wall extends as the posterior wall of the basilar sinus (Figs. 4.4 and 4.6). The configuration of the intercavernous sinuses connecting both CS around the sella is variable [2, 5]. These are related to the anterior, inferior, and posterior aspects of the pituitary gland and may form a circular sinus around the gland.

4.1.4 Venous Compartments of the CS

These are venous spaces within the CS between the intracavernous ICA and the CS walls [1, 2], which can be divided into the following four compartments: medial, anteroinferior, posterosuperior, and lateral (Figs. 4.4, 4.6, 4.9b, and 4.11). The medial compartment is lateral to the pituitary gland. The anteroinferior compartment is near the SOF receiving the superior and inferior ophthalmic veins separately or as a common trunk from both ophthalmic veins. The posterosuperior compartment is between the ICA and the posterior roof of the CS. This receives the basilar sinus. The lateral compartment is usually very narrow between the ICA and the lateral wall of the CS and contains the sixth nerve. The size of the compartments is determined by the course and tortuosity of the intracavernous ICA.

4.1.5 Associated Cranial Nerves

The third nerve reaches the CS roof at the oculomotor triangle. It goes through the dura at the centre of the triangle inferior to the ACP at a level just above the origin of the meningohypophyseal trunk off the intracavernous ICA (Figs. 4.1, 4.2, 4.3, 4.4, 4.5, 4.10, and 4.12). Its course in the inner aspect of the lateral wall of the CS in between the two dural leaves is above that of the fourth nerve along the inferior aspect of the ACP. It passes through the SOF within the annulus of Zinn, medial to the nasociliary nerve, and divides into a superior and an inferior division as it does so (Fig. 4.7) [1, 2, 6].

The fourth nerve initially pierces the dura of the roof of the CS at the posterolateral aspect of the oculomotor triangle. Initially its course is inferior to the third nerve in the lateral wall of the CS. Anteriorly at the base of the ACP where it joins the optic strut, the fourth nerve crosses the lateral aspect of the third nerve and passes medially to innervate the superior oblique muscle in the medial orbit. In doing so the fourth nerve passes through the lateral SOF outside the annulus of Zinn (Figs. 4.2, 4.3, 4.4, 4.5, 4.7, and 4.10) [1, 2, 6].

The sixth nerve after passing deep to Gruber's (petrosphenoid) ligament which is attached to the petrous apex and dorsum sellae, in the dural-lined Dorello's canal, then penetrates the inferior aspect of the posterior CS dural wall. The course of the sixth nerve is within the CS travelling to the lateral aspect of the ICA and medial to V1. It can be adherent to the ICA or V1. The distal part of its course before reaching the SOF joins the other nerves within the two layers of the dura of the lateral wall. It passes through the SOF and within the annulus of Zinn (Figs. 4.5, 4.6, 4.10, and 4.12). The sixth nerve receives some sympathetic fibres surrounding the ICA and then passes to V1 and eventually through long ciliary nerves passing through the ciliary ganglion [1, 2, 6].

The V1 nerve passes obliquely superiorly from the Gasserian ganglion and travels in the inferior aspect of the lateral wall of the CS until the SOF. The dura of the posterior part of the lateral wall of the CS also forms the medial wall of the upper aspect of Meckel's cave where V1 arises and hence courses in the lateral CS wall just above where it joins its medial wall (Figs. 4.3, 4.4, 4.5, and 4.10). Otherwise, most of Meckel's cave is below and lateral to the posterior aspect of the CS, and V2 does not travel in the lateral wall of the CS. The V1 divides into three branches, frontal, lacrimal, and nasociliary, prior to reaching the SOF. Both the frontal and lacrimal nerves pass through the SOF outside the annulus of Zinn, with the frontal nerve more medial whilst the nasociliary nerve passes within the annulus (Fig. 4.7) [1, 2, 6].

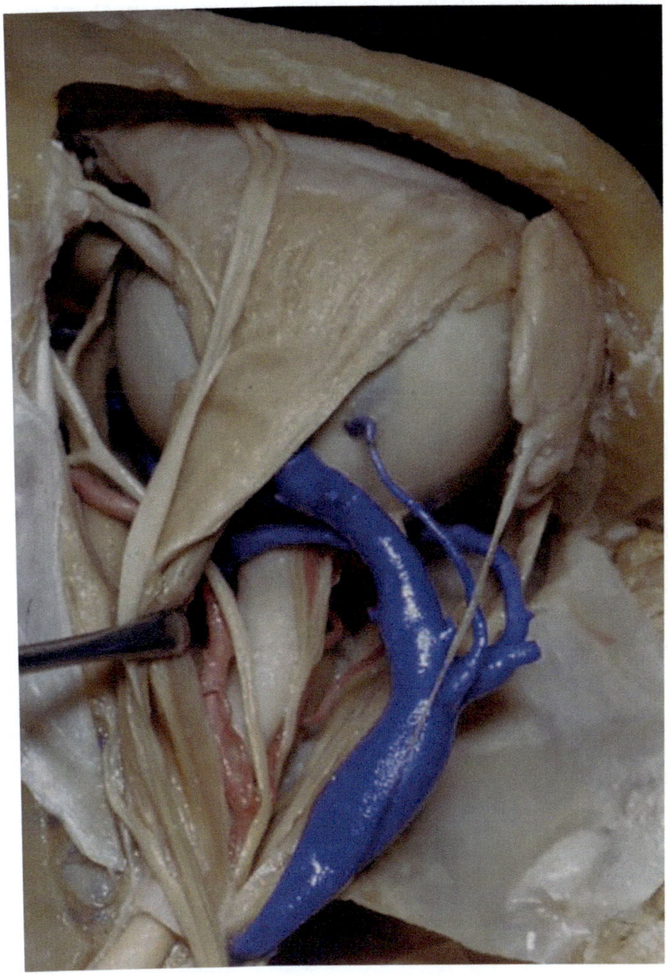

Fig. 4.7 The course of the SOV is from medial to lateral orbit, crossing over the optic nerve, and passing between the superior and lateral rectus muscles, through the SOF outside the annulus of Zinn and then inferior to V1 to join the CS. The superior and inferior divisions of the third nerve, sixth nerve, and the nasociliary branch of V1 are passing into the orbit within the annulus of Zinn. The other V1 branches, lacrimal and frontal, and the fourth nerve, shown to cross over the optic nerve just a few millimetres distally as it enters within the common tendinous origin from lateral to medial, are all outside the annulus of Zinn. The ophthalmic artery penetrates the optic sheath to give off the central retinal artery before giving off the other branches with the anterior ethmoidal artery shown

4.2 Anatomy of the Internal Carotid Artery

4.2.1 Course and Segments of ICA

A commonly used anatomical description of the segments of the proximal intracranial ICA at the skull base identifies a "petrous", "lacerum", "cavernous", "clinoidal", and "supraclinoidal" segments. The clinical implications are that by building a 3D concept of the orientation, course, and surrounding relationships, it becomes important in the management of the various pathological processes involving this region of the skull base. This facilitates the correlation with imaging and in particular the lateral views of carotid angiograms and MRI for localisation and preoperative planning (Fig. 4.8) [1, 2, 7].

The pharyngeal ICA enters the intracranial compartment through the carotid canal in the middle of the inferior aspect of the petrous bone, and initially its course follows the orientation of the long axis of the petrous pyramid. This course is directed horizontally, anteriorly, and medially—"horizontal petrous segment" (Figs. 4.8 and 4.10). This may have a thin

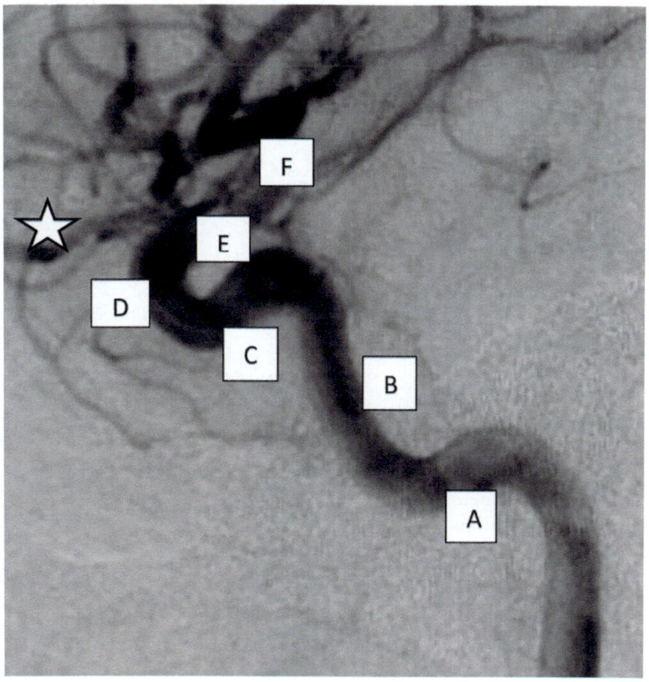

Fig. 4.8 Internal carotid angiogram—lateral view, showing the segments of ICA: "petrous" [A], "lacerum" [B], "cavernous" [B, C, D], "clinoidal" [E], and "supraclinoidal" [F] segments. The corresponding nomenclature used in the text is: "horizontal petrous segment" [A], "vertical petrosphenoid" [B], the "horizontal cavernous" [C] and the "syphon cavernous" [D], and "clinoidal" [E], to facilitate providing a 3D orientation and surrounding relationships concept. The distal portion of the "vertical petrosphenoid", the "horizontal cavernous", and the "syphon cavernous" segments constitute the cavernous ICA. The ophthalmic artery is marked by a star. Correlate with Fig. 4.10

shell of an overlying skull or even devoid of bone covering in parts. At the petrous apex, where it passes by the foramen lacerum, the ICA passes under the petrolingual ligament which is attached between the petrous apex and the lingua process of the sphenoid bone. At this point, it turns sharply superiorly in a vertical orientation and somewhat eventually anteriorly. This is the "vertical petrosphenoid segment" related to the sphenoid bone enclosing the sphenoid sinus and forming the superior part of the clivus (Figs. 4.5, 4.8, 4.9, 4.10, 4.11, and 4.12). The Gasserian ganglion at the petrous apex straddles the transition between the horizontal and vertical segments, in a 45° inclination on the coronal plane. The V2 is related to the initial vertical portion, whilst V1 enters the inferior aspect of the lateral wall of the CS more distally, i.e. superiorly. The V1 is parallel to the superior edge of the petrolingual ligament.

Just inferior to the V1 entrance, at the floor of the CS, this is where the ICA enters within the CS to become the "cavernous" segment. The course is vertically superiorly and slightly anterior. The sixth nerve within the CS is related to the lateral aspect of this portion of the ICA just medial to the course of V1 in the lateral wall. Distally the ICA sharply turns anteriorly as a "horizontal cavernous" segment with the origin of the meningohypophyseal trunk at the angle between the vertical and horizontal segments of the cavernous ICA (Figs. 4.5, 4.8, and 4.10). This is at the level of the inferior aspect of the sella, and the pituitary gland is medial to this horizontal segment. It is related to the carotid sulcus which is a shallow groove on the sphenoid bone. The third and fourth nerves are related to this segment. Historically, Parkinson's triangle was described to gain access to the cavernous ICA inferior to the fourth nerve and superior to V1 through the lateral wall of the CS. This is where the bend of the ICA and the origin of the meningohypophyseal trunk are located.

At the anterior end of the "horizontal cavernous" segment, the ICA smoothly turns supero-anteriorly in a C-shaped configuration, with the apex of the C being the most anterior point which is also slightly inclined away from the midline in the sagittal plane. At this point the course of the ICA continues supero-posteriorly until the exit of the cavernous ICA through the roof of the CS. This is the "syphon cavernous" ICA segment (Figs. 4.8, 4.9, 4.10, and 4.11). The cavernous ICA penetrates the roof of the CS surrounded by the proximal dural ring at the level of the floor of the sella. The proximal dural ring is attached to the inferior aspect of the ACP and to the optic strut, whilst the distal ring is attached to the superior surface of the ACP. The "clinoidal" segment of the

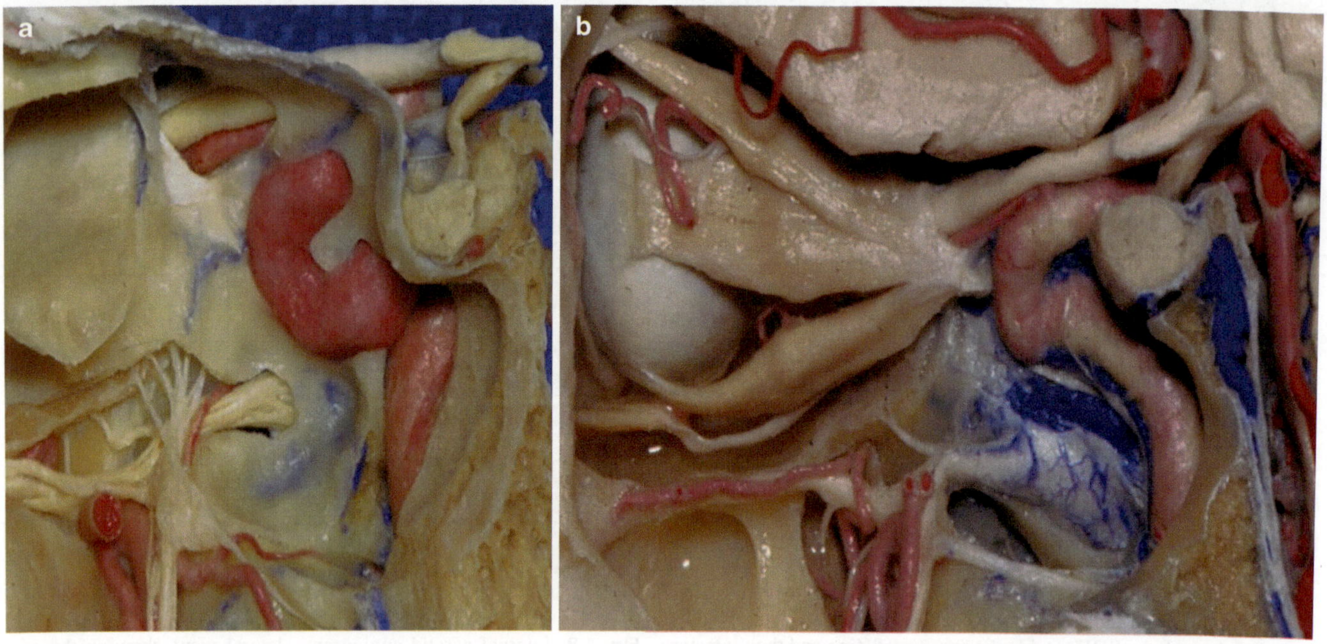

Fig. 4.9 (**a**) The wide opening of the SS and ethmoidectomy revealing the left cavernous ICA segments: vertical petrosphenoid or paraclival ICA, the horizontal cavernous, and the syphon cavernous or parasellar ICA, with relationship to SS, clivus, and sella harbouring the pituitary gland and stalk. The intact lamina papyracea is medial to the orbit. The course of the optic nerve and ophthalmic artery is visible through a bone window at the superolateral corner of the SS at the medial aspect of the distal optic canal prior to passing through the annulus of Zinn at a level adjacent to the anterior wall of the SS. V2 emerges through the foramen rotundum into the pterygopalatine fossa, associated with the maxillary artery, and gives the zygomatic, infraorbital branches and contribution through the sphenopalatine ganglion. (**b**) Similar view showing, in addition, the inferior extension and the medial CS venous compartment and the basilar venous sinus with the relationship with the cavernous ICA and sella. Endonasal endoscopic approaches allow access to orbital apex lesions extending to the medial CS. The V2 in the lateral recess of the SS and the annulus of Zinn with the recti muscles are clearly seen. The vidian canal at the floor of the SS inferomedial to V2

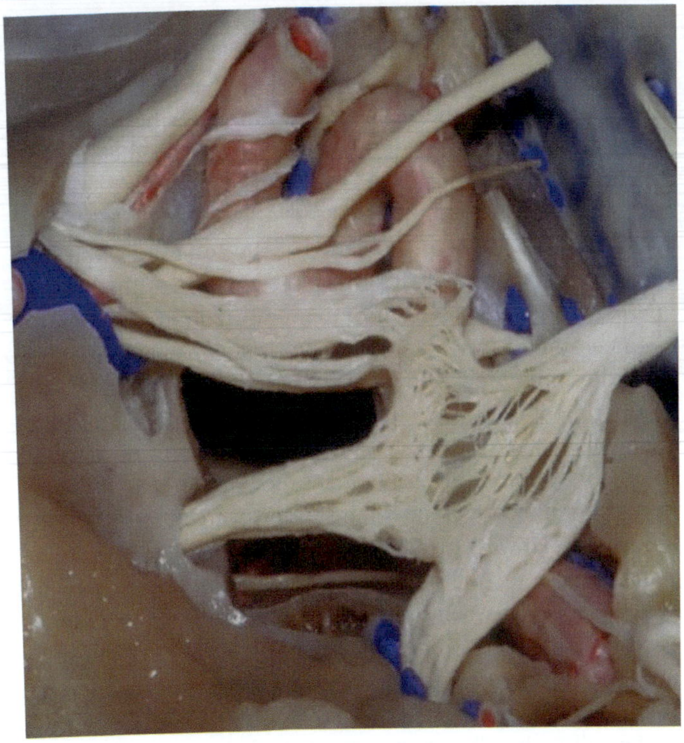

Fig. 4.10 A transcranial anatomical view from the left middle fossa and opening into the SS above and below V2. The geniculate ganglion of the seventh nerve gives the GSPN travelling on the surface of the horizontal petrous ICA segment being crossed over by V3 (mandibular division) to the foramen ovale and joined distally by the deep petrosal to from the vidian nerve shown in the vidian canal at the floor of the SS. The V2 division of the Gasserian ganglion which is straddling the junction between the horizontal petrous and the vertical petrosphenoid ICA segments is passing into the foramen rotundum. The relationship between the course of V2 and the SS explains the impression of V2 in lateral recess of well-aerated SS from a transsphenoidal view. The relationship between the vidian at the floor of the SS and the rotundum foramina at the pterygopalatine fossa is that the latter is superolateral to the former. The vertical petrosphenoid segment is seen from an endonasal approach as the paraclival ICA is shown with V1 and more medially VIth nerve passing to the SOF. The third nerve passes over the horizontal cavernous ICA segment in proximity to the meningohypophyseal trunk. The fourth nerve is cross over the IIIth nerve on approaching the SOF. The syphon cavernous segment seen as the parasellar ICA from an endonasal transsphenoidal route is at a more anterior plane than the paraclival ICA. The base of the optic strut is anterior to the clinoidal segment of ICA and separates the optic canal from the SOF. The proximal and distal dural rings are shown with the ophthalmic artery and optic nerve distally. Correlate with Fig. 4.8

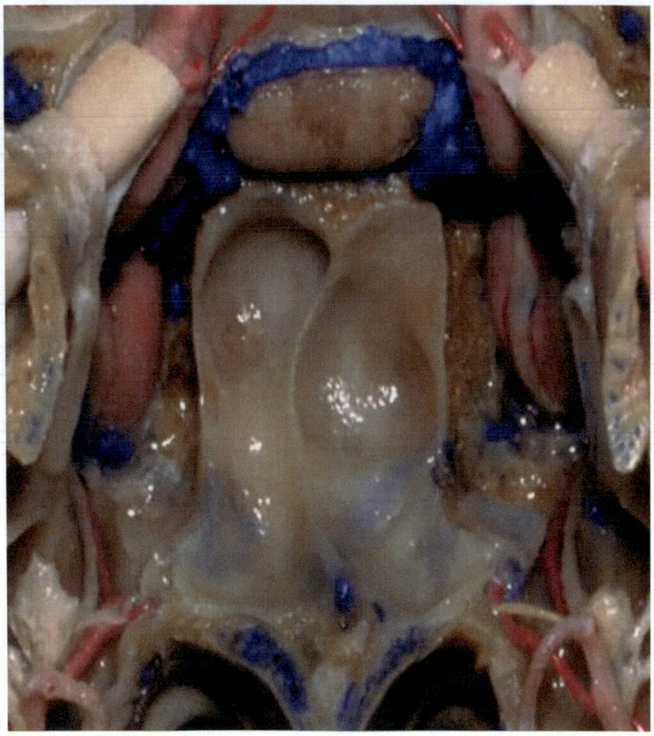

Fig. 4.11 An endonasal transsphenoidal anatomical view showing the paraclival ICA with the vidian canal at the level of the floor of the SS towards its junction with the horizontal petrous segment. The parasellar ICA are at either side of the sella, and the medial venous compartments of CS are joined by the superior and inferior anterior intercavernous sinuses. The optic nerve entering the annulus of Zinn and ophthalmic artery is seen

ICA is between these two rings (Figs. 4.6, 4.8, and 4.12). The optic strut is anterior to the "clinoidal" segment [2, 7].

Therefore, the cavernous ICA is formed by the distal portion of the "vertical petrosphenoid", the "horizontal cavernous", and the "syphon cavernous" segments of the ICA.

The branches of the cavernous ICA can be variable but include the meningohypophyseal trunk at the bend of the "horizontal cavernous" ICA giving inferior hypophyseal, tentorial, and dorsal meningeal branches, the inferolateral trunk more distally from the same ICA segment in proximity of the fourth nerve supplying the lateral wall of the CS, and finally an inconsistent capsular artery of McConnel to the pituitary gland and sella. In the rare cases of persistent trigeminal artery, this arises from the "vertical petrosphenoid" segment.

The ophthalmic artery in most cases originates off the clinoidal segment of the ICA and passes with the optic nerve into the optic canal to penetrate the optic sheath distally on its lateral aspect at the orbital apex (Figs. 4.8, 4.9, 4.10, 4.11, and 4.12).

4.2.2 Correlation Between Transcranial and Endonasal Anatomy of the Cavernous ICA

Endoscopic endonasal (EE) approaches to the skull base and orbit expose the anatomy of the cavernous ICA, some CS compartments, and the medial orbit and orbital apex from a basal extracranial point of view. The wide opening of the anterior wall of the sphenoid sinus (SS) allows visualisation "face on" and access to the sella and parasellar region and more inferiorly the upper part of the clivus (Figs. 4.8, 4.9,

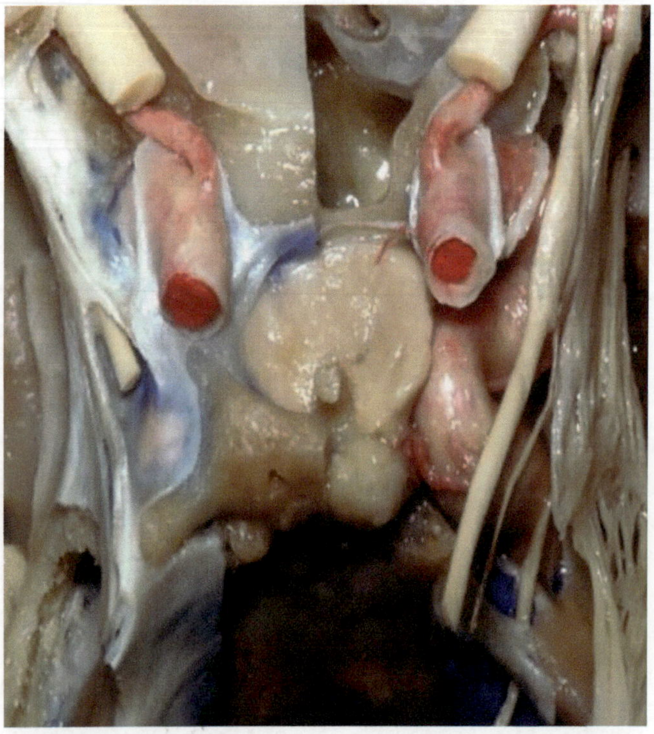

Fig. 4.12 The sixth nerve passes deep to Gruber's ligament in Dorello's canal, crossing the lateral aspect of the vertical petrosphenoid segment of the cavernous ICA and medial to the V1 division of the Gasserian ganglion which is straddling the junction of the horizontal petrous and vertical petrosphenoid ICA segments. Deeper and not shown, the petrolingual ligament demarcates the junction between these two segments. The third nerve is at the level of the origin of the meningohypophyseal trunk in proximity of the junction of the vertical petrosphenoid and the horizontal cavernous ICA segments. On the left the clinoidal segment of ICA emerges at the clinoidal triangle, whilst on the right the proximal and distal dural rings are diverging laterally with the optic strut anteriorly. It is giving off the ophthalmic branch and the superior hypophyseal distally

4.10, and 4.11). The lower limit of the exposure without further bone drilling is at the level of the floor of the SS.

In an aerated SS, the junction between the "horizontal petrous" and "vertical petrosphenoid" segments of the ICA is at a plane corresponding to the plane of the floor of the SS. From an EE view, the "vertical petrosphenoid" segment is named as the "paraclival" ICA in endoscopic terms. These, on either side, form the lateral limits for the endoscopic transclival approaches. Given that the vidian canal is located laterally at the level of the floor of the SS, the vidian nerve is valuable as a surgical landmark to the petrous ICA and apex of the petrous bone. The vidian foramen transmits the vidian nerve formed by the greater superficial petrosal nerve (GSPN) and the deep petrosal nerve containing the sympathetic nerve fibres around the petrous ICA to the pterygopalatine fossa. The foramen is at the base of the pterygoid process at the upper aspect of the pterygopalatine fossa and is inferior and medial to the foramen rotundum. It also contains a vidian artery. Hence, drilling the vidian canal and following the nerve will lead to the petrous apex with the junction of the "horizontal petrous" and "vertical petrosphenoid" segments of the ICA medial and inferior—as would be expected given the course of the GSPN on the superior aspect of the petrous ICA—and the Gasserian ganglion laterally.

However, with the prominence of the sella floor, the transition and junction between the "vertical petrosphenoid" or "paraclival" segment with the "horizontal cavernous" becomes at a deeper plane and is not readily visualised from an endoscopic view within the SS. The inferior medial CS compartment is between the superior of the "paraclival" ICA segment just below and lateral to the sella. In an well-aeriated SS, the V2 impression as it courses the paraclival ICA is seen in the lateral recess of the SS, just inferior to the inferior limit of the CS. However, during endoscopic surgery for sellar/pituitary lesions, the medial CS component adjacent to the ICA junction between the superior paraclival and horizontal cavernous segments may be accessed from within the sella, and the inferior hypophyseal artery may be encountered there (Figs. 4.9b and 4.11).

Distally the "syphon cavernous" segment becomes prominently visualised endoscopically on either side of the sella and hence named "parasellar" ICA. On occasions, the overlying bone is dehiscent [2, 5]. At the posterior roof of the SS, the ICA and optic nerve impressions define the lateral and medial optico-carotid recesses (OCR). The lateral OCR, which is occasionally well aeriated, represents the optic strut joining the sphenoid bone and separating the optic canal from the SOF. The medial extension of the SOF is lateral to the lateral OCR. This configuration reflects the fact that the anterior ICA syphon lies at the posterior surface of the optic strut and then emerges medial to the ACP. The medial OCR is at a plane just above the middle clinoid process, with the superior medial CS compartment, and is the "gateway" to the endoscopic corridor and access to the supraclinoid ICA.

4.2.3 Relevant Vascular Anatomic Variations

The ophthalmic artery arises from the cavernous ICA within the CS in 8% [2]. In that case it reaches the orbit through the SOF rather than the optic canal. Sometimes it is duplicated, being either of equal calibre or one dominant branch, one arising from the supraclinoid ICA in the subarachnoid space and passing through the optic canal whilst the other within the CS and passing through the SOF.

Rarely, the ophthalmic artery is replaced by a branch of the middle meningeal artery or a meningo-orbital branch passing through the lateral part of the SOF (Figs. 4.2, 4.3, and 4.4) [2, 8].

4.3 Relevance of CS Anatomy to the Management of Orbital Lesions

Anatomically the CS is located posterior to the orbital apex with neurovascular structures coursing through the SOF. This continuity determines the extension of pathological processes in this region and through further connections to other compartments. Furthermore, understanding the bony configuration, especially the ACP and optic strut with the proximity of the optic canal to the CS together with the dural attachments to the petrous and sphenoid bone and the ICA, is most important. This is mainly to determine individually tailored surgical approaches accessing the region around the orbital apex, optic canal, and SOF by knowing the exact need for bone drilling necessary to expose the pathological lesion extending between these compartments with minimal risk to the intimately related neurovascular structures.

4.3.1 Extension of Pathological Process Involving the Orbit

Given the anatomical proximity and connections between the orbit and CS, a number of neoplastic, infective, or vascular conditions involve both regions.

Schwannomas and nerve sheath tumours may extend along the course of the nerve of origin from the CS to the orbit (Fig. 4.13). Those related to both divisions of the third, nasociliary, and sixth nerves pass through the SOF within the annulus of Zinn. Further extensions for those involving the V1 branches namely the frontal, lacrimal, and nasociliary may even include the Meckel's cave. The adjacent Mekel's cave shares a dural wall with the posterolateral CS. Its superior aspect is just lateral to the posterior CS as the Mekel's cave is predominantly located inferior and lateral to the CS. Malignant tumours such as adenoid cystic carcinomas with the propensity for perineural spread may behave similarly.

Other lesions such as spheno-orbital meningiomas usually with hyperostotic involvement of the greater wing of sphenoid—forming part of the lateral orbital wall as well as part of the middle fossa—are associated with *en plaque* intradural meningioma mass involving the lateral wall of the CS.

Transvenous extension of infections between the orbit and CS is explained by their venous connections. In pathological situations, the anatomical boundaries of the CS are arbitrary as there are multiple venous connections, either through the pericavernous plexus or directly to other compartments. These venous connections explain the potential transvenous spread of infection or septic thrombosis to the orbit from adjacent regions via the CS such as the soft tissues of the face via the facial veins tributaries to the ophthalmic veins, retropharyngeal space via pterygoid plexus and emissary veins, and contralateral infection from one CS to the other via the intercavernous connections.

The effects of venous hypertension, manifesting by papilloedema or elevated intraocular pressure, can arise through the transmission of elevated venous pressure to the central retinal vein via a connection of the ophthalmic vein. This may occur, for example, from remote venous sinus thrombosis or a dural arterio-venous fistula involving the transverse sinus via the superior petrosal and the jugular bulb via the inferior petrosal sinus or the contralateral CS.

4.3.2 Implications for Operative Approaches

4.3.2.1 Transcranial Approaches

Anterolateral transcranial approaches with variations including pterional, modified orbitozygomatic, or supraorbital mini-craniotomies access widely the superolateral orbit and allow dealing with lesions extending from the orbital apex, optic canal, and SOF to the CS and other intracranial regions. This allows dealing with such extensions to the CS with extradural approaches.

During resection of orbital lesions extending to the parasellar region sometimes, it is possible to trace and distinguish lesions extending within the CS from those towards the Meckel's cave (Fig. 4.13). The latter will be surrounded by the pericavernous venous plexus which extends onto the rotundum and ovale foramina around V2 and V3 and haemorrhage from which would be easier to control as opposed to that from the CS.

Following the orbitotomy, the frontotemporal dura is adherent to the periorbita at the SOF, and an incision of the meningo-orbital band allows extradural separation of the dural layers of the lateral wall of the CS. Especially, with lesions expanding the sinus, "peeling" of the dural layers onto the potential space within the CS or lateral wall occupied by the lesion is facilitated.

The extent of drilling of the ACP, optic strut, and opening of the optic canal is tailored according to the extent of the lesion and the need to control the clinoidal segment of the ICA. Occasionally, a bony bridge between the middle clinoid and ACP forms a carotidoclinoidal foramen through which the ICA passes which needs to be drilled to mobilise this ICA segment, if needed, during transcranial approaches to the orbital apex.

4.3.2.2 Endoscopic Endonasal Approaches

Endonasal approaches access the medial orbit through the lamina papyracea and extended bone window. For lesions around the orbital apex, transsphenoidal extension is needed. The level of the junction of the anterior wall of the SS and its lateral wall is the approximate attachment of the annulus of Zinn. Therefore, drilling of the medial optic canal along the

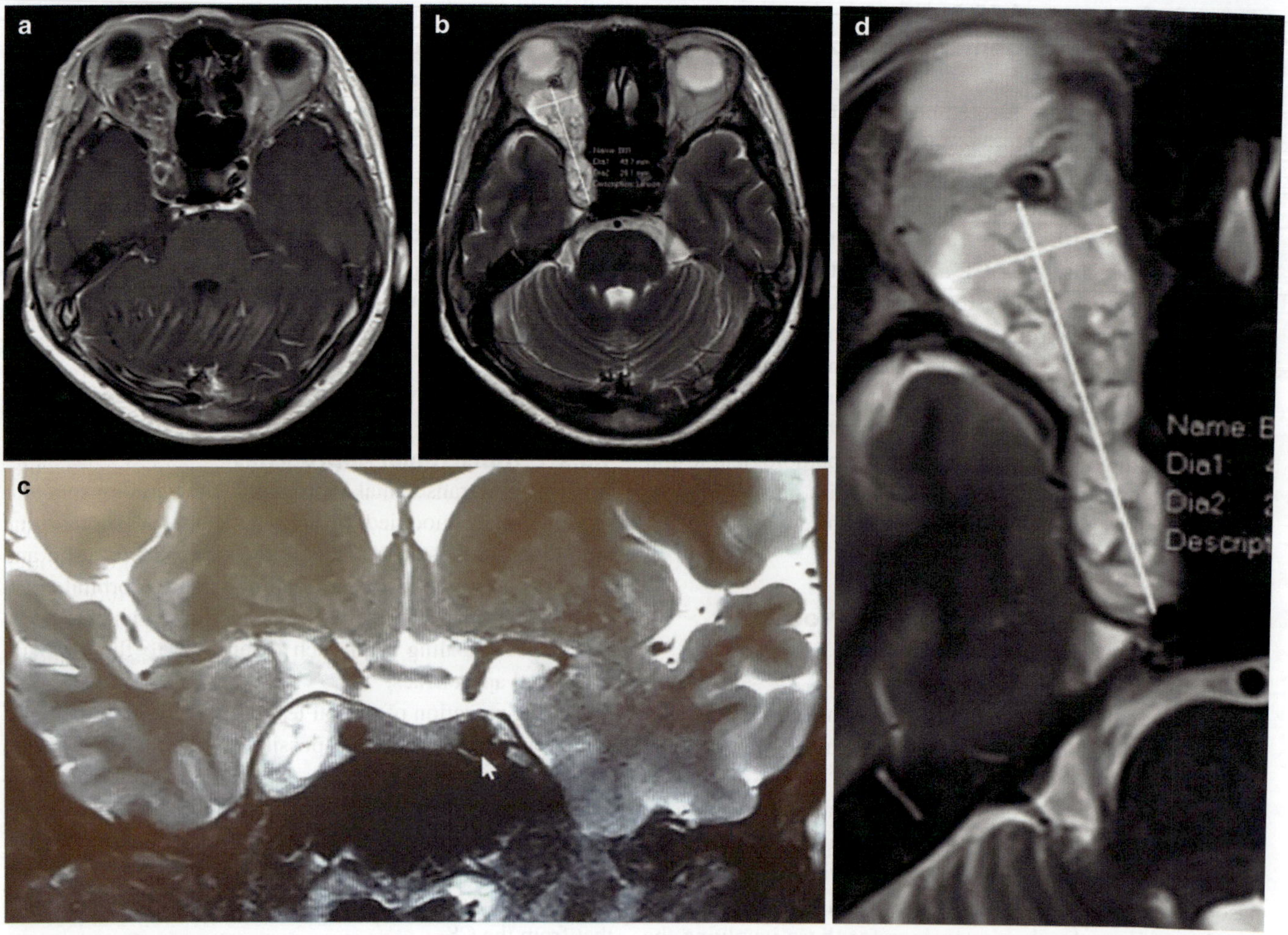

Fig. 4.13 Axial MRI, T1-weighted with gadolinium (**a**) and T2-weighted (**b**) sequences for a patient presenting with right-sided proptosis and severe compressive optic neuropathy showing an intraconal orbital schwannoma with heterogenous signal extending through the SOF to the CS. (**c**) Coronal T2-weighted MRI depicting the mixed signal intracavernous extension of the lesion expanding the CS on the right. An arrow is pointing to the contralateral ICA flow void for comparison. (**d**) Magnified axial T2-weighted MRI showing the course of the cisternal portion of the fifth nerve to the Meckel's cave which is clear and separated from the lesion extending to within the CS

lateral wall of the SS will access the medial orbital apex region proximal to the attachment of the annulus of Zinn (Fig. 4.9a). The medial CS venous compartment starts superior to the V2 impression on the SS lateral recess and medial to the paraclival ICA and more superiorly from within the sella between the pituitary gland and the ICA (Figs. 4.9b and 4.11).

4.3.3 Considerations for Potential Complications

In extended lesions with ICA encasement, thorough anatomical knowledge of the course, bony relationship, and dural attachment of the artery is imperative to avoid iatrogenic injury.

Awareness of anomalous arterial supply will mitigate potential complications. The ophthalmic artery branches within the orbit forming anastomosis with branches of the external carotid artery. Occlusion at its origin off the ICA does not necessarily result in blindness, but it is its first branch in the orbit which is the central retinal artery which is an end artery, and its occlusion will result in blindness. However, injury of the ophthalmic artery at surgery or through endovascular procedures may cause blindness through thromboembolic sequelae as the central retinal artery is of a small calibre. Unawareness of the possible variations of the ophthalmic artery such as those arising from the cavernous ICA may be coagulated erroneously during resection of orbital lesions extending through the SOF as in this variation the ophthalmic artery passes through the SOF rather than the optic canal.

Unrecognised postoperative infections after orbital surgery may result in septic thrombosis of the cavernous sinus with serious consequences if treatment is delayed.

Acknowledgement This chapter is predominantly based on the late Dr. Albert Rhoton publications on neurosurgical anatomy. The anatomical images are Dr. Rhoton's dissections [Courtesy of the Rhoton Collection, American Association of Neurological Surgeons (AANS)/ Neurosurgical Research and Education Foundation (NREF)].

References

1. Harris FS, Rhoton AL Jr. Anatomy of the cavernous sinus: a microsurgical study. J Neurosurg. 1976;45:169–80.
2. Rhoton AL Jr. The cavernous sinus, the cavernous venous plexus, and the carotid collar. Neurosurgery. 2002;51(Suppl 1):375–410.
3. Rhoton AL Jr, Hardy DG, Chambers SM. Microsurgical anatomy and dissection of the sphenoid bone, cavernous sinus and sellar region. Surg Neurol. 1979;12:63–104.
4. Rhoton AL Jr, Natori Y. The skull. In: Rhoton Jr AL, Natori Y, editors. The orbit and sellar region: microsurgical anatomy and operative approaches. New York: Thieme Medical Publishers, Inc.; 1996. p. 4–25.
5. Renn WH, Rhoton AL Jr. Microsurgical anatomy of the sellar region. J Neurosurg. 1975;43:288–98.
6. Rhoton AL Jr, Natori Y. Neural structures. In: Rhoton Jr AL, Natori Y, editors. The orbit and sellar region: microsurgical anatomy and operative approaches. New York: Thieme Medical Publishers, Inc.; 1996. p. 28–77.
7. Seoane ER, Rhoton AL Jr, de Oliveira EP. Microsurgical anatomy of the dural collar (carotid collar) and rings around the clinoid segment of the internal carotid artery. Neurosurgery. 1998;42:869–86.
8. Liu Q, Rhoton AL Jr. Middle meningeal origin of the ophthalmic artery. Neurosurgery. 2001;49:401–7.

Paranasal Sinuses

5

Hung Wai Cho

Abstract

The paranasal sinuses arise as evaginations from the nasal cavities. They are air-filled cavities lined with ciliated columnar respiratory epithelium with their ostia opening in the nasal cavities. Their development varies in time with the maxillary sinus being the first to develop, followed by ethmoid sinus, sphenoid sinus, and frontal sinus. The sinuses grow after birth till the early twenties with variable degrees of pneumatization [1]. The paranasal sinuses comprise five paired sinuses, namely, maxillary, frontal, anterior ethmoid, posterior ethmoid, and sphenoid. The maxillary, frontal, and anterior ethmoid sinuses are grouped as the anterior system with the final drainage pathway toward the osteomeatal complex. The posterior ethmoid and sphenoid sinuses are grouped as the posterior system which drains toward the sphenoethmoidal recess. The anatomy of the paranasal sinuses shows great individual variation, with different degrees of pneumatization and septation. A general understanding of the anatomy of the paranasal sinus creates the transnasal corridor to the orbit.

Keywords

Paranasal sinus · Maxillary sinus · Ethmoid sinus · Frontal sinus · Sphenoid sinus · Pneumatization · Septation

H. W. Cho (✉)
Department of Ear, Nose and Throat, United Christian Hospital, Hong Kong, China

Division of Rhinology, Department of Otorhinolaryngology, Head & Neck Surgery, Faculty of Medicine, The Chinese University of Hong Kong, Hong Kong, China
e-mail: chw553@ha.org.hk

5.1 The Maxillary Sinus

The maxillary sinus opens to the nasal cavity through its natural ostium on the medial wall. There may be accessory ostia, namely, anterior and posterior fontanelle. The roof of the maxillary sinus forms the majority of the orbital floor, and its posterior bony edge contributes to the inferior orbital fissure. The infraorbital nerve runs at the roof with bony dehiscence occasionally.

5.2 The Anterior and Posterior Ethmoid Sinuses

The ethmoid bone is extremely complex situated in the anterior base of the skull and contributes to the medial wall of the orbits, the roof and the lateral walls of the nasal cavity. The ethmoid sinus consists of 3–18 thin-walled cells [2]. The lateral wall, lamina papyracea, is the lateral limit of the nasal cavity as well as the medial orbital wall. The roof is constituted by the fovea ethmoidalis of the frontal bone. The uncinated process is a thin curved bar of bone from the ethmoid which is the door to the osteomeatal unit.

Anatomically, the anterior ethmoid and posterior ethmoid are separated by the ground lamella, which is attached to the middle turbinate. During surgery, the ground lamella is identified at the blind end between the bulla and middle turbinate. Radiologically, the ground lamella is at the junction of the middle turbinate and superior turbinate.

Supraorbital cells originate from the anterior ethmoid which extends superiorly over the orbit from the frontal recess. The anterior ethmoidal artery (AEA) lies posterior to the supraorbital cell, which can be a landmark for the identification of AEA [3].

Haller cells refer to the ethmoidal pneumatization at the superior aspect of the maxillary sinus and floor of the orbit [4]. Access to the maxillary sinus can be restricted by Haller cells. Recognition of Haller cells on preoperative computed tomography (CT) would aid in the dissection for identification of the

T. L. POON et al. (eds.), *Orbital Apex and Periorbital Skull Base Diseases*, https://doi.org/10.1007/978-981-99-2989-4_5

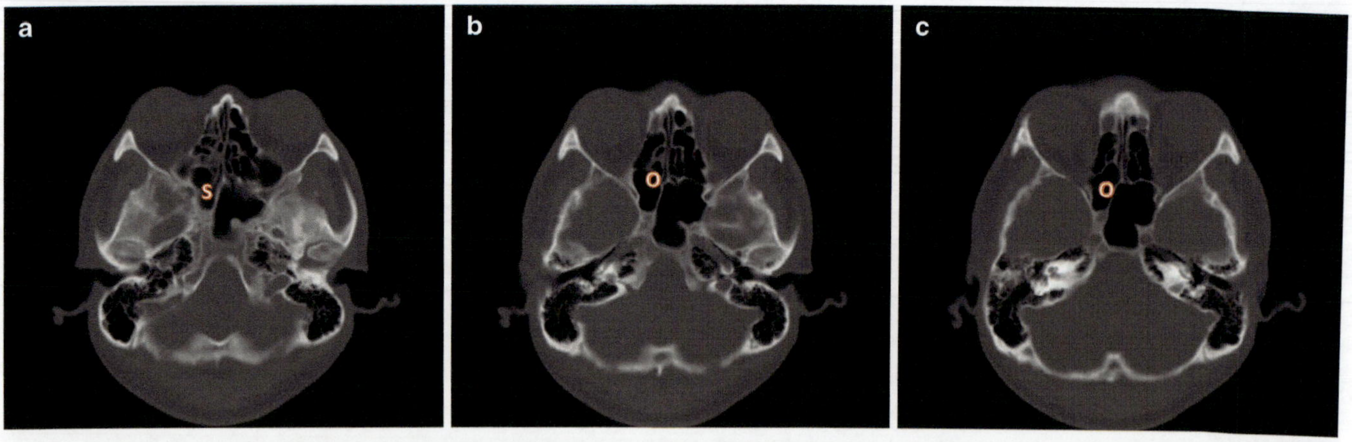

Fig. 5.1 Serial axial CT (from inferior to superior) showing a small right sphenoid sinus (**a**) and a large Onodi cell (**b** and **c**). The left sphenoid sinus is dominant in this patient. *S* sphenoid sinus, *O* Onodi cell

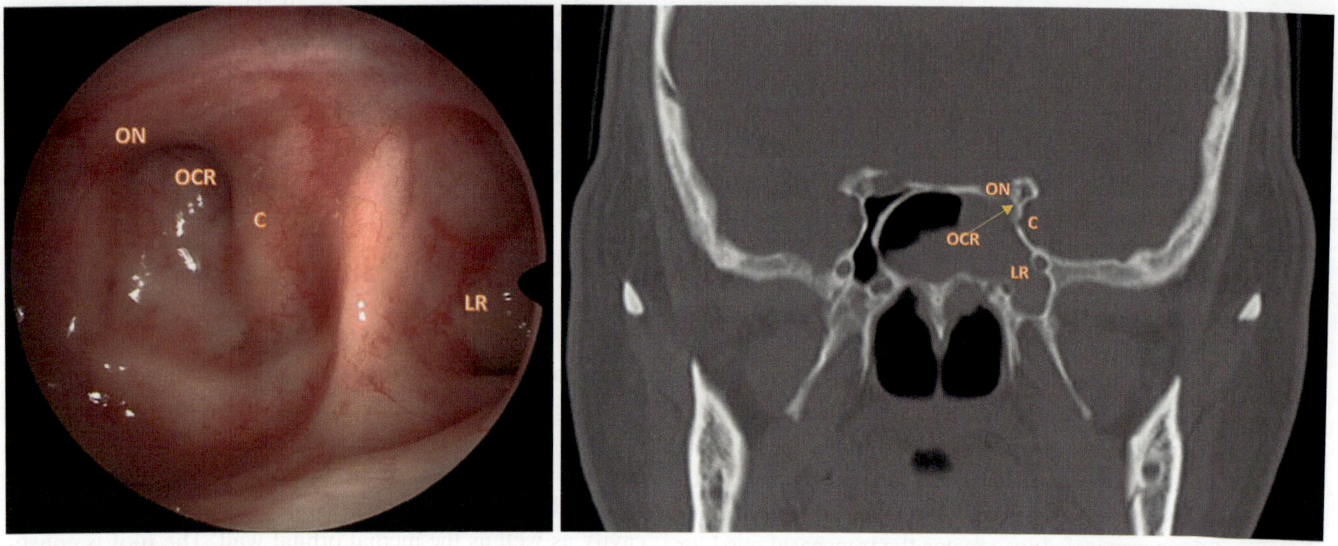

Fig. 5.2 Endoscopic picture of the left sphenoid sinus showing the optic nerve, carotid artery, opticocarotid recess, and lateral recess of the sphenoid sinus, with corresponding coronal CT images. *ON* optic nerve, *C* carotid artery, *OCR* opticocarotid recess, *LR* lateral recess

maxillary roof/orbital floor and the lamina papyracea. The floor of Haller cells can be mistaken as the floor of the orbit.

Onodi cells (sphenoethmoidal cells) are an anatomic variant of the most posterior ethmoid cells that pneumatized superiorly and laterally to the sphenoid sinus and are in close relation to the optic nerve (Fig. 5.1) [5]. Recognition of its relationship to the sphenoid sinus is important in dissection around the optic canal to avoid inadvertent injury.

5.3 The Sphenoid Sinus

The sphenoid sinuses are variable in size and often asymmetric with variable degrees of pneumatization into the greater wing, pterygoid processes, and rostrum. Several types of pneumatization are described, namely, conchal, presellar, sellar, and postseller, depending on the position of the sinus in relation to the sellar turcia [6]. The optic nerve prominence lies at the superior end on the lateral wall, with a variable relationship in the presence of Onodi cells. The intersphenoid septum and accessory septum can be attached to carotid prominence. The opticocarotid recess is the bony depression between the optic nerve and carotid artery. In the presence of pneumatization with a large lateral recess (Fig. 5.2), the transpterygoid approach may be required to reach the far lateral end.

5.4 The Frontal Sinus

The frontal sinus drainage pathway depends on the relative anatomy of uncinate process attachment and frontoethmoidal cells. The floor of the frontal sinus is shared with the anterior orbital roof. The orbital roof can be non-pneumatized, only the medial part pneumatized, the medial and a portion of the

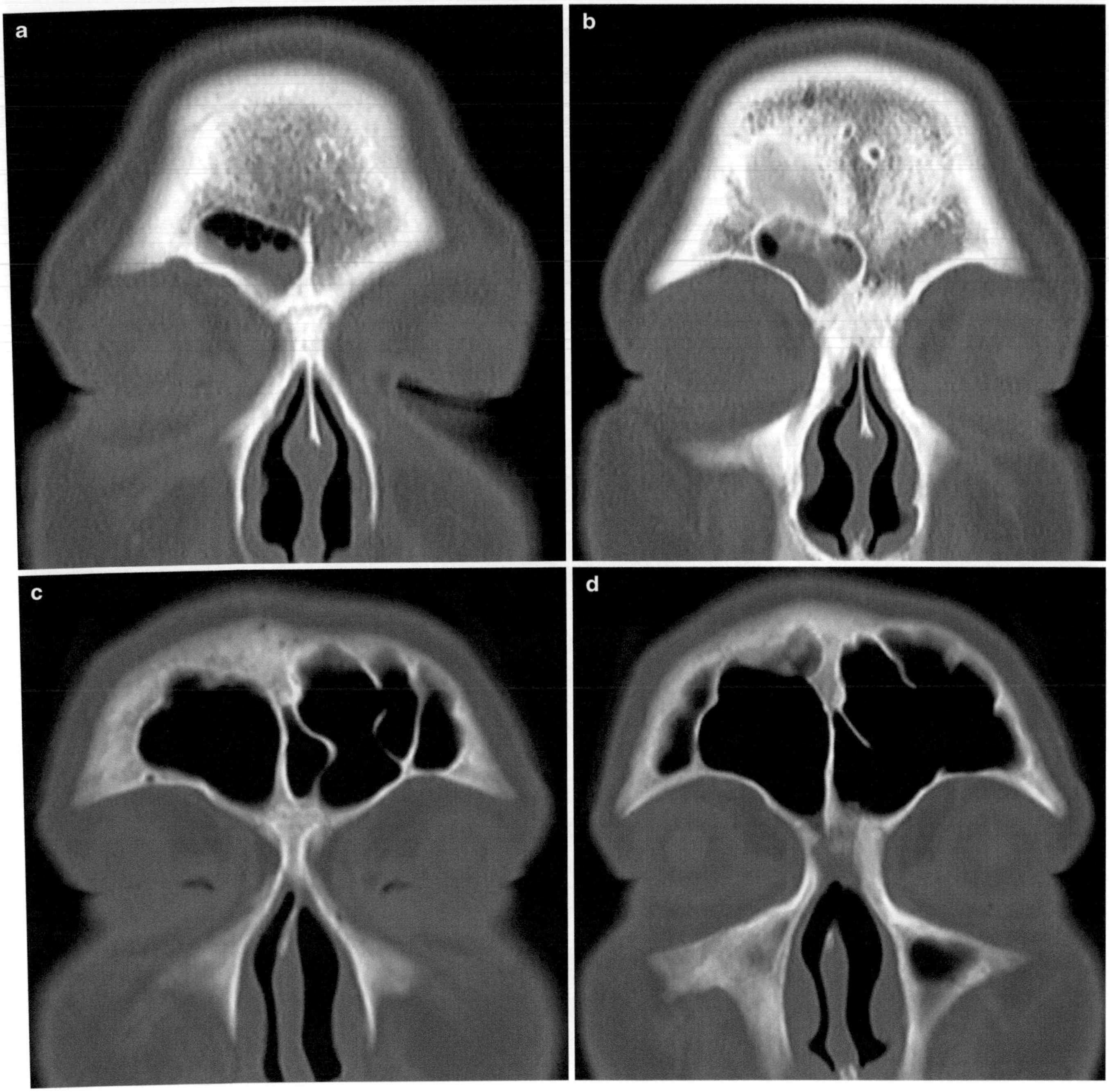

Fig. 5.3 Coronal CT images showing different degrees of pneumatization of frontal sinuses. Small right frontal sinus and absent left frontal sinus (**a** and **b**). Highly pneumatized frontal sinuses (**c** and **d**)

central part pneumatized, or roof predominantly pneumatized (Fig. 5.3) [7].

References

1. Maran AGD, Lund VJ. Clinical rhinology. New York: Thieme Medical Publishers, Inc.; 1990.
2. Başal Y, Başak S, Bedrosian JC. Surgical anatomy of the paranasal sinuses. In: Cingi C, Bayar Muluk N, editors. All around the nose. Cham: Springer; 2020.
3. Comer BT, Kountakis SE. The supraorbital ethmoid cell. In: Kountakis S, Senior B, Draf W, editors. The frontal sinus. Berlin: Springer; 2016.
4. Raina A, Guledgud MV, Patil K. Infraorbital ethmoid (Haller's) cells: a panoramic radiographic study. Dentomaxillofac Radiol. 2012;41:305–8.
5. Chmielik LP, Chmielik A. The prevalence of the Onodi cell – most suitable method of CT evaluation in its direction. Int J Pediatr Otorhinolaryngol. 2017;97:202–5.
6. Hamid O, Fiky LEI, Hassan O, et al. Anatomical variations of the sphenoid sinus and their impact on trans-sphenoid pituitary surgery. Skull Base. 2008;18:9–15.
7. Stokovic N, Trkulja V, Cukovic-Bagic I, et al. Anatomical variations of the frontal sinus and its relationship with the orbital cavity. Clin Anat. 2018;31:576–82.

Part II

Diagnosis and Radiology

History

6

Sai Lok Chu

Abstract

History is the first step in establishing the doctor-patient relationship. Both patients and doctors acquire the first impression of each other through this process. Through systematic inquiry, a list of differential diagnoses is formulated, and the door to a logical guessing game is opened.

Keywords

History · Chief complaint · Symptoms · Differential diagnosis · Etiology

6.1 Introduction

History is the first step in approaching a clinical problem. It is a fundamental skill in clinical medicine. The patient approaches the doctor with a chief complaint. After clarifying the problem in the history of present illness, we obtain the background information of the patient by taking the past medical history, family history, drug history, and social history. Most of the time, we will have an idea about the differential diagnosis. This guides the physical examination and investigations to reach a definitive diagnosis.

6.2 Chief Complaint

A chief complaint is the symptom that brings the patient to the doctor. This is the problem that the patient wants to solve. Our job is to clarify the complaint so that it suits the symptoms known. For presenting symptoms from periorbital skull base diseases, the main categories include neurological and ophthalmological symptoms, pain (periorbital pain, headache), and cosmetic problems. After clarifying the chief complaint, we can have a detailed inquiry into that and the other information associated.

6.3 History of Present Illness

6.3.1 Onset

Onset time should be the first question after clarifying the chief complaint. It gives us clues about the underlying etiology of the symptoms (Table 6.1). Sometimes, the description from the patient is not straightforward. Specific questioning will be needed to match their description to our framework so that we have a clearer direction for further questioning.

In the sudden onset group, acute trauma history is easy to elicit and usually volunteered by the patient. The vascular cause is usually due to acute arterial occlusion (seldom in periorbital skull base diseases) or rupture, e.g., in direct carotid cavernous fistula.

In the progressive-onset group, causes are more diverse. It is not easy to differentiate the causes with such little information at this stage. The exception is the vascular cause. Symptoms from the vascular cause can be prominent, which gives us a clearer direction in further questioning. Mucocele from paranasal sinuses enlarges slowly and behaves like a benign tumor.

Table 6.1 A rough guide between onset time and possible etiologies of the underlying diseases

Onset time	Descriptive term by patient	Etiology
Minutes to hours	Sudden	Vascular (arterial), trauma
Days to weeks	Progressive	Neoplasm, inflammatory, infection, vascular (venous), congenital/developmental

S. L. Chu (✉)
Department of Neurosurgery, Tuen Mun Hospital, Tuen Mun, New Territories, Hong Kong
e-mail: csl282@ha.org.hk

T. L. POON et al. (eds.), *Orbital Apex and Periorbital Skull Base Diseases*, https://doi.org/10.1007/978-981-99-2989-4_6

6.3.2 Duration

Duration of symptoms is clearer in sudden onset disease, as the patient can clearly define the duration lapsed before he/she presents. On the contrary, it is usually mixed with onset time in subacute or chronic problems. The progressive onset nature of these problems makes differentiation from onset and duration difficult. Practically, such differentiation is not mandatory in developing the list of differential diagnoses. Knowing the time frame from the appearance of symptoms to the presentation will be enough for history taking purposes.

6.3.3 Site, Radiation, and Character

These three items are mainly for the description of pain.

In periorbital pathology, the sites of pain are along the trigeminal territories, retrobulbar pain, or non-localizing headache. In the trigeminal territories, you will expect a higher incidence along the first and second divisions of the trigeminal nerve due to their close vicinity to orbit. These two branches go along the lower portion of the lateral wall of the cavernous sinus. The ophthalmic nerve (V1) runs into the orbit via the superior orbital fissure. The maxillary nerve (V2) runs into the pterygopalatine fossa via the foramen rotundum, and its terminal branch goes through the inferior orbital fissure into the floor of the orbit.

Asking about the radiation of pain is usually not useful. As pathological irritation usually comes from trigeminal territories, you will expect patient complaints of symptoms in the corresponding region. As a result, the site and radiation of pain are just the same. Another description from the patient will be radiation over the whole scalp or the vertex. This is nonspecific.

Wordings like pins and needles, ant crawling, stabbing, burning, and electric shock will be anticipated in patients in neuropathic pain, due to stimulation of the branches of the trigeminal nerves in the periorbital region. Though nonspecific, distending, bulging, or tension type of pain including headache can sometimes point to a space-occupying lesion. This is due to irritation of nerve fibers on the dura or periosteum and is mainly in the territories of the trigeminal nerve. However, most of the time, no lesion can be identified in patients with tension headache.

6.3.4 Severity

Subjective descriptions like mild, moderate, and severe are usually used in this part. This is the most common gauge for the disturbance of presenting symptoms to the patient. For pain, the visual analog scale can be included to allow comparison between different time frames (most useful) or between different individuals (sometimes useful as pain is subjective). Another aspect to reflect the severity is how it affects the patient's daily living. Some examples of daily activity concerns are sleeping, eating, job, and hobbies.

6.3.5 Precipitating, Aggravating, and Relieving Factors

This item hopes to find additional clues in formulating the differential diagnosis and the cause of the disease. Factors that we can explore include the timing of the day that affects the symptoms (e.g., morning, evening), Valsalva maneuver, history of recent infection, and history of old trauma.

Morning headache is a classical symptom of increased intracranial pressure but is not common. Valsalva maneuver leads to increased afterload, which increases the right atrial pressure and peripheral venous pressure. Symptoms due to venous congestion or increased intracranial pressure can be more prominent.

6.3.6 Associated Symptoms

A disease can cause multiple symptoms. Besides the presenting symptoms, other possibly related local symptoms should be screened (Table 6.2). Grouping of symptoms facilitates systematic questioning and documentation. The current system is not perfect. It is mainly anatomical, but cosmesis is more of a functional problem. Not surprisingly, you will expect some patients complaining of proptosis as a cosmetic problem. You can create your own system as long as it is helpful.

In addition to orbital and ophthalmological symptoms, screening intracranial neurological symptoms is sometimes helpful, especially in diseases causing disfiguring problems. As a lesion is big enough or affects cerebral circulation, cerebral symptoms will occur. With anatomical consideration, the frontal and temporal lobes will be most affected. The list of symptoms is numerous and can refer to neurology textbooks. Seizures may happen especially in pathology causing focal cerebral edema. Some patients complain of cognitive decline due to chronic increase in intracranial pressure.

Table 6.2 Examples of symptoms in periorbital skull base disease

Group	Symptoms
Orbital	Proptosis, periorbital pain
Ophthalmological	Visual blurring, diplopia
Neurological	Headache, facial numbness, dysphasia (frontal and temporal lobe), memory (temporal lobe)
Cosmesis	

6.3.7 System Review

This is recommended when your differential diagnosis includes potential systemic diseases, e.g., malignant tumor, hematological disease, inflammatory cause including sarcoidosis, and disseminated infection. Common symptoms in different body systems should be enquired about to define the cause and assess the extent of the disease.

6.4 Past Medical History

Medical comorbidities and a history of previous surgery is the focus of this part. Information from these can narrow down the list of differential diagnoses. These can also affect the management options, decision of anesthesia, and choice of surgical approaches.

History of disease in the periorbital area and history of paranasal sinus diseases should be enquired about. Other aspects that need particular attention include benign and malignant tumors or lesions including syndromes; hematological diseases, e.g., bleeding tendency and thrombophilia; inflammatory causes, e.g., IgG-4 disease and rheumatological disease; systemic or head and neck infection; and thyroid problem.

6.5 Family History

Patients should be asked if other family members have similar symptoms, periorbital diseases, or hereditary syndrome, e.g., neurofibromatosis. Other systemic diseases that may affect the periorbital area should also be asked, e.g., history of malignancy in the family.

6.6 Drug History

This part is straightforward. For prescribed medicine, patients usually can either remember them or show you the packages. On the other hand, we need to ask specifically for the use of over-the-counter medications, herbs, traditional Chinese medicine especially in Chinese ethnics, and health products. This is because for some patients, taking these is like a life routine. They cannot realize it unless you mention it specifically.

By knowing the variety of medications used for a particular disease, we can indirectly assess the severity of the disease. Compliance with medication may shed light on the degree of disease control.

Usually, the part of past medical history can explain why the patient is using the current medications, so using medication to provide clues to diagnosis is seldom needed. One exception is contraceptive pills. It can induce hypercoagulability and thrombosis in the cavernous sinus or its tributaries. However, this diagnosis is rare. Other causes of cavernous sinus thrombosis, e.g., facial infection, are more common.

6.7 Social History

Most of the information here may give some clues in establishing the diagnosis and tailoring the management plan later. Some time is worth spending on these few questions.

Occupation is the must-known information. This may tell us the etiology of the problem and formulate the plan. The same rationale is for asking about the patient's hobbies and recreational activities. Smoking and alcoholic history provides information for general health status and allows us to assess the risk of anesthesia when needed.

Living conditions and living companions are important pieces of information. We estimate the patient's social background and social support through them. These may also affect the patient's attitude to the disease. For diseases that will be debilitating in the future, we can provide some ways to the supporting groups or facilities later.

This is the last part of history taking. By this time, an impression of the patient's character is vaguely formed, e.g., anxious, introvert, optimistic. We may also know the reason why patients have such characteristics. Combining the character and background information from this part, we can individualize the plan of management. Then we can deliver the messages to our patients in a more palatable manner.

6.8 Conclusions

History is the gateway to establishing the doctor-patient relationship. By listening to the patient's story and asking specific questions, we paint a picture of his/her problem in our mind. This guides the planning of physical examinations and investigations to reach a definitive diagnosis. Furthermore, the background of the patient helps us to individualize the plan of management. By taking care of the biopsychosocial perspectives of the patient, holistic care can be achieved.

Physical Examination

7

Carmen K. M. Chan

Abstract

For patients with symptoms suggestive of orbital apex or periorbital skull base disease, a thorough examination should include an assessment of the ocular and periocular structures, afferent visual pathway (optic nerve function), and efferent visual pathway (pupils, eyelid position, and extraocular eye movement) as well as other cranial nerves. This allows us to localize the disease and shed light on the nature of the pathology and direct further investigations, including appropriate neuroimaging and blood tests. Quantification of any abnormities, e.g., by using automated visual field, optical coherence tomography, electrodiagnostics, prism cover tests, or Hess charts, allows us to assess the severity of the disease at baseline and monitor disease progress or response to treatment.

Keywords

Optic neuropathy · Extraocular movement · Visual field · OCT · Electrodiagnostics

7.1 Introduction

When a patient presents with symptoms which may suggest orbital apex or periorbital skull base disease, physical examination allows us to confirm the presence of pathology and assess its severity, so that it would guide the urgency and type of further investigations and management. This is especially important in low-resource settings, where investigations (e.g., neuroimaging or even visual field examination) are not readily available, and the clinician has a role to prioritize the patients according to their clinical urgency.

The surgical anatomy has been covered in detail in Chap. 1. To recap, the anatomical structures involved in the superior orbital fissure, orbital apex, and cavernous sinus syndromes [1], and the associated required examinations are summarized in Table 7.1. It is worth noting that while all those anatomical structures may be potentially involved, the actual involvement and physical signs depend on the disease severity, e.g., orbital apex syndrome may present with optic neuropathy alone.

In a busy clinic, it is impossible to perform the complete set of examinations for every patient, so the examination should be directed according to the symptoms. The neuro-ophthalmic examination for suspected orbital apex disease can be divided into the following parts:

(a) Inspection.
(b) Assessment of afferent visual pathway (including examination of ocular structures).
(c) Assessment of efferent visual pathway.
(d) Other cranial nerves and directed systemic examination.

Table 7.1 Anatomical structures involved in the superior orbital fissure, orbital apex, and cavernous sinus syndromes

	Syndromes			
Involved structures	Superior orbital fissure	Orbital apex syndrome	Cavernous sinus	Physical examination
CN II	x	✓	x	Afferent visual pathway
CN III	✓	✓	✓	Efferent visual pathway • Extraocular eye movement • Pupils • Lid position
CN IV	✓	✓	✓	
CN VI	✓	✓	✓	
Oculo-sympathetic fibers	x	x	✓	
CN V1	✓	✓	✓	Facial sensation
CN V2	x	±	✓	

C. K. M. Chan (✉)
Hong Kong Eye Hospital, Hong Kong SAR, China

Department of Ophthalmology and Visual Sciences, The Chinese University of Hong Kong, Hong Kong SAR, China
e-mail: carmen.chan@ha.org.hk

T. L. POON et al. (eds.), *Orbital Apex and Periorbital Skull Base Diseases*, https://doi.org/10.1007/978-981-99-2989-4_7

7.2 Inspection

Patients with orbital apex disease may have no external signs on inspection at all. However, they may also present with erythema or cellulitis of the periorbital skin, ptosis, proptosis, or eye redness, which may be unilateral or bilateral. For those with signs suggestive of cellulitis, it is important to distinguish whether it is superficial (pre-septal) or there is orbital involvement. Proptosis, ophthalmoplegia, and with or without eye redness would suggest orbital involvement. If proptosis is present, it should be quantified with an exophthalmometer (Fig. 7.1). While there are many causes of eye redness, and it usually takes an ophthalmologist to make the correct diagnosis with the aid of a slit-lamp (e.g., to rule out intraocular inflammation); the finding of eye redness due to cork-screw vessels (Fig. 7.2) is very suggestive of the presence of a carotid-cavernous fistula.

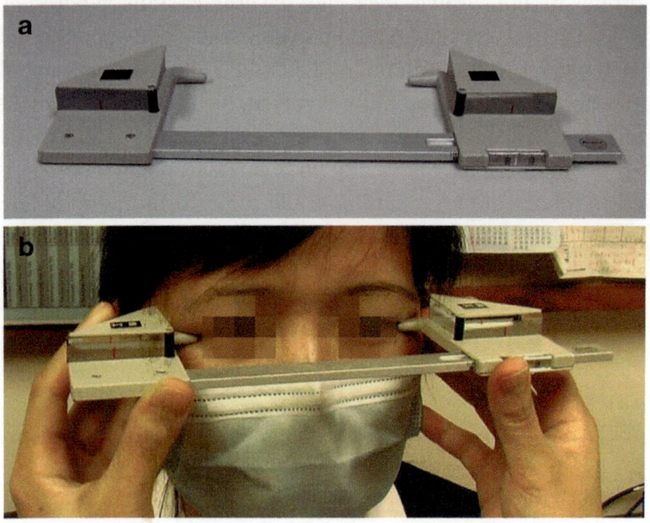

Fig. 7.1 Hertel's exophthalmometer (**a**) and its clinical application (**b**)

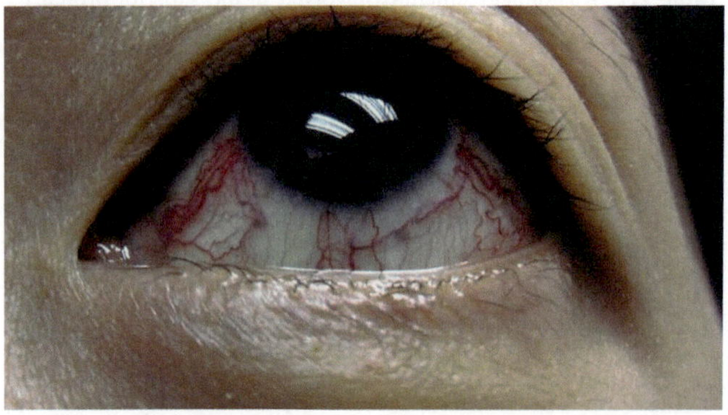

Fig. 7.2 Left eye of a patient with an indirect carotid-cavernous fistula, showing conjunctival corkscrew vessels

7.3 Afferent Visual Pathway

Ocular examination usually begins with visual acuity and intraocular pressure measurement. Visual acuity is one of the most important parameters in ocular examination. In the ideal situation, the best-corrected visual acuity (BCVA) of each eye should be documented individually using either a Snellen or Early Treatment of Diabetic Retinopathy Study (ETDRS) visual acuity chart. If BCVA is not possible, then visual acuity should be checked with the patient wearing appropriate spectacles and with the aid of a pinhole if the visual acuity is suboptimal. Uncorrected visual acuity alone is usually not sufficient.

The afferent visual pathway can be assessed in terms of its function and structure, as summarized in Table 7.2. Visual functions are assessed subjectively (dependent on the patient's responses) and objectively. In addition to visual acuity, subjective visual functions are usually also assessed in terms of color vision (using standardized tools like the Hardy Rand Rittler or Ishihara Pseudoisochromatic Plates) and visual field examination. In the absence of specialized equipment, confrontational visual field examination, if performed well, can give very useful information. The visual field can be further quantified and recorded with formal testing, e.g., with the Humphrey visual field analyzer (HVF 24-2/30-2 for the central visual field, FF-81 for the peripheral visual field) or the kinetic Goldmann perimeter (which is more operator dependent and fast becoming a lost art). Subjective brightness sensitivity and red desaturation (expressed as a subjective percentage of the diseased eye vs. normal fellow eye) and contrast sensitivity measurement (e.g. using Pelli-Robson chart), if available, may serve as adjunctive visual assessment parameters.

Objectively, the relative afferent pupillary defect (RAPD) is the most important clinical sign to elicit in patients with visual loss. It is performed on the basis that light stimulation of one eye causes simultaneous and equal constriction of both pupils. Therefore, by illuminating each eye alternately, one can gauge the integrity of the anterior visual pathway of one eye compared to the other. However, its utility is limited with patients with bilateral symmetrical visual loss or if the pupils of both eyes are not functional (e.g., bilateral CN3 palsy, damaged surgically or pharmacologically constricted/dilated). Even if one pupil is defective, checking for "reverse RAPD" is still possible using the fellow normal pupil. Quantification of the RAPD is feasible with neutral density filters or commercially available binocular pupillometers.

After checking the RAPD, it is conventional to examine the patient on the slit-lamp for any anterior segment pathology, then pharmacologically dilate both pupils to examine the posterior segment, particularly to rule out other intraocu-

Table 7.2 Assessment of afferent visual pathway

	Function		Structure
Subjective	1. Visual acuity	• Snellen Chart • ETDRS Charts	
	2. Color vision	• HRR Plates • Ishihara Plates	
	3. Visual field	• Confrontational • Humphrey • Goldmann	
	4. Brightness sensitivity/red desaturation		
	5. Contrast sensitivity	• Pelli Robson Chart	
Objective	1. Relative afferent pupillary defect (RAPD) 2. Visual electrodiagnostics, e.g., visual evoked potential		1. Optic disc photo 2. Ocular imaging: optical coherence tomography 3. Neuroimaging (CT/MRI)

ETDRS Early Treatment of Diabetic Retinopathy Study; *HRR* Hardy Rand Rittler

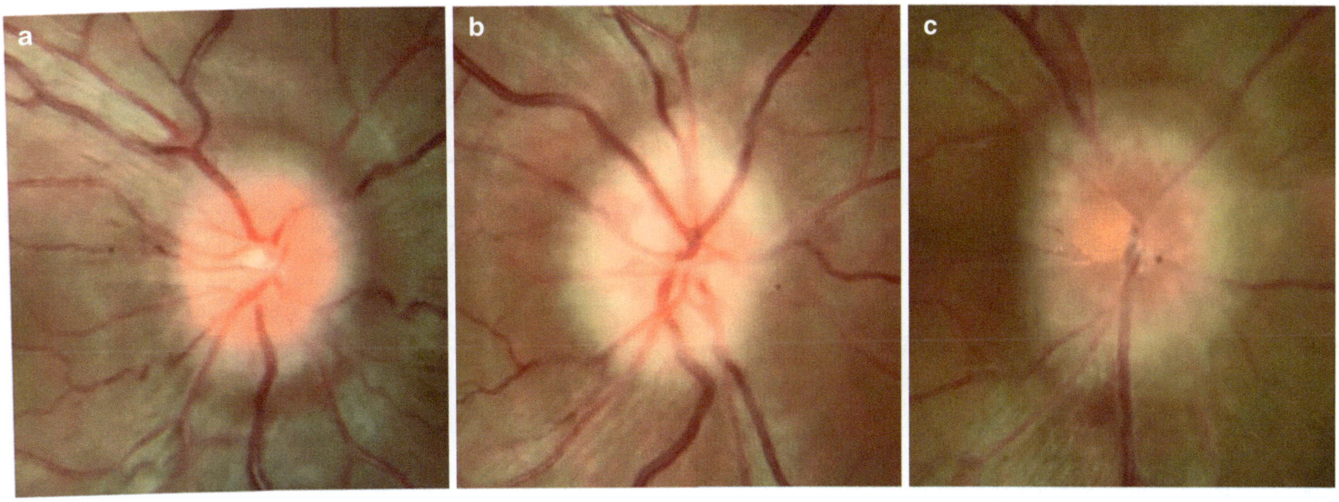

Fig. 7.3 Optic disc appearance of papilledema (**a**), optic neuritis with disc swelling (**b**), optic nerve sheath meningioma (**c**). It is usually not possible to determine the aetiology of the disc swelling by optic disc appearance alone

lar causes of visual loss and document the optic disc appearance. In orbital apex disease, the optic disc may appear normal but may also be swollen (with or without associated increased retinal vascular tortuosity) if there is orbital congestion or compression immediately behind the globe. With long-standing optic neuropathy (of at least 1 month duration), there may be clinically visible optic atrophy. While the disc appearance alone is seldom diagnostic of a particular pathology (Fig. 7.3), it is conventional to document any abnormal optic disc morphology by optic disc photography (stereoscopic photos preferred).

In recent years, there is an increasing trend to use optical coherence tomography (OCT) to assess and monitor optic neuropathies [2, 3]. OCT is widely used in ophthalmology to assess macular disease and glaucoma. In non-glaucomatous optic neuropathy, the peripapillary retinal nerve fiber layer thickness (pRNFL) can be used as a surrogate marker of optic disc swelling or optic atrophy. The optic nerve is made up of the axons of retinal ganglion cells which constitute one of the innermost layers of the retina. OCT scan of the macula can measure the thickness of the ganglion cell layer (GCL), usually together with the inner plexiform layer (IPL) due to a limitation of the OCT instrument's algorithm to delineate the two layers. The GCL-IPL thinning is another surrogate marker of optic atrophy, particularly useful in conditions where pRNFL thinning may be masked by disc swelling, e.g., in long-standing compressive optic neuropathy. Together with functional assessments, OCT pRNFL and GCL-IPL thickness can be used to quantitatively monitor optic neuropathy progression or response to treatment (see Fig. 7.4). It is worth noting that while visual acuity and visual field defects can recover and disc swelling (and pRNFL thickening) can resolve, pRNFL and GC-IPL thinning do not recover.

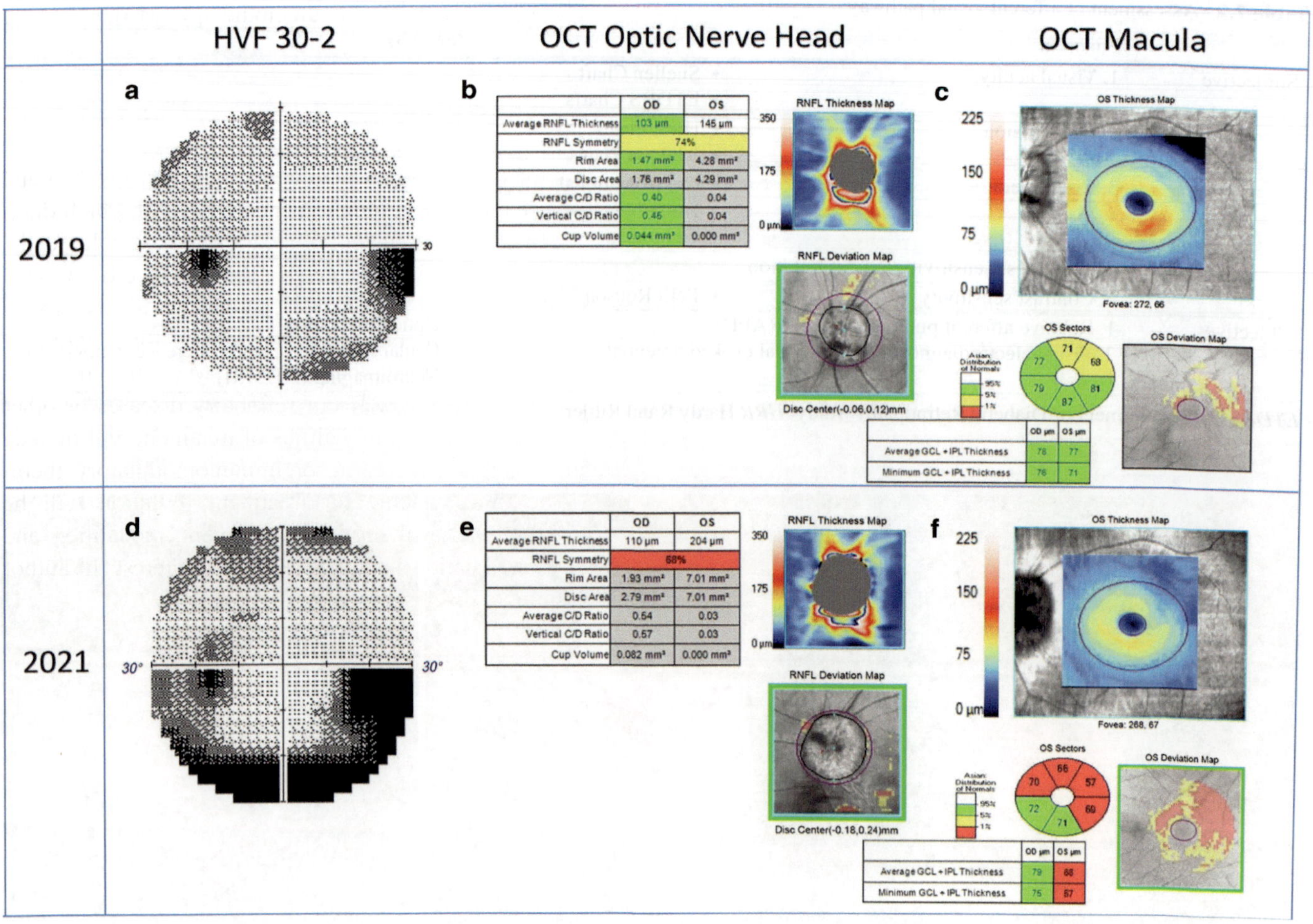

Fig. 7.4 The visual field (Humphrey 30-2) (**a**, **d**), Cirrus (Carl-Zeiss) optical coherence tomography (OCT) of optic nerve head (**b**, **e**) and macula (**c**, **f**) of a patient with left eye optic nerve sheath meningioma in 2019 (**a–c**) and 2021 (**d–f**), demonstrating disease progression in terms of inferior visual field defect enlargement, increase in retinal nerve fibre thickness (RNFL) (as an indirect measure of disc swelling) and thinning of ganglion cell layer-inner plexiform layer (GCL-IPL) (as an indirect measure of optic atrophy). Note how the pattern of GCL-IPL thinning corresponds topographically with the inferior visual field defect

Visual evoked potential (VEP) can be used to assess the function of the whole afferent visual pathway (from the cornea to the occipital cortex) objectively [4]; however, some clinicians only use it for patients who are unable to respond accurately (e.g., due to age or mental condition) or are unreliable (e.g., malingerers), because VEP results are affected by many factors (e.g., refractive error, maculopathy) and do not provide much information in addition to the examinations listed above in reliable patients. If VEP is deemed necessary, pattern VEP (performed with the patient wearing optimal spectacle/contact lens correction) is always preferable to flash VEP, which is much more variable.

7.4 Efferent Visual Pathway

The assessment of the efferent system consists of the evaluation of:

(a) Extraocular movement.
(b) Pupil size—look for anisocoria in light and dark conditions; reaction to light and accommodation (sympathetic and parasympathetic pathways).
(c) Eyelid position—look for ptosis and lid retraction (e.g., CN3 palsy or oculo-sympathetic pathway).

These three components should always be examined together if there is an abnormality with any one of them. Extraocular movement is controlled by six muscles in each eye, which are innervated by cranial nerves 3, 4, and 6. Space-occupying lesions in the orbit (e.g., enlarged extraocular muscles in thyroid eye disease) or orbital congestion may cause extraocular movement limitations in a restrictive pattern, not conforming to specific cranial nerve patterns. Ocular misalignment (e.g., convergent or divergent strabismus, hyper, or hypotropia), present with binocular diplopia, can be assessed with cover test and quantified with prism cover test (see Fig. 7.5) or HESS charts/Lees screen (Fig. 7.6) [5–7].

Pupil size and lid position (vertical palpebral fissure, levator function, marginal reflex distance) can be simply measured with a ruler.

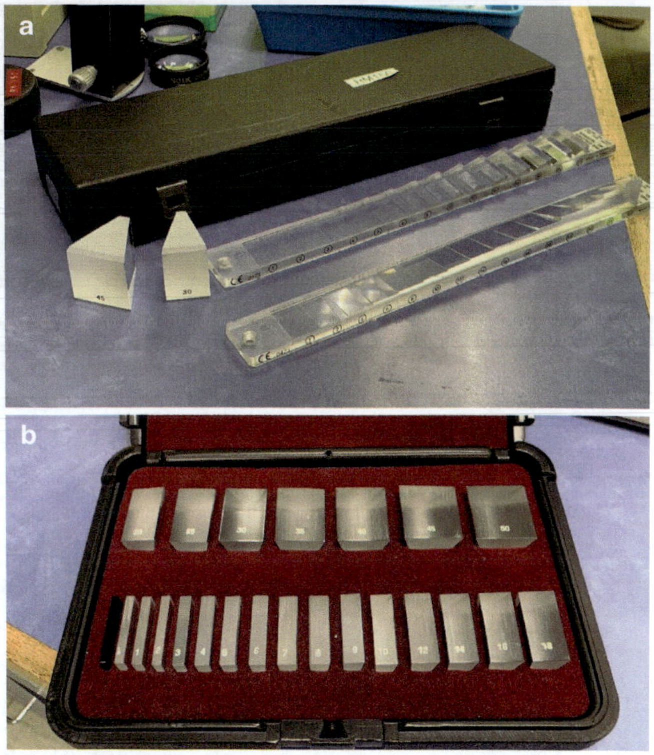

Fig. 7.5 Prism bars (**a**) or loose prisms (**b**) used for prism cover test

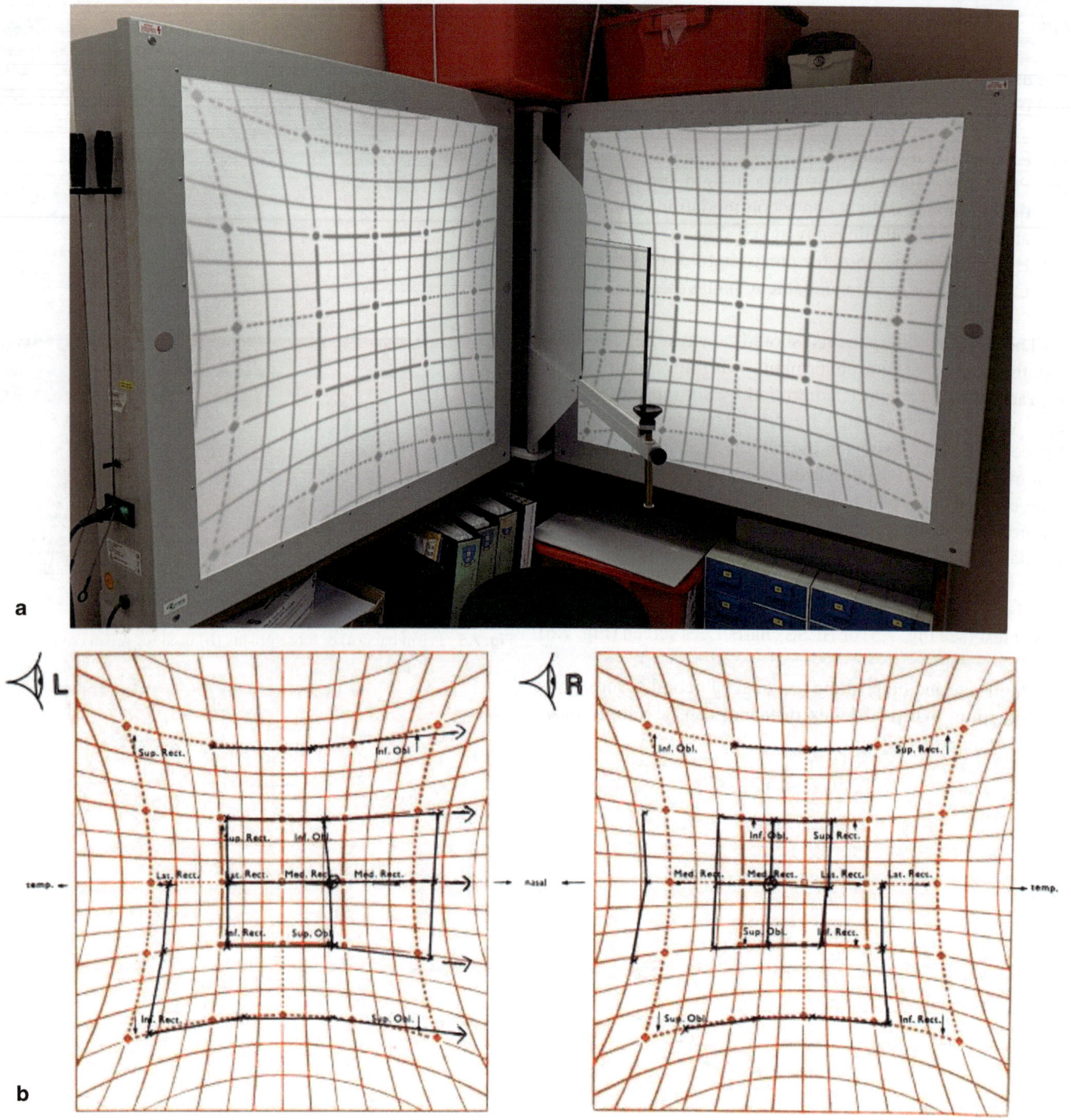

Fig. 7.6 Lees Screen (**a**). Hess chart (**b**) of a patient with right eye CN6 palsy (abduction defect)

7.5 Other Cranial Nerves and Directed Examination

Depending on the results of the above examinations, the function of other cranial nerves may need to be assessed. Corneal and facial sensation (CN V1–3), facial movement (CN VII), and hearing (CN VIII) are particularly relevant in patients with suspected orbital apex or skull base disease. Other directed examinations may include but are not limited to:

(a) Palpation for orbital masses, including lacrimal mass, when an orbital space-occupying lesion is suspected.
(b) Orbital auscultation for suspected carotid-cavernous fistula.
(c) Valsalva maneuver for suspected orbital vascular malformation.
(d) ENT examination for suspected nasopharyngeal carcinoma, particularly prevalent in Southern China.
(e) Systemic examination, e.g., body temperature (for fever associated with orbital infection), systemic signs of neurofibromatosis, thyrotoxicosis, or even acromegaly.

7.6 Investigations

The most important investigation in orbital apex and skull base disease is appropriate neuroimaging, which is covered in the next chapter. There are other systemic investigations which would help elucidate the nature of the pathology found in neuroimaging. These may include:

(a) Complete blood count with differential.
(b) Erythrocyte sedimentation rate, C-reactive protein.
(c) Lumbar puncture for cerebrospinal fluid composition, cytology, and culture.
(d) If infection is suspected: systemic sepsis workup including blood cultures, search for underlying risk factors like diabetes.
(e) If tuberculosis or sarcoidosis is suspected: chest X-ray, Mantoux testing, PCR for *Mycobacterium tuberculosis*, serum angiotensin-converting enzyme, interferon-gamma release assay.
(f) If noninfective inflammation is suspected: autoantibodies, baseline pre-steroid work-up.

These will be covered in more detail in the following chapters corresponding to specific pathology.

References

1. Badakere A, Patil-Chhablani P. Orbital apex syndrome: a review. Eye Brain. 2019;11:63–72.
2. Chan NCY, Chan CKM. The use of optical coherence tomography in neuro-ophthalmology. Curr Opin Ophthalmol. 2017;28(6):552–7.
3. Chan NCY, Chan CKM. The role of optical coherence tomography in the acute management of neuro-ophthalmic diseases. Asia Pac J Ophthalmol (Phila). 2018;7(4):265–70.
4. Marmoy OR, Viswanathan S. Clinical electrophysiology of the optic nerve and retinal ganglion cells. Eye (Lond). 2021;35(9):2386–405.
5. Thomas R, Braganza A, George T. Practical approach to diagnosis of strabismus. Indian J Ophthalmol. 1996;44(2):103–12.
6. Roper-Hall G. The hess screen test. Am Orthopt J. 2006;56:166–74.
7. Timms C. The lees screen test. Am Orthopt J. 2006;56:180–3.

Principles of Imaging for Orbital Apex Pathologies

8

Koel Wei Sum Ko and Wai Lun Poon

Abstract

Radiological assessment of the orbital apex is essential for diagnosing and depicting the extent of pathologies that can occur in this compact, strategically important location in the head and neck. This chapter aims to describe the radiological anatomy of the orbital apex, discuss the principle of imaging, and illustrate the diverse range of orbital apex pathologies commonly encountered in clinical practice.

Keywords

Orbital apex · Imaging anatomy · Principles of imaging

8.1 Introduction

Orbital apex pathologies and their radiological assessment have received relatively little literature attention in recent decades despite advances in imaging techniques, medical understanding of the pathologies, and advances in surgical techniques and expertise available for tackling these pathologies. A diverse range of pathologies can occur at the orbital apex, which often presents with overlapping symptomatology due to the anatomical compactness of this small but strategically important location in the head and neck region [1]. These pathologies include neoplasms, vascular lesions, inflammatory conditions, infections, traumatic injuries, and skull base lesions causing extrinsic compression to the orbital apex [2]. Cross-sectional radiological examinations are often crucial for characterizing the nature of orbital apex pathologies and delineating their extent. In this chapter, we aim to describe the radiological anatomy of the orbital apex region, discuss the principle of imaging, and illustrate a range of conditions afflicting the orbital apex region commonly encountered in clinical practice.

8.2 Anatomy

The orbital apex is a small, cone-shaped osseous tunnel at the posterior orbit, bound by the greater and lesser wings of the sphenoid bone. The superior orbital fissure is found over its lateral aspect, the optic canal is found at the center separated from the superior orbital fissure by the optic strut, and the posterior ethmoidal foramen is found on its medial aspect. The anterior clinoid process is found superolaterally, while the inferior orbital fissure and the opening of the foramen rotundum are found inferolaterally [3].

The orbital apex is at the crossroads between the orbit and the rest of the skull base. It communicates directly with the cavernous sinus over its posterior aspect. By way of the inferior orbital fissure, it is also connected to the pterygopalatine fossa, another important hub in the central skull base via the foramen rotundum and vidian canal, which permits access of lesions involving this area to the middle cranial fossa and foramen lacerum, respectively [4].

The orbital apex contains, or is in close proximity to, many neurovascular structures. Notably this includes multiple cranial nerves (optic, oculomotor, trochlear, abducens, nerves, and ophthalmic branch of the trigeminal nerve), and vascular structures (ophthalmic artery, superior ophthalmic vein, cavernous and ophthalmic segments of the internal carotid arteries, cavernous sinus, and periarterial sympathetic plexus) [5]. The orbital apex also houses the annulus of Zinn, a fibrous ring which serves as the insertions of six of the seven extraocular muscles (the four rectus muscles, the levator palpebrae superioris muscle, and the superior oblique muscle) [6, 7]. Routine orbital MRI is not able to clearly and completely depict this fibrous ring. The annulus of Zinn contains the optic nerve and ophthalmic artery which pass through the optic canal, as well as the cranial nerves III and VI and the nasociliary nerve which traverse the medial part of

K. W. S. Ko (✉) · W. L. Poon
Department of Radiology and Imaging, Queen Elizabeth Hospital, Hong Kong, People's Republic of China
e-mail: kws803@ha.org.hk; poonwl@ha.org.hk

T. L. POON et al. (eds.), *Orbital Apex and Periorbital Skull Base Diseases*, https://doi.org/10.1007/978-981-99-2989-4_8

the superior orbital fissure. These structures, which are within the confinement of the annulus of Zinn, are more susceptible to compression or shearing injury [8].

8.3 Principles of Imaging

Evaluation of orbital apex pathologies is primarily performed with magnetic resonance imaging (MRI) and computed tomography (CT). Secondary imaging modalities, such as fluoro-2-deoxy-D-glucose positron emission tomography/CT (FDG-PET CT), FDG-PET MRI, and additional MRI sequences, such as diffusion-weighted imaging (DWI), may offer additional imaging insights but are admittedly less commonly used in routine clinical practice [9]. For vascular lesions, noninvasive CT or MR angiography is often the first-line imaging of choice, with invasive digital subtraction angiogram (DSA) reserved as a gold standard modality for both diagnosis and endovascular treatment planning.

MRI is considered the imaging modality of choice due to superior soft tissue contrast for depicting the different orbital compartments (Fig. 8.1a) [10]. MRI examinations can be

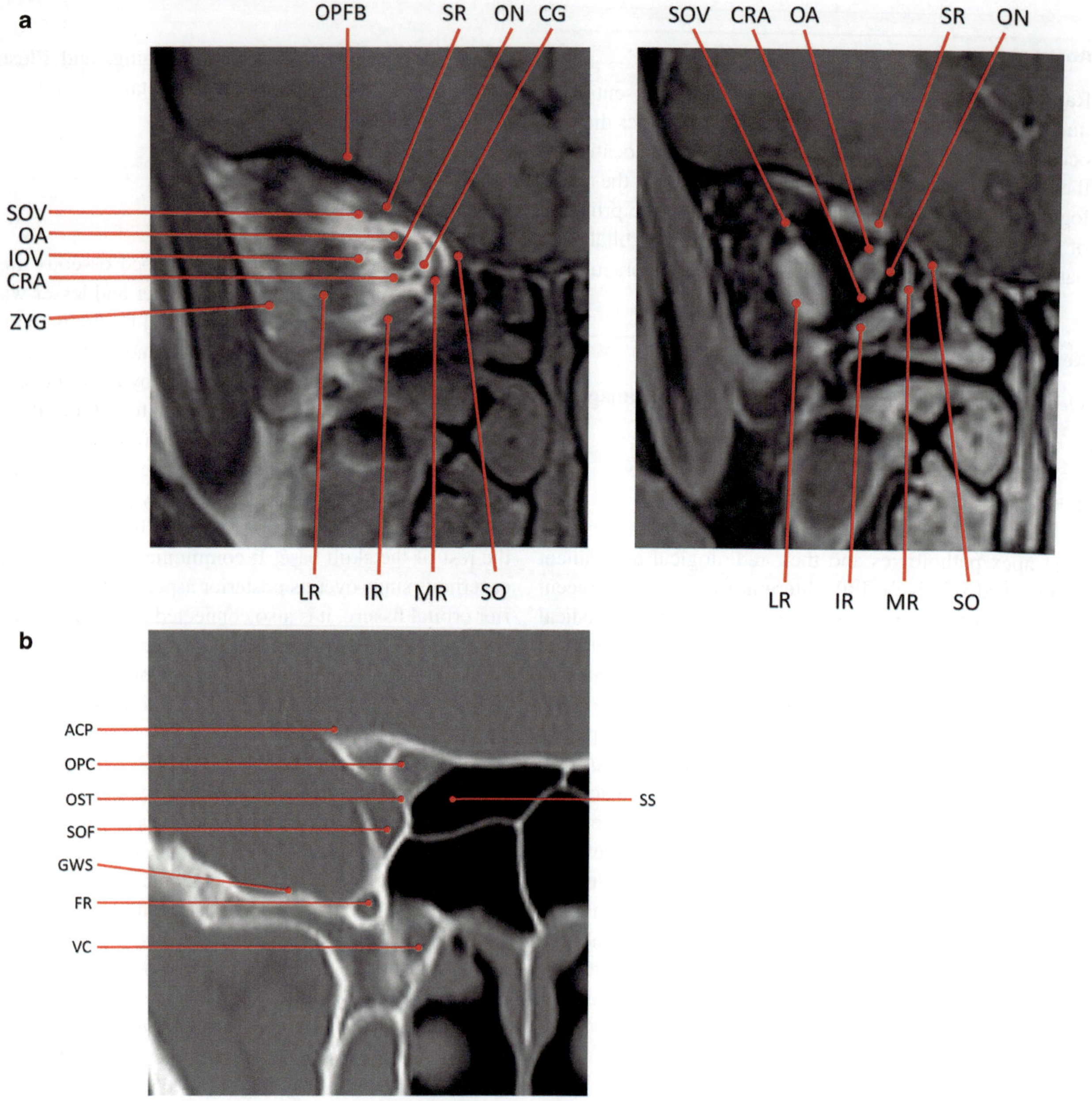

Fig. 8.1 (**a**) Coronal T1W non-contrast (left) and post-contrast fat-saturated (right) images at the level just anterior to the orbital apex and (**b**) coronal CT orbit of the bone window at the level of orbital apex for anatomical illustration. Abbreviations of anatomical structures are detailed as follows: *SOV* superior ophthalmic vein, *IOV* inferior ophthalmic vein, *OA* ophthalmic artery, *CRA* central retinal artery, *CG* ciliary ganglion, *ON* optic nerve, *ZYG* frontal process of the zygomatic bone, *OPFB* orbital plate of frontal bone, *SR* superior rectus, *IR* inferior rectus, *MR* medial rectus, *LR* lateral rectus, *SO* superior oblique, *ACP* anterior clinoid process, *OPC* optic canal, *OST* optic strut, *SOF* superior orbital fissure, *FR* foramen rotundum, *VC* vidian canal, *SS* sphenoid sinus, *GWS* greater wing of sphenoid

Table 8.1 A simple guide to selecting between MRI and CT for imaging of the orbital apex

	MRI	CT	PET-CT
Pros	• No ionizing radiation, i.e., lens friendly • High contrast resolution, better differentiation of soft-tissue structures/lesions • Allow multiplanar acquisition • Allow imaging of arteries without contrast injection • Assessment of some attributes of microscopic structures possible, e.g., diffusion-weighted imaging, diffusion tensor imaging	• High spatial resolution • Good delineation of the anatomy of bones • Fast scanning, ideal in an emergency • Imaging of choice to look for intraocular metallic foreign body	• All advantages of CT plus the metabolic activity of the concerned lesion
Cons	• Contraindicated if the presence of intraocular metallic foreign body is suspected, some models of pacemakers/cochlear implants, some metallic implants, or when patient is claustrophobic • Longer scanning time, prone to motion artifacts	• Risks related to ionizing radiation • No multiplanar acquisition capability. Spatial resolution of multiplanar reconstruction not as good as that of in plane	• Even higher radiation exposure to the patient compared to CT • Limited availability and expensive

performed on a 1.5 T or 3 T scanner using a combination of head or surface coils. The standard MRI protocol in our center comprises 2D axial T1W SE, axial STIR, coronal STIR, and both axial and coronal T1W SE sequences with fat saturation obtained after intravenous administration of gadolinium-based contrast agent. A slice thickness of 3 mm with a 512 × 512 matrix is used for these sequences in adults, and thinner slices are acquired for pediatric patients. For a better demonstration of the pathology at the orbital apex in relation to the optic nerve, dedicated 2D images along and perpendicular to the nerve at the orbital apex will also be acquired if necessary. In addition, a 3D T1W volumetric interpolated breath-hold examination (VIBE) sequence performed after intravenous contrast administration can be offered, with volumetric data sets permitting multiplanar reconstruction in any given plane and slide thickness in order to optimally delineate subtle findings. For better characterization of the orbital pathology, one of the more widely applied techniques is the addition of diffusion-weighted imaging (DWI) to the MRI scan of the orbits. DWI produces contrast on the basis of limited diffusivity of water molecules in different tissues, with lower apparent diffusion coefficient (ADC) values on ADC maps corresponding to more restriction of diffusion. In the setting of orbital apex pathologies, DWI shows promise in differentiating benign and malignant lesions, particularly infiltrative lesions that are difficult to diagnose in other modalities. It has been reported that an ADC value of $<1.0–1.15 \times 10^{-3}$ mm^2/s can be used as a threshold for differentiating lymphoma from orbital inflammatory disease with high sensitivity of 95%, specificity of 91%, and accuracy of 93% [11]. Despite potential benefits, the application of DWI is limited by susceptibility artifacts caused by bone, air, and soft tissue interfaces at the orbital apex region [12].

Complementary to MRI, CT is the modality of choice for evaluating orbital apex pathologies with osseous destruction, calcifications, or possible metallic foreign bodies (Fig. 8.1b). Thin slice CT scans with 1 mm thickness are often performed in this setting with the addition of intravenous iodinated contrast material [13]. Standard axial images with coronal and sagittal reconstructions are routinely obtained in soft tissue and bone windows for an optimal depiction of orbital apex pathologies.

Table 8.1 serves as a simple guide for ophthalmologists in choosing a suitable modality for imaging of suspected orbital apex pathology.

8.4 Radiological Features of Orbital Apex Pathologies

8.4.1 Neoplasms

A wide range of benign and malignant neoplasms arise from soft tissues within the orbital apex. Orbital neoplasms in general become more prevalent with age and have a higher probability of being malignant in the elderly population >60 years of age [14]. Extrinsic neoplasms compressing upon and extending into the orbital apex are dealt with at the end of this chapter.

Optic nerve sheath meningiomas commonly involve the orbital apex, accounting for up to 2% of all meningiomas [15], often presenting with proptosis and painless visual loss but normal-appearing optic disc on the ophthalmological exam [16]. On CT scan, optic nerve sheath meningiomas present as fusiform enlargement of the optic nerve with linear, granular, or plaque-like calcifications along the periphery. This signifies attenuation of the underlying optic nerve as opposed to expansion of the nerve in optic glioma. On MRI, the lesion is isointense on T1W and T2W images to grey matter and shows homogeneous contrast enhancement, producing the well-known “tram-track sign” with peripheral enhancing thickened nerve sheath surrounding the non-enhancing optic nerve at the center on post-contrast T1W MRI images (Fig. 8.2) [17].

Optic gliomas are the commonest neoplasms of the orbital apex, showing female predilection. They are most prevalent in young patients during the first two decades of life and are infamously associated with underlying neurofibromatosis type 1 (NF-1) [16]. Gliomas of the optic nerve often present similarly to meningiomas but with optic

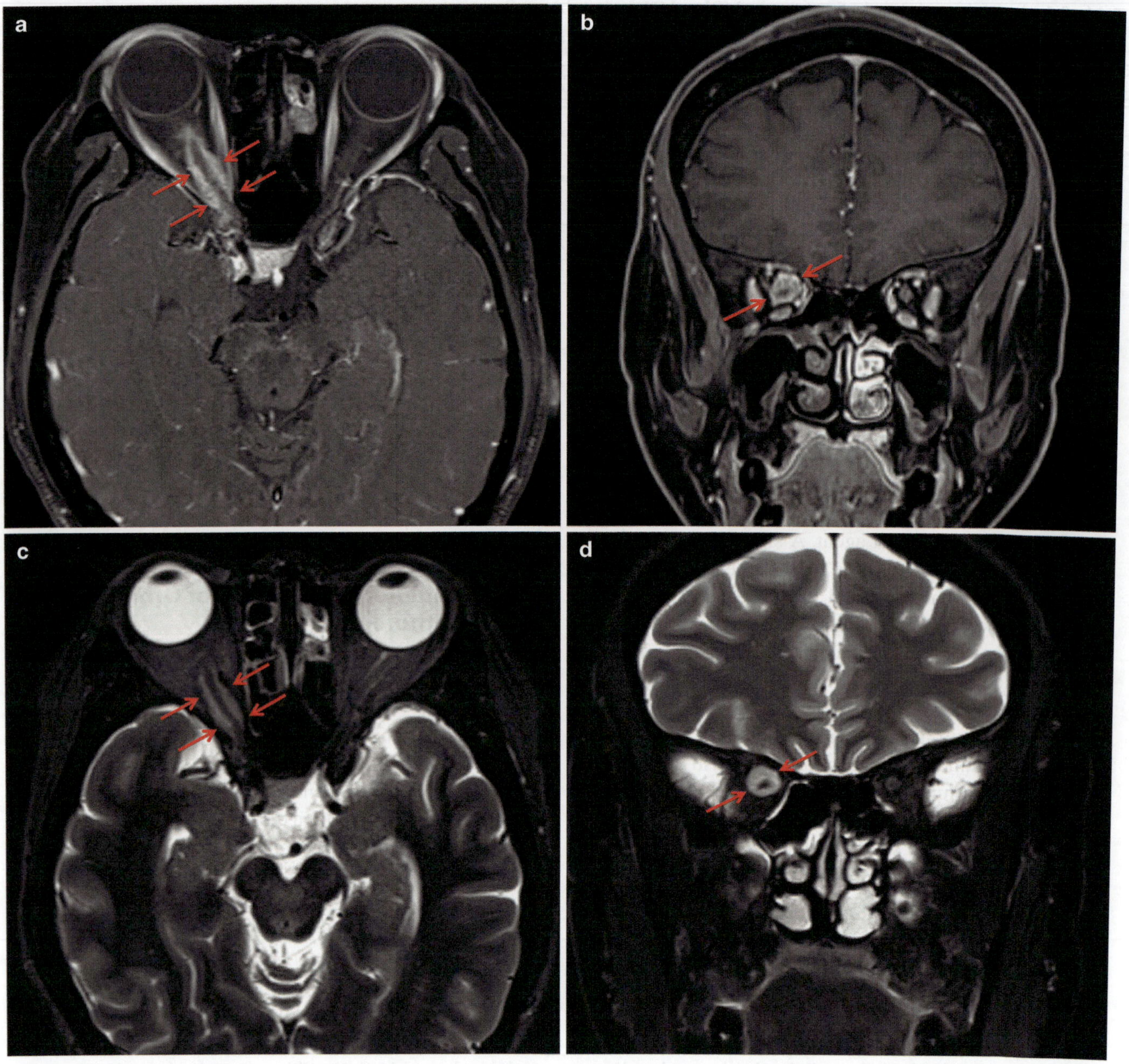

Fig. 8.2 A 55-year-old woman presents with blurring of vision for 6 months. (**a**) T1W fat-saturated post-contrast axial, (**b**) T1W fat-saturated post-contrast coronal, (**c**) T2W STIR axial, and (**d**) T2W fat-saturated coronal MRI images show T2W hyperintense optic nerve sheath thickening with intense homogeneous contrast enhancement involving mainly the intra-orbital and intracanalicular segments of the right optic nerve (arrows), findings typical of optic nerve sheath meningioma. The patient subsequently received intensity-modulated radiotherapy (IMRT) with mild improvement of right eye vision

disc pallor or swelling evident. Optic gliomas are usually histologically nonaggressive low-grade astrocytomas in NF-1 patients but can be aggressive in non-NF-1 cases [18]. Cross-sectional imaging shows enlargement, tortuosity, and kinking of the optic nerve, sometimes causing expansion of optic canal owing to chronicity of growth; MRI signal is variable but typically mildly hypointense on T1W and hyperintense on T2W images, with variable contrast enhancement (Fig. 8.3). In NF-1 patients, lesions are usually smaller, more homogeneous and involving the intra-orbital and intra-canalicular segments of the optic nerve; in non-NF-1 patients, lesions are larger and more mass-like, can contain more cystic components, and commonly involve optic chiasm and tracts [18]. Other primary tumors of the optic nerve including gangliogliomas and hemangioblastomas are much less common.

Schwannomas arise from the myelin sheath of peripheral nerves and are rare in the orbit, only accounting for 1% of

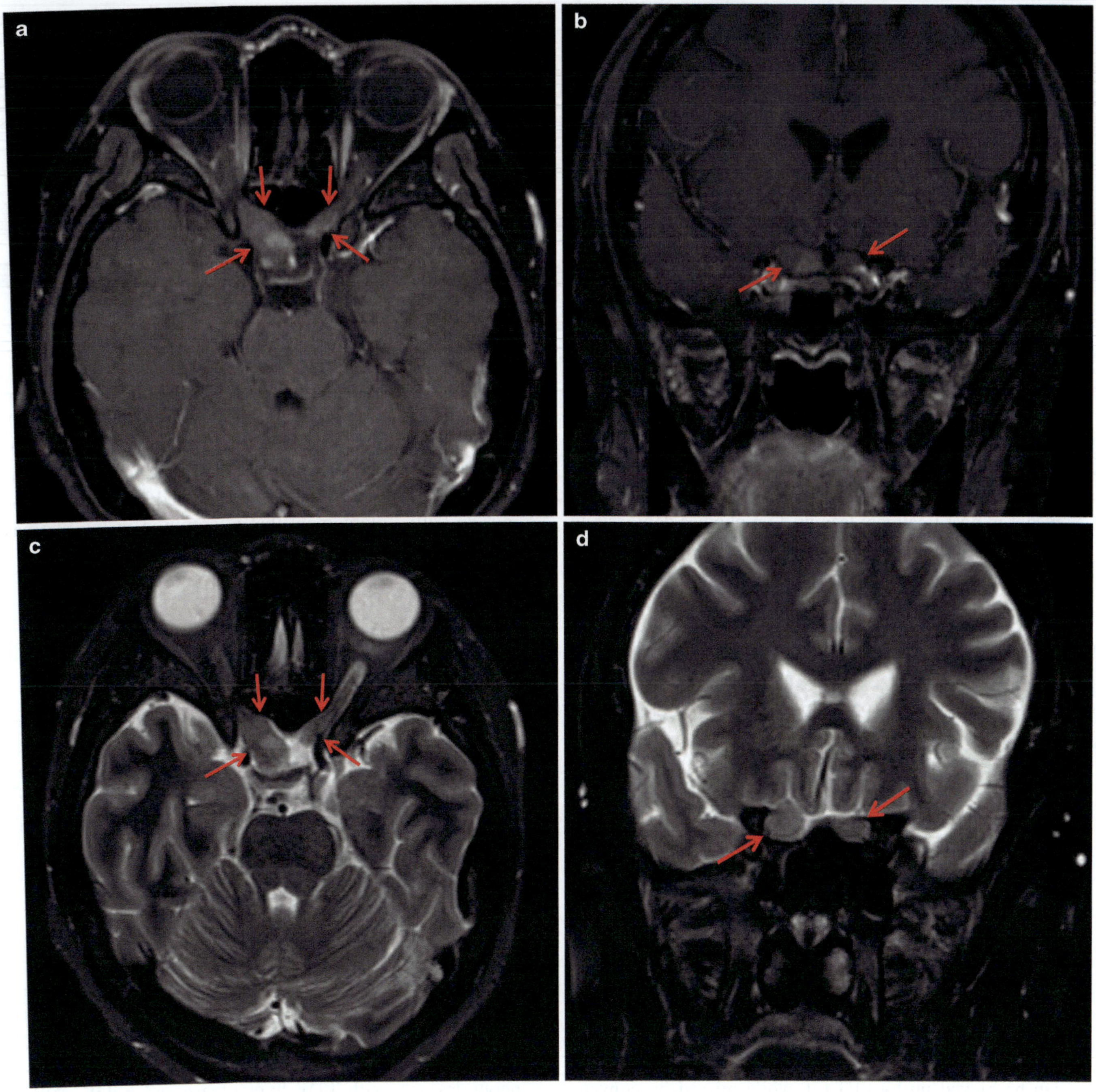

Fig. 8.3 A 31-year-old woman with a known history of neurofibromatosis type 1 (NF-1) with moderate visual impairment for more than 20 years. (**a**) T1W fat-saturated post-contrast axial, (**b**) T1W fat-saturated post-contrast coronal, (**c**) T2W STIR axial, and (**d**) T2W fat-saturated coronal MRI images demonstrate bilateral fusiform enlargement of intracanalicular and intracranial segments of optic nerves (arrows), which shows T2W intermediate signal and patchy contrast enhancement. Imaging appearance is classical of bilateral optic gliomas associated with NF-1

neoplasms in the orbit [19]. In the orbit they most commonly occur at the superior aspect and involve the orbital apex in up to 1/5 of cases [20]. Most orbital schwannomas arise from sensory nerves from branches of the ophthalmic division of the trigeminal nerve but may arise from the other cranial nerves in the orbit [21]. Orbital schwannomas are benign and slow-growing and are likely to conform to the shape of the orbital apex, appearing cone-shaped or dumbbell-shaped and extending along the longitudinal axis of the involved nerve, often causing smooth enlargement of superior orbital fissure [19]. Other differentiating imaging characteristics on MRI include peripheral ring-shaped enhancement with central hypointensity on T1W post-contrast images and peripheral hypointensity with central hyperintensity on corresponding T2W images [20].

Lymphoma is one of the commonest orbital apex lesions across all age groups (along with cavernous hemangiomas) but shows the highest incidence in the sixth to seventh decade of life [22, 23]. Lymphoid lesions in general constitute a spectrum of diseases ranging from benign hyperplasia to malignant lymphoma [24], which is of heterogeneous origin in the orbits, comprising of approximately 2% of non-Hodgkin lymphoma and 8% of extranodal mucosa-associated lymphoid tissue (MALT) lymphomas [25]. Lymphoma involves various compartments within the orbit, commonly the lacrimal gland; however, in the orbital apex, isolated extraocular muscle involvement and ill-defined multi-compartmental retro-orbital soft tissue infiltration are common patterns of radiological presentation [26].

On CT, lymphoma is characteristically hyperdense but rarely shows any intralesional calcification unlike meningiomas, except in post-treatment lesions. Lymphomas demonstrate variable patterns of osseous involvement from molding and insinuating along contours of orbital wall in low-grade lesions to permeative bone destruction and invasion of extra-orbital structures in high-grade lesions [27]. While MRI signal intensity is often nonspecific, orbital lymphomas characteristically show extremely low ADC values usually from 0.44 to 0.92×10^{-3} mm^2/s [28]. Certain studies even suggest that lymphoma can be differentiated from orbital pseudotumor with accuracy up to 100% using an ADC threshold of 1.0×10^{-3} mm^2/s [11] and similarly from IgG4-related disease [29] and orbital metastases [11].

Lymphoma is commonly a systemic disease with 2–5% of patients with systemic non-Hodgkin lymphoma showing orbital involvement and conversely 75% of patients with primary orbital lymphoma eventually developing systemic involvement [9]. Whole-body PET-CT is, therefore, indicated in the staging of orbital lymphoma despite the fact that low-grade MALT lymphoma may show relatively low FDG uptake, as studies have shown that systemic metastases of even low-grade orbital lymphomas can be picked up by PET-CT while missed by conventional CT or MRI [30, 31].

Notably, sarcoidosis can be extremely similar to lymphoma in all modalities including DWI, and the presence of hilar lymphadenopathies, lung lesions, elevated serum angiotensin-converting enzyme (ACE) levels, and ultimately histological examination may be necessary for diagnosis.

Rhabdomyosarcoma needs to be considered in the pediatric population as it is the commonest orbital malignancy before the age of 16 [18]. When involving the orbital apex, it often presents with rapid onset of ocular dysmotility, decrease in vision, and proptosis. In children the differential diagnoses are plethoric and include vascular malformations, neurofibromas, metastases, hematological malignancies, and ruptured dermoid cysts [18]. Radiological features are also quite non-specific, with hemorrhage, calcification, and necrosis uncommon on CT [32]. MRI may demonstrate a mass with T1W signal isointense to muscle, variable T2W hyperintensity, with extraocular muscles displaced or invaded but showing no muscle belly enlargement that is common in lymphoma or inflammatory lesions [18, 32].

8.4.2 Vascular Anomalies

Understanding and hence nomenclature of orbital vascular lesions had been confusing, resulting in occasions of misdiagnosis and mismanagement which could be catastrophic. Currently, many of these lesions are managed successfully by medications, surgery, radiological intervention, or a combination of these thanks to the gradual adoption of the International Society for the Study of Vascular Anomalies (ISSVA) classification [33] by different specialties after 2014. A simplified version of the latest ISSVA (2018) classification is summarized in Table 8.2.

Infantile hemangioma is the most common pediatric vascular tumor affecting the orbital apex. They usually progress during the first year of life and regress when the patient is about 5–7 years old [34]. They are lobulated heterogeneous lesions, with T1W hypointense and mildly T2W hyperintense signal on MRI, showing prominent

Table 8.2 A simplified version of the classification of vascular anomalies, adapted from ISSVA

Vascular anomalies				
Vascular tumors	Vascular malformations			
Infantile hemangioma Congenital hemangioma Other benign or malignant vascular tumors	Simple	Combined	Of major named vessels	Associated with other anomalies
	Capillary malformations Lymphatic malformations Venous malformations Arteriovenous malformations Arteriovenous fistula	CVM, CLM, LVM, CLVM, CAVM, CLAVM, others	"Channel type" or "truncal" vascular malformations	For example, Klippel-Trenaunay syndrome Parkes Weber syndrome Sturge-Weber syndrome

Abbreviations: *CVM* capillary venous malformation, *CLM* capillary lymphatic malformation, *LVM* lymphatic venous malformation, *CLVM* capillary lymphatic venous malformation, *CAVM* capillary arteriovenous malformation, *CLAVM* capillary lymphatic arteriovenous malformation intralesional flow voids and homogeneous intense contrast enhancement.

Venous malformation is the most common low-flow vascular malformation in the orbital apex. It is named as cavernous venous malformation by some and as cavernous hemangioma in the past. It occurs in isolation from the vascular system in the orbit [12]. It may be asymptomatic or present with slowly progressive proptosis, diplopia, and rarely decrease in visual acuity due to mass effect on the optic nerve. Venous malformations occur in the intraconal space and manifest as a hyperdense well-circumscribed lesion on CT, separate from the optic nerve and extraocular muscles. Phleboliths, when present, are highly suggestive of this diagnosis. On MRI the T1W signal is variable but usually hypointense, and the T2W signal is usually strongly hyperintense, with patchy T2W hypointensity that can be due to calcification or thrombosis [13]. Dynamic contrast-enhanced MRI shows patchy enhancement in early phases with homogeneous enhancement in delayed phase (Fig. 8.4) [35].

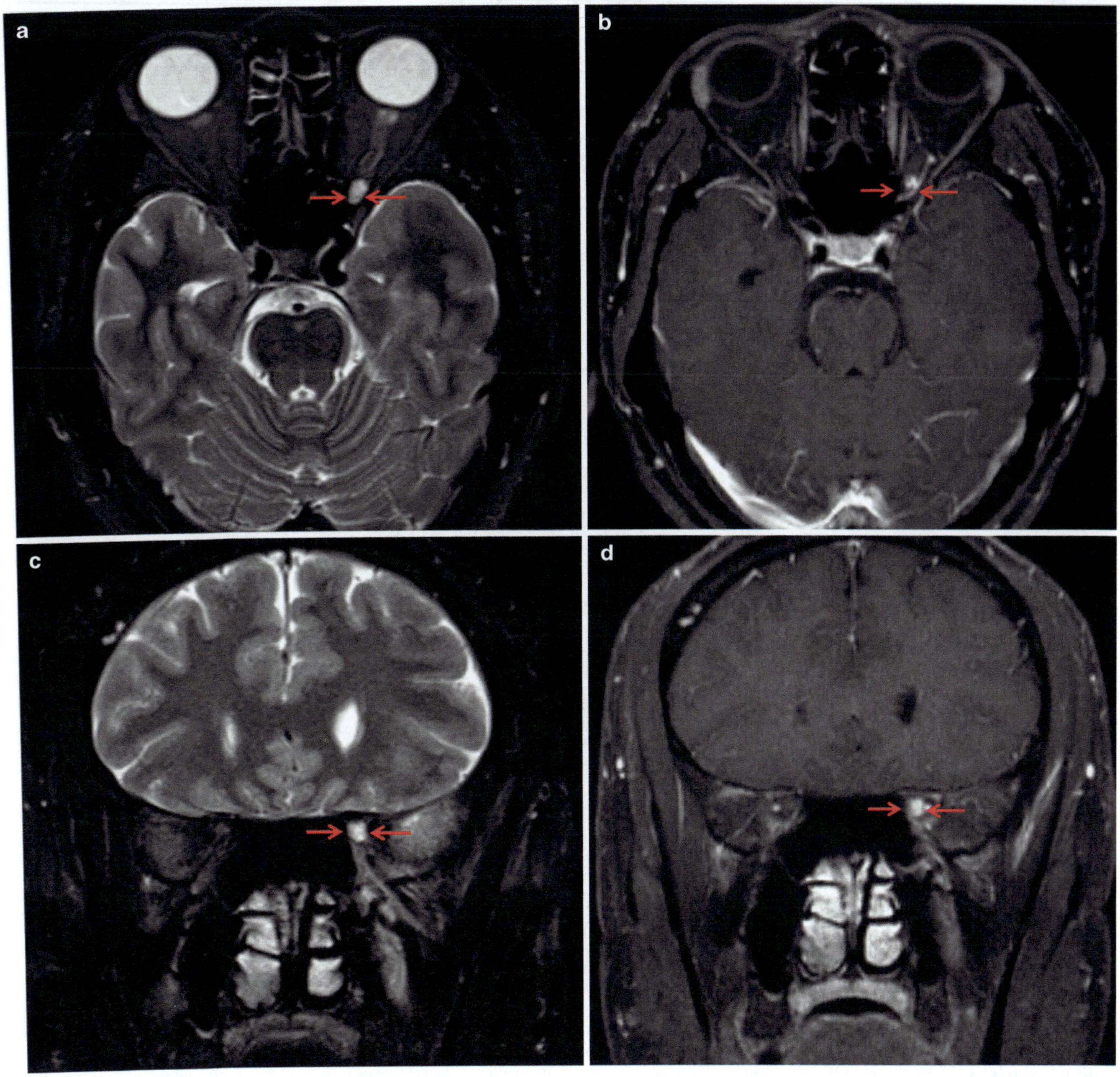

Fig. 8.4 A 39-year-old man with left eye visual deterioration for 2 months. (**a**) T2W STIR axial, (**b**) T1W fat-saturated post-contrast axial, (**c**) T2W fat-saturated coronal, (**d**) T1W fat-saturated post-contrast coronal MRI images show a 0.4 cm T2W strongly hyperintense nodule at the left orbital apex (arrows) lying just inferior to the intracanalicular segment of the left optic nerve causing compression. This nodule shows peripheral nodular contrast enhancement. The imaging features are suggestive of orbital cavernous venous malformation

Lymphatic malformation or lymphangioma in the past is a slow-growing, non-encapsulated lesion often presenting in infancy or childhood. On MRI, lymphatic malformations are diffuse and often insinuate between multiple compartments and are often strongly T2W hyperintense (Fig. 8.5). There can be variable hemorrhagic components which are usually T1W hyperintense, and episodes of previous hemorrhage classically give rise to blood-fluid levels which are considered pathognomonic [36]. The lymph within the lymphatic malformation shows no contrast enhancement. However, contrast enhancement is present in the walls and septa of the lesions.

Orbital varix can be primary or secondary. It can be considered as a type of vascular malformation affecting

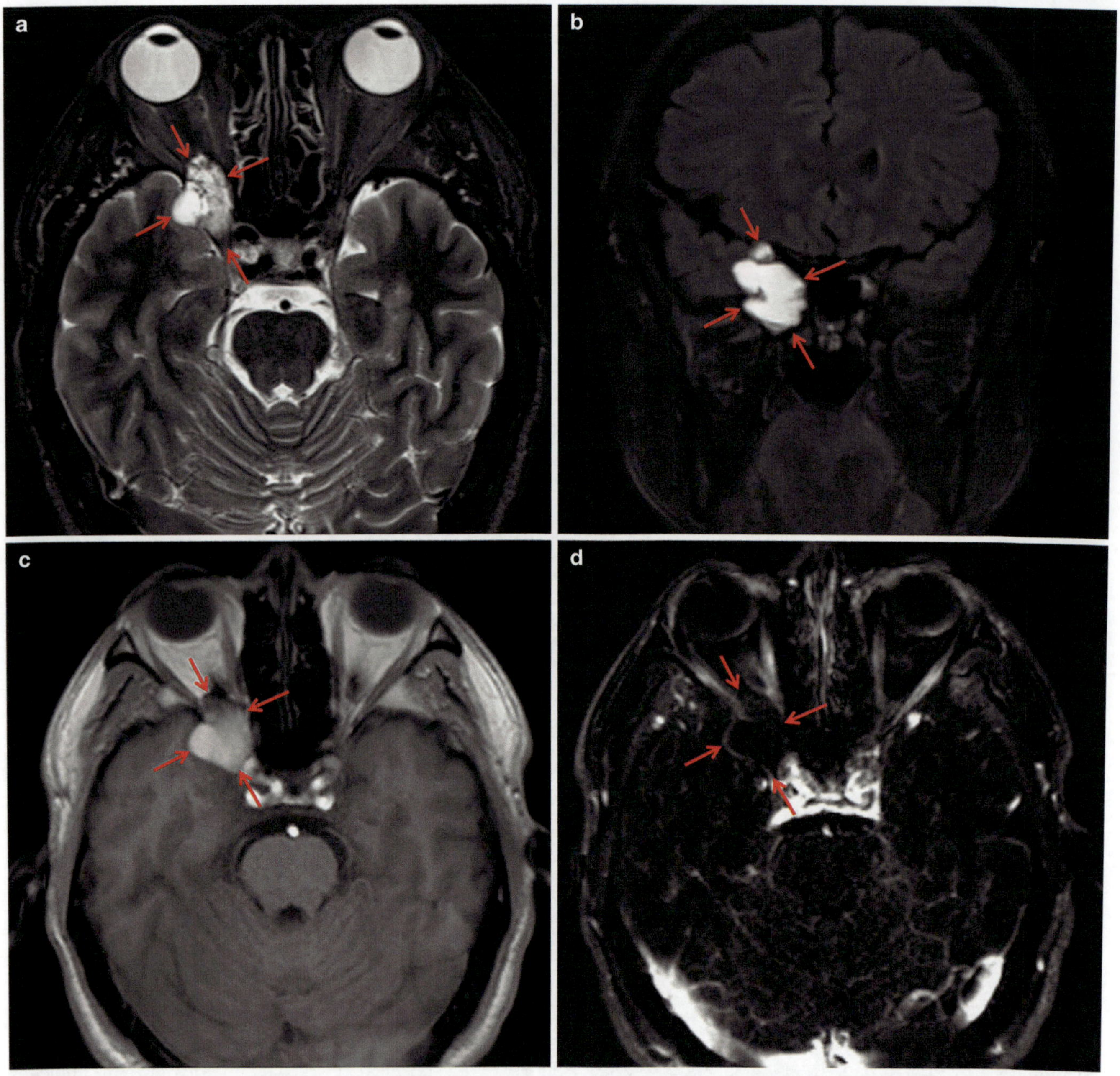

Fig. 8.5 A 48-year-old man with a known right orbital apex lesion incidentally discovered many years. (**a**) T2W STIR axial, (**b**) T2W STIR coronal, (**c**) T1W axial, (**d**) T1W post-contrast (with subtraction) axial MRI images show a lobulated well-defined lesion at the right orbital apex (arrows) involving superior and inferior orbital fissures and greater and lesser wings of the sphenoid bone. On T2W images it is avidly hyperintense with thin septations and some T2W intermediate signal components. On T1W images the lesion is homogeneously hyperintense suggestive of proteinaceous fluid content, and there is thin linear enhancement along the walls and septa only. Findings are that of an orbital lymphatic malformation

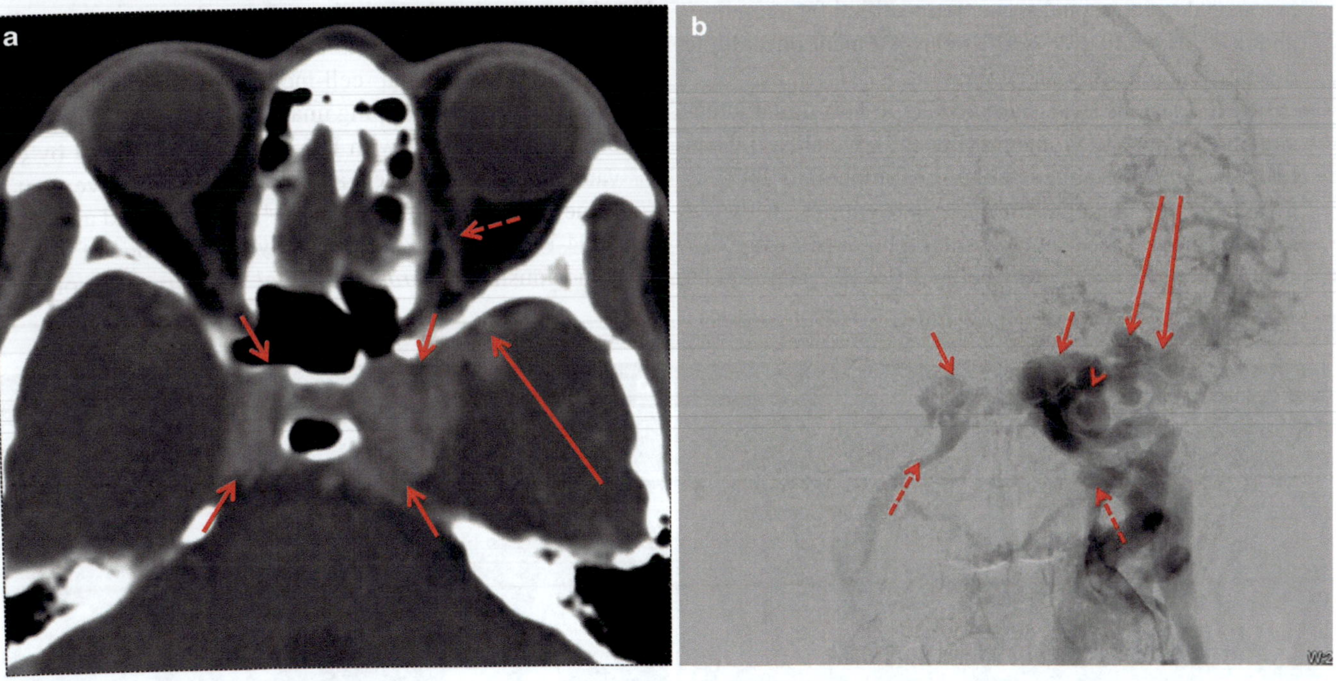

Fig. 8.6 A 39-year-old woman presents with left eye proptosis and redness for 2 months. (**a**) Axial contrast CT angiogram shows that bilateral cavernous sinuses are distended, more on the left side (short solid arrows); the left superior ophthalmic vein is also mildly dilated with increased contrast enhancement (dashed arrow); the left sphenoparietal sinus is tortuous and distended (long solid arrow). (**b**) Frontal view DSA of left internal carotid artery injection demonstrates early opacification of cavernous sinuses (short solid arrows), bilateral inferior petrosal sinuses (dashed arrows), dilated left superior ophthalmic vein (arrowhead), left sphenoparietal sinus (long arrows), and associated cortical venous reflux in the left cerebral hemisphere. Findings are that of a high-flow left carotico-cavernous fistula (CCF). Subsequent endovascular embolization is performed for the patient

"major named vessels" and with anomalies of vessel diameter. Primary orbital varix is thought to result from congenital weakness of venous walls, while secondary varices are related to arteriovenous shunting [37]. Primary orbital varix presents usually in young adulthood with proptosis that becomes more pronounced during maneuvers that induce higher venous pressure, such as Valsalva, coughing, or prone positioning [38]. On MRI, orbital varix is usually T1W and T2W hyperintense with intense contrast enhancement, unless complicated by thrombosis.

Carotid-cavernous fistula (CCF) is an arteriovenous fistula between the carotid arteries and cavernous sinus. It comprises direct (usually due to trauma or iatrogenic causes) and indirect types. Indirect CCF is a type of dural arteriovenous fistula. On CT or MRI angiograms, enlarged cavernous sinuses, superior ophthalmic veins, and other intracranial draining veins can be seen. On digital subtraction angiogram (DSA), early opacification of cavernous sinuses and superior ophthalmic veins can be observed, indicative of arteriovenous shunting (Fig. 8.6). The exact anatomy of CCF is highly variable, and DSA is indispensable for endovascular treatment planning.

8.4.3 Inflammatory Conditions

A diverse range of inflammatory conditions afflict the orbital apex region. Most of these conditions diffusely affect multiple orbital compartments. MRI is often essential for diagnosis and evaluation of treatment response for these conditions. Idiopathic orbital inflammation, thyroid eye disease, and optic neuritis are the commonest causes. Rarer causes in this locality such as vasculitis-related orbital inflammation (such as granulomatosis with angiitis) and orbital sarcoidosis are not dealt with in this chapter.

Idiopathic orbital inflammation (IOI), also known as orbital pseudotumor, is a non-granulomatous inflammatory process of unknown etiology causing myofibroblastic and spindle cell infiltrates affecting multiple compartments in the orbit [8]. Unilateral or bilateral asymmetrical painful proptosis is a common presentation.

Imaging features are variable and may involve multiple sites in the orbit, including myositis (fusiform enlargement of extraocular muscles without sparing of tendinous insertions), perineuritis affecting the optic nerve sheath, episcleritis affecting the anterior orbit, orbital apicitis affecting the posterior orbit, mass-like lesions in the extraconal or intraconal space, retro-orbital fat stranding, and dacryoadenitis [39]. Diffuse involvement of multiple orbital compartments is common.

On MRI, IOI lesions show intermediate to low signal intensity on T1W and T2W images (Fig. 8.7). Notably, IOI can be radiologically quite similar to lymphoma. DWI is invaluable for distinguishing the two entities, with IOI showing high ADC values and lymphoma showing low ADC values commonly way below 1.0×10^{-3} mm^2/s [11].

Notably, several pathological entities perhaps best treated as variants of IOI: *IgG4-related disease* (IgG4-RD) is characterized by plasma cell-mediated inflammation and shows widely overlapping imaging features and pattern of orbital involvement with IOI but is characterized by elevated serum IgG4 levels and multisystem involvement in some but not all of the patients [40]. In the head and neck, IgG4-RD is also characterized by the presence of chronic rhinosinusitis. *Sclerosing orbital inflammation*, or scle-

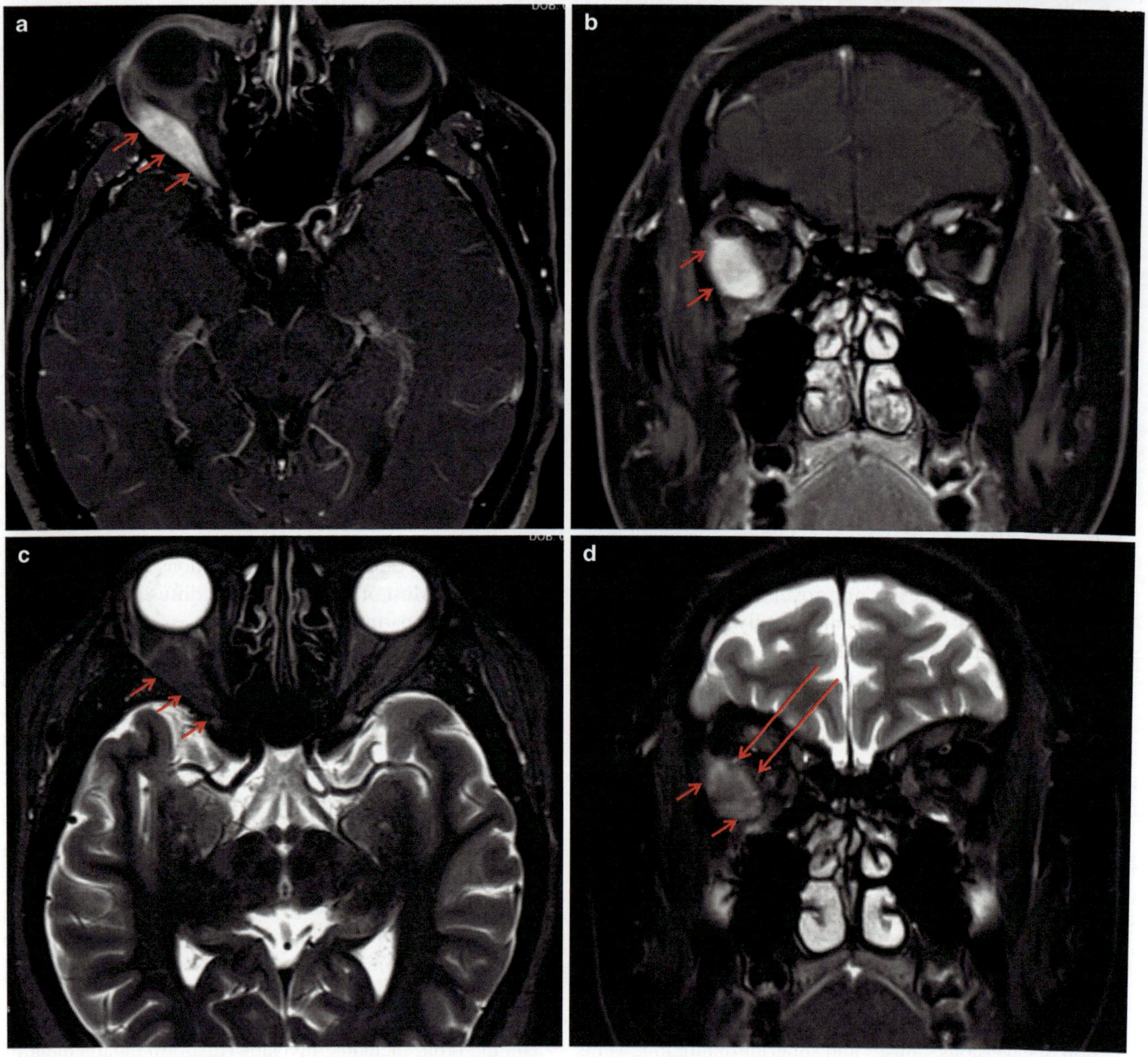

Fig. 8.7 A 39-year-old man presents with progressive right eye redness and diplopia. (**a**) T1W fat-saturated post-contrast axial, (**b**) T1W fat-saturated post-contrast coronal, (**c**) T2W STIR axial, and (**d**) T2W STIR coronal MRI images show fusiform enlargement of right lateral rectus muscle (short arrows) extending into the orbital apex and involving tendinous insertions, with T2W intermediate to high signal change and intense contrast enhancement. There is associated retrobulbar fat inflammatory stranding best seen on coronal T2W STIR image (long arrows). The findings are suggestive of idiopathic orbital inflammatory disease

rosing form of IOI, is characterized by chronic fibrosclerosis of orbital soft tissues with very low signal intensity on T2W images in MRI. *Tolosa-Hunt syndrome* (THS), otherwise known as the apical form of IOI, is characterized by unilateral meningeal and perineural inflammatory changes in the cavernous sinus with anterior extension to involve the orbital apex and superior orbital fissure [41, 42]. Although the MRI signal intensity of THS lesions is similar to that of IOI, it has been suggested that the presence of granulomatous inflammation is distinct from that seen in IOI and some authorities may treat THS as a distinct entity rather than a variant of IOI [43].

Thyroid orbitopathy is caused by mucopolysaccharide deposition in extraocular muscles from abnormal fibroblast activation due to autoimmune thyroid diseases, with Grave's disease and Hashimoto thyroiditis accounting for over 90% of cases [44]. On CT, thyroid eye disease often manifests as bilateral symmetrical extraocular muscle enlargement, increased volume of retro-orbital fat, and proptosis. On MRI, contrary to IOI, the T2W signal in extraocular muscle bellies is increased in acute thyroid orbitopathy, with sparing of the tendinous insertions. Retro-orbital fat also shows T2W hyperintensity reflecting edematous changes. A frequent pattern of involvement is a bilateral symmetric thickening of the inferior, medial, superior, and lateral rectus muscles in descending order of severity [45].

Optic neuritis is multifactorial but is commonly associated with demyelinating disease (multiple sclerosis and neuromyelitis optica spectrum disorders). Other causes include autoimmune diseases such as systemic lupus erythematosus, radiation, ischemia, and infection [46]. MRI is necessary for evaluation, showing optic nerve enhancement, and abnormal hyperintensity on fat-saturated T2W images. The nerve should only show minimal enlargement, contrary to findings in optic glioma [47].

8.4.4 Infection

Bacterial infection involving the orbital apex usually arises from direct posterior extension from post-septal orbital cellulitis, which in itself is multifactorial but most commonly due to extension from sinusitis, more commonly encountered in children than adults [48]. Other causes include penetrating injury, extension from dental, facial, or cavernous sinus infections, and hematogenous seeding. Extension from ethmoid sinus via lamina papyracea is commoner than sphenoid sinus due to the weaker periorbita at the medial orbital wall [48].

The early stage of infection is characterized by cellulitis and orbital phlegmon. Cellulitis appears as orbital fat stranding and extraocular muscle swelling on CT, with diffuse T2W hyperintensity with enhancement on MRI. Phlegmon is isodense to muscle on CT and appears intermediate signal on T1W and hyperintense on T2W images in MRI with contrast enhancement. Later stages of infection commonly involve subperiosteal abscesses along the medial extraconal space of the orbit adjacent to the involved paranasal sinus, appearing as a rim-enhancing lens-shaped hypodense collection on CT with a corresponding central T2W hyperintensity and peripheral rim enhancement on MRI [49].

A dreaded complication is cavernous sinus thrombosis, which can show up on CT as an enlarged cavernous sinus with a filling defect in post-contrast images. On MRI the cavernous sinuses can show T1W and T2W heterogeneous, non-enhancing areas corresponding to thrombus. The thrombosis may even extend into surrounding venous structures such as the superior ophthalmic vein [41].

Invasive fungal infection is predisposed by immunocompromised states, commonly uncontrolled diabetes (up to 80% of cases) [50]. Aspergillosis and mucormycosis are the commonest causes [49]. CT shows nodular mucosal thickening of the affected sinuses with sinus wall erosions. On MRI, thickened sinus mucosa and inflammatory masses characteristically show variable T2W hypointensity due to the presence of iron in fungal elements, with corresponding areas showing contrast enhancement [49]. Aggressive fungal invasions are often angioinvasive, and thrombosis of the internal carotid artery and cavernous sinus needs to be looked for. Perineural spread manifesting as a thickening and increased linear enhancement along the course of nerves is also common. MRI is also useful to assess complications such as mycotic aneurysms, cerebritis, and infarcts [51].

8.4.5 Extrinsic Compression

Metastases involving the orbit are rare, comprising only 1.5–7% of lesions in the orbit in general, with common primaries including the breast, lung, melanoma, prostate, kidney, and gastrointestinal tract [52]. Breast primaries are infamous for diffuse infiltrative involvement of retro-orbital fat and the muscle cone causing scirrhous and fibrotic reactions resulting in enophthalmos [53]; prostate cancer classically causes infiltrative sclerotic bone metastases; melanoma is known for involvement of extraocular muscle causing abnormal enlargement [54].

Nasopharyngeal carcinoma (NPC) and other aggressive head and neck tumors such as squamous cell carcinoma, sinonasal undifferentiated carcinoma, olfactory neuroblastoma, some pituitary macroadenomas, and minor salivary gland tumors such as adenocystic carcinoma

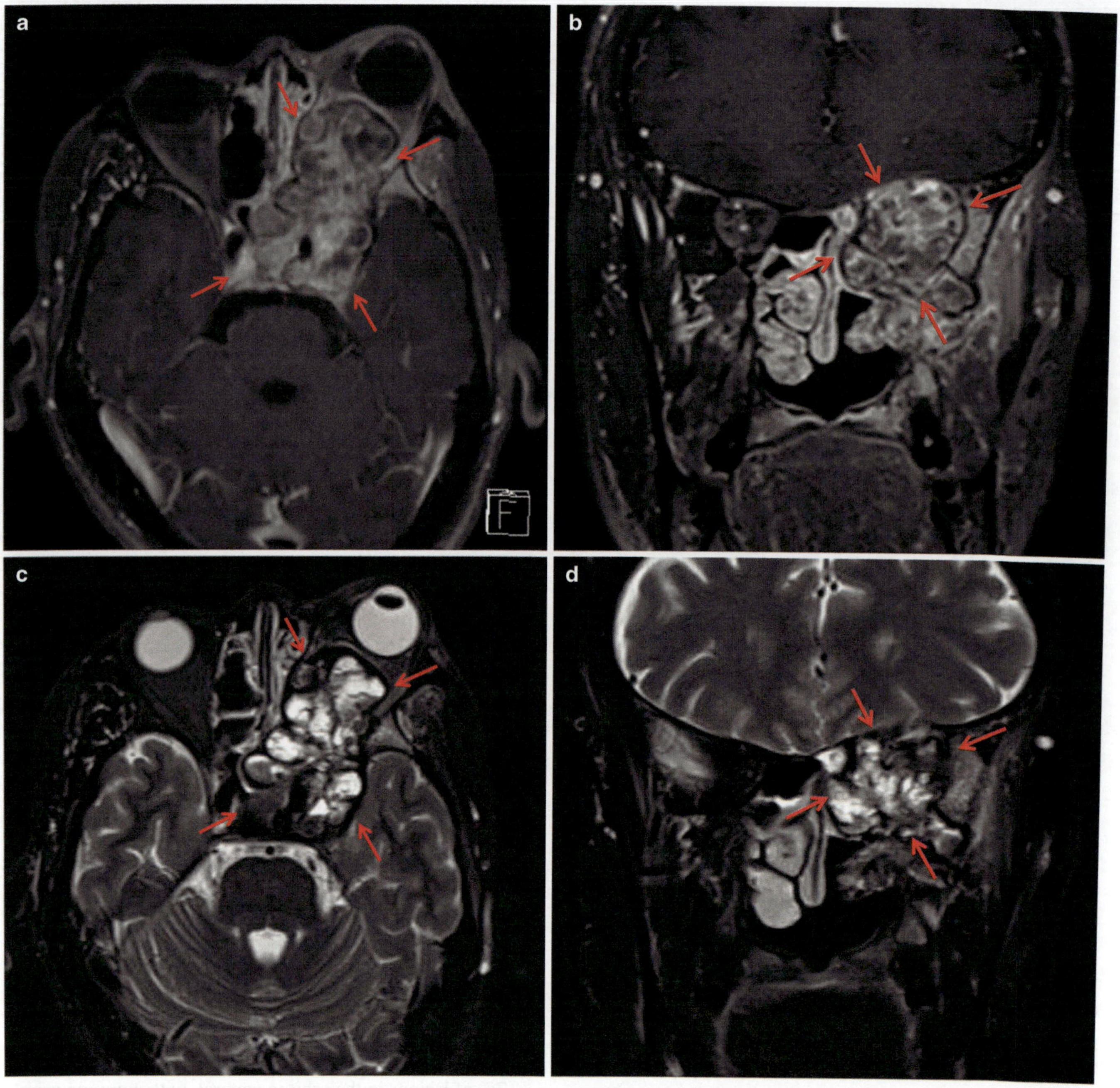

Fig. 8.8 A 63-year-old man with progressive visual loss in the left eye for 3 months. (**a**) T1W fat-saturated post-contrast axial, (**b**) T1W fat-saturated post-contrast coronal, (**c**) T2W STIR axial, and (**d**) T2W STIR coronal MRI images show a heterogeneous infiltrative mass involving the left orbit including the orbital apex (arrows). It shows a multicystic appearance with fluid levels on T2W images and heterogeneous contrast enhancement. The mass complete encases the left optic nerve, involves all extraocular muscles of the left orbit, and the left nasal cavity, left nasopharynx, left cavernous sinus, and pituitary fossa. Biopsy results confirm malignancy with histology shown to be adenocystic carcinoma

(Fig. 8.8) have a propensity for local invasion. Nasopharyngeal carcinoma is particularly common in South Asian males, and a common pattern of spread to orbital apex is via the pterygopalatine fossa into the inferior orbital fissure. On MRI, soft tissue thickening in the ipsilateral nasopharynx, with obliteration of fat signal and abnormal T2W intermediate signal soft tissue within the parapharyngeal space, pterygopalatine fossa, and inferior orbital fissure which show contrast enhancement, is suggestive of NPC invasion [55]. Perineural spread is a second common pattern of involvement, manifesting as enlargement and increased enhancement of the involved nerve on MRI and expansion of the involved canal or neural foramen on both CT and MRI [56].

Fibrous dysplasia (FD) is a congenital, indolent, progressive disorder of abnormal bone remodeling, where abnormal osteoblastic activity leads to the deposition of fibrous and immature osteoid tissue replacing normal cancellous bone [57, 58]. Skull base and facial bone involvement is observed in up to 50% of patients with polyostotic FD. The orbital apex is commonly involved with compression of the optic nerve and other cranial nerves necessitating surgical decompression. CT is the modality of choice for FD as it is a bone disease, with diffuse bony expansion with ground-glass matrix in 56% of patients, while homogeneous bony sclerosis occurs in 23% and cystic changes occur in 21% [59]. MRI appearance may be confusing, with T1W/T2W hypointense bony expansion more indicative of fibrous components but some FD cases demonstrate T1W intermediate and T2W hyperintense signal that may lead to confusion with soft tissue mass [59].

Mucocele is caused by obstruction of the sinus opening leading to the accumulation of mucoid secretion causing an expansion of the involved paranasal sinus, commonly frontal or anterior ethmoid sinus. In rare instances, mucoceles of the posterior ethmoid cell, sphenoid sinus, or an Onodi cell (variant posterior ethmoid cell extending into the optic strut, anterior clinoid process, or sphenoid sinus) may exert a mass effect upon the orbital apex and optic canal, leading to headache, diplopia, proptosis, and decreased vision [60, 61]. On CT, mucocele appears as an expansile hyperdense mass causing outward bulging and even pressure erosions of the walls of the involved sinus. Mucoceles show variable MRI signals due to their heterogeneous protein contents, with rim enhancement of the thickened mucosa and non-enhancement and sometimes abnormal restriction of diffusion in the contents of the mucocele [62].

Dermoid and epidermoid cysts are congenital, slow-growing benign lesions thought to arise from abnormal sequestration of the ectoderm during development. They can occur at suprasellar and parasellar regions, exerting mass effect on structures in the orbital apex and cavernous sinus [63]. On CT, the dermoid cyst shows up as a well-defined fat-containing cystic lesion, which may contain fluid and soft tissue densities as well as capsular calcifications; MRI demonstrates T1W and T2W hyperintense fat content. Epidermoid cyst on the other hand shows up as a well-defined homogeneous cystic lesion on both CT and MRI, with homogeneous fluid signal on T1W and T2W sequences, but characteristically shows abnormal restriction of diffusion on DWI. Both lesions can cause pressure erosion and scalloping of adjacent bone [64].

8.5 Conclusion

Orbital apex pathologies are diverse, and many lesions show variable and overlapping radiological features as detailed in this chapter. It is essential for physicians to have a thorough understanding of radiological anatomy and an appreciation of the powers and limitations of different modalities available in order to perform appropriate imaging assessments for patients with symptoms and signs pertaining to orbital apex pathologies.

References

1. Machleder DJ, Banik R, Rosenberg RB, Parikh SR. An unusual case of rhabdomyosarcoma presenting as orbital apex syndrome. Int J Pediatr Otorhinolaryngol. 2005;69:249–54.
2. Rootman J. Diseases of the orbit: a multidisciplinary approach. Philadelphia: Lippincott Williams & Wilkins; 2003.
3. Cho SW, Lee WW, Ma DJ, et al. Orbital apex lesions: a diagnostic and therapeutic challenge. J Neurol Surg B Skull Base. 2018;79(4):386–93.
4. Chong VF, Fan YF, Chan LL. Radiology of the orbital apex. Australas Radiol. 1999;43:294–302.
5. Daniels DL, Yu S, Pech P, Haughton VM. Computed tomography and magnetic resonance imaging of the orbital apex. Radiol Clin N Am. 1987;25:803–17.
6. Quiñones-Hinojosa A. Schmidek & Sweet operative neurosurgical techniques: indications, methods, and results. Elsevier; 2012.
7. Daniels DL, Mark LP, Mafee MF, et al. Osseous anatomy of the orbital apex. AJNR Am J Neuroradiol. 1995;16:1929–35.
8. Chen CT, Chen YR. Traumatic superior orbital fissure syndrome. Craniomaxillofac Trauma Reconstr. 2010;3:9–16.
9. Purohit BS, Vargas MI, Ailianou A, Merlini L, Poletti PA, Platon A, Delattre BM, Rager O, Burkhardt K, Becker M. Orbital tumours and tumour-like lesions: exploring the armamentarium of multiparametric imaging. Insights Imaging. 2016;7(1):43–68.
10. Lee AG, Johnson MC, Policeni BA, Smoker WR. Imaging for neuro-ophthalmic and orbital disease - a review. Clin Exp Ophthalmol. 2009;37:30–53.
11. Sepahdari AR, Aakalu VK, Setabutr P, Shiehmorteza M, Naheedy JH, Mafee MF. Indeterminate orbital masses: restricted diffusion at MR imaging with echo-planar diffusion-weighted imaging predicts malignancy. Radiology. 2010;256:554–64.
12. Rao AA, Naheedy JH, Chen JY, Robbins SL, Ramkumar HL. A clinical update and radiologic review of pediatric orbital and ocular tumors. J Oncol. 2013;2013:975908.
13. Heran F, Berges O, Blustajn J, et al. Tumor pathology of the orbit. Diagn Interv Imaging. 2014;95:933–44.
14. Becker M, Zaidi H. Imaging in head and neck squamous cell carcinoma: the potential role of PET/MRI. Br J Radiol. 2014;87:20130677.
15. Goldberg SH, Cantore WA. Tumors of the orbit. Curr Opin Ophthalmol. 1997;8:51–6.
16. Miller NR. Primary tumours of the optic nerve and its sheath. Eye. 2004;18:1026–37.
17. Jackson A, Patankar T, Laitt RD. Intracanalicular optic nerve meningioma: a serious diagnostic pitfall. AJNR Am J Neuroradiol. 2003;24:1167–70.

18. Mafee MF, Pai E, Philip B. Rhabdomyosarcoma of the orbit. Evaluation with MR imaging and CT. Radiol Clin N Am. 1998;36:1215–27.
19. Kapur R, Mafee MF, Lamba R, Edward DP. Orbital schwannoma and neurofibroma: role of imaging. Neuroimaging Clin N Am. 2005;15:159–74.
20. Wang Y, Xiao LH. Orbital schwannomas: findings from magnetic resonance imaging in 62 cases. Eye. 2008;22:1034–9.
21. Tezer MS, Ozcan M, Han O, Unal A, Ozlugedik S. Schwannoma originating from the infraorbital nerve: a case report. Auris Nasus Larynx. 2006;33:343–5.
22. Demirci H, Shields CL, Shields JA, Honavar SG, Mercado GJ, Tovilla JC. Orbital tumors in the older adult population. Ophthalmology. 2002;109:243–8.
23. Goh PS, Gi MT, Charlton A, Tan C, Gangadhara Sundar JK, Amrith S. Review of orbital imaging. Eur J Radiol. 2008;66:387–95.
24. Akansel G, Hendrix L, Erickson BA, et al. MRI patterns in orbital malignant lymphoma and atypical lymphocytic infiltrates. Eur J Radiol. 2005;53:175–81.
25. Stefanovic A, Lossos IS. Extranodal marginal zone lymphoma of the ocular adnexa. Blood. 2009;114:501–10.
26. Eckardt AM, Lemound J, Rana M, Gellrich NC. Orbital lymphoma: diagnostic approach and treatment outcome. World J Surg Oncol. 2013;11:73.
27. Sullivan TJ, Valenzuela AA. Imaging features of ocular adnexal lymphoproliferative disease. Eye. 2006;20:1189–95.
28. Kapur R, Sepahdari AR, Mafee MF, et al. MR imaging of orbital inflammatory syndrome, orbital cellulitis, and orbital lymphoid lesions: the role of diffusion-weighted imaging. AJNR Am J Neuroradiol. 2009;30:64–70.
29. Hiwatashi A, Yoshiura T, Togao O, et al. Diffusivity of intraorbital lymphoma vs. IgG4-related DISEASE: 3D turbo field echo with diffusion-sensitised driven-equilibrium preparation technique. Eur Radiol. 2014;24:581–6.
30. Hui KH, Pfeiffer ML, Esmaeli B. Value of positron emission tomography/computed tomography in diagnosis and staging of primary ocular and orbital tumors. Saudi J Ophthalmol. 2012;26:365–71.
31. Roe RH, Finger PT, Kurli M, Tena LB, Iacob CE. Whole body positron emission tomography/computed tomography imaging and staging of orbital lymphoma. Ophthalmology. 2006;113:1854–8.
32. Chung EM, Smirniotopoulos JG, Specht CS, Schroeder JW, Cube R. From the archives of the AFIP: pediatric orbit tumors and tumorlike lesions: nonosseous lesions of the extraocular orbit. Radiographics. 2007;27:1777–99.
33. International Society for The Study of Vascular Anomalies (ISSVA). https://www.issva.org.
34. Smoker WR, Gentry LR, Yee NK, Reede DL, Nerad JA. Vascular lesions of the orbit: more than meets the eye. Radiographics. 2008;28:185–204.
35. Mawn LA, Jordan DR, Gilberg SM. Cavernous hemangiomas of the orbital apex with intracranial extension. Ophthalmic Surg Lasers. 1998;29:680–4.
36. Sharma P, Sharma S, Gupta N, et al. Pott puffy tumor. Proc (Bayl Univ Med Cent). 2017;30:179–81.
37. Goyal P, Lee S, Gupta N, Kumar Y, Mangla M, Hooda K, Li S, Mangla R. Orbital apex disorders: imaging findings and management. Neuroradiol J. 2018;31(2):104–25.
38. Bhatti MT, Dutton JJ. Thyroid eye disease: therapy in the active phase. J Neuroophthalmol. 2014;34:186–97.
39. Narla LD, Newman B, Spottswood SS, Narla S, Kolli R. Inflammatory pseudotumor. Radiographics. 2003;23:719–29.
40. McNab AA, McKelvie P. IgG4–related ophthalmic disease. Part II: Clinical aspects. Ophthal Plast Reconstr Surg. 2015;31:167–78.
41. De Wyngaert R, Casteels I, Demaerel P. Orbital and anterior visual pathway infection and inflammation. Neuroradiology. 2009;51:385–96.
42. Schuknecht B, Sturm V, Huisman TA, Landau K. Tolosa-Hunt syndrome: MR imaging features in 15 patients with 20 episodes of painful ophthalmoplegia. Eur J Radiol. 2009;69:445–53.
43. Wasmeier C, Pfadenhauer K, Rosler A. Idiopathic inflammatory pseudotumor of the orbit and Tolosa-Hunt syndrome—are they the same disease? J Neurol. 2002;249:1237–41.
44. Fung S, Malhotra R, Selva D. Thyroid orbitopathy. Aust Fam Physician. 2003;32:615–20.
45. Bun RJ, Vissink A, Bos RR. Traumatic superior orbital fissure syndrome: report of two cases. J Oral Maxillofac Surg. 1996;54:758–61.
46. Grimm MA, Hazelton T, Beck RW, Murtagh FR. Postgadolinium enhancement of a compressive neuropathy of the optic nerve. AJNR Am J Neuroradiol. 1995;16:779–81.
47. Jacobs DA, Galetta SL. Neuro-ophthalmology for neuroradiologists. AJNR Am J Neuroradiol. 2007;28:3–8.
48. Swift AC, Charlton G. Sinusitis and the acute orbit in children. J Laryngol Otol. 1990;104:213–6.
49. Eustis HS, Mafee MF, Walton C, Mondonca J. MR imaging and CT of orbital infections and complications in acute rhinosinusitis. Radiol Clin N Am. 1998;36:1165–83.
50. Warwar RE, Bullock JD. Rhino-orbital-cerebral mucormycosis: a review. Orbit. 1998;17:237–45.
51. Eskey CJ, Whitman GJ, Chew FS. Invasive aspergillosis of the orbit. AJR Am J Roentgenol. 1996;167:1588.
52. Walrath JD, Lelli GJ Jr, Engelbert M, Kazim M. Metastatic endometrial carcinoma resulting in orbital apex compression. Ophthal Plast Reconstr Surg. 2007;23:250–1.
53. Ahmad SM, Esmaeli B. Metastatic tumors of the orbit and ocular adnexa. Curr Opin Ophthalmol. 2007;18:405–13.
54. Shields JA, Shields CL, Brotman HK, Carvalho C, Perez N, Eagle RC Jr. Cancer metastatic to the orbit: the 2000 Robert M. Curts Lecture. Ophthal Plast Reconstr Surg. 2001;17:346–54.
55. Luo CB, Teng MM, Chen SS, Lirng JF, Guo WY, Chang T. Orbital invasion in nasopharyngeal carcinoma: evaluation with computed tomography and magnetic resonance imaging. Zhonghua Yi Xue Za Zhi (Taipei). 1998;61:382–8.
56. Spitellie PH, Jordan DR, Brownstein S, Gooi P, Burns B. Sinonasal undifferentiated carcinoma with a frozen globe. Ophthal Plast Reconstr Surg. 2008;24:225–7.
57. Sammut SJ, Kandasamy J, Newman W, et al. Relief of severe retro-orbital pain and vision improvement after optic-nerve decompression in polyostotic fibrous dysplasia: case report and review of the literature. Childs Nerv Syst. 2008;24:515–20.
58. Rosa RH, Buggage R, Harocopos GJ, et al. Ophthalmic pathology and intraocular tumors: basic and clinical science course, Section 4. San Francisco, CA: American Academy of Ophthalmology; 2011. p. 5–45.
59. Chong VF, Khoo JB, Fan YF. Fibrous dysplasia involving the base of the skull. AJR Am J Roentgenol. 2002;178:717–20.
60. Lim CC, Dillon WP, McDermott MW. Mucocele involving the anterior clinoid process: MR and CT findings. AJNR Am J Neuroradiol. 1999;20:287–90.
61. Klink T, Pahnke J, Hoppe F, Lieb W. Acute visual loss by an Onodi cell. Br J Ophthalmol. 2000;84:801–2.
62. Van Tassel P, Lee YY, Jing BS, et al. Mucoceles of the paranasal sinuses: MR imaging with CT correlation. AJR Am J Roentgenol. 1989;153:407–12.
63. Orakcioglu B, Halatsch ME, Fortunati M, et al. Intracranial dermoid cysts: variations of radiological and clinical features. Acta Neurochir. 2008;150:1227–34.
64. Ahmed RA, Eltanamly RM. Orbital epidermoid cysts: a diagnosis to consider. J Ophthalmol. 2014;2014:508425.

Part III

Spectrum of Diseases

9 Optic Nerve Neoplasm

Noel C. Y. Chan

Abstract

This chapter will summarize different primary optic nerve neoplasms with the main focus on the more commonly encountered optic glioma and optic nerve sheath meningioma. Based on the published literature, this chapter will cover epidemiology, clinical presentations, histopathology, imaging characteristics, different treatment modalities, and management strategies. Up-to-date diagnostic and therapeutic options will also be discussed.

Keywords

Optic nerve · Optic glioma · Optic nerve sheath meningioma · Neurofibromatosis · Neuro-ophthalmology

9.1 Introduction

Optic nerve dysfunction is one of the common clinical manifestations and sequelae in optic nerve neoplasms regardless of its origin. Depending on its size and extent, some can also manifest with compressive orbitopathy, proptosis, squint, cranial nerve palsies, and nystagmus. Management has to be individualized depending on various factors including age, nature of the tumor, disease progression, visual complications, and prognosis. In this chapter we will be focusing on primary tumors arising from the optic nerve (ON) itself or from its surrounding optic nerve sheath (ONS). ON compression or infiltration secondary to other tumors in the periorbital region will be discussed in another chapter on periorbital skull base tumors.

N. C. Y. Chan (✉)
Department of Ophthalmology & Visual Sciences, Prince of Wales Hospital & Alice Ho Miu Ling Nethersole Hospital, Hong Kong SAR, China

Department of Ophthalmology & Visual Sciences, The Chinese University of Hong Kong, Shatin, Hong Kong SAR, China
e-mail: noelccy@fellow.hkam.hk

9.2 Primary Optic Nerve Tumors

9.2.1 Optic Glioma

Optic glioma (OG) refers to glial tumors involving the anterior visual pathway (i.e., optic nerves, optic chiasm, and optic tracts), and it accounts for 65% of all intrinsic ON tumors [1]. When the tumor is confined to only one ON, it is commonly known as optic nerve glioma (ONG) while optic chiasmal glioma (OCG) is used to describe a tumor involving the optic chiasm or optic tracts and/or the hypothalamus [2].

According to the World Health Organization (WHO), they are most often juvenile pilocytic astrocytoma (grade 1 or low-grade 2) or diffuse fibrillary astrocytoma (grade 2) [3]. There have been some controversies in the nomenclature of some ONGs due to their slow growth and lack of mitotic figures or anaplastic transformation [4]. They are sometimes called hamartoma which is a term to designate tumors that had the potential to grow in a self-limited form during the period of development and signifies a disorganized overgrowth of differentiated tissue normal to a site [5]. Immunohistochemical staining has however indicated that ONGs arise from type 1 astrocytes [6] and they shared identical molecular genetic makeup with low-grade astrocytomas elsewhere in the central nervous system (CNS). Thus, they are more commonly referred to as pilocytic astrocytoma [7, 8]. Measurements of tumor aggressiveness and proliferation can be performed using MIB-1 antibodies to the Ki-67 antigens [9].

ONGs comprise approximately 1% of all intracranial tumors [1]. Most of them are unilateral and occur in the first decade of life with a median age of 6.5 years and more frequently in females [10, 11]. More common than ONGs, OCGs represent less than 10% of all intracranial tumors in children and adults with a broader age group with no apparent sex predilection [12, 13]. In Dutton's review, 25% of OGs were isolated to ON alone, and 75% involved the chiasm. Among those OCGs, less than 10% were isolated to the chiasm while most extended to the ON, the hypothalamus, or

T. L. POON et al. (eds.), *Orbital Apex and Periorbital Skull Base Diseases*, https://doi.org/10.1007/978-981-99-2989-4_9

the third ventricle. Rarely do these tumors extend within the optic disc or globe [1].

For a better understanding of this tumor, the molecular genetic makeup of OGs had been explored in the recent decade [14]. Normally, there are two copies of the NF1 gene located on chromosome 17q11.2 which is responsible for the production of neurofibromin. Neurofibromin is an important protein for regulating the Ras-dependent intracellular signal pathway, and it is expressed in the cytoplasm of neurons, oligodendrocytes, Schwann cells, and astrocytes. Neurofibromatosis type 1 (NF-1) patients have a germline mutation giving rise to a nonfunctional copy of this gene in all cells of the body. OGs will develop when there is a complete loss of neurofibromin function due to somatic mutation of the remaining NF1 gene. Loss of neurofibromin will result in a low level of cyclic adenosine monophosphate (cAMP) and Ras hyperactivation, leading to loss of tumor growth inhibition and increased cellular proliferation through mitogen-activated protein (MAP) kinase, respectively [15, 16]. In sporadic OGs, activation of B-raf (BRAF) is observed instead while there is a rearrangement in the kinase portion of the serine/threonine-protein kinase BRAF gene due to a duplication at chromosome 7q34 [17].

Although there has been a clear genetic relationship between ONG and NF-1, most of the mutations are sporadic [18]. It can also occur in children with neurofibromatosis type 2 (NF-2), but it was a less frequent ocular manifestation [19]. In the literature, 10–70% of patients with ONG have NF-1 while 8% and 31% of NF-1 patients have clinical and radiological ONG, respectively [18, 20, 21]. For OCG, approximately 30% of patients with OCG have NF-1 while about 18% of patients with NF-1 have an OCG [1, 22].

Many NF-1-associated gliomas remain indolent with over 50% being asymptomatic while sporadic OG has a greater propensity to present symptomatically [23–25]. The majority of patients with ONGs have symptom onset in the first decade of life and up to 90% become symptomatic in the first two decades [26]. The tumor can give rise to anterior or posterior presentations depending on its extent and location. The anterior presentation includes ON dysfunction with optic disc swelling as well as proptosis which is more often axial but can also be associated with hypoglobus and strabismus. The posterior presentation comprises unilateral optic neuropathy with an apparent normal or pale optic disc. Orbital or ocular pain is not a common finding in ONGs. The visual loss is usually progressive and slow in nature unless there is an acute tumor hemorrhage [27] or occurrence of acute retinal vein occlusion [28].

Most patients with OCGs present with insidious visual loss bilaterally [29], which are sometimes discovered during routine examination. With minimally pale optic discs and invariably mild proptosis, they may be misdiagnosed as amblyopia or inorganic visual loss [12, 30]. Depending on the tissue involved, any type of visual field defect can be present in patients with OCGs, but bitemporal hemianopia is common. Acute visual loss can result from chiasmal apoplexy or similar pathologies as in ONG [31, 32].

Different types of nystagmus may occur in patients with OGs. For those with severe visual loss, the nystagmus can be secondary to the Heimann-Bielschowsky phenomenon which is always monocular, of low frequency, with variable amplitudes, and in a vertical direction. This type of nystagmus can also be found in other patients with acquired monocular visual loss. If the glioma involves the optic chiasm or the associated structures, apart from seesaw nystagmus, some patients may develop unilateral nystagmus of high frequency and low amplitude [33, 34]. This can sometimes be mistaken as spasmus nutans which is on the contrary a benign condition that is commonly resolved when the child reaches 3–4 years old. To avoid diagnostic delay, it is, therefore, important to perform neuroimaging in children who present with asymmetric spasmus nutans or those with atypical features such as lack of torticollis or head bobbing [35–37].

Nevertheless, some ONGs can be asymptomatic with patients enjoying clinically normal visual function [38]. In some of these patients, further ophthalmic investigations may reveal abnormal visual evoked potentials (VEPs) [39] or thinning of peripapillary retinal nerve fiber layer (pRNFL) [40] or macular ganglion cell/inner plexiform layer (mGCIPL) on optic coherence tomography (OCT) [41]. In the past, VEPs was considered a screening tool for detecting OGs before subjecting NF-1 patients to neuroimaging while some proposed its use in monitoring the progression of the glioma once detected [42, 43].

Apart from ophthalmic manifestations, patients with OCG may present with other neurological symptoms and signs such as precocious puberty, hypothalamic dysfunction, diencephalic syndrome, or raised intracranial pressure (ICP). In these circumstances, history taking is important in differentiating the types of OCG. Anterior-type OCGs originate from within the anterior visual system which may infiltrate the hypothalamus while posterior-type OCGs originate from the hypothalamic region and secondarily invades the optic chiasm and ON [13].

With a higher resolution, magnetic resonance imaging (MRI) is a better neuroimaging option than computer tomography (CT) in identifying intracranial extension and future monitoring of OGs. However, defining the tumor border can be difficult as ipsilateral enlargement of the optic canal may not necessarily signify intracranial extension while tumor cells can present beyond the apparent limits of MRI [44]. The typical imaging protocol is an MRI of the brain and orbits with thin cuts through the ONs which commonly shows a fusiform enlargement of the ON with T1 hypointensity/isointensity and T2 hyperintensity which is usually enhanced after injection of gadolinium contrast (see Figs. 9.1 and 9.2).

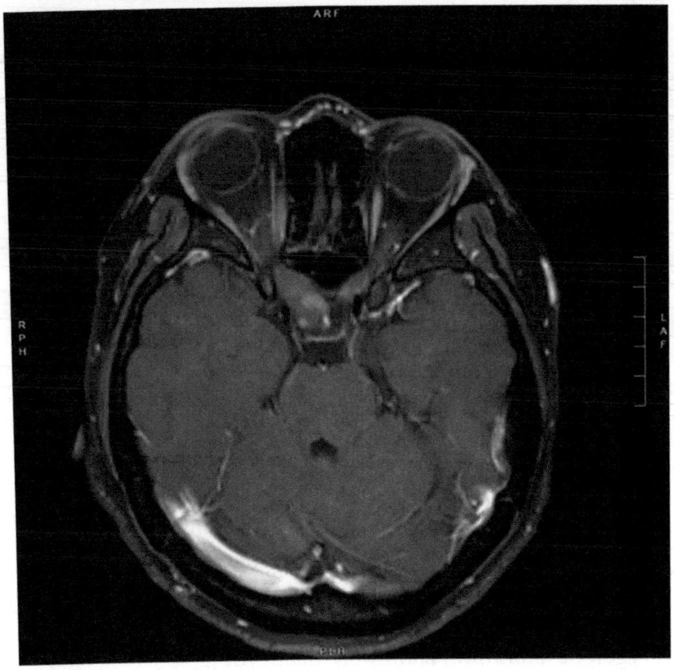

Fig. 9.1 MRI T1-weighted sequence with fat suppression showing fusiform enlargement of the bilateral optic nerve with T1 isointensity and intracranial extension on axial scan. (*Image Courtesy of Dr. Carmen Chan*)

While non-NF-1-associated ONGs tend to grow within the confinement of the neural tissue, some NF-1-associated ONGs can infiltrate leptomeninges [45]. In the presence of perineural gliomatosis [46], the tumor may rupture the pia and proliferate within the subarachnoid space resulting in a "pseudo-cerebrospinal fluid (CSF)" sign [47]. In some patients with NF-1, ONG will sometimes show up as a thickened kinked nerve with buckling or cystic areas within the nerve [22, 48]. More recently, optic nerve tortuosity on baseline MRI, but not thickening of nerve or sheath, was found to be associated with OG development in NF-1 patients [49]. Follow-up imaging will thus be warranted in these cases to distinguish this benign finding from tumor development.

The radiological appearance of OCGs varies with different levels of preservation of the original chiasmal macroarchitecture. Depending on the extent of the exophytic component, some OCGs appear as an enlargement of the chiasm while some appear as a poorly defined suprasellar mass replacing the chiasm. With the ability to show the orientation of the white matter tract, diffusion tensor imaging (DTI), and diffusion tensor tractography (DTT) can illustrate and trace the optic pathway clearly. However, DTI is technically difficult in the assessment of ONs due to susceptibility artifacts from neighboring bone or sinuses, and DTT can be

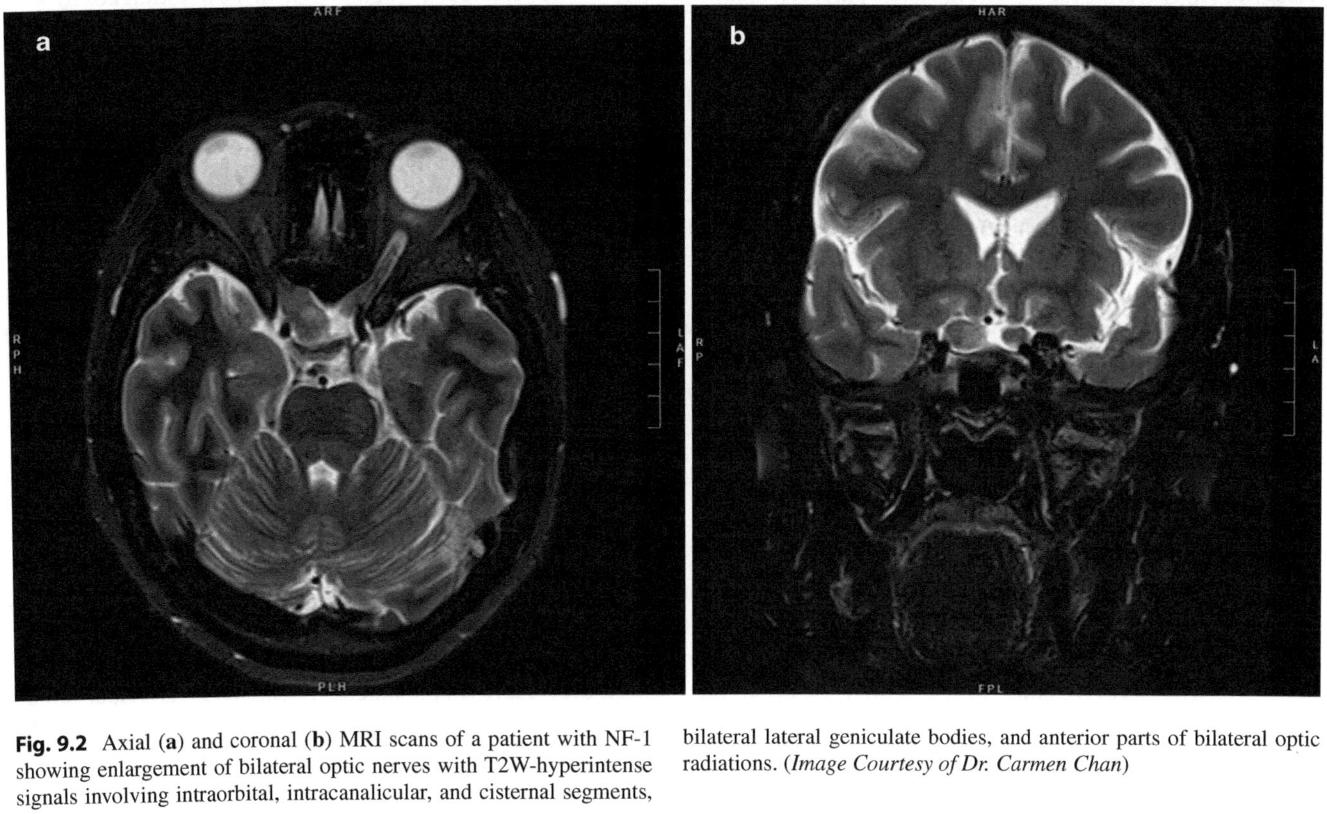

Fig. 9.2 Axial (**a**) and coronal (**b**) MRI scans of a patient with NF-1 showing enlargement of bilateral optic nerves with T2W-hyperintense signals involving intraorbital, intracanalicular, and cisternal segments, bilateral lateral geniculate bodies, and anterior parts of bilateral optic radiations. (*Image Courtesy of Dr. Carmen Chan*)

confounded by white matter decussations at the chiasmal region. It is therefore more suitable for evaluating the posterior visual pathway in selected cases. Although DTI carries the potential in predicting future visual loss, the correlation between imaged changes and visual dysfunction remains undetermined while results have to be replicated in larger trials [50].

Diagnosis of ONG is established with reasonable confidence using MRI, and biopsy is rarely indicated due to the potential risk of inadvertent damage resulting in the visual loss [51]. Secondly, ONGs may develop reactive leptomeningeal hyperplasia beyond the limits of the tumor, and biopsy may sometimes lead to an erroneous diagnosis of meningioma [52, 53]. Similarly, tissue diagnosis is usually not required for OCG with clearly defined borders as an intrinsic lesion with preservation of gross outline of the chiasm. However, in the settings of atypical clinical presentations (e.g., adults with diabetes insipidus), globular morphology on MRI or when there is uncertainty in defining if the suprasellar mass is intrinsic or extrinsic, a biopsy is recommended with either the stereotactic, endoscopic, or transcranial approach.

Monitoring disease progression in young patients with OG can be challenging in the presence of unreliable ophthalmic examinations and the lack of indicative biomarkers. Visual acuity (VA) is the most important parameter during follow-up, yet it is sometimes difficult to distinguish visual drop secondary to amblyopia from ON dysfunction. Depending on the age, Teller acuity testing, HOTV, and Lea optotypes may be used, and Snellen acuity should be attempted if feasible. Assessment with the same optotype as previously recorded is important to ensure standardization and particularly crucial upon detection of visual progression. Color vision testing with Ishihara pseudo-isochromatic plates or Hardy-Rand-Rittler color plates can be very helpful as ONGs tend to have poor color perception while color vision is preserved in amblyopia. Although there is no universally accepted guideline in defining visual deterioration in OGs, most experts would consider the worsening of two Snellen lines of acuity a significant change to suggest possible progression [54].

For patients who are not cooperative with subjective testing, OCT and VEP can be acceptable alternatives with a prior plan in the degree of change for the determination of progression [40, 55–57]. VEP has a high sensitivity in identifying OGs, but it is unable to distinguish symptomatic from asymptomatic OGs. Together with the high intervisit variability, need of skilled staff, and patient cooperation, VEP alone is not a good clinical biomarker for treatment decisions, but it serves as a good complementary tool [39]. OCT has gained considerable attention as a biomarker to assess structural changes upon visual pathway injury. Literature has demonstrated a good correlation between pRNFL thickness and concurrent visual loss in OGs while the availability of handheld OCT makes taking measurements practical and repeatable during sedation [57–59]. Although changes in pRNFL are uncertain in the prediction of impending visual loss and pRNFL decline may continue after visual loss has occurred, a normal pRNFL thickness (≥80 μm for example) may reassure the treating physician that visual loss is unlikely [40].

Current recommendations of surveillance intervals or methods are largely based on individual clinical experience and limited available evidence. Among patients with NF-1, the Optic Pathway Glioma Task Force in 1997 did not recommend serial screening with routine neuroimaging as early detection of these tumors does not reduce the rate of visual dysfunction nor affect therapeutic management [60, 61]. Although some advocate MRI screening in young children of age less than 15 months, this remains controversial as sedation is required for neuroimaging in this age group while it carries certain risks such as airway obstruction, aspiration, oxygen desaturation, and rarely death [62].

The most widely accepted screening for asymptomatic children with NF-1 is routine ophthalmic examinations. Annual comprehensive neuro-ophthalmic evaluation is warranted for children with NF-1 until 8 years old and then every other year until 18 years old or anytime when there is subjective visual change. In patients with newly diagnosed OG, neuro-imaging is recommended every 3 months for the first year. The frequency can be extended to every 6 months when there is no evidence of tumor progression or visual deterioration. Thereafter, annual neuroimaging can be arranged with interval neuro-ophthalmological assessments every 6 months. If clinically and radiologically stable, surveillance of known NF-1-associated OG can be discontinued after age 18 [63].

Treatment of OG is most commonly intended to reduce the risk of permanent, clinically significant visual dysfunction. However, given the high variability in growth patterns of individual tumors, there is currently no consensus on when to treat and when to observe [64]. Management of patients with OG has to be individualized according to the age at presentation, the patient's current vision or ocular morbidity, nature of the tumor (NF-1 or sporadic), its extent, and the risk of further progression.

For patients with good and stable vision, observation can be considered [29] given the slow-growing progress of this tumor, some enter a prolonged quiescent stage, and some may even regress spontaneously [65–68]. As visual deficit due to OGs may go unnoticed and sometimes precede the diagnosis of OGs, ophthalmological abnormalities found at tumor presentation which is thought to be chronic may not require treatment. Similar to ONG, in the absence of hypothalamic or other neurological manifestations, OCGs can be followed up clinically and with neuroimaging without intervention as they take similar slow-growing course. Precocious puberty should be treated with gonadotropin-releasing hormone antagonists while therapy for growth hormone excess related to OGs is controversial.

Nevertheless, some children may experience rapid growth of tumors. Local progression has been observed in 7 of 35 patients (20%) followed up without treatment [64]. In a study, 50% of the patients without initial chiasmal involvement progressed to chiasmal involvement during follow-up, most within 12 months and more so in those with NF-1 [69]. Yet, isolated growth of OG does not necessarily be an indication for treatment, and there have been different opinions in defining "disease progression." Radiological progression is often represented by an increase in tumor size, increased enhancement, or involvement of a greater proportion of the visual pathway or other CNS structures. However, one must note that MRI progression does not necessarily correlate with visual function deterioration and thus may not imply treatment initiation [70]. Yet, tumor growth definitely warrants increased surveillance of visual function and nonvisual morbidity given the potential risk of tumor infiltration to other intracranial structures. Therefore, apart from substantial radiological progression, the most frequent indication for treatment includes the presence of concomitant progressive visual loss (e.g., change of visual acuity of $\geq$0.2 logMar or new visual field deficit) or early visual compromise after almost complete visual loss in the contralateral eye [63]. Precocious puberty or neurohormonal changes are not indications for treatment initiation targeting at OGs.

Surgical resection or debulking is generally reserved for patients with severe visual loss and cosmetically unacceptable proptosis [71, 72]. Some have previously proposed resection of ONGs with close proximity to the optic chiasm with the intent to prevent chiasmal extension and contralateral involvement. However, it is important to note that tumor cells are often present beyond the apparent radiological limit in the MRI [73]. For patients undergoing debulking surgery, it is important to spare the orbital sensory nerve during the procedure to reduce the future risk of neurotrophic keratopathy. In selected cases, optic nerve sheath fenestration can be used to release trapped CSF or loose tumors during decompression [74, 75]. For ONG with a large orbital component resulting in severe visual loss, significant axial proptosis, and disfigurement, limited orbital debulking surgery via lateral orbitotomy has been proposed to improve cosmesis while minimizing the risk of other cranial nerve damage as compared to the transcranial approach [76]. In patients with OCGs, complete resection is almost impossible without sacrificing all vision or damaging the hypothalamus or surrounding structures. Partial excision or ultrasonic aspiration of the large exophytic component may occasionally be performed for temporary visual stabilization [77].

Radiotherapy can be considered in patients after puberty or in those above age of 5 as an alternative or adjunctive therapy [78]. To reduce adverse effects from conventional external beam radiotherapy, most radiation therapy performed nowadays acquire stereotactic fractionated techniques using photons as there is no long-term data on the use of proton beam therapy. Gamma knife radiosurgery has been reported in treating gliomas of the optic pathway and hypothalamus as well [79]. Although earlier studies had demonstrated the efficacy of radiotherapy in tumor shrinkage and stabilization of vision [80], long-term outcomes with newer techniques are still pending while some have reported a similar overall course as surgery or observation [29]. It is important to recognize potential radiation-related side effects in children including endocrinologic disturbances, vascular changes (e.g., moyamoya-like), behavioral problems, neurocognitive deficits, and secondary malignancies [81, 82]. Therefore, in current practice it is usually reserved for older patients or as a last resort in refractory cases.

Chemotherapy is considered the predominant treatment modality for OGs particularly in children below 5 years of age. Common choices of agents include vincristine, carboplatin, vinblastine, and temozolomide. The most common first-line combination of vincristine and carboplatin is generally well tolerated although 40% of patients may experience hypersensitivity to carboplatin. In a large cohort, secondary malignancies or treatment-related mortality had not been observed [83, 84]. In more recent years, monotherapies with vinblastine [85, 86], vinorelbine [87], or temozolomide [88] have been reported for progressive disease with positive results and low toxicity. Another chemotherapeutic regimen consisting of thioguanine, procarbazine, lomustine, and vincristine had also been reported [89]. However, this regimen should be used with caution given its associated risk of secondary leukemia [90]. As NF-1 patients are predisposed to leukemia, these agents may be useful for those with sporadic OG but should be avoided in NF-1 [91–93]. Chemotherapeutic agents (such as dabrafenib) that target MAP and extracellular signal-related kinase (ERK) pathways may have an edge in those with tandem duplication at the BRAF locus. In a prospective study looking at visual outcomes after chemotherapy for pediatric optic glioma in the UK, Falzon et al. have shown that better initial visual acuity, older age, absence of post-chiasmal tumor, and presence of NF-1 were associated with improved or stable vision after chemotherapy [94].

In general, children with NF-1-associated ONG had good long-term visual, anatomical, and overall outcome. Rarely do these patients die or develop neurological morbidity as a result of the tumor [29, 95]. In a study with a follow-up duration of 10 years or more, moderate to severe visual impairment was noted in approximately one third of the patients while good initial visual acuity while normal optic disc appearance at presentation may predict the final outcome.

Nevertheless, refractory cases still exist, and one tenth of these patients have severe visual loss bilaterally [96]. And in patients with untreated OCGs, despite an overall stable disease course, a substantial proportion did experience neurological/visual morbidity and mortality from the tumor [97]. It is also important to bear in mind that malignant transformation with or without metastasis of a previously benign lesion may develop in rare patients [98, 99]. Young age and hypothalamic involvement have been proposed to be worse prognostic indicators irrespective of association with NF1 [100–102]. Molecular-targeted therapy has therefore become an option for patients with progressive or refractory disease despite chemotherapy [103].

As OGs are often highly vascular with abnormally expressed vascular endothelial growth factor (VEGF), anti-VEGF monoclonal antibodies may be a viable option as an anti-angiogenic agent to control tumor growth [104]. Bevacizumab has shown some degree of efficacy in visual preservation in refractory cases as monotherapy or in combination with other traditional agents [105–108]. In cases of recurrence, retreatment with bevacizumab has also been shown to achieve good response [109]. Side effects of bevacizumab include fatigue, joint pain, hypertension, bleeding events, and proteinuria but are typically reversible [110]. A case series by Falsini et al. has also demonstrated the use of nerve growth factors to halt tumor growth resulting in VEPs improvement [111]. As activation of the mammalian target of the rapamycin (mTOR) pathway is being observed in low-grade gliomas in NF-1, a variety of mTOR inhibitors have been studied for their potential use in this group of patients. Phase 2 trials of mTOR inhibitors such as oral everolimus have yielded promising results in disease stabilization with well-tolerated toxicity profiles [112, 113].

Besides, a variety of MEK inhibitors (such as selumetinib, refametinib, trametinib, and cobimetinib) have demonstrated its ability in tumor shrinkage for children with NF-1 [114, 115]. Tandem duplication at the BRAF locus has been found in over 60% of optic glioma patients without NF-1. The BRAF gene normally produces a protein in the Ras/MAP kinase pathway, and increased BRAF will result in the activation of MEK and ERK proteins downstream and lead to the development of pilocytic astrocytoma [116, 117]. More recently, selumetinib which is a MEK inhibitor has obtained FDA approval for use in children with NF1 aged 2–18 who have inoperable plexiform neurofibromas [118]. Concerning treatment side effects, adverse ocular effects have been observed in adults and children upon the use of MEK inhibitors including retinal vein occlusion, uveitis, neurosensory retinal detachment, and MEK inhibitor-associated retinopathy [119–121]. However, as compared to adults, the toxicity is much less common and reversible for children [122].

Being the first drug specifically approved for NF-1 patients, this exciting breakthrough definitely shed light and opened new opportunities. With the development of biomarkers for vision, we expect more therapeutic options to emerge and become potential therapies for the future management of OG in NF-1 patients [123, 124]. And as we gain more knowledge on the molecular genetic makeup in OG, it is hopeful that gene therapy may as well be used in the future to prevent the development or growth of this tumor.

9.2.2 Malignant Optic Glioma

It is a rare and aggressive tumor which is classified as WHO grade III (anaplastic astrocytoma) or WHO grade IV (glioblastoma, gliosarcoma). In contrast to low-grade gliomas, they typically affect older adults ranging between 22 and 83 years old [1, 21, 125]. Its presentation depends on the site of the origin. For proximal tumors originating from the ONs, patients usually present with a rapidly progressive monocular visual loss with retrobulbar pain simulating acute optic neuritis. The red flags include rapid development of ischemic vascular occlusion, neovascular glaucoma, and bilateral involvement within 5–6 weeks. Tumors originating closer to the chiasm usually present with bilateral simultaneous visual loss and normal appearing or pale optic discs. Of the 77 cases of high-grade optic nerve glioblastoma reported in the literature, 1 had subretinal involvement while 1 described intravitreal seeding [126, 127]. MRI appearance is nonspecific and sometimes reveals a diffusely thickened nerve with heterogeneous enhancement [125, 128–130]. The biopsy will show characteristic histopathological features including infiltration to adjacent brain tissues, cellular pleomorphism, nuclear hyperchromatism, and scattered mitosis [131]. Despite treatment, it carries significant morbidity and death within 1–2 years of diagnosis [126, 127].

9.2.3 Ganglioglioma

This rare tumor comprises of both ganglion cells and astrocytes separated by connective tissue and had been reported to arise in the optic nerve [1, 21, 132–135]. Unlike OGs, they typically do not enhance on MRI after gadolinium injection and often require a biopsy to diagnose. There is minimal evidence on the use of chemotherapy in the treatment of this tumor in the literature, and most evidence is largely based on treatment of intracranial gangliogliomas which include surgical resection with or without adjuvant radiation [132].

9.2.4 Medulloepithelioma

Optic nerve medulloepithelioma has a similar clinical and radiological presentation to ONG, and the diagnosis is often made at the time of surgery with histological findings. Standard treatment is resection of the affected optic nerve with adjuvant radiotherapy, chemotherapy, or both to reduce the risk of recurrence or metastasis [21].

9.2.5 Hemangioblastoma

Optic nerve hemangioblastoma is a rare tumor which is sometimes considered a misnomer as they rarely infiltrate or metastasize [21]. Although it can occur sporadically, it is more commonly seen in patients with von Hippel-Lindau disease (VHL). In a recent review involving 35 reported cases, 71% had a diagnosis of VHL, and 5 of these cases had ON lesions being their first clinical presentation of the disease. Diagnosed at a mean age of 37 years, most lesions remain asymptomatic until adulthood, and the majority (73%) of these tumors were located in the intraorbital portion of the optic nerve. Although they have a similar clinical presentation as OGs, MRI with contrast can help differentiate it upon revealing flow voids, an absence of dural attachment as well as homogenous contrast enhancement. Histologically, they are well-circumscribed vascular lesions composed of stromal cells and vascular endothelial cells. Depending on the extent of intracranial involvement, surgical excision with preservation of the globe is well described via orbital, transsphenoidal, or transcranial approach. Given the indolent growing nature and the risks associated with surgical excision, a stepwise conservative approach is often adopted in the absence of severe symptoms. Surgery is usually indicated when there is rapid visual loss, pain, or unacceptable proptosis [136].

9.2.6 Oligodendroglioma

Constituting 4–12% of all intracranial tumors, this tumor mostly occurs in the cerebral hemisphere especially the frontal lobes and very rarely in the optic nerves [137]. There were only a handful of case reports [138, 139], and whether optic nerve oligodendrogliomas truly exist is unclear.

9.3 Mimickers of Primary Optic Nerve Tumors

9.3.1 Germ Cell Tumors

Intracranial germ cell tumor (GCT) is a rare type of tumor, and the majority are found in the suprasellar or pineal region. Primary, non-exophytic, isolated optic chiasm germ cell tumor is very rare with only a handful of case reports over the past decades [140–143]. The mean age of patients with ON involvement in these reports is 15.8 (range: 9–31), and all were male. Apart from progressive visual impairment, these patients usually suffered from coexisting endocrine abnormalities despite a negative neuroimaging finding on the hypothalamus. Neuroimaging typically shows a diffusely enhancing infiltrative lesion with the expansion of the affected nerve [140, 142, 143]. Given its juvenile onset, it may pose diagnostic challenges clinically and radiologically making it sometimes difficult to distinguish from ONGs with chiasmal involvement. However, histological dissection will demonstrate that this type of GCT is in fact sellar in origin with infiltration into the ON. A surgical exploration or biopsy in a suspicious case is therefore sometimes unavoidable as GCT has a very distinct treatment protocol from ONG.

9.4 Primary Optic Nerve Sheath Tumors

9.4.1 Optic Nerve Sheath Meningioma (ONSM)

In contrast to orbital tumors which are adherent to the ONS, primary ONSM arises from the cap cells of the arachnoid villi surrounding the intra-orbital or intracranial portion of the ON in the orbit. Secondary orbital meningiomas are caused by intraorbital extension of adjacent meningioma and usually arise from the sphenoidal ridge, anterior clinoid process, tuberculum sellar, and olfactory groove which subsequently extend through the superior orbital fissure, optic canal, or bones. Extending along the ONS, both types can involve the orbital, canalicular, and intracranial portions of the ON. In a review involving 5000 orbital meningiomas, 90% was found to be secondary with 10% being primary ONSM. Among those primary ONSM, 92% originates within the orbit, and the remaining arise from the optic canal [144]. All ONSM, primary and secondary, account for 2% of all orbital tumors [144–148].

Schick has proposed a classification of ONSM into three types. Type I refers to ONSM limited to the orbital portion with characteristic fusiform, tubular or globular appearance. Type II ONSM extends through optic canal or supraorbital fissure with or without extension to the cavernous sinus while type III involves more than 1 cm intracranial extension to the optic chiasm or across the planum sphenoidale to the contralateral ON [147].

Most primary ONSMs (95%) are unilateral with a slight predilection for the right ON [148]. Theoretically, it is possible to have contralateral spread but has not been reported. For bilateral ONSMs, they are either secondary in nature or are likely associated with NF-2 which is usually present in the first decade of life. In an epidemiological study of pediatric ONSM, almost one-third are diagnosed with NF-2 [149]. Therefore, for primary ONSM in children, one should also look for multifocal ONSM, aneurysms, or other intracranial diseases [150–153].

Primary ONSM can occur at any age, but similar to meningioma elsewhere in the CNS, they are most commonly found in middle-aged women with a peak incidence between 45 and 55 years old [144, 150]. An accelerated growth of meningioma has been reported during pregnancy, and some have postulated the effect of hormonal and hemodynamic changes during pregnancy as well as the presence of estrogen and progesterone receptors frequently expressed in meningioma cells [154–156].

Despite the benign and slow-growing nature, ONSM can cause progressive compression to pial vasculature leading to optic neuropathy and irreversible visual loss. Clinical presentation is similar to ONG with ON dysfunction where patients present with progressive painless visual loss or various types of visual field defects [150, 157]. Some experience transient visual obscuration secondary to ON ischemia upon compression at eccentric gaze which is normally termed as gaze-evoked amaurosis [158].

Depending on the location of the tumor and chronicity, optic disc morphology can be normal, swollen, or pale [144–146]. Unlike other inflammatory or demyelinating causes, the disc swelling may persist beyond 3 months. Of note, chronic disc edema may be associated with posteriorly located ONSMs causing dilatation of the perioptic subarachnoid space anteriorly where clinicians should think about possible ONSM upon persistent unilateral disc swelling [159]. About one-third of ONSM will develop an optociliary shunt at the optic nerve head which is a retinal-choroidal vessel that shunts venous blood from the retina due to compression of the central retinal vein. Though not pathognomonic, ONSM should be suspected in patients presenting with concomitant progressive visual loss [160–162].

The degree of proptosis depends on the volume of the lesion and its morphology. Fusiform and the rare globular type tend to have moderate proptosis while the tubular type may have no or minimal proptosis. Limitation of ocular motility has been reported, and it is more commonly associated with mechanical restriction from stiffened ONS rather than cranial nerve palsy [162]. Sporadically, patients with ONSM complain of orbital pain or headache resulting from apical meningiomas and associated sensory nerve compression [163]. ONSM can occasionally present atypically with acute visual loss upon tumor bleeding, thus masquerading as other diagnoses [164, 165].

These atypical features can impose diagnostic challenges, and misdiagnosis of ONSMs is not uncommon in real-life practice [165–169]. In a recent retrospective review by Kahraman-Koytak et al., 71.4% of ONSMs were misdiagnosed or had delayed diagnosis with the most frequent misdiagnosis being optic neuritis. They reported that the causes for misdiagnosis were clinician assessment failures in the presence of other ocular diseases and misinterpretation by radiologists due to the lack of training or errors in imaging orders [168].

CT scanning typically showed fusiform or tubular enlargement of the affected ON with thickened sheath which enhances. On axial sections and after intravenous contrast, 26% will yield a "tram-track" sign which is characterized by hyperdense enhanced meninges encasing the hypodense optic nerve [170]. Some cases will have partially calcified meninges creating this tram track appearance on pre-contrast soft tissue and bone-windowed CT as well [171]. Interestingly, noncalcified tumors have been shown to grow in volume and length up to six times more than calcified ones in volumetric studies [150].

MRI is currently the preferred imaging modality for the diagnosis of ONSM. In T1-weighted sequence with fat suppression and the use of gadolinium contrast, it is capable of revealing the hypointense ON which is in fact normal in diameter where the ONS is thickened and markedly enhanced which contributes to the overall enlarged ON (Fig. 9.3). On T2-weighted scans, ONSMs are hyperintense when compared to the brain or ON. And as opposed to the smooth dural outline in ONG, ONSM commonly shows small, thin extensions from the affected sheath into the orbit. The coronal cut will show concentric thickening of ON and "doughnut sign" (Fig. 9.4).

The diagnosis of ONSM can often be reached with the combination of clinical setting, history, examination findings, and imaging characteristics, rendering the need for a biopsy. As meningioma cells can express somatostatin receptor subtype 2, ONSM demonstrates high gallium-68-labeled dodecanetetraacetic acid-tyrosine-3-octreotate (^{68}Ga-DATATATE) uptake which is somatostatin receptor ligand, on positron emission tomography (PET)/CT scan [172, 173]. This characteristic and imaging modality is useful in assisting diagnosis in case of doubt. With the advent of modern neuroimaging while biopsy carries a risk of visual impairment, histological diagnosis is only indicated if there is atypical feature or upon aggressive disease course.

Histopathologically, ONSMs have similar histologic features to intracranial ones. The most frequently encountered subtype is the transitional type (50%) which is characterized by concentric whorls of spindle cells with interspersed hyalinized calcium deposits known as psammoma bodies. Sheets of polygonal cells separated by vascular trabeculae can be observed in meningothelial-type (19%) while the rest (31%) is mixed type [171, 174, 175]. According to WHO and based on their histologic and immunohistochemical characteristics, they can be further classified into benign (Grade I), anaplastic (Grade II), and malignant (Grade III).

The major morbidity of an ONSM is loss of vision in the affected eye. Therefore, similar to ONG, the management of ONSM must be tailored to individual patients, and treatment

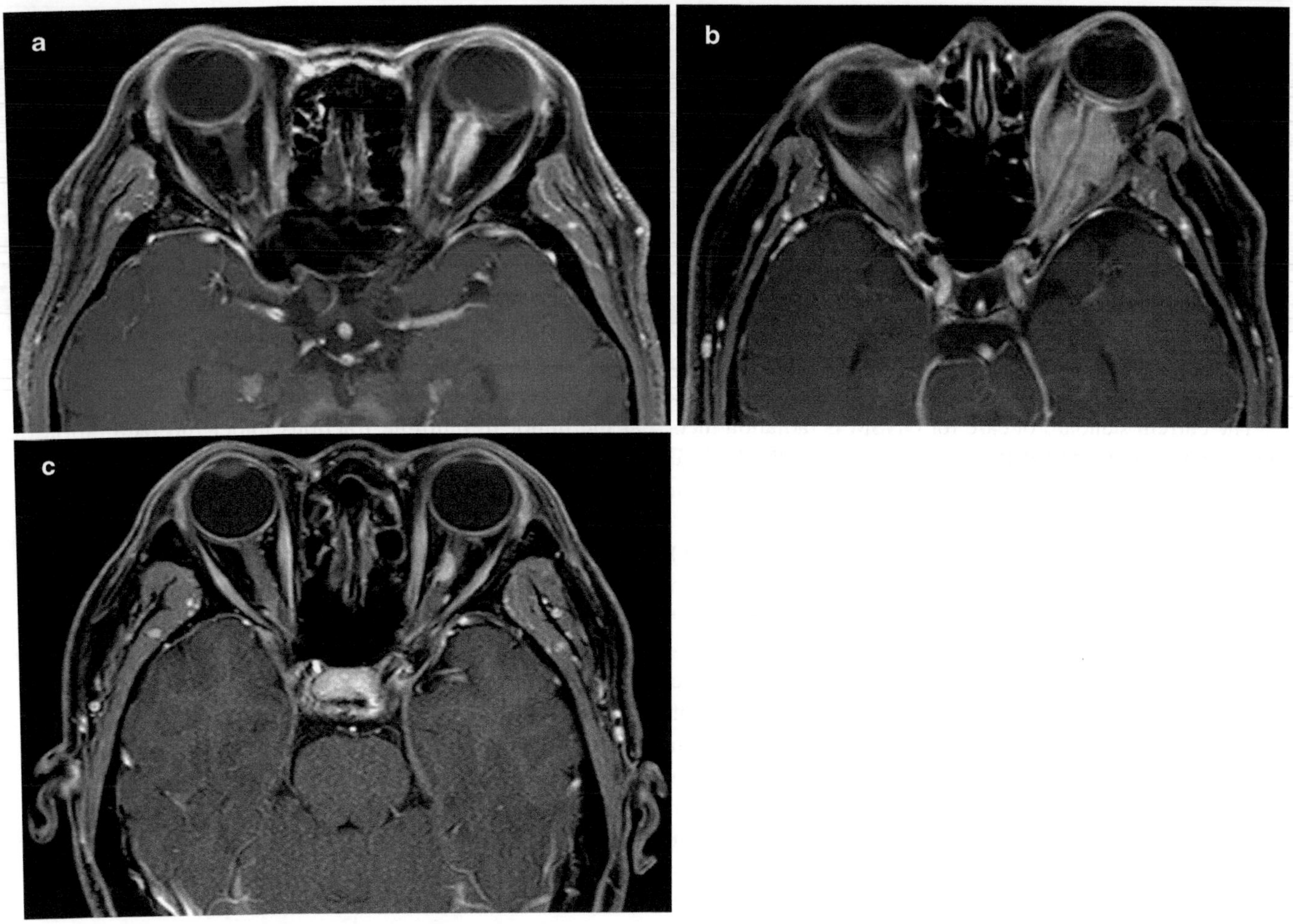

Fig. 9.3 MRI T1-weighted sequence with fat suppression and use of gadolinium contrast showing different morphologies of ONSMs: tubular form (**a**), fusiform form (**b**), focal (**c**). The hypointense ONs can be seen with normal diameter while the ONSMs show marked enhancement. In **b**, there is marked proptosis secondary to the fusiform tumor. (*Image Courtesy of Dr. Carmen Chan*)

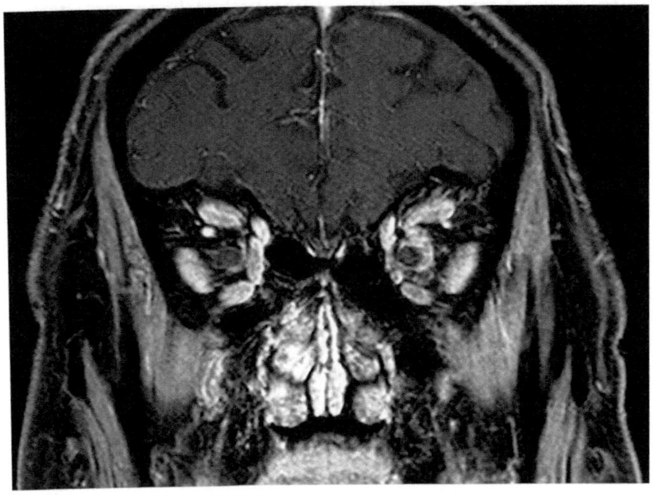

Fig. 9.4 The coronal cut of MRI showing "doughnut sign" in ONSM of the left orbit

options include conservative observation, radiation therapy, or rarely surgery along with radiation. Although ONSMs commonly show high estrogen or progesterone receptor expression, medical treatment like estrogen or progesterone antagonist (such as tamoxifen or mifepristone) had not been proven effective in the control of ONSMs [156].

As primary ONSM is not life-threatening and rarely extends intracranially to compromise the contralateral optic nerve, treatment is not required if there is no significant visual dysfunction, no clinical progression, or no intracranial extension. Given a high functional vision and variable progression, robust surveillance with clinical examination every 3–6 months and neuroimaging every 6–12 months should be arranged for this group.

With close proximity between most primary ONSM and the ON as well as its blood supply, surgical excision usually results in loss of vision in the affected eye. As a historical treatment of choice, 94% experienced visual drop postoperatively with 78% ending up with no light perception [144]. Therefore, surgical resection is only reserved for aggressive tumors with intracranial extension to prevent spread to contralateral ON or for cosmesis in a severely proptotic blind eye. Partial debulking can be considered in ONSMs which are primarily extradural where some of the tumor is left behind in the subdural or subarachnoid space surrounding the nerve. In cases presenting with acute visual loss, some recommend optic nerve decompression via opening up the ONS [150, 171]. This procedure should be followed by definitive radiation therapy to prevent the subsequent spread of the tumor throughout the orbit.

The current standard of care for ONSM is radiation therapy which is indicated if there is progressive ON damage where some have proposed a cutoff of VA of <20/40 or upon marked visual field constriction.

Conventional external beam radiotherapy (EBRT) involves high-energy radiation with linear accelerator to directly irradiate the tumor enclosing all extensions with liberal margins in a square radiation field including normal tissues in the treated area. It has been widely performed in the past, and it usually consists of 5000 cGy given in doses of 180–200 cGy daily fractions. The threshold for radiation damage to ON has been estimated to be 80–100 cGy for a single dose [176]. The advantage is the high availability by almost any radiation center, and it has been shown to result in a good long-term visual outcome as compared to observation, surgery or surgery, and radiotherapy [177]. However, it is no longer widely performed nowadays as the radiation damage to adjacent normal tissue can result in potentially serious complications including radiation-induced retinopathy, vascular occlusion, persistent uveitis, pituitary insufficiency, temporal lobe atrophy, and radiation-induced tumor.

3D conformal radiotherapy (3D-CRT) is the next advancement to EBRT which uses multiple radiation beams and beam-forming technology software to map the target tissue. This enables more precise delivery of radiation conforming to the target tissue volume. However, late radiation toxicities and ocular complications were still significantly observed and are therefore not recommended.

Intensity-modulated radiotherapy (IMRT) is the next evolution of 3D-CRT that further modifies the dose distribution within the target volume with an increased number of beam directions. Radiation beams are divided into grid-like patterns separating each big beam into numerous smaller beamlets. This allows radiation delivery of varying intensities, and special software is used to determine the optimal amount of radiation to the tumor itself while conforming more precisely to the shape of the tumor, sparing normal tissues. This technique is more time and labor-intensive during treatment planning. To ensure precise alignment of the target tissue, reacquisition of images at the time of therapy is also required for image-guided therapy. With promising results in treating ONSM, it has been shown to preserve or improve visual function. In particular, significant visual improvements have been demonstrated with early IMRT before the appearance of optic disc abnormalities and especially in patients with fusiform and globular growth [178, 179].

Stereotactic fractionated radiotherapy (SFRT) is one of the most widely reported radiation techniques for the treatment of ONSM. Also requiring complex planning, SFRT involves a large dose of radiation delivered to a single point where all the beams converge with high precision targeting at the tumor in multiple fractions under the facilitation of head immobilization, sophisticated software, and three-dimensional imaging. The usual treatment dosage for ONSM is 50–54 Gy in 180 cGy daily fractions, and literature has shown excellent short-term and long-term prognosis [180–188]. In general, visual improvement begins within 3 months after treatment. As we summarize the results from the published series to date, 86–100% of patients reported improvement or stability of their visual function. Although some tumors, particularly fusiform or globular ones, demonstrate a reduction in tumor volume after SFRT, the majority show no change in tumor size on posttreatment imaging. Current evidence has proved SFRT to be an effective treatment for primary ONSM with 90–100% radiological control [189].

Acute treatment side effects of SFRT include headache, nausea, local erythema, focal alopecia, endocrinological disturbance, and trigeminal nerve hypoaesthesia, but they tend to be mild or transient. In rare occasions, there can be transient optic neuritis which responds dramatically to systemic steroid. Despite the high degree of radiation conformity to the tumor, radiation toxicity has been reported in SFRT. A study has demonstrated that ONSM closest to the posterior pole of the eye needed a higher median total dose or radiation and was associated with higher complication rates [190].

Radiation-induced retinopathy (RR) can occur following a treatment dose of at least 50 Gy with a latency period of 6 months to 4 years. Visual comorbidity from RR can range from asymptomatic to loss of vision and ONSM involving the proximal part of the optic nerve adjacent to the globe are at greater risk of developing RR [191]. Therefore, this potential complication should be thoroughly discussed upon treating such patients. Although radiation optic neuropathy may occur especially in a radiation dose up to 54 Gy, it has rarely been reported, and it might be difficult to distinguish from visual deterioration secondary to tumor progression. Some other long-term ocular complications include dry eyes, cataract formation, and uveitis. Systemically, long-term side effects of SFRT include pituitary dysfunction and punctate white matter lesions in the cerebral hemisphere presumably from radiation effect on cerebral blood flow. Interval monitoring of pituitary hormonal function is mandated especially for those with posteriorly located ONSM after SFRT.

In a recent meta-analysis by Pintea et al. evaluating functional outcomes in patients with ONSM treated with SFRT, over 50% of cases had improvement of ophthalmic status with low morbidity and excellent control. They identified favorable prognostic factors being better pre-treatment visual acuity, shorter follow-up duration, and lower retinal dose. The authors advocated using SFRT as early as possible before vision deterioration occurs [192]. With improved imaging techniques and the latest long-term results from SFRT, the choice between observation and radiation therapy has become more difficult in patients with presumed ONSM and mild visual loss.

The value of robotic radiosurgery (RRS) for treating ONSM is still under evaluation [193]. Gamma knife radiosurgery is now rarely used in ONSM as the fixed frame required the dose to be applied in a single fraction which can easily exceed the dose tolerance of the visual pathway and result in visual morbidity [194, 195]. CyberKnife offers frameless irradiation and allows the dose to be divided into multiple fractions, thus referred to as hypofractionated radiosurgery. It consists of a 4- or 5-consecutive day regimen delivering a total dose of 200–250 cGy (50 cGy per session) to the tumor. As compared to SFRT, RRS can achieve tighter dose distribution and improved dose conformality with submillimeter accuracy. So theoretically it can reduce dose leaking over the retina or nearby structures, hence minimizing long-term radiation-induced toxicity [196]. Studies have also shown the effectiveness of this modality in tumor control in selected cases [197–200]. In the series of Marchetti et al., visual function was stabilized in 65% and improved in 35% of patients while no radiation-induced toxicity was observed in the mean follow-up duration of 30 months [200]. However, RRS for ONSM has only been performed in a few specialized institutions given its substantial technical requirements. Further studies, preferably multicenter are required to evaluate its long-term efficacy and safety [197–200].

Proton beam therapy (PBT) is a more confined way of radiation delivery with proton release within the tumor region resulting in a minimal dose beyond the tumor boundary. Theoretically it is less likely to produce damage to surrounding normal tissue because of the Bragg peak for protons as compared with photons. Moyal et al. reported the use of PBT as primary or adjunctive therapy in treating ONSM with 14 (out of 15 patients) attaining visual stability or improvement [201]. Despite encouraging preliminary data, there are only limited literature and small case series evaluating the efficacy of PBT in treating ONSM. As of today, the standard of care for patients with ONSM requiring treatment remained to be SFRT.

9.4.2 Optic Nerve Meningeal Hemangiopericytoma

Meningeal hemangiopericytoma is a rare tumor of mesenchymal origin which is believed to arise from the pericytes of the capillaries [202]. It accounts for less than 1% of all CNS tumors [203] but constitutes 2.7% of all primary orbital tumors [203–205]. Very rarely, it can arise from the optic nerve meninges and may clinically simulate ONSM [206–208]. This tumor is however notorious for its aggressive clinical course, infiltration, local recurrence, and distant metastasis [202, 203, 209]. Its terminology and classification had attracted discussion in the past decades, but advances in tissue diagnosis and immunohistochemical studies have separated its entity from meningioma [210]. Classical hemangiopericytomas are highly cellular with scanty intervening collagen and thin-walled branching vessels arranged in a stag-horn pattern. In contrast to the strong and diffused CD34-expression (80–100%) in solitary fibrous tumors, hemangiopericytoma has focal or absent CD34 reactivity (33%). Fibrous meningioma has positive expression of EMA (80%) and S-100 protein (80%) while these are negative for hemangiopericytoma [211, 212] The recommended treatment for hemangiopericytoma is complete excision with adjuvant radiotherapy and/or chemotherapy [213].

9.5 Conclusion

Among the diverse primary optic nerve neoplasms, OG and ONSM are the most commonly encountered of which diagnosis can often be made clinically and radiologically. However, a biopsy is warranted in the presence of atypical features or a rapidly progressive course. OG can usually be monitored while the mainstay of treatment for progressive OG is chemotherapy. Symptomatic ONSM on the other hand can be treated with SFRT. For refractory diseases or other optic nerve neoplasms, modalities of treatment will include radiation, surgical resection, or immunomodulatory therapies. The time window for treatment initiation will be affected by the evolving new treatment modalities and advances in radiation therapies.Conflict of InterestThe author has nothing to disclose.

References

1. Dutton JJ. Gliomas of the anterior visual pathway. Surv Ophthalmol. 1994;38:427–52.
2. Miller NR. Optic gliomas: past, present, future. J Neuroophthalmol. 2016;36:460–73.
3. Louis DN, Perry A, Reifenberger G, et al. The 2016 World Health Organization classification of tumors of the central nervous system: a summary. Acta Neuropathol. 2016;131:803–20.
4. Parsa CF, Givrad S. Juvenile pilocytic astrocytomas do not undergo spontaneous malignant transformation: grounds for designation as hamartomas. Br J Ophthalmol. 2008;92:40–6.
5. Parsa CF. Why optic gliomas should be called harmatomas. Ophthal Plast Reconstr Surg. 2010;26(6):497.
6. Cutarelli PE, Roessmann UR, Miller RH, et al. Immunohistochemical properties of human optic nerve glioma. Invest Ophthalmol Vis Sci. 1991;32:2521–4.
7. Miller NR. Optic pathway gliomas are tumors! Ophthal Plast Reconstr Surg. 2008;24:433.
8. Liu GT, Katowitz JA, Rorke-Adams LB, Fisher MJ. Optic pathway gliomas neoplasms, not hamartomas. JAMA Ophthalmol. 2013;131:646–50.
9. Bowers DC, Gargan L, Kapur P, et al. Study of the MIB-1 labeling index as a predictor of tumor progression in pilocytic astrocytomas in children and adolescents. J Clin Oncol. 2003;21:2968–73.
10. Nair AG, Pathak RS, Iyer VR, Gandhi RA. Optic nerve glioma: an update. Int Ophthalmol. 2014;34:999–1005.
11. Rush JA, Younge BR, Campbell RJ, et al. Optic glioma: long-term follow-up of 85 histologically verified cases. Ophthalmology. 1982;89:1213–9.
12. Binning MJ, Liu JK, Kestle JR, Brockmeyer DL, Walker ML. Optic pathway gliomas: a review. Neurosurg Focus. 2007;23:1–8.
13. Miller NR, Iliff WJ, Green WR. Evaluation and management of gliomas of the anterior visual pathways. Brain. 1974;97:743–54.
14. Rodriguez FJ, Lim KS, Bowers D, Eberhart CG. Pathological and molecular advances in pediatric low-grade astrocytoma. Annu Rev Pathol. 2013;8:361–79.
15. Houshmandi SS, Gutmann DH. All in the family: using inherited cancer syndromes to understand deregulated cell signaling in brain tumors. J Cell Biochem. 2007;102:811–9.
16. Warrington NM, Gianino SM, Jackson E, Goldhoff P, Garbow JR, Piwnica-Worms D, Gutmann DH, Rubin JB. Cyclic AMP suppression is sufficient to induce gliomagenesis in a mouse model of neurofibromatosis-1. Cancer Res. 2011;70:5717–27.
17. Helfferich J, Nijmeijer R, Brouwer OF, et al. Neurofibromatosis type 1 associated low grade gliomas: a comparison with sporadic low grade gliomas. Crit Rev Oncol Hematol. 2016;104:30–41.
18. Lewis RA, Gerson LP, Axelson KA, Riccardi VM, Whitford RP. Von Recklinghausen neurofibromatosis: II. Incidence of optic gliomata. Ophthalmology. 1984;91:929–35.
19. Dossetor FM, Landau K, Hoyt WF. Optic disk glioma in neurofibromatosis type 2. Am J Ophthalmol. 1989;108(5):602–3.
20. Di Mario FJ, Ramsby G, Greenstein R. Neurofibromatosis type I: resonance imaging findings. J Child Neurol. 1993;8:32–9.
21. Miller NR. Primary tumours of the optic nerve and its sheath. Eye. 2004;18:1026–37.
22. Prada CE, Hufnagel RB, Hummel TR, Lovell AM, Hopkin RJ, Saal HM, Schorry EK. The use of magnetic resonance imaging screening for optic pathway gliomas in children with neurofibromatosis type 1. J Pediatr. 2015;167:851–6.
23. Balcer LJ, Liu GT, Heller G, et al. Visual loss in children with neurofibromatosis type 1 and optic pathway gliomas: relation to tumor location by magnetic resonance imaging. Am J Ophthalmol. 2001;131:442–5.
24. Thiagalingam S, Flaherty M, Billson F, North K. Neurofibromatosis type 1 and optic pathway gliomas: follow-up of 54 patients. Ophthalmology. 2004;111:568–77.
25. Czyzyk E, Jozwiak S, Roszkowski M, Schwartz RA. Optic pathway gliomas in children with and without neurofibromatosis 1. J Child Neurol. 2003;18:471–8.
26. Chutorian AM, Schwartz JF, Evans RA, Carter S. Optic gliomas in children. Neurology. 1964;14:83–95.
27. Sharma A, Mohan K, Saini JS. Haemorrhagic changes in pilocytic astrocytoma of the optic nerve. Orbit. 1990;9:29–33.
28. Kozak I, Elkhamary SM, Bosley TM. Central retinal vein occlusion in a childhood optic nerve tumour. Neuroophthalmology. 2016;40:35–9.
29. Tow SL, Chandela S, Miller NR, et al. Long-term prognosis in children with gliomas of the anterior visual pathway. Pediatr Neurol. 2003;28:262–70.
30. Roh S, Mawn LA, Hedges TR. Juvenile pilocytic astrocytoma masquerading as amblyopia. Am J Ophthalmol. 1997;123:692–4.
31. Maitland CG, Abiko S, Hoyt WF, Wilson CB, Okamura T. Chiasmal apoplexy: report of four cases. J Neurosurg. 1982;56:118–22.
32. Hill JD, Rhee MS, Edwards JR, Hagen MC, Fulkerson DH. Spontaneous intraventricular hemorrhage from low-grade optic glioma: case report and review of the literature. Childs Nerv Syst. 2012;28:327–30.
33. Toledano H, Muhsinoglu O, Luckman J, Goldenberg-Cohen N, Michowiz S. Acquired nystagmus as the initial presenting sign of chiasmal glioma in young children. Eur J Paediatr Neurol. 2015;19(6):694–700.
34. Estrada M, Kelly JP, Wright J, Phillips JO, Weiss A. Visual function, brain imaging, and physiological factors in children with asymmetric nystagmus due to chiasmal gliomas. Pediatr Neurol. 2019;97:30–7.
35. Schulman JA, Shults WT, Jones JM Jr. Monocular vertical nystagmus as an initial sign of chiasmal glioma. Am J Ophthalmol. 1979;87(1):87–90.
36. Lavery MA, O'Neill JF, Chu FC, Martyn LJ. Acquired nystagmus in early childhood: a presenting sign of intracranial tumor. Ophthalmology. 1984;91(5):425–53.
37. Brodsky MC, Keating GE. Chiasmal glioma in spasmus nutans: a cautionary note. J Neuroophthalmol. 2014;34:274–5.
38. Campagna M, Opocher E, Viscardi E, Calderone M, Severino SM, Cermakova I, Perilongo G. Optic pathway glioma: long term visual outcome in children without neurofibromatosis type-1. Pediatr Blood Cancer. 2010;55:1083–8.
39. Kelly JP, Weiss AH. Detection of tumor progression in optic pathway glioma with and without neurofibromatosis type 1. Neuro Oncol. 2013;15:1560–7.
40. Avery RA, Liu GT, Fisher MJ, Quinn GE, Belasco JB, Phillips PC, Maguire MG, Balcer LJ. Retinal nerve fiber layer thickness in children with optic pathway gliomas. Am J Ophthalmol. 2011;151:542–9.
41. Gu S, Glaug N, Cnaan A, Packer RJ, Avery RA. Ganglion cell layer-inner plexiform layer thickness and vision loss in young children with optic pathway gliomas. Invest Ophthalmol Vis Sci. 2014;55:1402–8.
42. North K, Cochineas C, Tang E, Fagan E. Optic gliomas in neurofibromatosis type 1: role of visual evoked potentials. Pediatr Neurol. 1994;10(2):117–23.
43. Ng YT, North KN. Visual-evoked potentials in the assessment of optic gliomas. Pediatr Neurol. 2001;24(1):44–8.
44. Spicer GJ, Kazim M, Glass LR, et al. Accuracy of MRI in defining tumor-free margin in optic nerve glioma surgery. Ophthal Plast Reconstr Surg. 2013;29:277–80.

45. Stern J, Jakobiec FA, Housepian EM. The architecture of optic nerve gliomas with and without neurofibromatosis. Arch Ophthalmol. 1980;98:505–11.
46. Yeung SN, Heran MK, Smith A, White VA, Rootman J. Perineural gliomatosis associated with isolated optic nerve gliomas. Br J Ophthalmol. 2009;93:839–41.
47. Brodsky MC. The "pseudo-CSF" signal of orbital optic glioma on magnetic resonance imaging: a signature of neurofibromatosis. Surv Ophthalmol. 1993;38:213–8.
48. Imes RK, Hoyt WF. Magnetic resonance imaging signs of optic nerve gliomas in neurofibromatosis 1. Am J Ophthalmol. 1991;111:729–34.
49. Levin MH, Armstrong GT, Broad JH, et al. Risk of optic pathway glioma in children with neurofibromatosis type 1 and optic nerve tortuosity or nerve sheath thickening. Br J Ophthalmol. 2016;100:510–4.
50. Ge M, Li S, Wang L, et al. The role of diffusion tensor tractography in the surgical treatment of pediatric optic chiasmatic gliomas. J Neurooncol. 2015;122:357–66.
51. Revere KE, Katowitz WR, Katowitz JA, et al. Childhood optic nerve glioma: vision loss due to biopsy. Ophthal Plast Reconstr Surg. 2017;33:S107–9.
52. Zimmerman LE. Arachnoid hyperplasia in optic nerve glioma. Br J Ophthalmol. 1980;64:638–9.
53. Cooling RJ, Wright JE. Arachnoid hyperplasia in optic nerve glioma: confusion with orbital meningioma. Br J Ophthalmol. 1979;63:596–9.
54. Listernick R, Ferner RE, Liu GT, Gutmann DH. Optic pathway gliomas in neurofibromatosis-1: controversies and recommendations. Ann Neurol. 2007;61:189–98.
55. Kelly JP, Weiss AH. Comparison of pattern visual-evoked potentials to perimetry in the detection of visual loss in children with optic pathway gliomas. J AAPOS. 2006;10:298–306.
56. Chang BC, Mirabella G, Yagev R, et al. Screening and diagnosis of optic pathway gliomas in children with neurofibromatosis type 1 by using sweep visual evoked potentials. Invest Ophthalmol Vis Sci. 2007;48:2895–902.
57. Avery RA, Cnaan A, Schuman JS, et al. Longitudinal change of circumpapillary retinal nerve fiber layer thickness in children with optic pathway gliomas. Am J Ophthalmol. 2015;160:944–952.e941.
58. Fard MA, Fakhree S, Eshraghi B. Correlation of optical coherence tomography parameters with clinical and radiological progression in patients with symptomatic optic pathway gliomas. Graefes Arch Clin Exp Ophthalmol. 2013;251:2429–36.
59. Avery RA, Cnaan A, Schuman JS, Chen CL, Glaug NC, Packer RJ, Quinn GE, Ishikawa H. Reproducibility of circumpapillary retinal nerve fiber layer measurements using handheld optical coherence tomography in sedated children. Am J Ophthalmol. 2014;158:780–787.e1.
60. Listernick R, Louis DN, Packer RJ, Gutmann DH. Optic pathway gliomas in children with neurofibromatosis 1: consensus statement from the NF1 Optic Pathway Glioma Task Force. Ann Neurol. 1997;41:143–9.
61. Blanchard G, Lafforgue MP, Lion-Francois L, et al. Systematic MRI in NF1 children under six years of age for the diagnosis of optic pathway gliomas. Study and outcome of a French cohort. Eur J Paediatr Neurol. 2016;20:275–81.
62. Havidich JE, Beach M, Dierdorf SF, et al. Preterm versus term children: analysis of sedation/anesthesia adverse events and longitudinal risk. Pediatrics. 2016;137:e20150463.
63. de Blank PMK, Fisher MJ, Liu GT, et al. Optic pathway gliomas in neurofibromatosis type 1: an update: surveillance, treatment indications, and biomarkers of vision. J Neuroophthalmol. 2017;37(Suppl 1):S23–32.
64. Fisher MJ, Loguidice M, Gutmann DH, et al. Visual outcomes in children with neurofibromatosis type 1-associated optic pathway glioma following chemotherapy: a multicenter retrospective analysis. Neuro Oncol. 2012;14:790–7.
65. Parsa CF, Hoyt WF, Lesser RL, et al. Spontaneous regression of optic gliomas. Thirteen cases documented by serial neuroimaging. Arch Ophthalmol. 2001;119:516–29.
66. Liu GT, Lessell S. Spontaneous visual improvement in chiasmal gliomas. Am J Ophthalmol. 1992;114:193–201.
67. Perilongo G, Moras P, Carollo C, Battistella A, Clementi M, Laverda A, Murgia A. Spontaneous partial regression of low-grade glioma in children with neurofibromatosis-1: a real possibility. J Child Neurol. 1999;14:352–6.
68. Piccirilli M, Lenzi J, Delfinis C, Trasimeni G, Salvati M, Raco A. Spontaneous regression of optic pathways gliomas in three patients with neurofibromatosis type I and critical review of the literature. Childs Nerv Syst. 2006;22:1332–7.
69. Gayre GS, Scott IU, Feuer W, et al. Long-term visual outcome in patients with anterior visual pathway glioma. J Neuroophthalmol. 2001;21:1–7.
70. Aquilina K, Daniels DJ, Spoudeas H, et al. Optic pathway glioma in children: does visual deficit correlate with radiology in focal exophytic lesions? Childs Nerv Syst. 2015;31:2041–9.
71. Wolter JR. Large optic nerve glioma removed by the transconjunctival approach. J Pediatr Ophthalmol. 1973;10:142–6.
72. Althekair FY. Debulking optic nerve gliomas for disfiguring proptosis: a globe-sparing approach by lateral orbitotomy alone. Presented as a poster at the 42nd Annual Meeting of the North American Neuro-Ophthalmology Society, Tucson, AZ, February 28, 2016.
73. Spicer GJ, Kazim M, Glass LR, Harris GJ, Miller NR, Rootman J, Sullivan TJ. Accuracy of MRI in defining tumor-free margin in optic nerve glioma surgery. Ophthal Plast Reconstr Surg. 2013;29:277–80.
74. Vanderveen DK, Nihalani BR, Barron P, Anderson RL. Optic nerve sheath fenestration for an isolated optic nerve glioma. J AAPOS. 2009;13:88–90.
75. Chen A, Yoon MK, Haugh S, et al. Surgical management of an optic nerve glioma with perineural arachnoidal gliomatosis growth pattern. J Neuroophthalmol. 2013;33:51–3.
76. Farazdaghi MK, Katowitz WR, Avery RA. Current treatment of optic nerve gliomas. Curr Opin Ophthalmol. 2019;30:356–63.
77. Goodden J, Pizer B, Pettorini B, Williams D, Blair J, Didi M, Thorp N, Mallucci C. The role of surgery in optic pathway/hypothalamic gliomas in children. J Neurosurg Pediatr. 2014;13:1–12.
78. Marwaha G, Macklis R, Singh AD. Radiation therapy: orbital tumors. Dev Ophthalmol. 2013;52:94–101.
79. El-Shehaby AM, Reda WA, Abdel Karim KM, et al. Single-session Gamma Knife radiosurgery for optic pathway/hypothalamic gliomas. J Neurosurg. 2016;125(Suppl 1):50–7.
80. Taveras JM, Mount LA, Wood EH. The value of radiation therapy in the management of glioma of the optic nerves and chiasm. Radiology. 1956;66:518–28.
81. Pierce SM, Barnes PD, Loeffler JS, et al. Definitive radiation therapy in the management of symptomatic patients with optic glioma. Survival and long term effects. Cancer. 1990;65:45–52.
82. Grill J, Couanet D, Cappelli C, et al. Radiation-induced cerebral vasculopathy in children with neurofibromatosis and optic pathway glioma. Ann Neurol. 1999;45:393–6.
83. Lafay-Cousin L, Sung L, Carret AS, et al. Carboplatin hypersensitivity reaction in pediatric patients with low-grade glioma: a Canadian Pediatric Brain Tumor Consortium experience. Cancer. 2008;112:892–9.

84. Yu DY, Dahl GV, Shames RS, Fisher PG. Weekly dosing of carboplatin increases risk of allergy in children. J Pediatr Hematol Oncol. 2001;23:349–52.
85. Bouffet E, Jakacki R, Goldman S, et al. Phase II study of weekly vinblastine in recurrent or refractory pediatric low-grade glioma. J Clin Oncol. 2012;30:1358–63.
86. Lassaletta A, Scheinemann K, Zelcer SM, et al. Phase II weekly vinblastine for chemotherapy-naive children with progressive low-grade glioma: a Canadian Pediatric Brain Tumor Consortium Study. J Clin Oncol. 2016;34:3537–43.
87. Cappellano AM, Petrilli AS, da Silva NS, et al. Single agent vinorelbine in pediatric patients with progressive optic pathway glioma. J Neurooncol. 2015;121:405–12.
88. Gururangan S, Fisher MJ, Allen JC, et al. Temozolomide in children with progressive low-grade glioma. Neuro Oncol. 2007;9:161–8.
89. Ater J, Holmes E, Zhou T, et al. Abstracts from the thirteenth international symposium on pediatric neuro-oncology: results of COG protocol A9952-a randomized phase 3 study of two chemotherapy regimens for incompletely resected low-grade glioma in young children. Neuro Oncol. 2008;10:451–2.
90. Leone G, Mele L, Pulsoni A, et al. The incidence of secondary leukemias. Haematologica. 1999;84:937–45.
91. Maris JM, Wiersma SR, Mahgoub N, et al. Monosomy 7 myelodysplastic syndrome and other second malignant neoplasms in children with neurofibromatosis type 1. Cancer. 1997;79: 1438–46.
92. Stiller CA, Chessells JM, Fitchett M. Neurofibromatosis and childhood leukaemia/lymphoma: a population-based UKCCSG study. Br J Cancer. 1994;70:969–72.
93. Shannon KM, O'Connell P, Martin GA, et al. Loss of the normal NF1 allele from the bone marrow of children with type 1 neurofibromatosis and malignant myeloid disorders. N Engl J Med. 1994;330:597–601.
94. Falzon K, Drimtzias E, Picton S, Simmons I. Visual outcomes after chemotherapy for optic pathway glioma in children with and without neurofibromatosis type 1: results of the International Society of Paediatric Oncology (SIOP) Low-Grade Glioma 2004 trial UK cohort. Br J Ophthalmol. 2018;102(10):1367–71.
95. Hamideh D, Hoehn ME, Harreld J, Klimo PD, Gajjar Am Qaddoumi I. Isolated optic nerve glioma in children with and without neurogibromatosis: retrospective characterization and analysis of outcomes. J Child Neurol. 2018;33(6):375–82.
96. Kinori M, Armarnik S, Listernick R, Charrow J, Zeid JL. Neurofibromatosis type 1-associated optic pathway glioma in children: a follow-up of 10 years or more. Am J Ophthalmol. 2021;221:91–6.
97. Imes RK, Hoyt WF. Childhood chiasmal gliomas: update on the fate of patients in the 1969 San Francisco Study. Br J Ophthalmol. 1986;70:179–82.
98. Wilson WB, Feinsod M, Hoyt WF, Nielsen SL. Malignant evolution of childhood chiasmal pilocytic astrocytoma. Neurology. 1976;26:322–5.
99. Nishio S, Takeshita I, Fukui M, Yamashita M, Tateishi J. Anaplastic evolution of childhood optico-hypothalamic pilocytic astrocytoma: report of an autopsy case. Clin Neuropathol. 1988;7: 254–8.
100. Dodgshun AJ, Elder JE, Hansford JR, Sullivan MJ. Long-term visual outcome after chemotherapy for optic pathway glioma in children: site and age are strongly predictive. Cancer. 2015;121:4190–6.
101. Gan HW, Phipps K, Aquilina K, Gaze MN, Hayward R, Spoudeas HA. Neuroendocrine morbidity after pediatric opticgli omas: a longitudinal analysis of 166 children over 20 years. J Clin Endocrinol Metab. 2015;100:3787–99.
102. El Beltagy MA, Reda M, Enayet A, Zaghloul MS, Awad M, Zekri W, Taha H, El-Khateeb N. Treatment and outcome in 65 children with optic pathway gliomas. World Neurosurg. 2016;89:525–34.
103. Packer RJ, Vezina G. New treatment modalities in NF-related neuroglial tumors. Childs Nerv Syst. 2020;36:2377–84.
104. Machein M, Plate K, Machein M, Plate K. VEGF in brain tumors. J Neurooncol. 2000;50:109–20.
105. Avery RA, Hwang EI, Jakacki RI, Packer RJ. Marked Recovery of vision in children with optic pathway gliomas treated with bevacizumab. Arch Ophthalmol JAMA Ophthalmol. 2014;132(1):111–4.
106. Gorsi HS, Khanna PC, Tumblin M, et al. Single-agent bevacizumab in the treatment of recurrent or refractory pediatric low-grade glioma: a single institutional experience. Pediatr Blood Cancer. 2018;65:e27234.
107. Gururangan S, Fangusaro J, Poussaint TY, et al. Efficacy of bevacizumab plus irinotecan in children with recurrent low-grade gliomas – a pediatric brain tumor consortium study. Neuro Oncol. 2014;16:310–7.
108. Zhukova N, Rajagopal R, Lam A, et al. Use of bevacizumab as a single agent or in adjunct with traditional chemotherapy regimens in children with unresectable or progressive low-grade glioma. Cancer Med. 2019;8:40–50.
109. Kalra M, Heath JA, Kellie SJ, et al. Confirmation of bevacizumab activity, and maintenance of efficacy in retreatment after subsequent relapse, in pediatric low-grade glioma. J Pediatr Hematol Oncol. 2015;37:e341–6.
110. Hwang EI, Jakacki RI, Fisher MJ, et al. Long-term efficacy and toxicity of bevacizumab-based therapy in children with recurrent low-grade gliomas. Pediatr Blood Cancer. 2013;60:776–82.
111. Falsini B, Chiaretti A, Barone G, et al. Total nerve growth factor as a visual rescue strategy in pediatric optic gliomas: a pilot study including electrophysiology. Neurorehabil Neural Repair. 2011;25:512–20.
112. Ullrich NJ, Prabhu SP, Reddy AT, et al. A phase II study of continuous oral mTOR inhibitor everolimus for recurrent, radiographic-progressive neurofibromatosis type 1-associated pediatric low-grade glioma: a Neurofibromatosis Clinical Trials Consortium study. Neuro Oncol. 2020;22(10):1527–35.
113. Wright KD, Yao X, London WB, et al. A POETIC Phase II study of continuous oral everolimus in recurrent, radiographically progressive pediatric low-grade glioma. Pediatr Blood Cancer. 2021;68(2):e28787.
114. Banerjee A, Jackacki R, Onar A, et al. A phase I trial of the MEK inhibitor selumetinib (AZD6244) in pediatric patients with recurrent or refractory low-grade glioma: a Pediatric Brain Tumor (PBTC) Study. Neuro Oncol. 2017;19(8):1135–44.
115. Fangusaro J, Onar-Thomas A, Young Poussaint T, et al. Selumetinib in paediatric patients with BRAF-aberrant or neurofibromatosis type 1-associated recurrent, refractory, or progressive low-grade glioma: a multicenter, phase 2 trial. Lancet Oncol. 2019;20(7):1011–22.
116. Pfister S, Janzarik WG, Remke M, et al. BRAF gene duplication constitutes a mechanism of MAPK pathway activation in low-grade astrocytomas. J Clin Invest. 2008;118:1739–49.
117. Rodriguez FJ, Ligon AH, Horkayne-Szakaly I, Rushing EJ, Ligon KL, Vena N, Garcia DI, Cameron JD, Eberhart CG. BRAF duplications and MAPK pathway activation are frequent in gliomas of the optic nerve proper. J Neuropathol Exp Neurol. 2012;71: 789–94.
118. Gross AM, Wolters PL, Dombi E, Baldwin A, Whitcomb P, Fisher MJ, et al. Selumetinib in children with inoperable plexiform neurofibromas. N Engl J Med. 2020;382(15):1430–42.
119. McCannel TA, Chmielowski B, Finn RS, et al. Bilateral subfoveal neurosensory retinal detachment associated with MEK inhibitor use for metastatic cancer. JAMA Ophthalmol. 2014;132:1005–9.

120. Nolan DP, Lewis S, Hariprasad SM. Retinal toxicity associated with MEK inhibitor use for metastatic cancer: a rising trend in ophthalmology. Ophthalmic Surg Lasers Imaging Retina. 2016;47:398–402.
121. Mendez-Martinez S, Calvo P, Ruiz-Moreno O, et al. Ocular adverse events associated with MEK inhibitors. Retina. 2019; https://doi.org/10.1097/IAE.0000000000002451.
122. Avery RA, Trimboli-Heidler C, Kilburn LB. Separation of outer retinal layers secondary to selumetinib. J AAPOS. 2016;20:268–71.
123. Brosseau J-P, Liao C-P, Le LQ. Translating current basic research into future therapies for neurofibromatosis type 1. Br J Cancer. 2020;123(2):178–86.
124. Galvin R, Watson AL, Largaespada DA, Ratner N, Osum S, Moertel CL. Neurofibromatosis in the era of precision medicine: development of MEK inhibitors and recent successes with selumetinib. Curr Oncol Rep. 2021;23(4):45.
125. Spoor TC, Kennerdell JS, Martinez Z, et al. Malignant gliomas of the optic nerve pathways. Am J Ophthalmol. 1980;89:284–92.
126. Traber GL, Pangalu A, Neumann M, Costa J, Weller M, HunaBaron R, Landau K. Malignant optic glioma—the spectrum of disease in a case series. Graefes Arch Clin Exp Ophthalmol. 2015;253:1187–94.
127. Cimino PJ, Sychev Y, Gonzalez-Cuyar LF, et al. Primary gliosarcoma of the optic nerve: a unique adult optic pathway glioma. Ophthal Plast Reconstr Surg. 2017;33:e88–92.
128. Brodovsky S, ten Hove MW, Pinkerton RM, et al. An enhancing optic nerve lesion: malignant glioma of adulthood. Can J Ophthalmol. 1997;32:409–13.
129. Taphoorn MJB, de Vries-Knoppert WAEJ, Ponssen H, et al. Malignant optic glioma in adults. Case report. J Neurosurg. 1989;70:277–9.
130. Woiciechowsky C, Vogel S, Meyer R, Lehmann R. Magnetic resonance imaging of a glioblastoma of the optic chiasm. J Neurosurg. 1995;83:923–5.
131. Nagaishi M, Sugiura Y, Takano I, et al. Clinicopathological and molecular features of malignant pathway glioma in an adult. J Clin Neurosci. 2015;22:207–9.
132. Rolston JD, Han SJ, Cotter JA, et al. Gangliogliomas of the optic pathway. J Clin Neurosci. 2014;21:2244–9.
133. Gritzman MCD, Snyckers FD, Proctor NS. Ganglioglioma of the optic nerve. A case report. S Afr Med J. 1983;63:863–5.
134. Bergin DJ, Johnson TE, Spencer WH, et al. Ganglioglioma of the optic nerve. Am J Ophthalmol. 1988;105:146–9.
135. Sadun F, Hinton DR, Sadun AA. Rapid growth of an optic nerve ganglioglioma in a patient with neurofibromatosis 1. Ophthalmology. 1996;103:794–9.
136. McGrath LA, Mudhar HS, Salvi SM. Hemangioblastoma of the optic nerve. Surv Ophthalmol. 2019;64:175–84.
137. McLendon RE, Kros JM, Bruner J, et al. Oligodendrogliomas. In: McLendon RE, Rosenblum MK, Bigner DD, editors. Russell and Rubinstein's pathology of tumors of the nervous system. 7th ed. London: Hodder Arnold; 2006. p. 167–86.
138. Lucarini C, Tomei G, Gaini SM, et al. A case of optic nerve oligodendroglioma associated with an orbital non-Hodgkin's lymphoma in adult. Case report. J Neurosurg Sci. 1990;34:319–21.
139. Offret H, Gregoire-Cassoux N, Frau E, et al. Solitary oligodendroglioma of the optic nerve. Apropos of a case. J Fr Ophtalmol. 1995;18:158–63.
140. DiLuna ML, Two AM, Levy GH, et al. Primary, non-exophitic, optic nerve germ cell tumors. J Neurooncol. 2009;95:437–43.
141. Wilson JT, Wald SL, Aitken PA, Mastromateo J, Vieco PT. Primary diffuse chiasmatic germinomas: differentiation from optic chiasm gliomas. Pediatr Neurosurg. 1995;23:1–5.
142. Iizuka H, Nojima T, Kadoya S. Germinoma of the optic nerve: case report. Noshuyo Byori. 1996;13:95–8.
143. Nadkarni TD, Fattepurkar SC, Desai KI, Goel A. Intracranial optic nerve germinoma. J Clin Neurosci. 2004;11:559–61.
144. Dutton JJ. Optic nerve sheath meningiomas. Surv Ophthalmol. 1992;37:167–83.
145. Miller NR. New concepts in the diagnosis and management of optic nerve sheath meningioma. J Neuroophthalmol. 2006;26:200–8.
146. Shapey J, Sabin HI, Danesh-Meyer HV, et al. Diagnosis and management of optic nerve sheath meningiomas. J Clin Neurosci. 2013;20:1045–56.
147. Schick U, Dott U, Hassler W. Surgical management of meningiomas involving the optic nerve sheath. J Neurosurg. 2004;101:951–9.
148. Ortiz O, Schochet SS, Kotzan JM, Kostick D. Radiologic-pathologic correlation meningioma of the optic nerve sheath. Am J Neuroradiol. 1996;17:901–6.
149. Levin LA, Jakobiec FA. Optic nerve tumors of childhood: a decision-analytical approach to their diagnosis. Int Ophthalmol Clin. 1992;32:223–40.
150. Saeed P, Rootman J, Nugent RA, et al. Optic nerve sheath meningiomas. Ophthalmology. 2003;110:2019–30.
151. Bosch MM, Wichmann WW, Boltshauser E, et al. Optic nerve sheath meningiomas in patients with neurofibromatosis type 2. Arch Ophthalmol. 2006;124:379–85.
152. Germano IM, Edwards MS, Davis RL, Schiffer D. Intracranial meningiomas of the first two decades of life. J Neurosurg. 1994;80:447–53.
153. Douglas KA, Douglas VP, Cestari DM. Neuro-ophthalmic manifestations of the phakomatoses. Curr Opin Ophthalmol. 2019;30:434–42.
154. Luis EA, Scheithauer BW, Yachnis AT, et al. Meningiomas in pregnancy: a clinicopathologic study of 17 cases. Neurosurgery. 2012;71:951–61.
155. Laviv Y, Ohla V, Kasper EM. Unique features of pregnancy-related meningiomas: lessons learned from 148 reported cases and theoretical implications of a prolactin modulated pathogenesis. Neurosurg Rev. 2018;41:95–108.
156. Thom M, Martinian L. Progesterone receptors are expressed with higher frequency by optic nerve sheath meningiomas. Clin Neuropathol. 2002;21:5–8.
157. Sibony PA, Krauss HR, Kennerdell JS, et al. Optic nerves sheath meningiomas: clinical manifestations. Ophthalmology. 1984;91:1313–26.
158. Orcutt JC, Tucker WM, Mills RP, Smith CH. Gaze-evoked amaurosis. Ophthalmology. 1987;94:213–8.
159. Arnold AC, Lee AG. Dilation of the perioptic subarachnoid space anterior to optic nerve sheath meningioma. J Neuroophthalmol. 2021;41(1):e100–2.
160. Hollenhorst RW, Hollenhorst RW, MacCarty CS. Visual prognosis of optic nerve sheath meningiomas producing shunt vessels on the optic disk: the Hoyt–Spencer syndrome. Trans Am Ophthalmol Soc. 1978;75:141–63.
161. Frisen L, Hoyt WF, Tengroth BM. Optociliary veins, disc pallor and visual loss: a triad of signs indicating spheno-orbital meningioma. Acta Ophthalmol. 1973;51(2):241–9.
162. Wilson WB. Meningiomas of the anterior visual system. Surv Ophthalmol. 1981;26:109–27.
163. Swenson SA, Forbes GS, Younge BR, Campbell RJ. Radiologic evaluation of tumors of the optic nerve. Am J Neuroradiol. 1982;3:319–26.
164. Holan C, Homer NA, Epstein A, Durairaj VD. Atypical acute presentation of an optic nerve sheath meningioma. Am J Ophthalmol Case Rep. 2020;20:100951.

165. Alroughani R, Behbehani R. Optic nerve sheath meningioma masquerading as optic neuritis. Case Rep Neurol Med. 2016;2016:5419432.
166. Kalen BD, Hess RA, Abi-Aad KR, et al. Addressing misdiagnosis of optic nerve sheath meningiomas. World Neurosurg. 2020;133:419–20.
167. Mao JF, Xia XB, Tang XB, Zhang XY, Wen D. Analyses on the misdiagnoses of 25 patients with unilateral optic nerve sheath meningioma. Int J Ophthalmol. 2016;9(9):1315–9.
168. Kahraman-Koytak P, Bruce BB, Peragallo JH, et al. Diagnostic errors in initial misdiagnosis of optic nerve sheath meningiomas. JAMA Neurol. 2019;76:326–32.
169. Jackson A, Patankar T, Laitt RD. Intracanalicular optic nerve meningioma: a serious diagnostic pitfall. Am J Neuroradiol. 2003;24:1167–70.
170. Jakobiec FA, Depot MJ, Kennerdell JS, et al. Combined clinical and computed tomographic diagnosis of orbital glioma end meningioma. Ophthalmology. 1984;91:P137–55.
171. Turbin RE, Pokorny K. Diagnosis and treatment of orbital optic nerve sheath meningioma. Cancer Control. 2004;11: 334–41.
172. Klingenstein A, Haug AR, Miller C, Hintschich C. Ga-68-DOTA-TATE PET/CT for discrimination of tumors of the optic pathway. Orbit. 2015;34(1):16–22.
173. Yarmohammadi A, Savino PJ, Koo SJ, Lee RR. Case report 68Ga-DATATATE of optic nerve sheath meningioma. Am J Ophthalmol Case Rep. 2021;22:101048.
174. Jain D, Ebrahimi KB, Miller NR, Eberhart CG. Intraorbital meningiomas a pathologic review using current world health organization criteria. Arch Pathol Lab Med. 2010;134:766–70.
175. Marquardt MD, Zimmerman LE. Histopathology of meningiomas and gliomas of the optic nerve. Hum Pathol. 1982;13:226–35.
176. Parsons JT, Bova FJ, Fitzgerald CR, et al. Radiation optic neuropathy after megavoltage external-beam irradiation: analysis of time-dose factors. Int J Radiat Oncol Biol Phys. 1994;30:755–63.
177. Turbin RE, Thompson CR, Kennerdell JS, et al. A long-term visual outcome comparison in patients with optic nerve sheath meningioma managed with observation, surgery, radiotherapy, or surgery and radiotherapy. Ophthalmology. 2002;109:890–9.
178. Sasano H, Shikishima K, Aoki M, Sakai T, Tsutsumi Y, Nakano T. Efficacy of intensity-modulated radiation therapy for optic nerve sheath meningioma. Graefes Arch Clin Exp Ophthalmol. 2019;257:2297–306.
179. Inoue T, Mimura O, Ikenaga K, et al. The rapid improvement in visual field defect observed with weekly perimetry during intensity-modulated radiotherapy for optic nerve sheath meningioma. Int Cancer Conf J. 2019;8:136–40.
180. Liu JK, Forman S, Hershewe GL, et al. Optic nerve sheath meningiomas: visual improvement after stereotactic radiotherapy. Neurosurgery. 2002;50:950–7.
181. Andrews DW, Faroozan R, Yang BP, et al. Fractionated stereotactic radiotherapy for the treatment of optic nerve sheath meningiomas: preliminary observations of 33 optic nerves in 30 patients with historical comparison to observation with or without prior surgery. Neurosurgery. 2002;51:890–902.
182. Narayan S, Cornblath WT, Sandler HM, et al. Preliminary visual outcomes after three dimensional conformal radiation therapy for optic nerve sheath meningioma. Int J Radiat Oncol Biol Phys. 2003;56:537–43.
183. Baumert BG, Villa S, Studer G, et al. Early improvements in vision after fractionated stereotactic radiotherapy for primary optic nerve sheath meningioma. Radiother Oncol. 2004;72:169–74.
184. Richards JC, Roden D, Harper CS. Management of sight-threatening optic nerve sheath meningioma with fractionated stereotactic radiotherapy. Clin Exp Ophthalmol. 2005;33:137–41.
185. Pitz S, Becker G, Schiefer U, et al. Stereotactic fractionated irradiation of optic nerve sheath meningioma: a new treatment alternative. Br J Ophthalmol. 2002;86:1265–8.
186. Lesser RL, Knisely JP, Wang SL, et al. Long-term response to fractionated radiotherapy of presumed optic nerve sheath meningioma. Br J Ophthalmol. 2010;94:559–63.
187. Metellus P, Kapoor S, Kharkar S, et al. Fractionated conformal radiotherapy of optic nerve sheath meningiomas: long-term outcomes of tumor control and visual function at a single institution. Int J Radiat Oncol Biol Phys. 2011;80:185–92.
188. Pacelli R, Cella L, Conson M, Tranfa F, Strianese D, Liuzzi R, Solla R, Farella A, Salvatore M, Bonavolontà G. Fractionated stereotactic radiation therapy for orbital optic nerve sheath meningioma—a single institution experience and a short review of the literature. J Radiat Res. 2011;52:82–7.
189. Ratnayake G, Oh T, Mehta R, Hardy T, Woodford K, Haward R, et al. Long-term treatment outcomes of patients with primary optic nerve sheath meningioma treated with stereotactic radiotherapy. J Clin Neurosci. 2019;68:162–7.
190. Abouaf L, Girard N, Lefort T, et al. Standard-fractionated radiotherapy for optic nerve sheath meningioma: visual outcome is predicted by mean eye dose. Int J Radiat Oncol Biol Phys. 2012;82:1268–77.
191. Subramanian PS, Bressler NM, Miller NR. Radiation retinopathy after fractionated stereotactic radiotherapy for optic nerve sheath meningioma. Ophthalmology. 2004;111:565–7.
192. Pintea B, Boström A, Katsigiannis S, Gousias K, Pintea R, Baumert B, Boström J. Prognostic factors for functional outcome of patients with optic nerve sheath meningiomas treated with stereotactic radiotherapy-evaluation of own and meta-analysis of published data. Cancers (Basel). 2021;13(3):522.
193. Senger C, Kluge A, Kord M, Zimmermann Z, Conti A, Kufeld M, Kreimeier A, Loebel F, Stromberger C, Budach V, Vajkoczy P, Acker G. Effectiveness and safety of robotic radiosurgery for optic nerve sheath meningiomas: a single institution series. Cancers (Basel). 2021;13(9):2165.
194. Kwon Y, Bae JS, Kim JM, et al. Visual changes after gamma knife surgery for optic nerve tumors. Report of three cases. J Neurosurg. 2005;102(Suppl):43–6.
195. Adeberg S, Welzel T, Rieken S, Debus J, Combs SE. Prior surgical intervention and tumor size impact clinical outcome after precision radiotherapy for the treatment of optic nerve sheath meningiomas (ONSM). Radiat Oncol. 2011;6:117.
196. Romanelli P, Bianchi L, Muacevic A, Beltramo G. Staged image guided robotic radiosurgery for optic nerve sheath meningiomas. Comput Aided Surg. 2011;16:257–66.
197. Metellus P, Kapoor S, Kharkar S, Batra S, Jackson JF, Kleinberg L, Miller NR, Rigamonti D. Fractionated conformal radiotherapy for management of optic nerve sheath meningiomas: long-term outcomes of tumor control and visual function at a single institution. Int J Radiat Oncol. 2011;80:185–92.
198. Klink DF, Miller NR, Williams J. Preservation of residual vision 2 years after stereotactic radiosurgery for a presumed optic nerve sheath meningioma. J Neuroophthalmol. 1998;18:117–20.
199. Romanelli P, Wowra B, Muacevic A. Multisession CyberKnife radiosurgery for optic nerve sheath meningiomas. Neurosurg Focus. 2007;23:E11–6.
200. Marchetti M, Bianchi S, Milanesi I, et al. Multisession radiosurgery for optic nerve sheath meningiomas—an effective option: preliminary results of a single-center experience. Neurosurgery. 2011;69:1116–22.
201. Moyal L, Vignal-Clermont C, Boissonnet H, et al. Results of fractionated targeted proton beam therapy in the treatment of optic nerve sheath meningioma. J Fr Ophtalmol. 2014;37: 288–95.

202. Spitz FR, Bouvet M, Pisters PW, et al. Hemangiopericytoma: a 20-year single-institution experience. Ann Surg Oncol. 1998;5:350–5.
203. Mena H, Ribas JL, Pezeshkpour GH, et al. Hemangiopericytoma of the central nervous system: a review of 94 cases. Hum Pathol. 1991;22:84–91.
204. Enzinger FM, Smith BH. Hemangiopericytoma: an analysis of 106 cases. Hum Pathol. 1976;7:61–82.
205. Fountas KN, Kapsalaki E, Kassam M, et al. Management of intracranial meningeal hemangiopericytomas: outcome and experience. Neurosurg Rev. 2006;29:145–53.
206. Boniuk M, Messmer EP, Font RL. Hemangiopericytoma of the meninges of the optic nerve. A clinicopathologic report including electron microscopic observation. Ophthalmology. 1985;92:1780–7.
207. Schwent BJ, Wojino TH, Grossniklaus HE. Hemangiopericytoma of the optic nerve sheath. Am J Ophthalmol. 2007;143:904–6.
208. Manjandavida PF, Honavar SG, Gowrishankar S, et al. Optic nerve meningeal hemangiopericytoma: a clinicopathologic case report. Surv Ophthalmol. 2013;58:341–7.
209. Galanis E, Buckner JC, Scheithauer BW, et al. Management of recurrent meningeal hemangiopericytoma. Cancer. 1998;82:1915–20.
210. Furusato E, Valenzuela IA, Fanburg-Smith JC, et al. Orbital solitary fibrous tumor: encompassing terminology for hemangiopericytoma, giant cell angiofibroma, and fibrous histiocytoma of the orbit: reappraisal of 41 cases. Hum Pathol. 2011;42:120–8.
211. Kim JH, Jung H, Kim Y. Meningeal hemangiopericytomas: long-term outcome and biological behavior. Surg Neurol. 2003;59:47–54.
212. Perry A, Scheithauer BW, Nascimento AG, et al. The immunophenotypic spectrum of meningeal hemangiopericytoma: a comparison with fibrous meningioma and solitary fibrous tumor of meninges. Am J Surg Pathol. 1997;21:1353–60.
213. Staples JJ, Robinson RA, Wen BC, et al. Hemangiopericytoma—the role of radiotherapy. Int J Radiat Oncol Biol Phys. 1990;19:445–51.

Orbital Apex Vascular Disease

10

Affan Permana Priyambodo
and Zharifah Nafisah Fauziyyah

Nadya Zaragita and Kania Indriani

Abstract

The orbital apex is a complex anatomical region and the narrowest part of the orbit. Critical structures inside are only millimeters apart. Several etiologies can cause clinical manifestation, and one of them is vascular disease. Anatomical knowledge is very important to project the location of the lesion and the structure involved. Even some diseases behind the orbital apex also can cause orbital apex syndrome, constituted by the involvement of the optic nerve, oculomotor nerve, trochlear nerve, abducens nerve, and first division of the trigeminal nerve. Several vascular diseases can happen in the orbital apex including arteriovenous malformations, arteriovenous fistula, ophthalmic artery aneurysm, hemangiopericytoma of the orbit, carotid cavernous fistula, cavernous sinus thrombosis, and carotid cavernous aneurysm.

Keywords

Orbital apex · Vascular disease · AVM · CCF · Aneurysm
Hemangiopericytoma · Cavernous sinus thrombosis

10.1 Introduction

The orbital cavity in humans is pyramid-shaped with the orbital apex directed posteriorly. This is a complex region anatomically with the interactions of bone, vascular, and neural structures [1]. The orbital apex is the narrowest part of the orbit, and critical structures inside are only millimeters apart [2]. Any involvement of various structures in this area will progress to several signs and symptoms called orbital apex syndrome. Several etiologies such as inflammation, infection, trauma, iatrogenic, vascular, endocrine, tumor, and others can lead to these clinical manifestations of orbital apex syndrome [1].

10.2 Orbital Apex Anatomy

The orbital apex bone area is the narrowest part of the orbit (Fig. 10.1). Bones forming this structure are the lesser wing of the sphenoid bone at the roof, the ethmoid sinus at the medial, the greater wing of the sphenoid wings at the lateral, and the orbital palate at the floor. The optic canal (OC) is bordered by sphenoid bone, superior by the lesser wing, inferolateral by the optic strut, and medial by the body. The superior orbital fissure is located inferolateral to the OC, separated by the optic strut and bordered by the lesser wing of the sphenoid superior-medially, by the greater wing of the sphenoid bone laterally, and by the orbital process of the palatine bone inferiorly [2].

A. P. Priyambodo · Z. N. Fauziyyah (✉)
Department of Neurosurgery, Faculty of Medicine, Universitas Indonesia, dr. Cipto Mangunkusumo National General Hospital, Jakarta, Indonesia

T. L. POON et al. (eds.), *Orbital Apex and Periorbital Skull Base Diseases*, https://doi.org/10.1007/978-981-99-2989-4_10

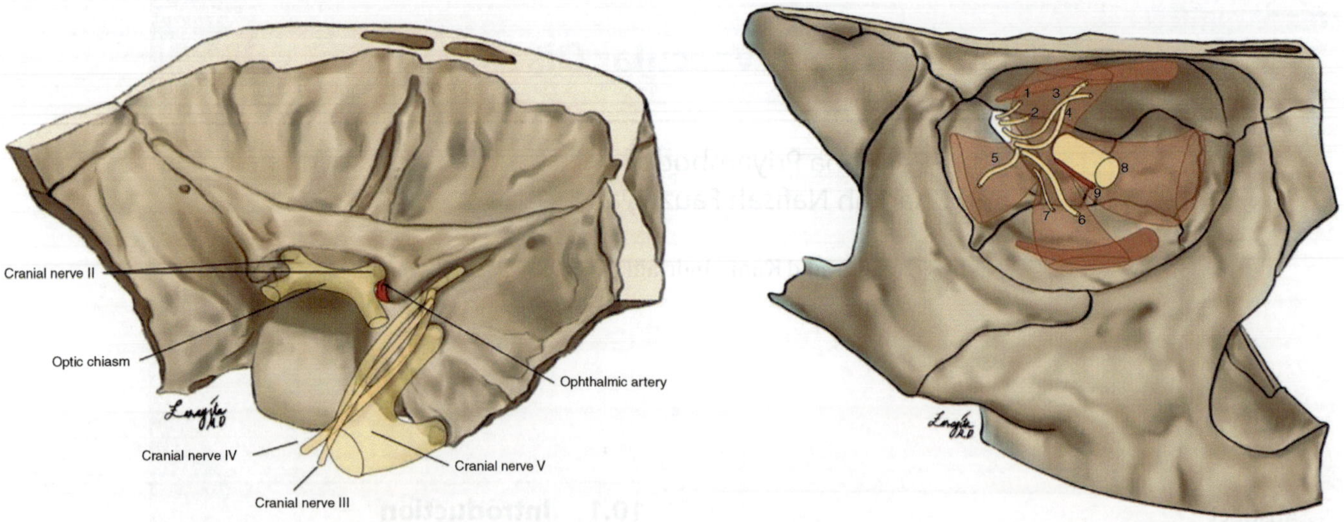

Fig. 10.1 Important anatomy structure of the orbital apex (1) Lacrimal nerve, (2) frontal nerve, (3) trochlear nerve, (4) superior division of oculomotor nerve, (5) abducens nerve, (6) inferior division of oculomotor, (7) nasociliary nerve, (8) optic nerve, (9) ophthalmic artery

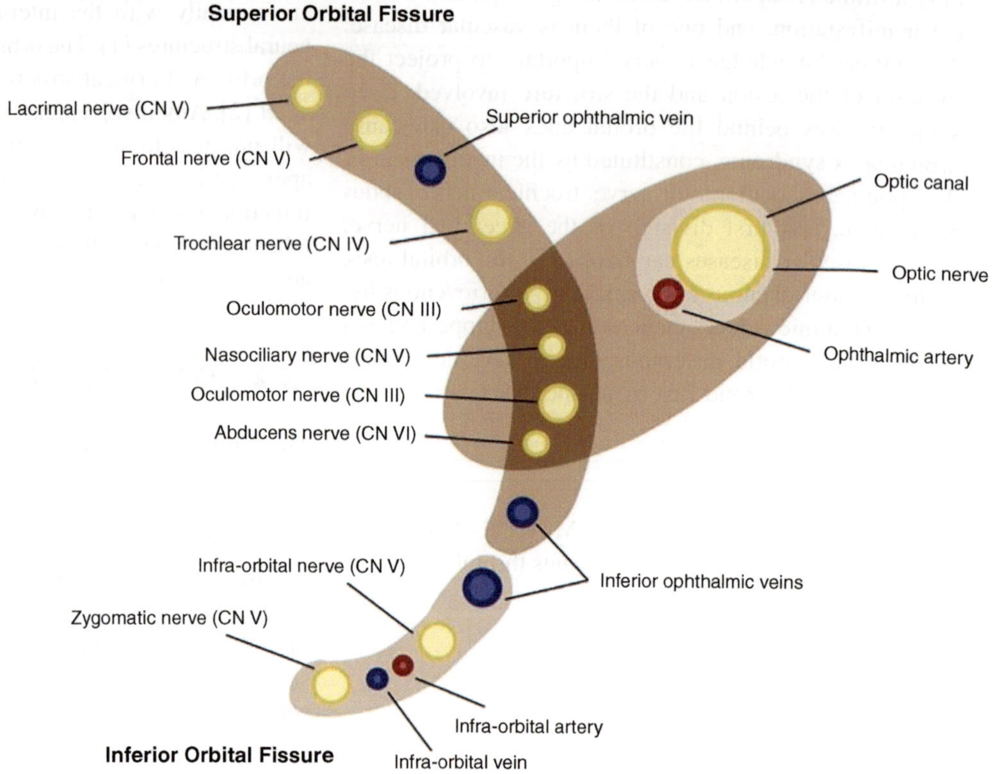

Fig. 10.2 Anatomical structure inside the orbital apex [1]

10.3 Orbital Apex Syndrome

The involvement of disease in the orbital apex region (Fig. 10.2), which results in a set of symptoms and signs, is called orbital apex syndrome. These structures include the rectus muscles (superior, inferior, medial, and lateral), and they originate from the tendinous annulus of Zinn. Ophthalmic artery, and optic nerve pass through the optic canal inside the annulus of Zinn together with the oculomotor nerve, the abducens nerve, and the nasociliary nerve in the middle portion of the superior orbital fissure. This syndrome is constituted by the involvement of the optic nerve (II C.N), oculomotor nerve (III C.N), trochlear nerve (IV C.N), abducens nerve (VI C.N), and the first division of the trigeminal nerve (ophthalmic division of V C.N) [1].

10.3.1 Clinical Features

Several etiologies can affect the orbital apex, and the prominence and severity of clinical symptoms can be variable. The most common clinical feature in the orbital apex is painful vision disturbance and eye movement (ophthalmoplegia). The clinical sign and symptoms can lead to a certain location of the lesion as shown in Table 10.1 [1].

10.3.2 Etiopathogenesis

Several etiologies can cause orbital apex syndrome such as inflammatory, infections, traumatic, iatrogenic, vascular, endocrine, tumors, or other diseases (Table 10.2).

10.4 Orbital Apex Vascular Disease

10.4.1 Ophthalmic Arteriovenous Malformations (AVMs)

Intraorbital AVMs are rare lesions (Fig. 10.3), usually congenital in origin. These lesions are high-flow communications between arteries and veins that enlarge progressively and bypass normal capillary beds. They usually have multiple feeder arteries, a central nidus, and several dilated draining veins. On initial examinations, the appearance can be variable and may rarely show symptoms in childhood. Their growth was stimulated by menarche, pregnancy, and trauma. Common signs and symptoms found were periocular pain, dilated corkscrew vessels on the globe extending to the limbus, proptosis, pulsating lesion, bruit, and raised intraocular pressure [3]. They can also cause visual disturbance, diplopia, discoloration, and episcleral congestion [4]. Orbital AVMs are diagnosed through angiographic findings that showed an engorged, rapidly filling proximal arterial system, a malformation, and a distal venous outflow. Histopathology examination can find irregularity of the muscularis layer thickness in the affected feeder arteries and draining veins and also the presence of a partial elasticity in other vessels [3].

The diagnosis can be also supported by clinical history and noninvasive imaging studies, such as flow Doppler ultrasound, CT angiography, or MR angiography, to highlight the expansion of the lesions. This lesion should be considered as a differential diagnosis of other orbital vascular lesions with similar features such as carotid cavernous fistulas (CCF), dural cavernous sinus fistulas, orbital arteriovenous fistulas (AVFs), and cerebral AVMs with drainage into orbital veins. Orbital AVF is the only possible condition that had the most similar appearance on radiology and angiography examination. However, either traumatic or spontaneous AVF are limited to the orbit, and have no connection to the cavernous sinus. AVFs demonstrate a direct arteriovenous connection without nidus. Management of orbital AVMs should be done with a multidisciplinary approach. The primary treatment is surgical excision with or without prior embolization. Other modalities such as radiotherapy with new techniques that focus on radiation to the lesion (linear accelerator, proton

Table 10.1 Signs and symptoms of the cranial nerve involved in the disease at the orbital apex area [1]

Cranial nerves involved	Sign and symptoms
II C.N	Vision disturbance/loss Pupillary abnormalities (relative afferent pupillary defect—RAPD) Optic disc edema or optic atrophy Choroidal folds
III C.N	Pupillary abnormalitics (anisocoria)
III, IV, VI C.N	Ophthalmoplegia (eye movement)
V_1 C.N	Pain around the orbit or the skin Presence/absence of corneal sensations and corneal reflex

Table 10.2 Etiopathogenesis and disease causing orbital apex syndrome [1]

Etiology	Disease
Inflammatory	Sarcoidosis
	Tolosa-Hunt syndrome
	Systemic lupus erythematosus
	Microscopic polyangiitis
	Granulomatosis with polyangitis
	Churg-Strauss syndrome
	IgG4-related variant form
	Nonspecific orbital inflammation
Infections	Bacterial
	Fungal
	Viral
	Parasitic
Traumatic	Cranial-maxillo-facial injuries
Iatrogenic	Postorbital and sino-nasal surgeries
Vascular (most frequently present as cavernous sinus syndrome)	Cavernous sinus thrombosis
	Carotid cavernous fistula
	Carotid artery aneurysm
Endocrine	Thyroid orbitopathy
Tumors	Head and neck tumors
	Nasopharyngeal carcinoma
	Adenoid cystic carcinoma
	Head and neck tumors with perineural spread
	Metastases (breast, lung, renal carcinoma)
	Hematologic (Burkitt's lymphoma, non-Hodgkin's lymphoma, leukemia)
Others	Neurofibromatosis
	Fibrous dysplasia
	Mucocele

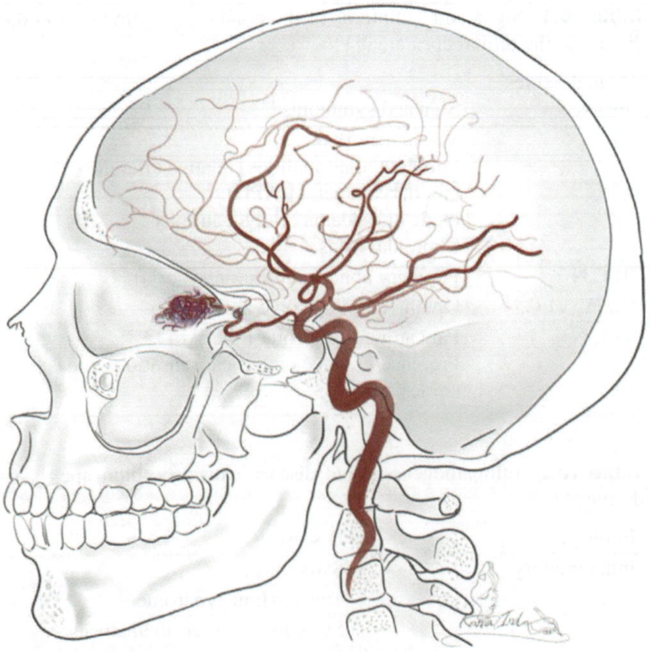

Fig. 10.3 AVM in the orbital apex with a feeding artery from the ophthalmic artery

beam, or Gamma Knife) can also be a choice for AVMs. Radiation will induce thrombosis inside the lumen; however, this method has not been used for orbital lesions. Several studies show that incomplete excision or partial embolization alone will cause recurrences. Intervention should be done immediately when there is visual compromise and persistent or progressive patient discomfort [3]. Other adjunctive therapies that can be given before intervention are sclerotherapy, direct intralesional injections, and laser treatments. Multidisciplinary care involves oculoplastic surgeons and craniofacial plastic surgeons, and neuroradiologist post-resection surgery is also needed [4, 5].

From the case series of Warrier et al. including ten intraorbital AVM cases, 70% were fed by ophthalmic artery, 80% were embolized, and 60% were followed by surgical resection. One patient was treated using Gamma Knife treatment. The outcomes of using a multidisciplinary approach are usually good, with few recurrences reported during follow-up. The main cause of poor management outcomes is perioperative hemorrhage [3].

10.5 Arteriovenous Fistulas (AVFs)

Dural arteriovenous fistulas (dAVFs) are abnormal direct connections between arteries and veins in the dura mater. The most common location of the fistule is with the cavernous sinus, the symptoms were chemosis, diplopia, and ptosis. The prevalence of intraorbital AVF who received DSA suspected of cavernous sinus dAVF is only 1 out of 350 patients [6]. Intraorbital AVFs usually have a direct connection between the superior or inferior ophthalmic vein and intraorbital arteries such as the ophthalmic artery and its branches (Fig. 10.4), such as the central retinal artery. Intraorbital AVFs can cause a severe decrease in visual acuity and visual field defect [7]. Clinical presentation is usually indistinguishable from CCF with predominantly ocular findings. The manifestations are chemosis, a decreased visual acuity, exophthalmos, and extraocular symptoms [8].

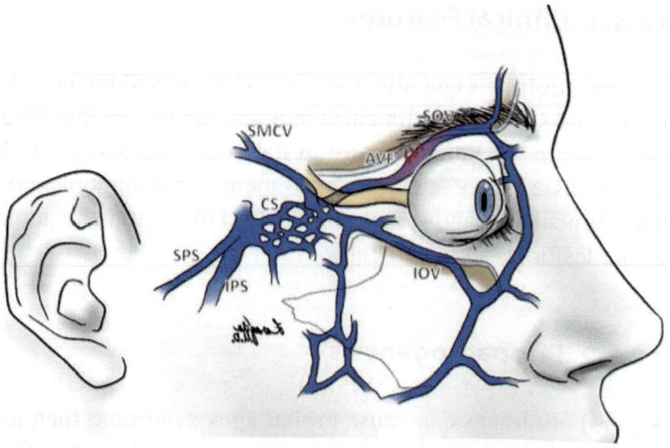

Fig. 10.4 Intraorbital arteriovenous fistula formed from the branches of meningeal arteries

Conservative treatment for intraorbital AVF consists of clinical observation and measurement of ocular pressure. Treatment should be given to patients with progressive symptoms or intractable ocular pressure with medication [8]. Endovascular intervention for dAVFs is usually categorized based on the approach, either transarterial or transvenous embolization. Transarterial embolization could be dangerous since the ophthalmic artery has a potential anastomosis with the anteromedial branch of the inferolateral trunk (ILT) that runs through the superior orbital fissure, especially for embolization using liquid materials. The transarterial embolization from the branches of the meningeal media artery (MMA) also has a high risk of retinal ischemia because of the anastomosis between the MMA branches, recurrent meningeal artery, meningo-lacrimal artery, and lacrimal artery [6]. Direct surgical ligation through the extradural transcranial approach is where the roof of the orbit is opened, the superior rectus muscle is retracted to visualize the superior ophthalmic vein, and then the vein is ligated. Intraoperative angiography is needed to confirm complete obliteration of the fistula after the SOV was ligated [8]. Williamson et al. reported the treatment of intraorbital AVF through retrograde transvenous catheterization and embolization with coils to the fistula through an IPS route [8].

10.6 Intraorbital Ophthalmic Artery Aneurysm

Intraorbital ophthalmic artery (OA) aneurysms are rare; however, this is a serious threatening condition. Internal carotid artery (ICA) branches become OA as they pass from the cavernous sinus and then enter the orbit via the optic canal, forming the intraorbital segment of the OA (Fig. 10.5). It is divided into three sections, in the direction from the orbit, the first run inferolateral to the optic nerve, the second superomedial to the optic nerve, and the third lies medial to the optic nerve [9].

The symptoms caused by an intraorbital OA aneurysm are caused by the mass effect and chronic pulsation. The aneurysm location determines the symptoms. Distal intraorbital OA aneurysms may be asymptomatic, while the proximal aneurysm can cause paresis of the extraocular muscles innervated by the oculomotor and abducens nerve. Ruptured aneurysms will rapid onset proptosis and visual loss due to hemorrhage. The most common presentations include visual loss, exophthalmos, and severe headache [9]. Compared with other sites, large and giant aneurysms are more commonly found in OA aneurysms. Large-sized aneurysms have been reported to cause compression injury [10].

Unruptured OA aneurysms can be treated with three methods: conservative medication, endovascular intervention, or microsurgical clipping. Conservative treatment is only suggested for unruptured ophthalmic artery aneurysms with a low risk of rupture [11]. However, Kumon et al. proposed to treat all unruptured asymptomatic ophthalmic segment aneurysms to prevent the risk of rupture. In contrast, De Jesus et al. suggested only patients with a life expectancy of more than 10 years should be treated and if the aneurysm size was more than 4 mm [12]. Reported treatments for OA aneurysms include occlusion of the OA, clipping of the aneurysm, or aneurysm resection or trapping [9]. Endovascular coiling and surgical clipping are two common forms of treatment for intracranial aneurysms [13]. Microsurgical clipping of OA aneurysms can be done with several risks such as visual loss, intraoperative ruptures, and stroke. A study in the Hospital of Qingdao University, China, showed there were two independent risk factors for poor outcome of surgical clipping of OA aneurysms: age more than 60 (OR 5.877; 95% CI 1.039–33.254, $p = 0.045$) and aneurysm size more than 10 mm (OR 9.417; 95% CI 1.476–60.072, $p = 0.018$). Retracting the optic nerve close to the aneurysm during surgery risks the problem of visual acuity and visual field defect, and retraction can be reduced by cutting the falciform ligament to displace the nerve. Opening the ICA dural ring and drawing the dura mater towards the orbital roof can expose the ICA, OA, and aneurysm neck broadly. Removing the anterior clinoid process can be necessary to expand the exposure of the anterior edge of the aneurysm neck if it cannot be fully separated from the optic nerve [10].

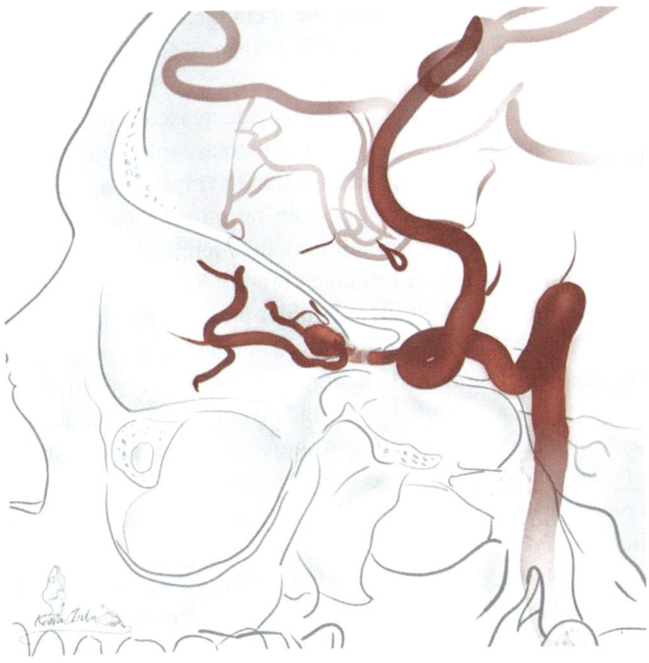

Fig. 10.5 Intraorbital aneurysm of the ophthalmic artery [9]

Endovascular treatment should be chosen for moderate-sized aneurysms. The current choice modalities that have been recently used were coiling and flow diverter [11]. Other options available include sole coils embolization, balloon-assisted coils, stent-assisted coil, or flow diversion. Several factors such as dual antiplatelet therapy during the perioperative period can cause a high risk of bleeding, and other risks such as in-stent thrombosis and stent malposition during stent-assisted coils embolization or flow diversion implant can lead to poor prognosis after the procedure. Balloon-assisted coiling can create significant technical stress for the aneurysm wall and parent vessel. Stents were used for wide-necked or complex aneurysms. The complication of in-stent thrombosis can be caused by antiplatelet drug resistance or a defect on the wall attachment of the stent [12]. Recent evidence shows that flow diverters could achieve better occlusion compared to coiling, fewer neurological complications, and a lower risk of death. The occlusion rate of the flow diverter is up to 64% within 6 months and 94% within 3 years postimplantation compared with coiling. Dual antiplatelet must be administered for a minimum of 6 months after implantation to prevent in-stent thromboembolic events. The flow diverter is recommended for moderate- to large-sized aneurysms in large arteries and can be the best choice for aneurysms in locations presenting serious complications such as blindness [11].

10.7 Hemangiopericytoma of the Orbit

Hemangiopericytoma is a tumor composed of cells that resemble the vascular pericyte, first delineated by Stout and Murray as a distinctive vascular tumor of soft tissue [14, 15]. Hemangiopericytomas are a rare entity that accounts for only 1% of all intracranial tumors. Commonly, HP is acknowledged as a dura-based, subdural tumor originating from Zimmermann's pericytes [16]. Hemangiopericytoma counts for 1–3% of all orbital lesions [17]. Hemangiopericytoma can occur anywhere capillaries are found and is rarely found in orbits [18]. It can resemble other common tumors of the orbit such as lymphangiomas and hemangiomas from clinical or radiological examination, and therapy for these patients is challenging. The distinction must be made between other differential diagnoses such as vascular malformations and hemangiomas [17]. Hemangiopericytomas are usually found in the fourth to fifth decade of life, with 80% diagnosed in the range of 20–70 years old. The etiology is still unknown. However, trauma has been suggested as one possible risk factor, since several reports of orbital hemangiopericytomas have a history of trauma prior to clinical complaints. Clinical signs and symptoms found were proptosis, pain, diplopia, decreased visual acuity, eye swelling, and ecchymosis of the eyelids due to the mass effect. The tumor can be located anywhere around the orbit including intraconal, extraconal, lacrimal gland, lacrimal sac, meninges of the optic nerve, conjunctiva, eyelid, and intraocular, but the most common location is in the superior orbit. The tumor is typically slow-growing and encapsulated, but sometimes we can find pseudocapsules [18]. The orbital margins are usually indistinct, and they appear to invade the surrounding tissue that can be found in CT and MRI. There can be also erosions of adjacent bony structures and contrast enhancement. Angiography will show significant blush in all three phases, without prominent arteriovenous shunting [18].

Hemangiopericytoma considerably compressed the optic nerve. For the tumor, total resection should be achieved to reduce the chance of recurrence, malignant transformation, and the possibility of reoperation [16, 17]. The effectiveness of radiotherapy for hemangiopericytoma is not well determined, and it is usually not administered immediately after resection. Radiotherapy as adjuvant treatment should be carefully determined the time and dose case-by-case according to the tumor location and extent of resection. Stereotactic radiosurgery can be an alternative option for local recurrence; however, it also can cause distant metastases regardless of the histological grades [16]. With incomplete removal, these tumors tend to recur and have a malignant transformation that is more infiltrative and difficult to be removed. Metastasis most commonly occurs to the lung [18].

Hemangiopericytomas are often brittle and tend to cause bleeding [18]. Intraoperative hemorrhage can be massive in these cases; therefore, preoperative embolization was suggested in several reports. The methods of embolization included the use of polyvinyl alcohol, Onyx, and particulate embospheres [17]. After endovascular embolization, the surgery should be more secure compared to other cases that did not have prior embolization, and wide surgical excision can be performed with minimal bleeding [18, 19].

10.8 Carotid Cavernous Fistula (CCF)

Carotid cavernous fistulas (CCFs) are abnormal connections between the carotid arteries and the cavernous sinus. CCFs are classified into two main subtypes, direct high-flow CCF and indirect low-flow CCF. Direct CCFs result from defects in the intracavernous carotid artery wall, causing direct communication around the cavernous sinus. This type is usually caused by trauma and most common in young men. The second subtype, indirect CCF, or also called as dural arteriovenous fistulas, are pathological connections between the branches of the carotid artery within the dura mater and the cavernous sinus. This type is seen more commonly in postmenopausal women. Both types of CCF result in a rise of flow and pressure within the cavernous sinus, resulting in late flow draining into the orbital veins. CCFs can also be divided into four types: (1) type A where there is a direct high-flow shunt between ICA and cavernous sinus (traumatic and spontaneous due to aneurysm rupture); (2) type B, indirect fistula from the meningeal branches of the ICA; (3) type C, indirect fistula from the meningeal branches of the ECA; and (4) type D, indirect fistula from meningeal branches of both ICA and ECA.

The clinical presentations include decreased visual acuity, proptosis, chemosis, diplopia, and increase intraocular pressure [20] (Fig. 10.6). Other signs and symptoms are orbital and/or retroorbital pain, pulsatile proptosis, ocular and/or cranial bruit, pupillary dilation, ophthalmoplegia, neovascularization of the iris or retina, and rarely SAH. Indirect CCF has a more gradual onset and milder presentation than direct CCF [21]. MRI and CT usually demonstrate proptosis and showed serpiginous and engorged intraocular vessels including the superior ophthalmic vein and convexity of the lateral wall of the cavernous sinus. Angiography will show a shunt of blood flow from ICA into the cavernous sinus. Rapid opacification of the petrosal sinus and/or ophthalmic vein may be seen (Fig. 10.7) [21].

Indirect CCF can close spontaneously (20–50%) through thrombosis. Therefore, conservative management is given as long as visual acuity is stable and intraocular pressure is

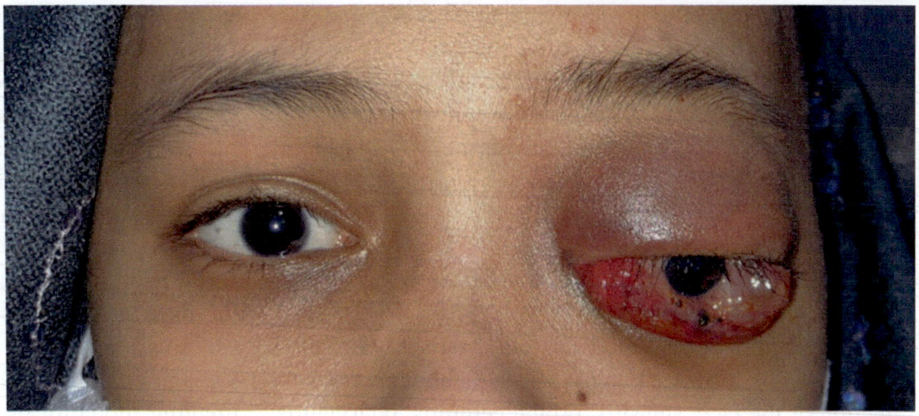

Fig. 10.6 Clinical presentation of patient with direct CCF of left ICA: exophtalmus and ophtalmoparesis of left eye (*Courtesy of Department of Neurosurgery, Dr. Cipto Mangunkusumo National General Hospital*)

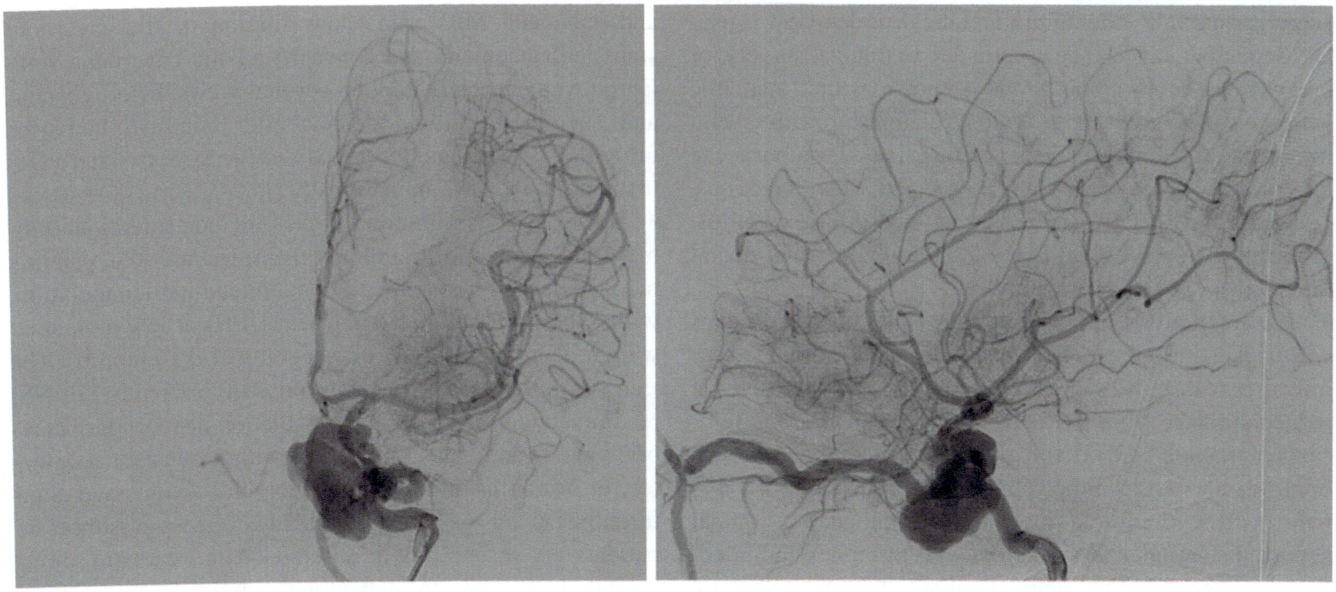

Fig. 10.7 Digital Subtraction Angiography of left CCF showed direct communication between cavernous segment of ICA to the cavernous sinus (AP view), and dilatation of superior ophtalmic vein (lateral view) (*Courtesy of: Department of Neurosurgery, dr. Cipto Mangunkusumo National General Hospital*)

under 25. The indication for treatment is for symptomatic high-flow CCFs, either embolization by an endovascular interventional or trapping using surgical clips. Endovascular interventions are the most preferable choice and can be done through arterial or venous approaches. Embolization can be done using platinum coils, detachable coils, detachable balloons, and liquid or particle embolic agents. For direct CCFs, the transcranial route is preferred; however, for indirect CCFs, tortuous arterial branches are very difficult to reach. Embolization of the CCFs via the superior ophthalmic vein (SOV), inferior ophthalmic vein (IOV), and medial ophthalmic vein (MOV) has been successfully reported in a variety of studies. Traditionally the cavernous sinus is approached via the inferior petrosal sinus (IPS). Orbital approaches are considered to have more risk due to increase the chance of hemorrhages because of the fragility of the ophthalmic veins and damage to nearby orbital structures such as the trochlear and optic nerves. An orbital approach to the SOV is the most commonly used to access the orbital vessel. The incision in the upper eyelid continued with blunt dissection of the orbital fat. Then, the orbicularis oculi muscle must be divided with the orbital septum opened into an area where there is a branch of the SOV as the supratrochlear vein. This branch can be followed to the main arterialized trunk of the SOV, which can be cannulated. This approach direct via the orbital vein can reduce the net distance and catheter manipulations but can cause complications such as infection, glaucoma, and orbital hematoma. If an attempt at a percutaneous SOV puncture fails and the SOV is ruptured, the risk of raised venous pressure within the orbit increases, which causes visual disturbances and the development of conditions such as glaucoma. The transvenous IOV and MOV approaches were not as commonly used because the size is smaller, and they generally do not act as primary drainage pathways from the orbital region and are not as dilated as the SOV in patients with symptomatic CCF [20, 21].

10.9 Cavernous Sinus Thrombosis

Cavernous sinus thrombosis (CST) is a rare disease but a life-threatening disorder because it can complicate to cause infection of the face, sinusitis, orbital cellulitis, pharyngitis, or otitis. It usually happened following traumatic injury or surgery, especially after thrombophilic disorder. CST is usually septic but can also be aseptic due to trauma, surgery, or pregnancy. The cavernous sinus is known as the "anatomic jewel box" because it shares a close relationship with several important structures. Septic cavernous sinus thrombosis can be occurred because of local spread, adjacent infections, facial cellulitis or abscess, periorbital and orbital cellulitis, pharyngitis, tonsilitis, otitis media, mastoiditis, and dental infections [22].

The assembly of bacteria and other infectious organisms will trigger thrombosis which then leads to entrapment of infection within the cavernous sinus. This thrombosis will reduce drainage from the facial vein and superior and inferior ophthalmic vein. It will manifest to facial and periorbital edema, ptosis, proptosis, chemosis, discomfort, and pain with eye muscle movement, papilledema, retinal venous distention, and visual loss. The thrombus and infection can spread to the contralateral side because there is a communication between the right and left cavernous sinuses via the intercavernous sinuses, anterior and posterior to the sella. Local compression due to thrombosis and inflammation of cranial nerves cause symptoms of partial or complete cranial neuropathies such as diplopia due to partial or complete ophthalmoplegia of abducens, oculomotor and trochlear nerves, nonreactive pupil caused by damage to autonomic fibers, numbness or parethesia and loss of corneal blink reflex due to ophthalmic nerve neuropathy, and facial pain, paresthesias, or numbness from compression of the maxillary branch of the trigeminal nerves. In physical examination, Horner syndrome that consist of ptosis, miosis, and anhidrosis can be present [22]. The most common imaging modality used was MRI (42%) followed by contrast-enhanced CT brain (23%) [23]. Evaluation using CTV and enhanced MRV can show dilation of the cavernous sinus, enhancement, and convexity of the cavernous sinus lateral wall especially seen in coronal views, heterogeneous and asymmetric filling defects after contrast, increased orbital fat density, and thrombosis of the SOV or other veins that lead to the cavernous sinus [22].

Because the common etiologies include infection, antimicrobial and antithrombotic therapies are the primary management. Most experts recommend anticoagulation, with either unfractionated heparin (UFH) or low molecular weight heparin (LMWH) for several weeks to months. The European Federation of Neurological Societies (EFNS) recommended the use of anticoagulation in secondary cerebral venous and sinus thrombosis with a transient risk factor for 3 months and idiopathic cerebral venous and sinus thrombosis for 6–12 months. However, in a subset of patients not responding despite adequate treatment, direct thrombolysis or thrombectomy may be performed (Fig. 10.8) [22, 24].

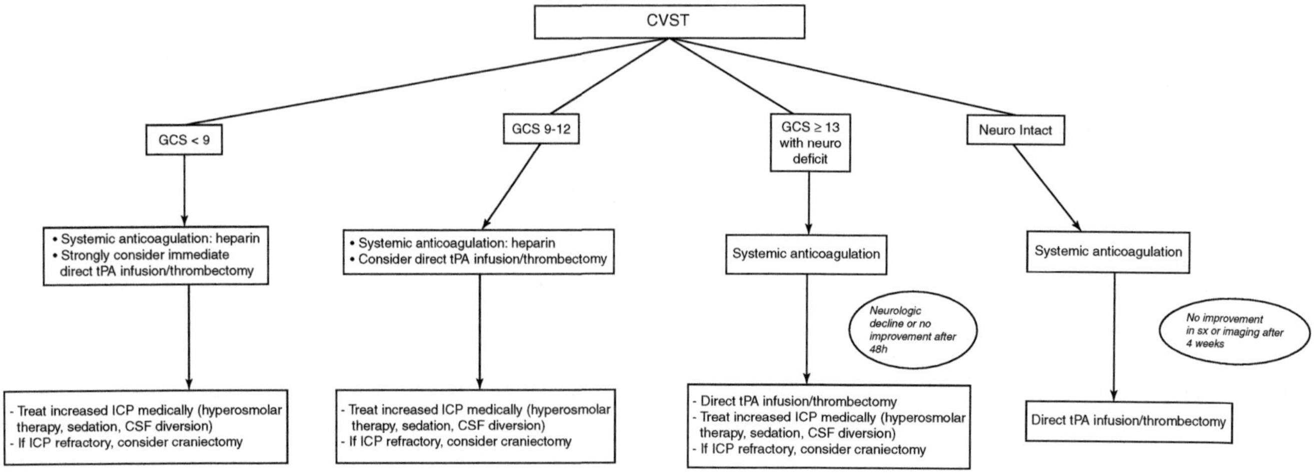

Fig. 10.8 Algorithm for CVST treatment [24]

10.10 Carotid Cavernous Aneurysm

Carotid cavernous aneurysms (CCAs) account for 2–9% of all intracranial aneurysms and 15% were originated from the ICA. The etiology of CCA can be due to trauma, infection, or idiopathic. The risk of rupture can cause carotid cavernous fistula, compressive cranial neuropathy, progressive worsened headache, and erosions of the sphenoid sinus. The rupture risk of asymptomatic lesions that are less than 13 mm is 0% over 5 years. Conservative management can be considered in cases of pain, asymptomatic patients, and simple cranial neuropathy. The decision to treat CCAs is always a challenge since to treat the patient, we need to weigh the risks and benefits of the intervention. CCAs can be originated from any segment of the cavernous carotid artery (Fig. 10.9) but most commonly are from the horizontal segment and then projected anterolaterally with the superior orbital fissure, under the anterior clinoid process. A combination of high wall shear stress and a high gradient predisposes to cerebral aneurysm formation. CCAs frequently created symptoms as a consequence of nerve compression, more specific for abducens (n. VI) lesion due to its position within the cavernous sinus. In a multicenter series, complications occurred in 5% of untreated CCAs [25].

Thromboembolic events and cerebral infarcts were identified in up to 2–13% of asymptomatic and untreated CCA. Surgical complications can happened up to 37% of all cases. Therefore, indication of treatment for such aneurysms should be evaluated (Table 10.3). One of the most common complications caused by the endovascular technique is thromboembolism since both the catheters and coil mass became a thromboembolic source. Other complications that can occur are perforation and rupture of the aneurysm, parent artery occlusion, cerebral embolisms, coil rupture and migration, and vasospasm. The mortality and morbidity of treatment have decreased significantly in recent years, partly as the result of improved pre-treatment screening with other techniques such as temporary balloon occlusion of the ICA to treat a CCA [25].

Coiling aneurysms are preferred for small aneurysms with a small or intermediate neck size. Carotid artery occlusion test should be considered first for large and giant aneurysms. If test occlusion indicated nontolerance, the choice is either conservative therapy or bypass surgery, depending on clinical presentation, patient age, comorbidity, and patient or family expectation. Balloon occlusion test of the ICA should be performed when the patient is awake, and angiography of

Table 10.3 Indication for treatment of cavernous carotid aneurysms [26]

Asymptomatic aneurysms	Symptomatic aneurysms
Extension of an aneurysm into the subarachnoid space	Subarachnoid hemorrhage
Extension of an aneurysm into the sphenoid sinus	Epistaxis
Origin from the anterior genu of the cavernous carotid	Unbearable ipsilateral face or retro-orbital pain
Radiographic enlargement of an aneurysm	Progressive ophthalmoplegia or visual loss
	Sudden, severe ophthalmoplegia

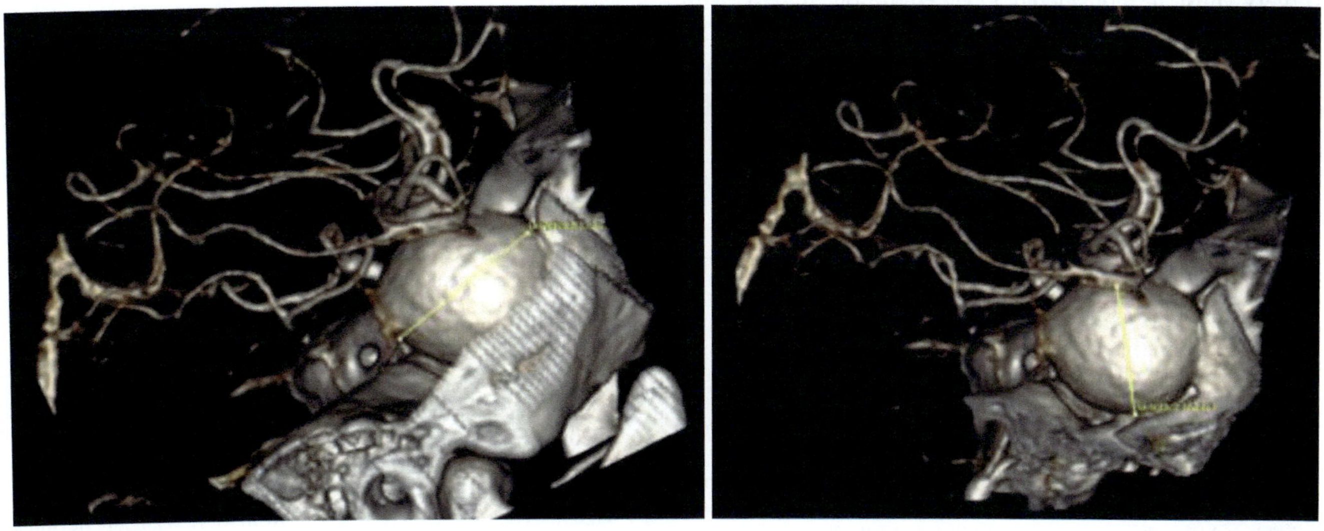

Fig. 10.9 CTA of the giant cavernous part of a carotid aneurysm. (*Courtesy of Department of Neurosurgery, Dr. Cipto Mangunkusumo National General Hospital*)

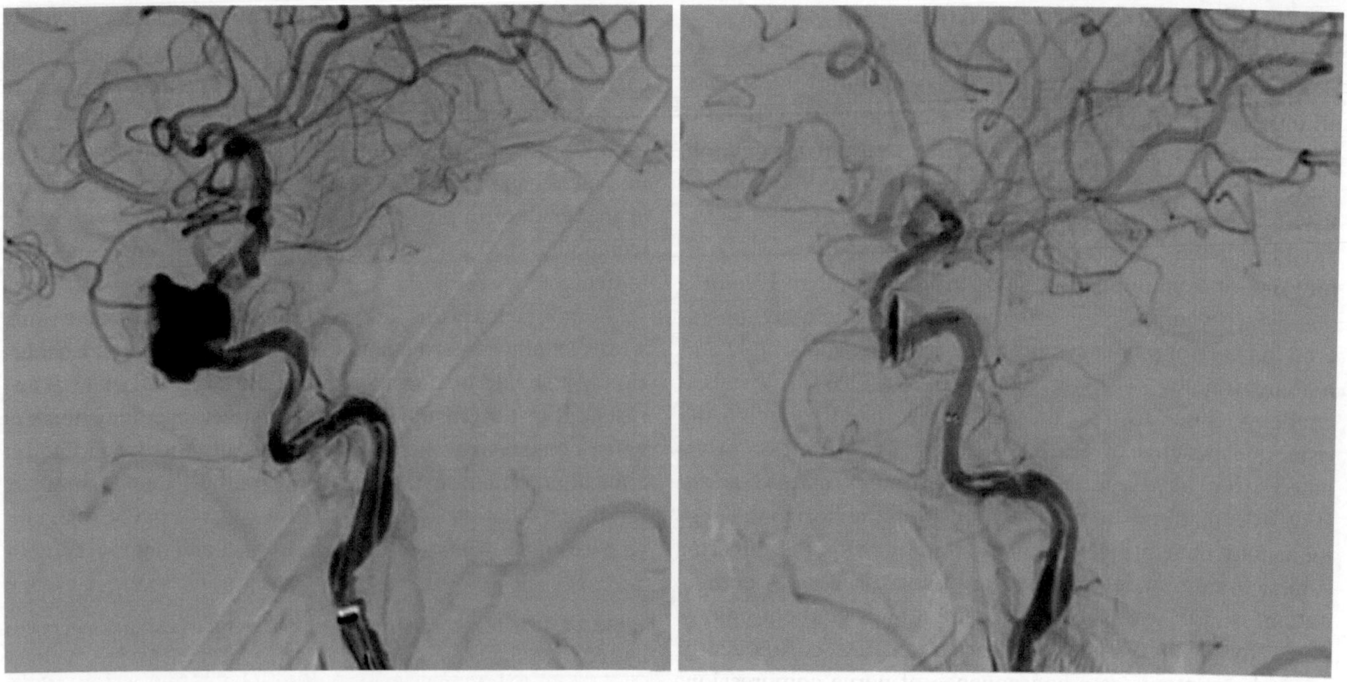

Fig. 10.10 Digital subtractional angiography of a giant cavernous carotid aneurysm before (left) and after placement of flow diverter (right). (*Courtesy of Neurosurgery Department, Dr. Cipto Mangunkusumo National General Hospital*)

the contralateral carotid artery and/or vertebral artery is performed to view the collateral flow via the anterior and posterior communicating arteries. Endovascular intervention such as coiling or flow diverter placement (Fig. 10.10) should be performed under general anesthesia. Wide-neck aneurysms can also be coiled with balloon or stent assistance. In symptomatic patients with wide-neck large or giant aneurysms who could not tolerate carotid artery occlusion, bypass surgery must be considered [27]. High-flow bypass with proximal occlusion of ICA (without trapping) seems to be the first choice treatment for large and giant CCA to reduce the mass effect, because aneurysm thrombosis is of high rate and its symptoms can significantly improve [26].

References

1. Badakere A, Patil-Chhablani P. Orbital apex syndrome: a review. Eye Brain. 2019;11:63–72.
2. Engin Ö, Adriaensen GFJPM, Hoefnagels FWA, Saeed P. A systematic review of the surgical anatomy of the orbital apex. Surg Radiol Anat. 2021;43(2):169–78.
3. Warrier S. Orbital arteriovenous malformations. Arch Ophthalmol. 2008;126(12):1669.
4. Wu CY, Kahana A. Immediate reconstruction after combined embolization and resection of orbital arteriovenous malformation. Ophthal Plast Reconstr Surg. 2017;33(3S):S140–3.
5. Xie J, Xu S, Shi Y, Li T, Jia R, Fan X. Comprehensive treatment of primary orbital arteriovenous malformation. J Craniofac Surg. 2017;28(6):e557–9.
6. Yamamoto Y, Yamamoto N, Satomi J, Yamaguchi I, Korai M, Kanematsu Y, et al. Dural arteriovenous fistula in the superior orbital fissure: a case report. Surg Neurol Int. 2018;9(1):95.
7. Akamatsu Y, Kubo Y, Chida K, Matsumoto Y, Ogasawara K. Intraorbital arteriovenous fistula presenting with impaired extraocular movement after a provocation test at the third segment of the ophthalmic artery. World Neurosurg. 2019;131:1–5.
8. Williamson RW, Ducruet AF, Crowley RW, McDougall CG, Albuquerque FC. Transvenous coil embolization of an intraorbital arteriovenous fistula. Neurosurgery. 2013;72(1):E130–4.
9. Garala P, Virdee J, Qureshi M, Gillow T. Intraorbital aneurysm of the ophthalmic artery. BMJ Case Rep. 2019;12(4):e227044.
10. Lu D, Xiong J, Liu H, Zhou H, Cheng J, Yue Y, et al. Surgical clipping of ophthalmic artery aneurysms: a single center series. Br J Neurosurg. 2021;35(2):157–60.
11. Hidayat R, Asmaniar F, Priambodo A, Mesiano T, Kurniawan M, Rasyid A, et al. Endovascular treatment of an unruptured ophthalmic artery aneurysm with a flow diverter: a case report. Med J Indones. 2021;30(4):297–300. https://mji.ui.ac.id/journal/index.php/mji/article/view/4899
12. Chaohui L, Yu ZG, Kai H. Balloon-assisted coils embolization for ophthalmic segment aneurysms of the internal carotid artery. Front Neurol. 2021;15(12):658661.
13. Feng G-J, Gao F, Huang X-Y, Hati P, Yang X-P, Wu H-X. Efficacy and safety of endovascular coiling vs surgical clipping for patients with ruptured carotid-ophthalmic aneurysm: a protocol for systematic review and meta-analysis. Medicine (Baltimore). 2020;99(47):e23235.
14. Croxatto JO, Font RL. Hemangiopericytoma of the orbit: a clinicopathologic study of 30 cases. Hum Pathol. 1982;13(3):210–8.
15. Jakobiec FA, Howard GM, Jones IS, Wolff M. Hemangiopericytoma of the orbit. Am J Ophthalmol. 1974;78(5):816–34.
16. Tsutsumi S, Adachi S, Ishii H, Yasumoto Y. Atypical epidural hemangiopericytoma presenting with visual disturbance. Surg Neurol Int. 2018;9(1):69.

17. Wallace KM, Alaraj A, Aakalu VK, Aletich V, Setabutr P. Endovascular preoperative embolization of orbital hemangiopericytoma with n-butyl cyanoacrylate glue. Ophthal Plast Reconstr Surg. 2014;30(4):e97–100.
18. Pihlblad MS, Schaefer DP. Percutaneous embolization of an orbital hemangiopericytoma with onyx facilitates its surgical excision. Ophthal Plast Reconstr Surg. 2012;28(6):e147–9.
19. Takahasi Y, Terasaki M, Maruiwa H, Tokutomi T, Shigemori M. Orbital hemangiopericytoma: a case report. Neurol Med Chir. 1997;37:688–91.
20. Phan K, Xu J, Leung V, Teng I, Sheik-Ali S, Maharaj M, et al. Orbital approaches for treatment of carotid cavernous fistulas: a systematic review. World Neurosurg. 2016;96:243–51.
21. Greenberg MS. Handbook of neurosurgery. 8th ed. New York: Thieme; 2016.
22. Plewa W, Tadi P, Gupta M. Cavernous sinus thrombosis. StatPearls Publishing; 2020.
23. Weerasinghe D, Lueck CJ. Septic cavernous sinus thrombosis: case report and review of the literature. Neuroophthalmology. 2016;40(6):263–76.
24. Rahman M, Mocco J. Direct thrombolysis for cerebral venous sinus thrombosis. Neurosurg Focus. 2009;27:8.
25. Rosi Junior J, Welling LC, Yeng LT, Caldas JG, Schafranski M, Teixeira MJ, et al. Cavernous carotid artery aneurysms: epidemiology, natural history, diagnostic and treatment. An experience of a single institution. Clin Neurol Neurosurg. 2014;125:32–5.
26. Sriamornrattanakul K, Sakarunchai I, Yamashiro K, Yamada Y, Suyama D, Kawase T, et al. Surgical treatment of large and giant cavernous carotid aneurysms. Asian J Neurosurg. 2017;12(3):382.
27. van Rooij WJ. Endovascular treatment of cavernous sinus aneurysms. Am J Neuroradiol. 2012;33(2):323–6.

Orbital Apex Infective Diseases

11

Matthew C. W. Lam and Carmen K. M. Chan

Abstract

Orbital apex infections are uncommon conditions which can be caused by a wide range of organisms. In particular, bacterial and fungal involvement of the orbital apex can have life-threatening and sight-threatening consequences if not diagnosed in time and properly managed.

Keywords

Orbital apex syndrome · Orbital apex infection · Orbital cellulitis · Mucormycosis · Herpes zoster ophthalmicus · Orbital cysticercosis

11.1 Introduction

Orbital apex syndrome is characterised by optic neuropathy (CN II) and the involvement of multiple other cranial nerves, including the oculomotor (CN III), trochlear (CN IV), abducens (CN VI), and the ophthalmic branch of the trigeminal (CN V_1) nerves. This should be distinguished from cavernous sinus syndrome and superior orbital fissure syndrome, which share similar features.

In cavernous sinus syndrome, the optic nerve is usually unaffected; in addition to CN III, CN IV, CN V_1 and CN VI, the sympathetic fibres and the maxillary branch of the trigeminal nerve (CN V_2) could also be involved. In superior orbital fissure syndrome, palsy of CN III, CN IV, CN V_1 and CN VI may occur, but the optic nerve is generally spared.

The orbital apex is an uncommon site of infection. Infective causes should be suspected when patients with orbital apex syndrome have a fever and rapidly progressive signs/symptoms or are immunocompromised (e.g. diabetes, haematological malignancy, iatrogenic immunosuppression) [1]. Infections can be caused by bacteria, fungi, viruses, or parasites.

Generally, the diagnosis of orbital apex infections can be aided by neuroimaging, in particular magnetic resonance imaging (MRI) with gadolinium contrast and fat suppression sequences of the brain and orbit. After ruling out other inflammatory or neoplastic causes, further specific investigations can be directed towards the potential infective agents. It is crucial to distinguish between inflammatory and infective causes of orbital apex syndrome as steroids and/or immunosuppressants directed towards inflammatory causes can have severe, if not fatal, consequences in bacterial or fungal infections.

11.2 Bacterial Infections

Bacterial infection of the orbital apex can occur as part of generalised orbital cellulitis; however, cases which present with isolated orbital apex syndrome have been reported [1] (Fig. 11.1). As with orbital cellulitis, infection commonly spreads from adjacent sinusitis; occasionally, infection can follow functional endoscopic sinus surgery. Common infective agents include *Staphylococcus* spp., *Streptococcus pneumoniae* and Gram-negative bacilli (e.g. *Pseudomonas aeruginosa*, *Klebsiella* spp. and *Proteus* spp.). *Pseudomonas* causes tissue destruction via enzymes and toxins and destroys bones via osteoclastogenic lipopolysaccharides [2]. In endemic areas, the possibility of mycobacterial infections (e.g. *M. tuberculosis*, *M. leprae*) should be borne in mind [3].

Patients are usually immunocompromised and generally present with poor visual acuity, facial hypoesthesia and ophthalmoplegia. The progression of signs and symptoms can be rapid. Imaging may demonstrate bony destruction and non-specific soft tissue inflammatory changes [2]. Nasal endos-

M. C. W. Lam · C. K. M. Chan (✉)
Hong Kong Eye Hospital, Hong Kong SAR, China

Department of Ophthalmology and Visual Sciences, The Chinese University of Hong Kong, Hong Kong SAR, China
e-mail: carmen.chan@ha.org.hk

T. L. POON et al. (eds.), *Orbital Apex and Periorbital Skull Base Diseases*, https://doi.org/10.1007/978-981-99-2989-4_11

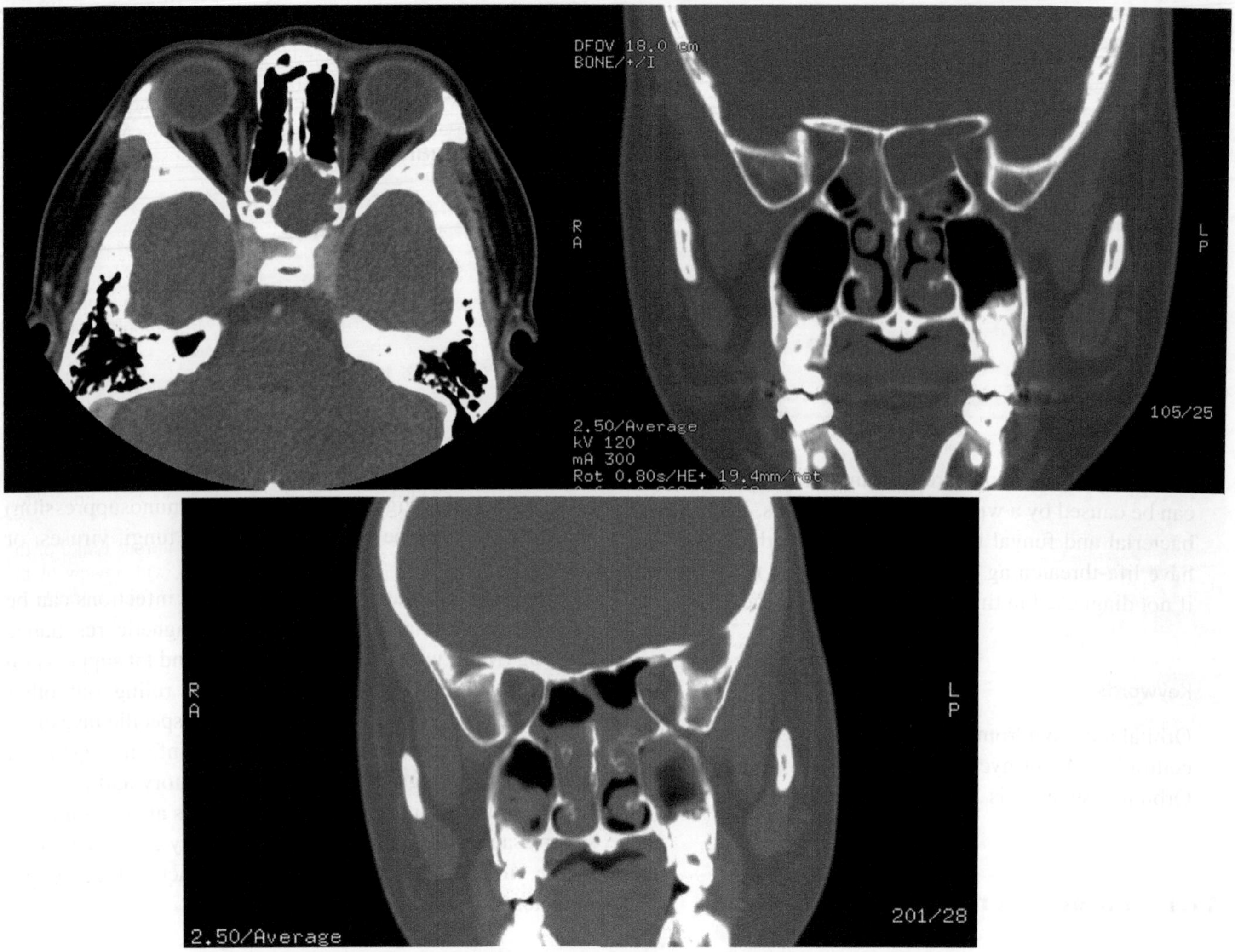

Fig. 11.1 (Upper panel) Computed tomography (CT) brain images (axial and coronal) showing opacified sphenoid sinus in a 17-year-old girl of good past health, who presented with isolated left optic neuropathy. She was initially misdiagnosed as having 'optic neuritis'. Functional endoscopic sinus surgery (FESS) was performed to drain the sphenoid sinus, yielding mucous which was positive for diphtheroids. The patient had a good visual recovery after the surgery. (Lower panel) Coronal CT images after FESS. (Photo courtesy of Dr. Andrew C.Y. Mak)

copy may be necessary to biopsy infected tissues for microscopy and culture to differentiate bacterial from invasive fungal infections. A blood culture may also be positive for the culprit bacterial agent. Chest X-ray, Mantoux test and/or interferon-gamma release assay may be considered if tuberculosis is suspected.

Early initiation of broad-spectrum antibiotics and antifungals can prevent further extension of the infection to intracranial structures and can be potentially lifesaving [1, 2]. Antimicrobial therapy should subsequently be tailored according to culture and sensitivity results. Urgent endoscopic surgical decompression of the orbital apex with or without debridement of infected tissues has a role in obtaining tissue samples and may relieve pressure on the optic nerve. Unfortunately, despite treatment, visual prognosis is poor with few patients retaining useful vision [1, 2].

11.3 Fungal Infections

Rhino-orbito-cerebral mucormycosis is an aggressive and often fatal fungal infection. Hyperglycaemia and ketoacidosis nourish fungal colonies; fungi are angioinvasive, and their hyphae tend to grow into vessel lumens, resulting in endothelial dysfunction and thrombosis. Mucormycosis should be suspected in any immunocompromised or diabetic patient who presents with orbital apex syndrome, orbital cellulitis or sinusitis (Fig. 11.2) [4].

Mucormycosis present very similarly to bacterial orbital apex infection, and progression is typically rapid. Imaging may demonstrate tissue necrosis with lack of enhancement of the sinonasal mucosa (Fig. 11.3); infarction of the brain and optic nerve manifests as restricted diffusion on MRI [2]. Nasal endoscopy sometimes reveals hyphae in sinuses

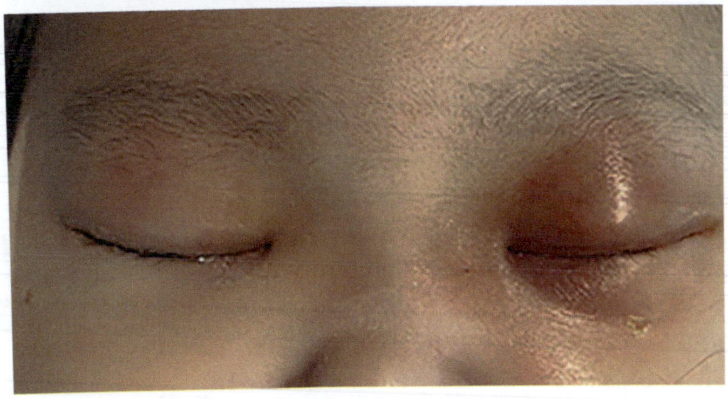

Fig. 11.2 Clinical photo showing orbital mucormycosis in an infant with underlying leukaemia, showing a dusky colour of left periorbital skin. (Photo courtesy of Prof. H.K. Yuen)

and biopsy can be taken to confirm the diagnosis (Figs. 11.4 and 11.5).

Patients with aggressive orbital apex infection should be empirically started on antifungal and broad-spectrum antibiotics. Intravenous amphotericin B is effective against mucormycosis but carries a risk of nephrotoxicity. The underlying hyperglycaemia or immunocompromised state should be addressed as soon as possible. Surgical debridement is often necessary apart from adequate antimicrobial coverage; some patients require orbital exenteration. Prior use of steroids significantly worsens the disease, which can become uncontrolled with intracranial extension. Even with appropriate and timely treatment, the disease has a poor visual prognosis and extremely high mortality [4, 5].

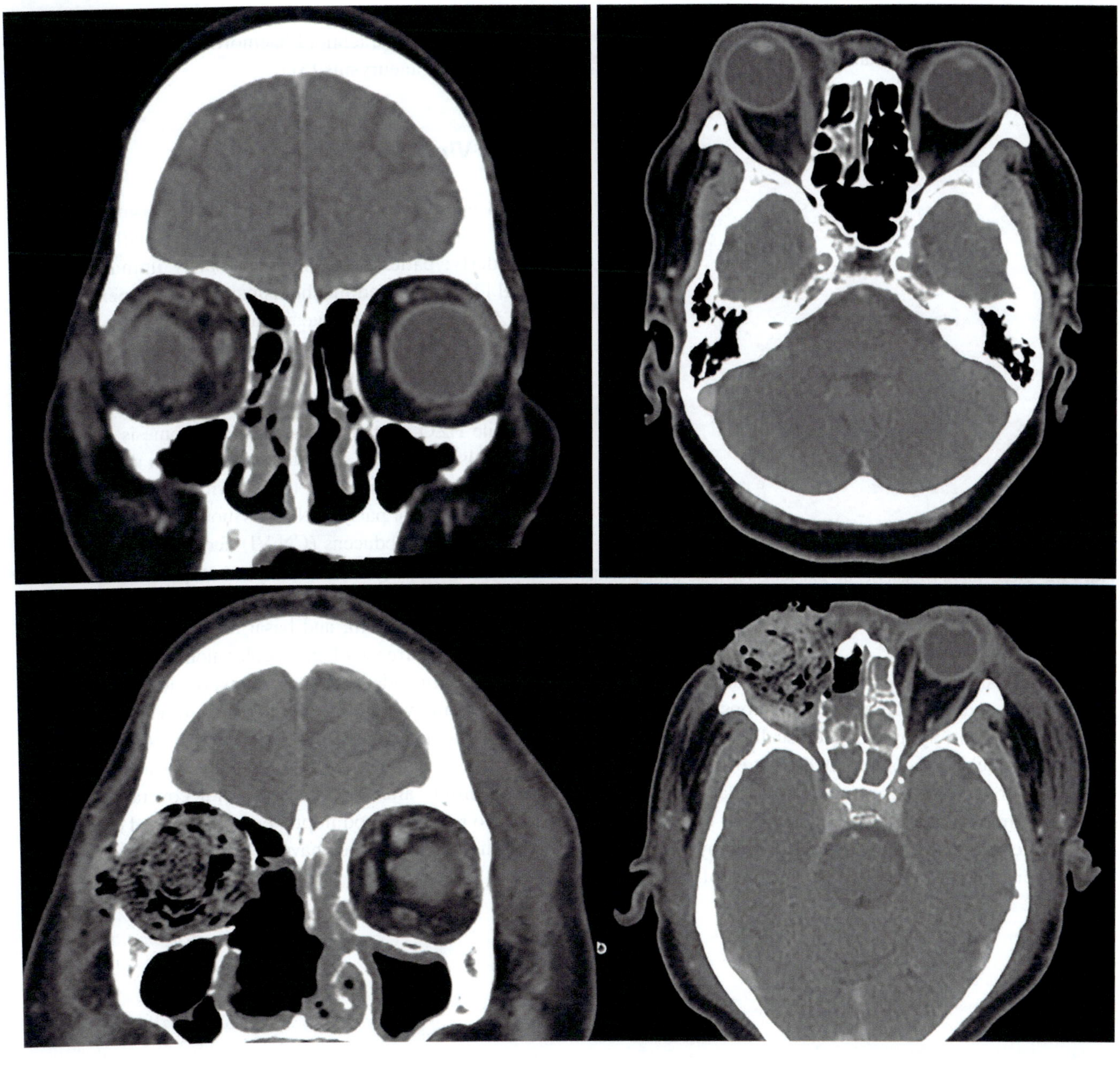

Fig. 11.3 (Upper panel) CT images with contrast of orbit showing right rhino-orbital mucormycosis, demonstrating right eye proptosis, increased stranding in the right orbit and opacification of the right nasal cavity and ethmoidal sinuses. (Lower panel) CT images of the same patient after right orbital exenteration, bilateral anterior ethmoidectomy and debridement of the nasal cavity

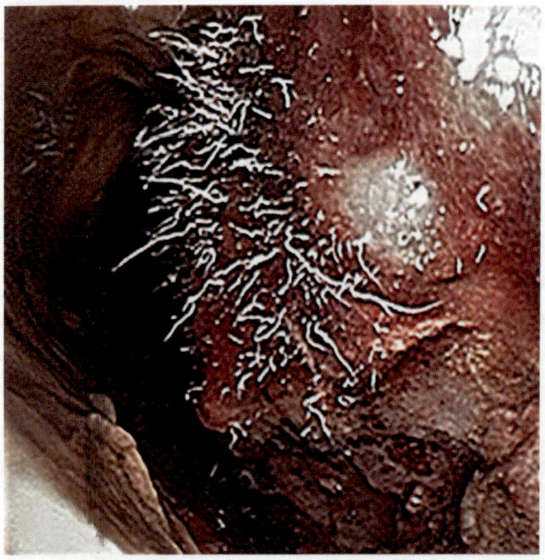

Fig. 11.4 Intraoperative endoscopic photo showing fungal hyphae in the nasal cavity of a patient with rhino-orbital mucormycosis. (Photo courtesy of Prof. H.K. Yuen)

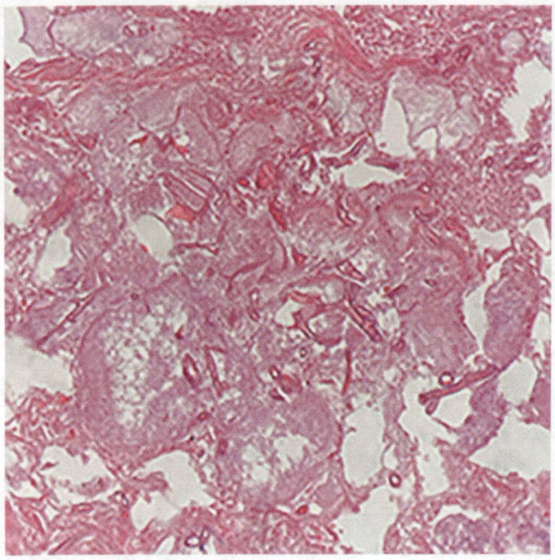

Fig. 11.5 H&E 400×. Broad, ribbon-like fungal hyphae with irregular branching are seen amongst necrotic tissue, consistent with mucormycosis. (Photo courtesy of Dr. M.N. Hau)

Aspergillosis is another cause of fungal infection at the orbital apex and most frequently develops after sphenoid sinus involvement. Symptoms are usually of subacute onset in terms of weeks and commonly consist of unilateral vague headache or periorbital pain, with visual disturbances. Similarly, immunocompromised status (e.g. diabetes mellitus, chronic steroid use, systemic chemotherapy) is an important association; however, more than half of the reported cases did not have immunocompromising risk factors [5]. *Aspergillus* infection in immunocompetent patients may present with a fungal ball that simulates a mass, i.e. an aspergilloma.

In suspected cases, empirical antifungal therapy should be started, and tissue biopsy obtained as soon as possible. Diagnosis may be confirmed with polymerase chain reaction (PCR) testing if histopathology turned out to be negative. Serum testing of β-D glucan may be useful in diagnosing invasive fungal infections in biopsy-negative cases [5, 6].

Aspergillosis should be treated with a prolonged course of systemic voriconazole or amphotericin B, and serial clinical and radiographic monitoring for treatment response is necessary. If left untreated, potentially serious complications can occur, such as intracranial extension, cerebral arterial occlusion and subarachnoid haemorrhage secondary to ruptured mycotic aneurysms [5].

11.4 Viral Infections

Orbital apex syndrome is an uncommon complication of herpes zoster ophthalmicus (HZO) and usually occurs in the elderly; patients are not necessarily immunocompromised [7]. Postulated mechanisms of orbital apex infection in HZO include extensive inflammation with soft tissue oedema, direct spread of the varicella zoster virus from CN V to other cranial nerves with resultant cytopathic effect, and occlusive vasculitis induced by viral infection [7, 8].

While HZO-related orbital apex syndrome is rare, ocular motor palsies in HZO are not that uncommon and may occur in up to one-third of those with newly diagnosed HZO. Oculomotor palsy (CN III) is more common than trochlear (CN IV) or abducens (CN VI) nerve involvement; bilateral ophthalmoplegia has also been reported. Apart from orbital apex involvement, extension of infection to the cavernous sinus or brainstem, and basal meningoencephalitis may explain the occurrence of extraocular motility defects [8].

It is recommended to treat HZO with 1 to 2 weeks of systemic antiviral, which is preferably started within 72 h of the onset of cutaneous vesicular rash. Early treatment has been shown to correlate with better outcomes. The addition of systemic steroids after adequate antiviral coverage has been shown to result in good improvement, provided that clinical and radiological features have ruled out bacterial or fungal causes [7].

Visual prognosis of HZO-related orbital apex infections is generally better than their bacterial and fungal counterparts. Nevertheless, there are a few reported cases with resultant optic atrophy and no residual useful vision. Ophthalmoplegia has been shown to resolve in a few months in the majority, but this may take up to 1.5 years [7, 8].

Cytomegalovirus (CMV)-related sinusitis with resultant orbital apex infection is exceedingly rare and has only been reported in immunocompromised hosts. The clinical course is subacute to chronic. Bacterial and fungal infections are important differentials to consider. Biopsy of infected tissues may reveal intranuclear and cytoplasmic inclusion bodies in CMV infection; immunostaining can be confirmatory [9].

11.5 Parasitic Infections

Cysticercosis refers to an infestation of the cyst form of *Taenia solium*. When the cyst is present in the posterior orbit, optic neuropathy and extraocular dysmotility can occur. Imaging with CT or MRI is vital, showing a cystic lesion with a central spot/nodule that represents the scolex. Treatment is with antihelminthic medication and steroids to control the inflammatory reaction secondary to the death of the parasite [10].

References

1. Pfeiffer ML, Merritt HA, Bailey LA, Richani K, Phillips ME. Orbital apex syndrome from bacterial sinusitis without orbital cellulitis. Am J Ophthalmol Case Rep. 2018;10:84–6.
2. Leung V, Dunn H, Newey A, O'Donnell B. Orbital apex syndrome in Pseudomonas sinusitis after functional endoscopic sinus surgery. Ophthalmic Plast Reconstr Surg. 2018;34(5):e166–e8.
3. El Beltagi AH, El-Nil H, Alrabiah L, El Shammari N. Orbital apex syndrome due to trigeminal perineural spread of sinonasal leprosy: a case report. Clin Imaging. 2012;36(2):142–5.
4. Anders UM, Taylor EJ, Martel JR, Martel JB. Acute orbital apex syndrome and rhino-orbito-cerebral mucormycosis. Int Med Case Rep J. 2015;8:93–6.
5. Yuan M, Tandon A, Li A, Johnson E, Greer C, Tooley A, et al. Orbital apex syndrome secondary to invasive Aspergillus infection: a case series and literature review. J Neuroophthalmol. 2020;41:e631.
6. Theel ES, Doern CD. Beta-D-glucan testing is important for diagnosis of invasive fungal infections. J Clin Microbiol. 2013;51(11):3478–83.
7. Lim JJ, Ong YM, Wan Zalina MZ, Choo MM. Herpes zoster ophthalmicus with orbital apex syndrome-difference in outcomes and literature review. Ocul Immunol Inflamm. 2018;26(2):187–93.
8. Marsh RJ, Dulley B, Kelly V. External ocular motor palsies in ophthalmic zoster: a review. Br J Ophthalmol. 1977;61(11):677–82.
9. Nomura JH, Eichhorn K, Cao TM, Sahebi F. Cytomegalovirus sinusitis complicated by orbital apex syndrome in an immunocompromised host. Transpl Infect Dis. 2016;18(6):957–9.
10. Chaugule P, Varma DR, Patil Chhablani P. Orbital apex syndrome secondary to optic nerve cysticercosis. Int Ophthalmol. 2019;39(5):1151–4.

Orbital Apex Inflammatory and Infectious Diseases

12

Yuk Fai Cheung

Abstract

Infectious disease is one of the numerous causes of orbital apex disorders. In this chapter, the author will discuss the clinical features, diagnosis, and treatment of several infectious conditions which are associated with significant visual morbidity and **even** mortality. The impact of the COVID-19 pandemic will also be highlighted.

Keywords

Orbital apex syndrome · Bacterial sinusitis · Aspergillosis · Mucormycosis · COVID-19 · Herpes zoster ophthalmicus

Orbital apex disorders can be divided into superior orbital fissure syndrome, cavernous sinus syndrome, and orbital apex syndrome (OAS). All three syndromes share common characteristics of damage to the oculomotor nerve, trochlear nerve, and abducens nerve, along with the ophthalmic division of the trigeminal nerve. Patients with cavernous sinus syndrome also exhibit hypoesthesia in the distribution of maxillary division of the trigeminal nerve and Horner's syndrome due to involvement of sympathetic chain next to the cavernous segment of the internal carotid artery. On the other hand, patients with OAS experience visual disturbance additionally as a consequence of optic nerve dysfunction. With disease progression, superior orbital fissure syndrome can evolve into either OAS or cavernous sinus syndrome [3, 21]. Orbital apex disorders can be caused by a wide range of disease entities, infection affecting the orbital structures is one of them. The pathogens include bacteria, fungi, viruses, spirochetes, mycobacterium, and parasites. Making a prompt and accurate diagnosis with administration of appropriate treatment is crucial to save the vision and lives of patients. In this chapter we will discuss some of these conditions.

12.1 Bacterial Infections

Orbital apex syndrome commonly occurs as a complication of bacterial sinusitis. It is usually associated with orbital cellulitis. Orbital infection can be classified, with respect to the orbital septum, into preseptal (periorbital) and post-septal (orbital) infection [7]. The orbital septum works as a barrier against the spread of periorbital infection into the orbit; therefore, orbital apex disorder is unlikely to happen as a complication of preseptal cellulitis. Pansinusitis or ethmoid sinusitis occurs frequently in 86–98% of cases of orbital cellulitis. Other causes of orbital cellulitis are surgery, anesthesia, trauma, dental infection, and middle ear infection. Apart from causing orbital cellulitis, sinusitis can lead to other serious complications like orbital abscess and subperiosteal abscess [50]. Further extension of the infection into intracranial structures may lead to meningitis, subdural empyema, epidural abscess, or septic cavernous sinus thrombophlebitis [66].

OAS originating from isolated bacterial sinusitis without concurrent orbital cellulitis is less common. It is presumably because the pathogens can penetrate more readily through the thin sinus walls adjacent to the anterior orbit instead of the thick ethmoidal and sphenoidal walls [14]. Several case examples are listed below.

A 63-year-old woman with a history of metastatic breast cancer and diabetes mellitus (DM) presented with initial involvement of the trigeminal and abducens nerves, which had rapidly progressed to involve the optic and oculomotor nerves. Her visual acuity further declined to no perception of light despite appropriate antibiotics and surgical interven-

Y. F. Cheung (✉)
Division of Neurology, Department of Medicine, Queen Elizabeth Hospital, Hong Kong SAR, China
e-mail: cyfz02@ha.org.hk

T. L. POON et al. (eds.), *Orbital Apex and Periorbital Skull Base Diseases*, https://doi.org/10.1007/978-981-99-2989-4_12

tion. Magnetic resonance imaging (MRI) of the orbit showed pansinusitis and enhancement of the optic nerve. Cultures of blood and surgical specimens yielded methicillin-sensitive *Staphylococcus aureus* [64].

Kusunoki et al. reported a 60-year-old woman with diabetic nephropathy and heart disease who was diagnosed as OAS due to pansinusitis with *Pseudomonas aeruginosa* infection [36].

Colson and Daily described a 49-year-old man, with a history of DM and chronic sinusitis, who developed OAS and cavernous sinus thrombosis concomitantly due to mixed infection with *Staphylococcus aureus* and *Pseudomonas aeruginosa*. His affected optic nerve demonstrated microinfarctions due to arterial thrombosis [14]. Another case with mixed growth of bacteria occurred in a 58-year-old diabetic man who was hospitalized for right herpes zoster ophthalmicus and methicillin-sensitive *Staphylococcus aureus* osteomyelitis of his toe. During the course of treatment, he developed left OAS secondary to left sphenoid sinusitis. Subsequent MRI of the orbit demonstrated extension of inflammatory soft tissues towards the orbital apex and cavernous sinus, with enhancement of retro-orbital fat, rectus muscles, and optic nerve. Computed tomography (CT) showed bony erosion of the lateral wall of the sphenoid sinus. Sphenoidotomy with drainage yielded methicillin-resistant *Staphylococcus aureus* (MRSA) and *Pseudomonas aeruginosa*. This man unfortunately died because of multi-organ failure [87].

The last example is a 68-year-old woman with acute myelogenous leukemia and migraine who complained of severe headache around 2 weeks after chemotherapy. With a CT angiogram and MRI showing mucosal thickening of ethmoid and sphenoid sinuses, which was initially thought to be insignificant, she was treated as a migraine attack. Two weeks later, she presented with typical features of OAS. She was found to have an interval progression of the mucosal thickening and bony erosion into the orbital apex. Erosion into the cavernous segment of the internal carotid artery resulted in thrombosis. She was treated with broad-spectrum antibiotics and antifungals. Sinus drainage finally revealed *Streptococcus viridans* [6].

These case examples illustrate a few crucial points. First, susceptible patients are often immunocompromised like having DM or malignancy. Second, prognosis can be very guarded despite appropriate interventions. Pfeiffer et al. have reviewed six analogous case reports [64]. Five patients presented with no light perception and only one patient made minimal visual recovery, from no light perception to hand motion. Third, presentation can be insidious and clinical signs and radiographic findings can be subtle, so that a high index of suspicion is necessary. Actually previous case reports have suggested that among patients with OAS secondary to sinusitis, the absence of overt orbital pathology on imaging or at surgery portends a better visual prognosis than patients who have apparent masses at the orbital apex [14]. Once bacterial infection is suspected, parenteral broad-spectrum antibiotics which cover *Staphylococcus aureus* (including MRSA), streptococci, and gram-negative bacilli such as *Pseudomonas aeruginosa* should be initiated promptly. Management should also include endoscopic nasal surgery and biopsy for histopathology and culture. Finally, it is essential to rule out invasive fungal infection because it shares similar clinical features and carries significant morbidity and mortality. Empirical antifungal therapy might be considered while waiting for the laboratory results.

12.2 Fungal Infections

Similar to bacterial infections, orbital apex disorders caused by fungi usually come after paranasal sinus infection. Fungal rhinosinusitis can be divided into two broad categories, namely, invasive and noninvasive, depending on the potential of the fungal hyphae to invade the adjacent tissues through the epithelium. Besides, further subdivision can be made based on the chronicity of the illness—acute (less than 4 weeks) and chronic (more than 4 weeks). Hence, fungal rhinosinusitis can be classified into six subgroups [18].

1. *Noninvasive fungal rhinosinusitis*
   (a) Saprophytic fungal infestation
   (b) Fungal ball
   (c) Allergic fungal rhinosinusitis
2. *Invasive fungal rhinosinusitis*
   (a) Acute invasive fungal rhinosinusitis
   (b) Chronic invasive fungal rhinosinusitis
   (c) Chronic granulomatous invasive fungal rhinosinusitis

Lee et al. reported a case series of 30 patients with orbital mycoses encountered in an Australian subtropical population over three decades. Most patients (87%) had invasive diseases, often with poor visual and survival outcomes. OAS was initially observed in 27% of patients. Common causative pathogens included *Mucorales* ($N = 16$) and *Aspergillus* ($N = 8$). Common risk factors included hematological disorders (myelodysplastic syndrome and aplastic anemia), hematological malignancies, neutropenia, corticosteroids use, and DM [39].

Fungal spores are abundant in the atmosphere. In normal subjects, inhaled fungal spores form part of the normal sinonasal flora without causing overt diseases, because these fungi are killed by neutrophils, monocytes, and macrophages. In immunocompromised individuals, a more fulminant and invasive disease may emerge. In immunocompetent individuals, *Aspergillus* tends to cause noninvasive fungal rhinosinusitis. However, there are a number of exceptions reported in the literature. From 2000 to 2011, 11 cases of rhino-orbital-cerebral mucormycosis (ROCM) affecting immunocompetent hosts have been published. Among them, nine cases were due to *Apophysomyces elegans* [71].

12.2.1 Aspergillosis

Sino-orbital aspergillosis is a relatively uncommon cause of orbital apex disorders, but it remains an important differential diagnosis due to its aggressive clinical course. Inhalation of fungal spores released into the atmosphere is the typical route of infection. Paranasal sinuses are the usual portal of entry. *Aspergillus fumigatus* is the most frequent species isolated in human infections, followed by *A. flavus* [17]. As mentioned before, aspergillosis can be divided into invasive and noninvasive forms.

Invasive aspergillosis can either follow a fulminant or an indolent course. The fungal hyphae invade the sinus mucosa, orbital tissue, and spread along the skull base. It may produce bony destruction, hematogenous spread to other organs by vascular invasion, and intracranial extension via the orbital fissures or the optic canal. Cases of permanent blindness have been reported even with immediate antifungal therapy. Fatal outcomes can occur when the condition is complicated by central nervous system infection or subarachnoid hemorrhage (SAH) secondary to ruptured mycotic aneurysms. For example, Yip et al. reported a 73-year-old woman, who was maintained on long-term corticosteroids for her rheumatoid arthritis and presented with OAS. Massive fatal SAH suddenly occurred 5 days after endoscopic removal of the orbital apex lesion, due to a ruptured mycotic aneurysm [88]. Huang and Gui described a DM patient with simultaneous orbital apex and cavernous sinus invasions who was treated with voriconazole, surgery, and anticoagulant [26]. Perineural spread along the optic nerve to involve the optic chiasm has also been reported [42].

Immunocompromised individuals are typically more susceptible to invasive aspergillosis. Prolonged neutropenia, use of corticosteroids or other immunosuppressive agents, malignancies, allogeneic hematopoietic stem cell transplantation, and solid organ transplantation are the major risk factors for aspergillosis. DM, acquired immunodeficiency syndrome, severe burns, prosthetic devices, trauma, excessive environmental exposure, residence in endemic areas, drug abusers, alcoholics, liver cirrhosis, and elderly are other risk factors [41, 42]. Though less common, invasive aspergillosis can also be found in immunocompetent hosts [42, 49, 60].

Fungal ball, also known as aspergilloma, is one manifestation in patients with noninvasive aspergillosis. Typically, this happens in patients with intact immunity. Nevertheless, when host defenses are weakened, noninvasive aspergillosis can turn itself into an invasive form [13, 56]. Because of its nonspecific clinical and radiographic appearance as well as its potentially invasive and aggressive nature, misdiagnosis of aspergilloma as primary malignancy [60, 90] or metastasis [12] can occur. It can also mimic orbital pseudotumor [8] when the commencement of corticosteroid therapy may cause worsening rather than beneficial effects. Chang et al. reported a 61-year-old woman with uncontrolled DM whose MRI initially suggested paranasal sinus tumor. Tissue biopsy subsequently revealed *Aspergillus* and chronic granulomatous inflammation. Her vision was permanently damaged despite treatment with voriconazole and surgery. The authors have also conducted a systematic literature review from 1970 to 2017 and identified five case reports of OAS caused by aspergilloma [10].

Imaging is of great importance for establishing an anatomical diagnosis. CT may reveal intraluminal calcifications which are almost pathognomonic for aspergillosis, but it is present in only 50% of patients [40, 41]. In MRI, aspergillosis appears as iso- to hypointense signals on T1-weighted images, iso- to extremely hypointense signals on T2-weighted images, and intense homogenous (and rarely ring) enhancement on post-contrast T1-weighted images [74].

Tissue biopsy remains the gold standard for definitive diagnosis. Direct microscopy, preferably using optical brighteners, histopathology, and culture, are all recommended [79]. Septate fungal hyphae branching at 45° angle are typical of aspergillosis. These are best visible using periodic acid-Schiff (PAS) or Grocott-Gomori methenamine silver (GMS) stains. Unfortunately, the sensitivity of microscopy is rather low, between 33% and 50%, and repeated biopsy may be necessary. Serological markers such as serum galactomannan and (1→3)-β-D-glucan can be helpful, but their reliability can be limited by false-positive results. Polymerase chain reaction (PCR) provides a high sensitivity and specificity, hence reducing the need for repeated biopsies. Furthermore, PCR can hasten the initiation of the appropriate therapy. It can also be utilized to identify genetic mutations that confer resistance to triazole therapy [40].

Treatment of sino-orbital aspergillosis has evolved substantially over decades. In the past, radical surgical resection of the affected tissues or even orbital exenteration was considered the standard of therapy. However, radical surgery guarantees neither disease control nor patient survival. Recently, reports of satisfactory outcomes using combinations of less radical surgery and systemic antifungal therapy have been published [58]. Functional endoscopic sinus surgery with debridement is currently advised. It is also recommended to reverse the immunosuppression if possible.

Systemic antifungal agents consist of polyenes, triazoles, and echinocandins. The overall response rate to antifungal therapy is 40–60%. Amphotericin B is widely used, but due to its nephrotoxicity, it is getting out of favor. Other antifungals such as voriconazole and itraconazole can also be considered alone or combined with amphotericin B. Voriconazole showed a high efficacy, low-toxicity profile, and its availability in both intravenous and oral formulations which allows for more management flexibility [24]. Reports of successful treatment with voriconazole monotherapy have been published [53]. The Infectious Disease Society of America (IDSA) recommends triazoles as preferred agents for the treatment of invasive aspergillosis. Echinocandins are recommended as salvage therapy, either alone or in combination, but not as primary treatment [62].

12.2.2 Mucormycosis

Mucormycosis is another acute fulminating, visual- and life-threatening opportunistic fungal infection. It is classified into different forms based on the organ systems involved, the most common clinical presentation of which is rhino-orbital-cerebral infection (ROCM). In a review of 175 patients of sino-orbital mucormycosis, males were more commonly affected (68.5%), and the overall mean age was 43 years. The overall survival rate was 59.5% [80]. The initial symptoms are rather nonspecific. Patients usually present with acute sinusitis—fever, nasal congestion, rhinorrhea, ocular pain, facial pain, and headache. OAS represents an emergency as it signifies neuromuscular infarction and a threat to cavernous sinus extension. The following red flags have been proposed in DM patients to facilitate early recognition, testing, and intervention: cranial nerve palsy, diplopia, sinus pain, proptosis, periorbital swelling, OAS, and palatal ulcer [16].

Mucormycosis is caused by fungi belonging to the class *Zygomycetes* and the order *Mucorales*, which comprise *Rhizopus*, *Mucor*, *Rhizomucor*, *Lichtheimia* (*Absidia*), *Apophysomyces*, *Cunninghamella*, *Saksenaea*, *Cokeromyces*, *Actinomucor*, *Mortierella*, and *Syncephalastrum* [65, 76]. These organisms are ubiquitous in the environment, particularly in soil and decaying organic matter. The first four genera are the most commonly reported pathogens in humans [43], and *Rhizopus arrhizus* (formerly *Rhizopus oryzae*) accounts for 90% of ROCM.

Poorly controlled DM, with or without diabetic ketoacidosis (DKA), is the leading predisposing factor for mucormycosis globally, especially in Asian and African countries. In a meta-analysis of 851 cases, DM is reported as the commonest underlying condition and an independent risk for ROCM (odds ratio 2.49), with an overall mortality of 46% [28]. Other risk factors include prolonged neutropenia, hematological malignancies, other malignancies, allogeneic bone marrow transplantation, solid organ transplantation, corticosteroids and other immunosuppressive agents, open wounds, burns, illicit intravenous drug use, chronic malnutrition, AIDS, liver disease, chronic kidney disease, and post-pulmonary tuberculosis [5, 70, 71, 76]. Iron overload and deferoxamine treatment for iron chelation are other specific risk factors, because some fungi like *Rhizopus* can bind to deferoxamine which supplies the organism with extra iron for its growth [18, 27]. Hematological malignancies and transplantation are more prevalent risk factors among patients in Western countries [76].

Like aspergillosis, mucormycosis usually begins in the paranasal sinuses through inhalation of spores into the oral and nasal cavities. These fungal hyphae are angioinvasive and cause necrotizing vasculitis and thrombosis, resulting in extensive infarction and necrosis of host tissues (hence the name "black fungus" because it turns tissues black). The disease can spread to the orbit by direct extension, via hematogenous route or via nasolacrimal duct. Intracranial extension may give rise to grave conditions like cavernous sinus thrombosis, sagittal sinus thrombosis, carotid artery occlusion, cerebral infarction, cerebral aneurysm, and brain abscesses.

Because clinical diagnosis has a low sensitivity and specificity, laboratory testing remains an invaluable tool. Direct microscopy of specimens obtained from the nasal cavity and paranasal sinuses show broad ribbon-like nonseptate or pauci-septate hyphae forming right-angle branching. Culture in Sabouraud's dextrose agar shows typical findings of cottony white or grayish black colonies. Histopathology by hematoxylin and eosin (H&E), PAS, or GMS stains can demonstrate the characteristic fungal hyphae. It is indispensable by showing necrotizing vasculitis with invasion of vessel walls by fungal hyphae. Alternative techniques for tissue diagnosis include immunohistochemistry, PCR, and in situ hybridization [22, 76].

The management of ROCM requires early diagnosis and high index of suspicion. Due to its rapid progression and destructive nature, empirical antifungal therapy should be started once the diagnosis is considered. A delay of even 6 days in initiating treatment is associated with a doubling of 30-day mortality from 35% to 66%. Antifungal therapy consists of systemic conventional or liposomal amphotericin B or combination therapy with amphotericin B and posaconazole or caspofungin. Isavuconazole can be used as salvage therapy. Reversal of predisposing risk factors if possible and control of systemic conditions like hyperglycemia and DKA are essential.

The global guidelines for diagnosis and management of mucormycosis in 2019 by the European Confederation of Medical Mycology (ECMM) and Mycoses Study Group Education and Research Consortium (MSGERC) recommends an early surgical intervention in addition to systemic antifungal treatment [15]. Surgical debridement of infected and necrotic tissue, with drainage of infected parental sinuses should be performed. It reduces the fungal load in the tissue and allows for better penetration of intravenous drugs.

Medical management alone with antifungal is ineffective because extensive vascular thrombosis and ischemic necrosis prevent entry of antifungal in adequate concentrations.

Some centers advocate aggressive surgical debridement of sinuses with orbital exenteration. However, there are reports of success with a more conservative approach with limited or no surgical intervention in the orbit [22]. There remains a lack of consensus regarding the indications for exenteration. A retrospective study concluded that there was no added survival benefit. Some series have even found exenteration to be detrimental because it allows for further dissemination of the infection [52].

Various treatment modalities have been employed to avoid orbital exenteration [63]. Frozen section monitoring of the surgical margin has been utilized with success. Drug-soaked packing of the affected orbit and sinuses and direct irrigation with amphotericin B via percutaneous catheters might enhance direct drug delivery to the infected tissues. Hirabayashi et al. have reported a successful case managed with retrobulbar injections of amphotericin B [25]. Hyperbaric oxygen therapy has been tried to improve survival rate through several mechanisms such as promoting the fungicidal effect of neutrophils and macrophages.

In a review of 145 patients by Yohai et al., the following factors were associated with a lower survival rate: delayed diagnosis and treatment, hemiparesis or hemiplegia, bilateral sinus involvement, leukemia, renal disease, and treatment with deferoxamine [89].

12.2.2.1 COVID-19-Associated Mucormycosis (CAM)

The coronavirus disease 2019 (COVID-19) first documented in Wuhan, China, has rapidly become a global public health crisis. COVID-19 is caused by a novel coronavirus SARS-CoV-2. As of this writing, 181 million confirmed COVID-19 cases were reported worldwide, with more than 3.9 million deaths [84]. Patients with COVID-19 are at increased risk of a wide range of secondary bacterial and fungal infections which complicate their clinical course. Fungal infections are more likely to develop during the middle and later stages of COVID-19 infection. The mortality rate is higher among COVID-19 patients with secondary fungal infections (53% vs. 31%).

Ismaiel et al. in Egypt have reported a threefold rise in the incidence of acute invasive fungal rhinosinusitis in 2020 compared to those of the previous 3 years. Sixty-two percent of these patients suffered from COVID-19. The most common organisms were *Rhizopus arrhizus*, *Aspergillus fumigatus*, and *Absidia mucor* [27]. In India, there was an explosion of cases [20], with an estimated number of cases of over 4000 in May 2021 [57]. Patel et al. conducted a nationwide, retrospective multicenter study across India between September and December 2020. They found a 2.1-fold increase in mucormycosis cases when compared with the corresponding study period in 2019. Among the total 287 patients with mucormycosis, 65.2% had CAM [61].

Multiple factors may contribute to the vulnerability of COVID-19 patients to secondary fungal infections:

- Hypoxia due to acute respiratory distress syndrome (ARDS), hyperglycemia (corticosteroid-induced or pre-existing DM), and acidosis facilitate the germination of fungal spores.
- SARS-CoV-2 can infect the beta cells of the pancreas with the possibility of causing hyperglycemia.
- Iron overload. The binding of iron to ferritin and transferrin is reduced in acidosis.
- Shared pre-existing comorbid risk factors for COVID-19 and invasive fungal rhinosinusitis. DM is an independent risk factor for both COVID-19 and mucormycosis.
- Hypoxia may exacerbate the tissue infarction caused by angioinvasion of fungal hyphae.
- SARS-CoV-2 also induces endothelialitis and microvascular thrombosis in the pulmonary and extrapulmonary vascular beds [32].
- Damage to the lung tissues by SARS-CoV-2 puts the patients vulnerable to develop invasive fungal infections [5].
- Immune dysregulation with decreased number of CD4+ and CD8+ T lymphocytes, overexpression of inflammatory cytokines, and reduced phagocytic activity of white blood cells.
- Widespread and inappropriate use of corticosteroids.
- Liberal and empirical use of broad-spectrum antibiotics may suppress normal bacterial flora allowing fungi to colonize.
- ICU admission, long duration of hospital stay, mechanical ventilation.

Ashour et al. published a radiological case series of acute invasive fungal rhino-orbital-cerebral sinusitis (AIFS) patients. At least six out of the eight cases were mucormycosis. Symptoms of fungal sinusitis started 12–35 days after the COVID-19 diagnosis. There was moderate to severe mucosal thickening of variable sinuses. Their cases illustrated that the imaging findings associated with COVID-19 infection were not different from those reported in non-COVID-19 cases. However, these patients had numerous features commonly identified at an aggressive late stage. These included panophthalmitis, orbital compartment syndrome, optic nerve infiltration, osteonecrosis of the hard palate, and nasal septum. Intracranial complications included perineural spread along the trigeminal nerve, meningeal infiltration, cavernous sinus thrombosis, vasculitis/thrombosis of the cavernous segment of the internal carotid artery, mycotic aneurysm, cerebral abscess, and cerebral infarction.

Their mortality and long-term morbidity were 37.5% and 100%, respectively [2].

Mucormycosis can develop during the course of COVID-19 or during the recovery phase.

Werthman-Ehrenreich first reported a 33-year-old woman with concurrent new onset DKA, COVID-19, ROCM, and orbital compartment syndrome. She presented with cough, shortness of breath, and vomiting followed by altered mental status. An emergent lateral canthotomy was performed due to raised intraocular pressure. MRI of the brain revealed evidence of cerebral infarction which later evolved to bifrontal brain abscesses. The patient succumbed on day 26 [83].

Another 24-year-old obese woman who presented with facial pain, facial numbness, and lid swelling was similarly diagnosed with new onset DKA, rhino-orbital mucormycosis, and COVID-19. Fungal culture revealed *Lichtheimia* (*Absidia*). There was a rapid progression of eschar on her face over a few days. She died of septic shock and multi-organ failure eventually [82].

Karimi-Galougahi et al. reported a 61-year-old female with good past health who was hospitalized with COVID-19 for 2 weeks. She was treated with remdesivir, interferon-alpha, and corticosteroid during hospitalization. She did not require mechanical ventilation. One week later she developed symptoms of invasive mucormycosis including facial pain, facial numbness, and visual loss. On examination, there was an eschar over the nasal, malar, and periorbital regions on top of the typical signs of OAS. Blood glucose levels were elevated. CT and MRI showed acute maxillary and ethmoid sinusitis and intraorbital fat involvement. Unfortunately she required orbital exenteration despite treatment with insulin, systemic antifungals, and endoscopic debridement. This is a case of new-onset DM and immunosuppression induced by systemic corticosteroids [32].

Another 60-year-old male, long-standing DM patient received meropenem, oseltamivir, methylprednisolone, dexamethasone, and tocilizumab for the treatment of COVID-19. Rhino-orbital mucormycosis started on the right side on day 10. On the next day, the left eye appeared fixed, and the left pupil was dilated and nonreactive to light, with the authors suggesting that it was either due to the spread of infection or COVID-19 coagulopathy. He was treated with amphotericin B and enoxaparine. This man unfortunately died on day 6 [47].

Sen et al. presented a case series of six consecutive patients managed at their centers in India over 4.5 months. Their mean age was 60.5 (range: 46.2–73.9) years. All patients were male with DM, and two of them were newly diagnosed. Three had DKA during hospitalization for COVID-19. All but one received systemic corticosteroid treatment for COVID-19 and developed symptoms of rhino-orbital mucormycosis after recovering from COVID-19, with a time lag of 15.6 ± 9.6 days (range: 3–42 days) from the diagnosis of COVID-19. Intracranial extension was common and visual recovery was poor. Two underwent orbital exenteration, and all six patients were alive at their last follow-up [70].

Bayram et al. evaluated 11 patients from Turkey over 9 months [4]. Their mean age was 73.1 (range: 61–88) years. Nine were male, eight had uncontrolled DM, and 63.6% developed OAS. Three had cerebral involvement. All patients had received corticosteroids for the treatment of ARDS. The mean time interval between diagnosis of COVID-19 and mucormycosis was 14.4 ± 4.3 days. Despite treatment with intravenous and retrobulbar/intravitreal liposomal amphotericin B and radical surgical debridement, the mortality was 63.6% with a mean duration of follow-up of 51.2 (range: 15–153) days.

Singh et al. conducted a systematic review of case reports and case series published up to May 13, 2021. They found a total of 101 cases of mucormycosis in COVID-19 patients have been reported. Most cases (81.2%) were from India. DM was present in 80% of cases (DKA 14.9%). Corticosteroids were given for COVID-19 in 76.3% of cases. Mucormycosis was predominantly seen in males (78.9%), both in people who were active (59.4%) or recovered (40.6%) from COVID-19. Mucormycosis involving the nose and sinuses (88.9%) was most common followed by rhino-orbital (56.7%) and ROCM (22.2%). Mortality was noted in 30.7% of cases [75].

These case examples and systematic review highlight the importance of considering mycotic co-infection in COVID-19 patients. Given the rapid upsurge in the incidence of CAM, the Pan American Health Organization/World Health Organization has issued an alert and guidance to its member states to prepare for this devastating crisis [57]. In fact, diagnostic and management challenges of CAM are even greater than those of mucormycosis without COVID-19, given the critical conditions that many patients are suffering with ARDS, hemodynamic instability, and multi-organ dysfunction. These preclude timely diagnostic imaging, testing, and surgical debridement.

12.2.3 Herpes Zoster Ophthalmicus

Herpes zoster ophthalmicus (HZO) refers to herpes zoster affecting the ophthalmic branch of the trigeminal nerve, which accounts for 10–20% of overall herpes zoster occurrence [44]. HZO develops after the reactivation of latent varicella zoster virus (VZV) infection in the trigeminal ganglion. Most patients belong to the older age group, over the age of 50, when VZV-specific cell-mediated immunity declines. During the pre-antiviral era, 50% of HZO patients developed ocular complications [23], for example, blepharitis, keratoconjunctivitis, anterior uveitis, and scleritis. Furthermore, it may give rise to acute phthisis bulbi, central retinal artery occlusion, acute retinal necrosis, cataract, or secondary glaucoma. Ophthalmoplegia with involvement of the oculomotor nerve, trochlear nerve, or abducens nerve has been documented in 3.5% and 9.8% of HZO cases in the Mayo Clinic series and the Moorfields Eye Hospital series, respectively [46, 85]. OAS is a rare but serious vision-threatening complication of HZO.

Multiple mechanisms have been proposed in the pathogenesis of OAS secondary to HZO. Different pathogenic mechanisms may be associated with different prognoses:

1. In many reported cases, HZO-induced optic neuritis in immunocompetent patients. It points towards an immune-mediated mechanism of damage. The immune response is both humoral and cell-mediated.
2. Naumann et al. described chronic inflammatory cell infiltration along the long posterior ciliary nerves and vessels in 21 enucleated eyes affected by HZO. Ocular ischemia due to extensive inflammation around the posterior ciliary nerves and vessels has been postulated to contribute to optic nerve dysfunction [51].
3. Orbital soft tissue edema or myositis produces a compressive effect on the surrounding cranial nerves.
4. Direct viral cytopathic effect caused by dissemination of VZV from trigeminal nerve to the neighboring cranial nerves, due to their close proximity at the orbital apex, superior orbital fissure, or cavernous sinus.
5. Demyelination of the cranial nerves with perivascular monocytic infiltrates of the vessels supplying these nerves [37].

A literature search for articles published in English from 1997 to 2020, and review of these cases showed that the mean age of patients was 67.4 years (range: 29–84 years). In addition, 48% were male (Table 12.1). Nine of these previously reported cases had backgrounds of immunocompromised state. One had chronic lymphocytic leukemia for 19 years treated with pulse chemotherapy [11]. Saxena et al. reported a 29-year-old patient newly diagnosed with human immunodeficiency virus (HIV) infection. HIV was suspected due to her atypical age, severity of presentation, and the presence of soft exudates in the retina. Her ocular motility and visual acuity improved by the end of the fourth week after treatment. The authors attributed her favorable outcome to the prompt initiation of highly active antiretroviral therapy (HAART) and judicious use of systemic corticosteroids with rapid tapering over 10 days [69]. Another patient had a history of multiple myeloma and had recently received a course of chemotherapy. Despite treatment with intravenous acyclovir and oral steroids, he made a minimal recovery at 8 months. The authors suspected ischemic vasculitis to be the cause of irreversible damage [19]. Another six patients had diabetes mellitus (Table 12.1).

The diagnosis of OAS secondary to HZO is primarily based on clinical assessment. Patients typically present with rash, swelling of eyelids, visual loss, periorbital pain, and headache. Systemic symptoms like fever, anorexia, nausea, vomiting, malaise, and dizziness may occur [38, 45, 48]. On examination, periocular edema, conjunctival injection, chemosis, ptosis, proptosis, reduced visual acuity, complete ophthalmoplegia, reduced sensation in the territory of the ophthalmic division of the trigeminal nerve, diminished corneal sensation, anisocoria, and relative afferent pupillary defect may be observed. Swollen optic disc may be found [19, 81]. Intraocular pressure can be elevated [19, 29, 77]. Ophthalmoplegia and optic nerve involvement usually manifest within the first 2 weeks following the appearance of herpetic skin eruptions [30, 38]. By definition, visual acuity was always impaired, from 0.4 to no perception of light (Table 12.1).

Crusted and vesiculopustular skin eruptions in the dermatome of the ophthalmic nerve (upper eyelid, forehead, and tip and side of the nose) are almost always present. Dermatomal involvement can be minimal as compared to the ocular manifestations. It highlights the fact that the severity of cutaneous involvement may not correlate well with that of ophthalmic involvement [30]. Even a single lesion in the territory of the nasociliary nerve (Hutchinson's sign—lesions at the tip, side, or root of the nose) should alert the clinicians owing to its strong prediction of ocular inflammation and corneal denervation.

CT scan of the orbit shows exophthalmos, soft tissue swelling, and myositis with enlargement of the extraocular muscles [19, 48]. Unlike bacterial and fungal causes of OAS, there is no paranasal sinus involvement.

The characteristic MRI findings were first described by Krasnianski et al. and Shirato et al. [34, 73]. Contrast-enhanced MRI with gadolinium and fat suppression sequences demonstrate exophthalmos, enhancing soft tissue swelling of periorbital tissues [1, 38], orbital myositis with swollen extraocular muscles [1, 9, 29, 30, 34, 38, 59, 69, 77, 78, 81], and retrobulbar fat stranding causing crowding at the orbital apex [29, 33, 69]. It is very common to detect enhancement of the retrobulbar optic nerve sheath [9, 29, 30, 33, 35, 38, 54, 59, 67, 78, 81] as well as the optic nerve [9, 34, 69, 77, 81]. Prominent superior ophthalmic veins can occasionally be present [1, 29].

Paraskevas et al. reported an interesting case with increased T2 signal intensity along the spinal trigeminal tract and nucleus within the medulla oblongata and pons, suggesting an anterograde transsynaptic spread of the virus with high neurotropism [59]. Xiao et al. mentioned another patient with concurrent T2 lesions in the ipsilateral temporo-occipital lobe and cerebellar hemisphere with dural enhancement, suggestive of meningoencephalitis [86]. Other associated intracranial involvements can sometimes be

Table 12.1 Reported cases of OAS secondary to HZO

	Gender/age	Comorbidities	Treatment	Ptosis/ocular motility recovery	Visual recovery
Chang-Godinich et al. [11]	F/72	Chronic lymphocytic leukemia	Oral acyclovir for several days followed by IV acyclovir for 6 days (for rash). Oral acyclovir for 3 months, oral prednisolone with tapering for 8 weeks	2 mm residual ptosis, mild adduction, and elevation deficits after 8 weeks of treatment	VA 0.1–0.8 after 8 weeks of treatment
Krasnianski et al. [34]	F/67	–	IV acyclovir for 10 days, IV prednisolone then oral taper	–	VA 0.3–0.6 within 2 weeks
Shin et al. [72]	M/70	–	IV acyclovir for 3 days. IM dexamethasone for 10 days followed by oral prednisolone tapered over 4 weeks	Ptosis and ophthalmoplegia recovered except adduction 6 months after the onset of herpes zoster	–
Dhingra et al. [19]	M/63	Multiple myeloma recently completed a course of chemotherapy	IV acyclovir followed by oral, stopped within 2 weeks. Oral prednisolone tapered over 2 months	Complete ptosis, minimal ocular movement 8 months after presentation	VA 0.1 to HM 8 months after presentation; disc pale
Shirato et al. [73]	M/71	Colonic carcinoma	Oral prednisolone at the 22nd day after the onset of periocular pain	Ptosis and abduction palsy after 291 day	0.06 after the 22nd day, did not improve during the 10 month follow-up period; optic atrophy
Saxena et al. [69]	F/29	HIV infection	HAART, oral acyclovir. Oral prednisolone 5 days later. By the tenth day, steroids were tapered over the next 10 days HAART and acyclovir were continued	Ocular motility and ptosis improved at the end of 4 weeks	VA 0.03–0.8 at the end of 4 weeks
Ugarte et al. [77]	F/80	Migraine, HT, hypercholesterolemia	Oral acyclovir for 1 week (for rash). Ten days later, oral acyclovir and prednisolone (with tapering) for 2 months	Ocular motility: near complete recovery 6 months later	VA HM to 0.67 6 months later
Kurimoto et al. [35]	F/81	–	IV vidarabine and betamethasone. Vidarabine and IV prednisolone about 17 days later, followed by tapering	Ptosis had recovered by 11 weeks after the start of treatment, limited abduction at 20 weeks	VA 0.4–1.0 at 12 weeks after onset
Arda et al. [1]	M/75	HT	Oral fluocortolone switched to oral valacyclovir and then switched to IV acyclovir. Tapering dose of oral prednisolone after acute symptoms improved	Partial improvement in ptosis and ocular motility at the end of 5 month follow-up period	HM to CF from 1.5 months (did not significantly improve because of cataract and choroidal detachment)
Paraskevas et al. [59]	F/67	–	Oral acyclovir for 1 week (for HZO). About 4 weeks later, IV acyclovir for 10 days, IVMP for 5 days	Slow saccades 5 months later	VA 0.2 to marked improvement
Merino-Iglesias et al. [48]	M/61	–	IV acyclovir for 7 days followed by oral antiviral. Oral methylprednisolone for 7 days then tapered over 10 weeks	Ocular motility was completely restored	VA CF from 1 month to 1.0 after 1 year
Ugurlu et al. [78]	F/49	No chronic illness	Oral brivudine (for HZO). IV acyclovir and oral prednisolone and then oral acyclovir and prednisolone both tapered over 3 months	Complete recovery of extraocular motility	VA 0.1–0.67 at 5 months after presentation
Lee et al. [38]	M/78	DM, chronic obstructive pulmonary disease	IV acyclovir for 15 days, oral prednisolone for 4 days followed by monthly taper over 12 weeks	Limitation of abduction and paralysis of the upper eyelid at 180 days	VA 0.05–0.2

Table 12.1 (continued)

	Gender/age	Comorbidities	Treatment	Ptosis/ocular motility recovery	Visual recovery
Xiao et al. [86]	F/65	(Immunocompetent)	IV ganciclovir. IV dexamethasone. Oral prednisolone tapered over 6 weeks	Persistent ophthalmoplegia 3 months later	Persistent blindness 3 months later
Kalamkar et al. [30]	M/65	–	IVMP for 3 days followed by oral steroid tapered over 2 months. Oral acyclovir	Limited abduction at 6 month follow-up	Light perception (no improvement) at 6 month follow-up; optic atrophy
Verhaeghe et al. [81]	M/80	Bilateral cataract surgery, myocardial infarction, atrial fibrillation, corneal foreign body (removed)	Oral acyclovir for 1 week (for keratitis), followed by IV acyclovir for 14 days. IVMP for 15 days after 7 days of IV acyclovir. Then oral valacyclovir and prednisolone, tapered over 2 months	Ptosis had resolved and ocular motility had improved at 5 months	VA CF to 0.4 at 5 months; optic disc pale
Chandrasekharan et al. [9]	F/60	HT, DM	IVMP for 3 days followed by oral prednisolone tapered over 4 weeks. Oral acyclovir	Mild ptosis. -1 limitation of adduction, elevation, and depression	HM to 0.5 at 3 months; optic disc pallor
Lim et al. [45]	F/77	HT	Oral acyclovir for 2 months. Oral prednisolone tapered over 2 months	Full extraocular movements at 2 months Partial ptosis	Light perception at 2 months (remained poor due to extensive vascularization and scarring of the cornea)
Lim et al. [45]	M/65	DM	Oral acyclovir for 10 days	Mild ptosis and full eye movements at 6 weeks	VA 0.033–0.25 at 6 weeks (worsening of nuclear sclerosis)
Othman et al. [55]	F/59	HT, DM, asthma	Oral acyclovir followed by IV acyclovir and oral prednisolone for 2 weeks, then oral acyclovir for 12 weeks and oral prednisolone tapered over 6 weeks	Full ocular motility at 6 weeks later	Light perception to 0.16 (hyphema) 6 weeks later
Jun et al. [29]	M/67	HT, DM, hyperlipidemia, ischemic heart disease	Oral acyclovir (for HZO) followed by IV acyclovir for 22 days, followed by oral valacyclovir for 4 weeks	Complete ophthalmoplegia 9 months later	No perception of light 9 months later; optic atrophy
Kocaoğlu et al. [33]	M/67	HT, DM	Oral valacyclovir. Pulse prednisolone for 5 days followed by oral prednisolone tapered over 4 months	Ptosis and ophthalmoplegia regressed at 2 months after diagnosis of OAS	VA 0.2–0.4 at 2 months after diagnosis of OAS (permanent); temporal disc pallor
Ruiz-Arranz et al. [67]	F/84	Hypothyroidism, multinodular goiter, asthma, pulmonary hypertension, nocturnal apnea syndrome, congenital dyserythropoietic hemolytic anemia type II, bilateral pseudophakia, age-related macular degeneration	Oral acyclovir (for rash) Oral valacyclovir IV acyclovir and IVMP for 10 days, followed by prednisolone tapered over 10 weeks and oral valacyclovir	Slight abduction limitation	VA 0.05–0.2; slight papillary pallor

CF counting fingers, *DM* diabetes mellitus, *HAART* highly active antiretroviral therapy, *HM* hand movements, *HT* hypertension, *IV* intravenous, *IVMP* intravenous methylprednisolone, *VA* visual acuity detected including cavernous sinus involvement [29, 35, 67], extension to Meckel's cave [67], diffusion abnormalities in the frontal and frontoparietal regions [1], and transverse sinus thrombosis [33].

Laboratory tests including complete blood count with differential, erythrocyte sedimentation rate, and C-reactive protein are usually normal [9, 30, 69, 77]. Cerebrospinal fluid analysis may reveal lymphocytic pleocytosis and elevated protein level [9, 29, 35, 59, 86]. VZV DNA by polymerase chain reaction can be positive [29]. Positive IgG antibodies against VZV in the blood or CSF were reported in three cases [35, 55, 59].

Visual evoked potentials have been performed in several patients. They were either not recordable [31, 69, 73] or with reduced amplitude and delayed latency [34].

Optimal therapy for OAS secondary to HZO has not been studied with a randomized controlled trial, and there is no standard regimen. In most reported cases, a core combination of systemic corticosteroids and systemic antivirals, either oral or intravenous, was employed (Table 12.1). For the best results, antiviral treatment should be started within 72 h of the onset of rash. Options for antivirals include acyclovir, valacyclovir, and famciclovir. Systemic corticosteroids are used to mitigate the inflammatory response to VZV and are usually given in the form of intravenous methylprednisolone or oral prednisolone. Duration of corticosteroid treatment varies in literature from 2 weeks to 6 months.

As stated in the case reports, there were variable improvements in ptosis, ocular motility, and visual function. As discussed, different pathogenic mechanisms involved may affect the prognosis. Orbital myositis may cause temporary compression on the structures at the orbital apex and carry a better outcome as the congestion resolves. On the other hand, occlusive vasculitis may cause permanent damage and irreversible visual loss [19]. From Table 12.1, we can appreciate that 15 patients (68%, one missing data) showed some recovery of visual acuity, but a complete resolution was rather uncommon (8.7%) [35, 48]. Overall, complete or near resolution of ophthalmoplegia secondary to HZO has been reported to occur in 65% of cases and may take between 2 weeks and 1.5 years to achieve (mean: 4.4 months) [68].

References

1. Arda H, Mirza E, Gumus K, Oner A, Karakucuk S, Sirakaya E. Orbital apex syndrome in herpes zoster ophthalmicus. Case Rep Ophthalmol Med. 2012;2012:1–4.
2. Ashour MM, Abdelaziz TT, Ashour DM, Askoura A, Saleh MI, Mahmoud MS. Imaging spectrum of acute invasive fungal rhino-orbital-cerebral sinusitis in COVID-19 patients: a case series and a review of literature. J Neuroradiol. 2021; https://doi.org/10.1016/j.neurad.2021.05.007.
3. Badakere A, Patil-Chhablani P. Orbital apex syndrome: a review. Eye Brain. 2019;11:63–72.
4. Bayram N, Ozsaygılı C, Sav H, Tekin Y, Gundogan M, Pangal E, Cicek A, Özcan İ. Susceptibility of severe COVID-19 patients to rhino-orbital mucormycosis fungal infection in different clinical manifestations. Jpn J Ophthalmol. 2021;65:515–25. https://doi.org/10.1007/s10384-021-00845-5.
5. Bhatt K, Agolli A, Patel MH, Garimella R, Devi M, Garcia E, Amin H, Domingue C, Guerra Del Castillo R, Sanchez-Gonzalez M. High mortality co-infections of COVID-19 patients: mucormycosis and other fungal infections. Discoveries (Craiova). 2021;9(1):e126.
6. Bodily L, Yu J, Sorrentino D, Branstetter B. Invasive Streptococcus viridans sphenoethmoiditis leading to an orbital apex syndrome. Am J Ophthalmol Case Rep. 2017;8:4–6.
7. Chandler JR, Langenbrunner DJ, Stevens ER. The pathogenesis of orbital complications in acute sinusitis. Laryngoscope. 1970;80(9):1414–28.
8. Chandra P, Ahluwalia BK, Chugh TD. Primary orbital aspergilloma. Br J Ophthalmol. 1970;54(10):693–6.
9. Chandrasekharan A, Gandhi U, Badakere A, Sangwan V. Orbital apex syndrome as a complication of herpes zoster ophthalmicus. BMJ Case Rep. 2017;2017:bcr2016217382.
10. Chang YM, Chang YH, Chien KH, Liang CM, Tai MC, Nieh S, Chen YJ. Orbital apex syndrome secondary to aspergilloma masquerading as a paranasal sinus tumor. A case report and literature review. Medicine (Baltimore). 2018;97(30):e11650.
11. Chang-Godinich A, Lee AG, Brazis PW, Liesegang TJ, Jones DB. Complete ophthalmoplegia after zoster ophthalmicus. J Neuroophthalmol. 1997;17(4):262–5.
12. Cheko A, Jung S, Teuber-Hanselmann S, Oseni AW, Tsogkas A, Scholz M, Petridis AK. Orbital apex syndrome caused by aspergilloma in an immunocompromised patient with cutaneous lymphoma: a case report of a rare entity. S Afr Med J. 2016;106(4):46–7.
13. Cho SH, Jin BJ, Lee YS, Paik SS, Ko MK, Yi HJ. Orbital apex syndrome in a patient with sphenoid fungal balls. Clin Exp Otorhinolaryngol. 2009;2(1):52–4.
14. Colson AE, Daily JP. Orbital apex syndrome and cavernous sinus thrombosis due to infection with Staphylococcus aureus and Pseudomonas aeruginosa. Clin Infect Dis. 1999;29:701–2.
15. Cornely OA, Alastruey-Izquierdo A, Arenz D, et al. Global guideline for the diagnosis and management of mucormycosis: an initiative of the European Confederation of Medical Mycology in cooperation with the Mycoses Study Group Education and Research Consortium. Lancet Infect Dis. 2019;19(12):e405–21.
16. Corzo-León DE, Chora-Hernández LD, Rodríguez-Zulueta AP, Walsh TJ. Diabetes mellitus as the major risk factor for mucormycosis in Mexico: epidemiology, diagnosis, and outcomes of reported cases. Med Mycol. 2018;56(1):29–43.
17. Denning DW. Invasive aspergillosis. Clin Infect Dis. 1998;26(4):781–803.
18. Deutsch PG, Whittaker J, Prasad S. Invasive and non-invasive fungal rhinosinusitis — a review and update of the evidence. Medicina (Kaunas). 2019;55(7):319.
19. Dhingra S, Williams G, Pearson A. Severe permanent orbital disease in herpes zoster ophthalmicus. Orbit. 2008;27(4):325–7.
20. Gandra S, Ram S, Levitz SM. The "black fungus" in India: the emerging syndemic of COVID-19-associated mucormycosis. Ann Intern Med. 2021;174:1301. https://doi.org/10.7326/M21-2354.
21. Goyal P, Lee S, Gupta N, Kumar Y, Mangla M, Hooda K, Li S, Mangla R. Orbital apex disorders: imaging findings and management. Neuroradiol J. 2018;31(2):104–25.
22. Gupta S, Goyal R, Kaore NM. Rhino-orbital-cerebral mucormycosis: battle with the deadly enemy. Indian J Otolaryngol Head Neck Surg. 2020;72(1):104–11.

23. Harding S, Lipton J, Wells J. Natural history of herpes zoster ophthalmicus: predictors of postherpetic neuralgia and ocular involvement. Br J Ophthalmol. 1987;71(5):353–8.
24. Herbrecht R, Denning DW, Patterson TF, et al. Voriconazole versus amphotericin B for primary therapy of invasive aspergillosis. N Engl J Med. 2002;347(6):408–15.
25. Hirabayashi KE, Kalin-Hajdu E, Brodie FL, Kersten RC, Russell MS, Vagefi MR. Retrobulbar injection of amphotericin B for orbital mucormycosis. Ophthal Plast Reconstr Surg. 2017;33(4):e94–7.
26. Huang Y, Gui L. Cavernous sinus-orbital apex aspergillus infection in a diabetic patient. A case report. Medicine. 2019;98:e15041.
27. Ismaiel WF, Abdelazim MH, Eldsoky I, Ibrahim AA, Alsobky ME, Zafan E, Hasan A. The impact of COVID-19 outbreak on the incidence of acute invasive fungal rhinosinusitis. Am J Otolaryngol. 2021;42(6):103080.
28. Jeong W, Keighley C, Wolfe R, Lee WL, Slavin MA, Kong DC, Chen SCA. The epidemiology and clinical manifestations of mucormycosis. A systematic review and meta-analysis of case reports. Clin Microbiol Infect. 2019;25(1):26–34.
29. Jun LH, Gupta A, Milea D, Jaufeerally FR. More than meets the eye: varicella zoster virus-related orbital apex syndrome. Indian J Ophthalmol. 2018;66(11):1647–9.
30. Kalamkar C, Radke N, Mukherjee A, Radke S. A rare case of orbital apex syndrome in herpes zoster ophthalmicus. J Clin Diagn Res. 2016;10(6):ND04–5.
31. Kalamkar et al: https://pubmed.ncbi.nlm.nih.gov/27504322/.
32. Karimi-Galougahi M, Arastou S, Haseli S. Fulminant mucormycosis complicating coronavirus disease 2019 (COVID-19). Int Forum Allergy Rhinol. 2021;11(6):1029–30.
33. Kocaoğlu G, Utine CA, Yaman A, Men S. Orbital apex syndrome secondary to herpes zoster ophthaimicus. Turk J Ophthalmol. 2018;48(1):42–6.
34. Krasnianski M, Sievert M, Bau V, Zierz S. External ophthalmoplegia due to ocular myositis in a patient with ophthalmic herpes zoster. Neuromuscul Disord. 2004;14(7):438–41.
35. Kurimoto T, Tonari M, Ishizaki N, Monta M, Hirata S, Oku H, Sugasawa J, Ikeda T. Orbital apex syndrome associated with herpes zoster ophthalmicus. Clin Ophthalmol. 2011;5:1603–8.
36. Kusunoki T, Kase K, Ikeda K. A case of orbital apex syndrome due to Pseudomonas aeruginosa infection. Clin Pract. 2011;1:e127.
37. Lavin PJM, Yonkin SG, Kori SH. The pathology of ophthalmoplegia in herpes zoster ophthalmicus. Neuroophthalmology. 1984;4:75–80.
38. Lee CY, Tsai HC, Lee SSJ, Chen YS. Orbital apex syndrome: an unusual complication of herpes zoster ophthalmicus. BMC Infect Dis. 2015;15:33.
39. Lee AS, Lee PWY, Allworth A, Smith T, Sullivan TJ. Orbital mycoses in an adult subtropical population. Eye. 2020;34(9):1640–7.
40. Lever M, Wilde B, Pförtner R, Deuschl C, Witzke O, Bertram S, Eckstein A, Rath PM. Orbital aspergillosl: a case report and review of the literature. BMC Ophthalmol. 2021;21(1):22.
41. Levin LA, Avery R, Shore JW, Woog JJ, Baker AS. The spectrum of orbital aspergillosis: a clinicopathological review. Surv Ophthalmol. 1996;41(2):142–54.
42. Leyngold I, Olivi A, Ishii M, Blitz A, Burger P, Subramanian PS, Gallia G. Acute chiasmal abscess resulting from perineural extension of invasive sino-orbital aspergillosis in an immunocompetent patient. World Neurosurg. 2014;81(1):203.e1–6.
43. Liang KP, Tleyjeh IM, Wilson WR, Roberts GD, Temesgen Z. Rhino-orbitocerebral mucormycosis caused by Apophysomyces elegans. J Clin Microbiol. 2006;44:892–8.
44. Liesegang TJ. Herpes zoster ophthalmicus: natural history, risk factors, clinical presentation, and morbidity. Ophthalmology. 2008;115(2 Suppl):S3–S12.
45. Lim JJ, Ong YM, Zalina MZW, Choo MM. Herpes zoster ophthalmicus with orbital apex syndrome - difference in outcomes and literature review. Ocul Immunol Inflamm. 2018;26(2):187–93.
46. Marsh RJ, Cooper M. Ophthalmic herpes zoster. Eye (Lond). 1993;7(Pt 3):350–70.
47. Mehta S, Pandey A. Rhino-orbital mucormycosis associated with COVID-19. Cureus. 2020;12:e10726.
48. Mo-Iglesias A, Montero JA, Calabuig-Goena M, Giraldo-Agudelo LF. Orbital apex syndrome secondary to herpes zoster virus infection. BMJ Case Rep. 2014;2014:bcr2013203200. https://pubmed.ncbi.nlm.nih.gov/24614776/.
49. Mody KH, Ali MJ, Vemuganti GK, Nalamada S, Nail MN, Honavar SG. Orbital aspergillosis in immunocompetent patients. Br J Ophthalmol. 2014;98(10):1379–84.
50. Mograbi AE, Ritter A, Najjar E, Soudry E. Orbital complications of rhinosinusitis in the adult population: analysis of cases presenting to a tertiary medical center over a 13-year period. Ann Otol Rhinol Laryngol. 2019;128(6):563–8.
51. Naumann G, Gass JD, Font RL. Histopathology of herpes zoster ophthalmicus. Am J Ophthalmol. 1968;65(4):533–41.
52. Nithyanandam S, Jacob MS, Battu RR, Thomas RK, Correa MA, D'Souza O. Rhino-orbito-cerebral mucormycosis. A retrospective analysis of clinical features and treatment outcomes. Indian J Ophthalmol. 2003;51(3):231–6.
53. Ohlstein DH, Hooten C, Perez J, Clark CL III, Samy H. Orbital aspergillosis: voriconazole – the new standard treatment? Case Rep Ophthalmol. 2012;3(1):46–53.
54. Othman et al: https://pubmed.ncbi.nlm.nih.gov/28061417/.
55. Othman K, Evelyn-Tai LM, Raja-Azmi MN, Julieana M, Liza-Sharmini AT, Tharakan J, Besari AM, Zunaina E, Shatriah I. Concurrent hyphema and orbital apex syndrome following herpes zoster ophthalmicus in a middle aged lady. Int J Surg Case Rep. 2017;30:197–200.
56. Oto R, Katada A, Bandoh N, Takahara M, Kishibe K, Hayashi T, Harabuchi Y. A case of invasive paranasal aspergillosis that developed from a non-invasive form during 5-year follow-up. Auris Nasus Larynx. 2010;37(2):250–4.
57. Pan American Health Organization/World Health Organization. Epidemiological alert: COVID-19 associated Mucormycosis. Washington, DC: PAHO/WHO; 2021.
58. Panda NK, Saravanan K, Chakrabarti A. Combination antifungal therapy for invasive aspergillosis: can it replace high-risk surgery at the skull base? Am J Otolaryngol. 2008;29(1):24–30.
59. Paraskevas GP, Anagnostou E, Vassilopoulou S, Spengos K. Painful ophthalmoplegia with simultaneous orbital myositis, optic and oculomotor nerve inflammation and trigeminal nucleus involvement in a patient with herpes zoster ophthalmicus. BMJ Case Rep. 2012;2012:bcr2012007063.
60. Parija S, Banerjee A. Invasive fungal disease misdiagnosed as tumour in association with orbital apex syndrome. BMJ Case Rep. 2021;14:e237626.
61. Patel A, Agarwal R, Rudramurthy SM, Shevkani M, Xess I, Sharma R, Savio J, Sethuraman N, Madan S, Shastri P, Thangaraju D, Marak R, Tadepalli K, Savaj P, Sunavala A, Gupta N, Singhal T, Muthu V, Chakrabarti A, MucoCovi Network. Multicenter epidemiologic study of coronavirus disease-associated mucormycosis, India. Emerg Infect Dis. 2021;27(9):2349. https://doi.org/10.3201/eid2709.210934.
62. Patterson TF, Thompson GR III, Denning DW, Fishman JA, Hadley S, Herbrecht R, Kontoyiannis DP, Marr KA, Morrison VA, Nguyen MH, Segal BH, Steinbach WJ, Stevens DA, Walsh TJ, Wingard JR, Young JAH, Bennett JE. Practice guidelines for the diagnosis and management of aspergillosis: 2016 update by the Infectious Diseases Society of America. Clin Infect Dis. 2016;63(4):e1–60.
63. Pelton RW, Peterson EA, Patel BCK, Davis K. Successful treatment of rhino-orbital mucormycosis without exenteration. The

use of multiple treatment modalities. Ophthal Plast Reconstr Surg. 2001;17(1):62–6.
64. Pfeiffer ML, Merritt HA, Bailey LA, Richani K, Phillips ME. Orbital apex syndrome from bacterial sinusitis without orbital cellulitis. Am J Ophthalmol Case Rep. 2018;10:84–6.
65. Rao SP, Kumar KR, Rokade VR, Khanna V, Pal C. Orbital apex syndrome due to mucormycosis caused by Rhizopus microsporum. Indian J Otolaryngol Head Neck Surg. 2006;58(1):84–7.
66. Ronen JA, Malik FA, Weichmann C, Kolli S, Nwojo R. More than meets the eye: aspergillus-related orbital apex syndrome. Cureus. 2020;12(7):e9352.
67. Ruiz-Arranz C, Reche-Sainz JA, de Uña-Iglesias MC, Ortueta-Olartecoechea A, Muñoz-Gallego A, Ferro-Osuna M. Orbital apex syndrome secondary to herpes zoster ophthalmicus. Arch Soc Esp Oftalmol (Engl Ed). 2021;96(7):384–7.
68. Sanjay S, Chan EW, Gopal L, Hegde SR, Chang BCM. Complete unilateral ophthalmoplegia in herpes zoster ophthalmicus. J Neuroophthalmol. 2009;29(4):325–37.
69. Saxena R, Phuljhele S, Aalok L, Sinha A, Menon V, Sharma P, Mohan A. A rare case of orbital apex syndrome with herpes zoster ophthalmicus in a human immunodeficiency virus-positive patient. Indian J Ophthalmol. 2010;58(6):527–30.
70. Sen M, Lahane S, Lahane TP, Parekh R, Honavar SG. Mucor in a viral land: a tale of two pathogens. Indian J Ophthalmol. 2021;69(2):244–52.
71. Shatriah I, Mohd-Amin N, Tuan-Jaafar TN, Khanna RK, Yunus R, Madhavan M. Rhino-orbito-cerebral mucormycosis in an immunocompetent patient: case report and review of literature. Middle East Afr J Ophthalmol. 2012;19(2):258–61.
72. Shin HM, Lew H, Yun YS. A case of complete ophthalmoplegia in herpes zoster ophthalmicus. Korean J Ophthalmol. 2005;19(4):302–4.
73. Shirato S, Oshitari T, Hanawa K, Adachi-Usami E. Magnetic resonance imaging in case of cortical apex syndrome caused by varicella zoster virus. Open Ophthalmol J. 2008;2:109–11.
74. Siddiqui AA, Bashir SH, Shah AA, Sajjad Z, Ahmed N, Jooma R, Enam SA. Diagnostic MR imaging features of craniocerebral Aspergillosis of sino-nasal origin in immunocompetent patients. Acta Neurochir. 2006;148(2):155–66.
75. Singh AK, Singh R, Joshi SR, Misra A. Mucormycosis in COVID-19: a systemic review of cases reported worldwide and in India. Diab Metab Syndr Clin Res Rev. 2021;15:102146. https://doi.org/10.1016/j.dsx.2021.05.019.
76. Skiada A, Pavleas I, Drogari-Apiranthitou M. Epidemiology and diagnosis of mucormycosis: an update. J Fungi (Basel). 2020;6(4):265.
77. Ugarte M, Dey S, Jones CA. Ophthalmoplegia secondary to herpes zoster ophthalmicus. BMJ Case Rep. 2010;2010:bcr1220092532.
78. Ugurlu S, Atik S, Imre SS. Orbital apex syndrome secondary to herpes zoster ophthalmicus. Neuroophthalmology. 2014;38(5):260–3.
79. Ullmann AJ, Aguado JM, Arikan-Akdagli S, et al. Diagnosis and management of Aspergillus diseases: executive summary of the 2017 ESCMID-ECMM-ERS guideline. Clin Microbiol Infect. 2018;24(Suppl 1):e1–e38.
80. Vaughan C, Bartolo A, Vallabh N, Leong SC. A meta-analysis of survival factors in rhino-orbital-cerebral mucormycosis-has anything changed in the past 20 years? Clin Otolaryngol. 2018;43(6):1454–64.
81. Verhaeghe F, Villain M, Labauge P, Daien V. Orbital apex syndrome secondary to herpes zoster ophthalmicus. J Neuroophthalmol. 2016;36(2):147–51.
82. Waizel-Haiat S, Guerrero-Paz JA, Sanchez-Hurtado L, Calleja-Alarcon S, Romero-Gutierrez L. A case of fatal rhino-orbital mucormycosis associated with new onset diabetic ketoacidosis and COVID-19. Cureus. 2021;13(2):e13163.
83. Werthman-Ehrenreich A. Mucormycosis with orbital compartment syndrome in a patient with COVID-19. Am J Emerg Med. 2021;42:264.e5–8.
84. WHO Coronavirus (COVID-19) Dashboard. 2021. https://covid19.who.int. Accessed 30 Jun 2021.
85. Womack LW, Liesegang TJ. Complications of herpes zoster ophthalmicus. Arch Ophthalmol. 1983;101(1):42–5.
86. Xiao Z, Lu Z, Pan S, Liang J, Liu Z. Orbital apex syndrome and meningoencephalitis: a rare complication of herpes zoster. Int J Clin Exp Med. 2015;8(8):14260–3.
87. Xiong M, Moy WL. Orbital apex syndrome resulting from mixed bacterial sphenoid sinusitis. Eur J Case Rep Intern Med. 2018;5:000905.
88. Yip CM, Hsu SS, Liao WC, Chen JY, Liu SH, Chen CH. Orbital apex syndrome due to aspergillosis with subsequent fatal subarachnoid hemorrhage. Surg Neurol Int. 2012;3:124.
89. Yohai RA, Bullock JD, Aziz AA, Markert RJ. Survival factors in rhino-orbital-cerebral mucormycosis. Surv Ophthalmol. 1994;1(39):3–22.
90. Zafar MA, Waheed SS, Enam SA. Orbital aspergillus infection mimicking a tumour: a case report. Cases J. 2009;2:7860.

13 Periorbital Skull Base Neoplasms

Ehsan Dowlati, Max Fleisher, and Walter C. Jean

Abstract

The anatomical relationship of the orbit and specifically the orbital apex to the skull base makes it vulnerable to neoplastic invasion or extension by skull base and primary periorbital tumors. These lesions, although rare, provide a challenge in terms of diagnosis and treatment given their location. Patients may present with proptosis, ophthalmoplegia, and/or vision loss. Workup involves imaging and biopsy in many cases. They can range from benign histology such as meningiomas to neoplastic pathologies such as aggressive sarcomas. Surgery remains the primary treatment modality in most cases. Characteristics of several tumors and neoplasms that may involve the orbit or orbital apex are discussed in this chapter including sphenoid wing meningiomas, trigeminal schwannomas, sellar region tumors, sinonasal tumors, cavernous angiomas, lymphangiomas, lymphomas, soft tissue neoplasms, and metastases.

Keywords

Skull base neoplasms · Orbital apex · Meningioma · Schwannoma · Sinonasal tumors · Metastases · Periorbital lesions

E. Dowlati
Department of Neurosurgery, MedStar Georgetown University Hospital, Washington, DC, USA

M. Fleisher
Department of Neurosurgery, George Washington University Hospital, Washington, DC, USA

W. C. Jean (✉)
Department of Neurosurgery, Lehigh Valley Health Network, Allentown, PA, USA

Department of Neurosurgery and Brain Repair, University of South Florida, Tampa, FL, USA
e-mail: Walter.Jean@lvhn.org

13.1 Introduction

Many types of neoplasms can involve the periorbital region, and whereas some originate in the orbit, the majority of these arise elsewhere in the skull base and involve the orbit secondarily by extension. The orbital apex consists of the pyramidal-shaped posterior orbit. It contains the Annulus of Zinn, a fibrous ring encompassing the ophthalmic artery and nasociliary nerve, and an attachment point for cranial nerves II, III, and VI. Invasion into the orbit or orbital apex can be further subdivided into transosseus extension, which is comparatively rare and invasion through bony apertures such as the superior orbital fissure and optic foramen. Although typically benign in nature, these tumors can be locally aggressive and most of them require surgical management. Tumors of the nasal cavity and paranasal sinuses can grow to involve the periorbital region and most of these are malignant. In this chapter, we will review various types of periorbital neoplasms, their characteristics, diagnosis and assessment pathways, and management strategies.

13.2 Clinical Presentation and Evaluation

Because of the slow-growing nature of most periorbital tumors, they may escape diagnosis until they are quite large. Similarly, tumors of the paranasal sinuses, although malignant, can grow silently and expand in the sinuses without being symptomatic. By the time these tumors are large enough to cause nasal obstruction and epistaxis, they frequently involve the orbit.

Lesions of this region can present with orbital apex syndrome, defined by compression and/or damage to neurovascular structures traversing the superior orbital fissure and optic foramen. It manifests as painful proptosis, ophthalmoplegia, and ocular vision loss. Since the orbit is a confined structure with limited space, large tumors cause proptosis, the most common presenting symptom seen in 60% of cases.

T. L. POON et al. (eds.), *Orbital Apex and Periorbital Skull Base Diseases*, https://doi.org/10.1007/978-981-99-2989-4_13

Diplopia, the second most common finding, is mostly related to compression of the nerves involved in oculomotility. Direct tumor invasion of these nerves is relatively rare. Decreased visual acuity is typically a late finding and indicates proximity to the orbital apex or optic nerve [1]. Commonly accompanying these symptoms, periorbital pain is what frequently motivates the patients to seek medical attention.

Magnetic resonance imaging (MRI) with and without gadolinium contrast provides the most detailed information about the anatomical relationship among the extraocular muscles, the cranial nerves, the globe, and the skull base, as well as an idea of the state of tumor borders and potential encapsulation. Fat-saturation sequences are often useful for tumors that may be hidden by periorbital fat. MRI can also inform the pattern of growth and whether there is bone marrow or intra-axial involvement. Computed tomography (CT) is used to assess the relationship of the lesion to the surrounding bones and sinuses and may provide critical information regarding transosseous spread or bony remodeling/erosion perpetrated by the neoplasms. Tumor histology can significantly influence management, especially for malignant disease. Since most of the malignant neoplasms in this region also involve the paranasal sinuses, endoscopic biopsy can yield valuable information. Finally, angiography, whether noninvasive (e.g., CTA, MRA) or through a catheter, can help design the best treatment for vascular tumors or those that distort the circle of Willis.

13.3 Meningiomas

Meningiomas are the most common neoplasm that invade the periorbital region, and any meningioma of the medial anterior and middle fossa, whether they arise from the tuberculum sellae, medial sphenoid wing, clinoid process, even olfactory groove, can extend to the orbital apex. Many of these will cause hyperostosis of the bony orbit, which leads to proptosis and pain. These tumors typically affect people in their sixth decade of life and women four times more frequently than men [2]. They invade the orbit in different ways, entering through the optic canal, the superior fissure, or directly through bone (Fig. 13.1). Visual loss is present in 37% of patients [3].

Cavernous sinus meningiomas neighbor the carotid artery and multiple cranial nerves. Progression of these lesions can involve the orbital apex, transosseous expansion, and invasion into the orbit via the superior orbital fissure (Fig. 13.2). Most of these present with ophthalmoplegia, mainly by compression, but sometimes by direct invasion, of cranial nerves III, IV, and VI. Finally, optic nerve sheath meningiomas contact the optic nerve and partially or completely surround it. These patients present with a gradual decrease in visual acuity by atrophy. The major risk from progression is extension through the orbital canal to the intracranial compartment and involvement of the contralateral optic nerve [4].

Meningiomas are homogeneously enhancing on MRI, and their appearances are quite typical even without calcification or dural tail. The treatment for most symptomatic or progressive periorbital meningiomas is surgical removal. Meningiomas of the orbital apex and cavernous sinus present a number of surgical challenges given their deep location, proximity to eloquent structures, and hyperostosis that is typically seen. For those that extend through bony foramina, additional drilling steps such as clinoidectomy or opening the superior orbital fissure or optic canal may be necessary. Gonen et al. propose a surgical algorithm that involves an extradural stage followed by an intradural then intraorbital stage for best results. They had a 51.8% rate of complete tumor resection. The extent of resection was limited by invasion of the cavernous sinus (61.5%) and the superior orbital fissure (84%) [3]. Most common neurologic complications included oculomotor nerve palsy and trigeminal neuropathy in 6.4% and 28%, respectively [5].

Cavernous sinus meningiomas may also be approached through the anterolateral corridor, and extradural or intradural approaches to the cavernous sinus can be done [6]. The goal of surgery is typically decompression of the neural elements and orbital compartment. For residual tumor, radiation therapy has been recommended but others reserve radiation therapy for patients with tumor progression on follow-up or after a second re-operation [7, 8]. More recently, endoscopic approaches to the orbit have been developed. These will be discussed in detail in ensuing chapters.

The prognosis for periorbital meningioma is good, with mortality rates from 0 to 14%, with most studies citing no mortality [9]. There is, however, a high recurrence rate following surgical resection, ranging from 4% to 60%, which is a major factor in prognosis [10]. Survival rates depend on histopathology and intracranial extent of involvement. There have been small case series showing efficacy of radiosurgery in the treatment of orbital apex meningiomas [11]. No effective chemotherapeutic treatment has been established. Kiyofuji et al. determined that visual field defect other than a central scotoma was the only variable on multivariate analysis to independently predict improvement [5].

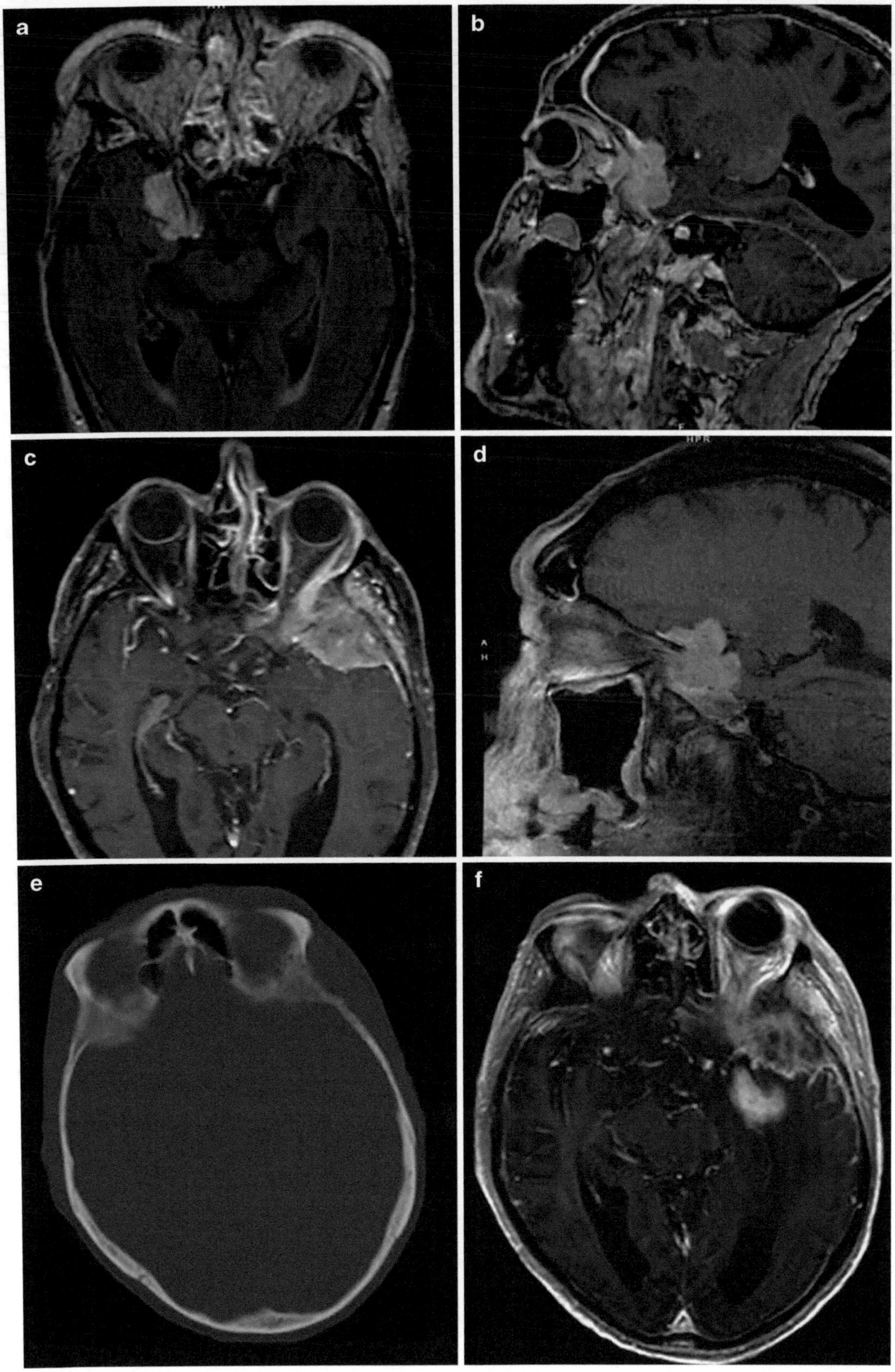

Fig. 13.1 Sphenoid wing meningiomas. A 69-year-old male presenting with right eye diplopia found to have a medial sphenoid wing meningioma on the right with extension into the orbital apex on (**a**) axial and (**b**) sagittal T1-weighted MRI with gadolinium. Patient underwent surgical resection followed by radiation. A 73-year-old male with a history of thyroid carcinoma presenting with painless vision loss in the left eye and left ptosis. (**c**) Axial and (**d**) sagittal views of a brain MRI demonstrated a left sphenoid wing meningioma with lateral orbital involvement. (**e**) Notable hyperostosis along the lateral orbital wall and sphenoid wing noted on CT. He underwent a frontotemporal craniotomy for tumor resection, and he underwent Cyberknife treatment for the residual tumor. (**f**) Post treatment MRI at 6-month follow-up demonstrated surgical and radiation induced changes

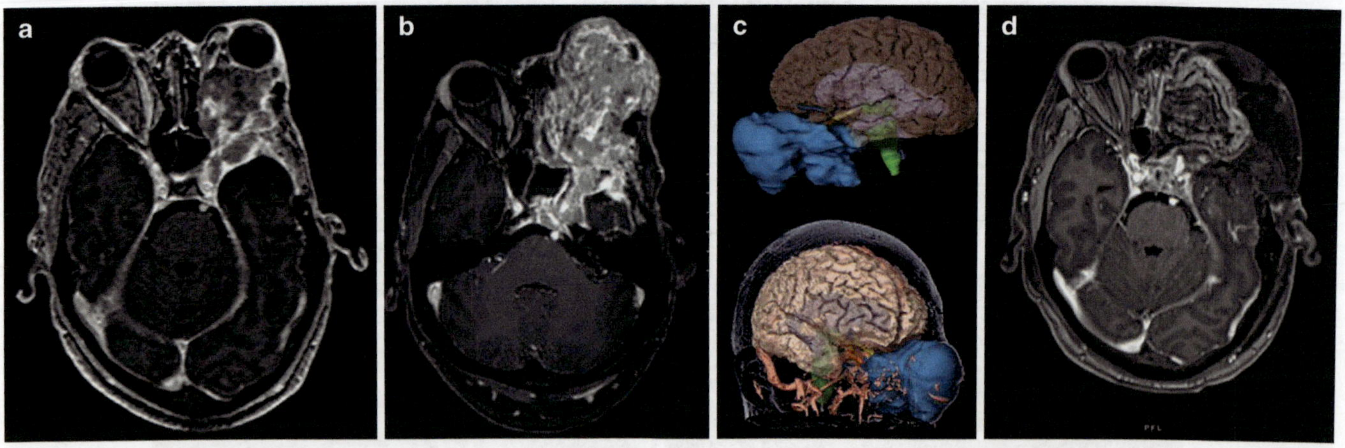

Fig. 13.2 Cavernous sinus meningioma. A 58-year-old male with history of left cavernous meningioma with orbital extension presenting with ophthalmoplegia and L orbital proptosis. (**a**) Preoperative T1-weighted MRI with gadolinium demonstrating tumor with extensive orbital involvement and proptosis. He had undergone surgical resection and radiation therapy and subsequently left globe enucleation. (**b**) Two years later, he presents with recurrent meningioma with further orbital involvement as demonstrated on the axial T1-weighted MRI with gadolinium. (**c**) Three-dimensional reconstruction of the MRI demonstrating tumor and adjacent structures involved. Patient underwent frontotemporal craniotomy for resection of recurrent tumor and vascular flap reconstruction over the orbit with plastics and oculoplastic surgery. (**d**) T1-weighted MRI with gadolinium demonstrating postoperative changes

13.4 Schwannomas

Schwannomas are benign, slow-growing, encapsulated peripheral nerve sheath tumors that arise from myelin. Trigeminal schwannomas are second to vestibular schwannomas as the most common intracranial schwannomas, but they only account for 0.07–0.36% of all intracranial tumors [12]. These tumors typically occur sporadically, however, there is an association with neurofibromatosis type 2. Typical origin sites include the trigeminal nerve at the cerebellopontine angle and the Gasserian ganglion at the cavernous sinus or Meckel's cave [13]. The most frequent tumor location is the middle cranial fossa (50%), followed by posterior fossa (30%) and dumbbell (20%) tumors [14]. Extension into the cavernous sinus and orbit is common. As they grow larger, they spread into extracranial compartments through the foramina in the skull, extending into the orbit, cavernous sinus, and paranasal sinuses (Fig. 13.3) [15, 16]. Although much less common, facial and vidian nerve schwannomas have been reported with orbital involvement [17].

Trigeminal sensory dysfunction (hypesthesia, dysesthesia, anesthesia) is the most common presenting symptom of trigeminal schwannomas. In addition to loss of facial sensation, keratitis can be seen due to diminished corneal reflex. Motor symptoms involving muscles of mastication may be present, although rare. Patients may present with facial pain at any of the three divisions. Finally, symptoms may present from mass effect on the surrounding neural structures, including cranial nerves including the oculomotor or abducens nerve leading to diplopia, or from compression on the globe resulting in exophthalmos-related diplopia. Diplopia is the initial symptom in about 15% of patients.

Schwannomas sharply enhance on post-gadolinium MRI, and they may have cystic components [18]. Close relationship with cranial nerves may be apparent, and the involvement of Meckel's and cavernous sinus can be further clues on MRI. A CT is useful for defining the bony anatomy of the skull base and any resultant bony erosion. Overall, trigeminal schwannomas vary significantly in their size, shape, and location. The operative approach and difficulty of resection are highly dependent on the location of the tumor along the trigeminal nerve. Various skull base approaches for trigeminal schwannomas have been described in the literature but still remain a challenge [13, 19]. Classically, these tumors are resected via a retrosigmoid craniectomy if they are localized to the trigeminal root and middle fossa craniotomy for subtemporal, or combined petrosal approaches for dumbbell shaped tumors [20]. Similar to vestibular schwannomas, recurrence is common with partial resection, and a gross total resection is the goal.

Orbitocavernous schwannomas require anterior clinoidectomy, and orbital and cavernous components can be removed separately. Monitoring of oculomotor, trochlear, and abducens nerves can be done to identify normal anatomy around the tumor. Recent advancements in endoscopic surgery provide a more minimally invasive and direct route for tumors in and around Meckel's cave, including the endoscopic endonasal approach (EEA) [21, 22] and endoscopic transpalpebral, transorbital approach [23]. EEA is ideal in cases where the tumor is medial to the optic nerve. A case series of 25 patients who underwent endoscopic approaches

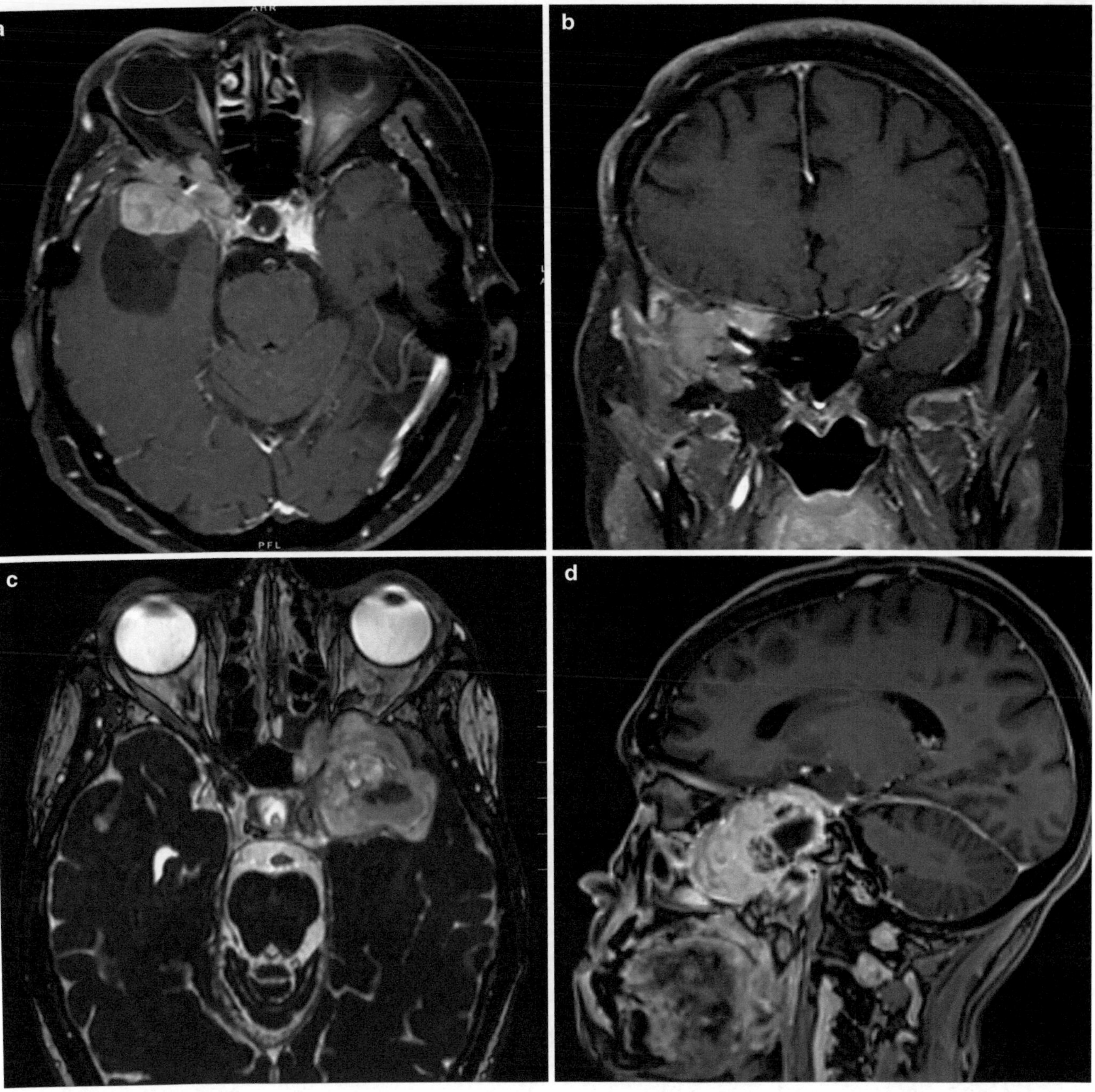

Fig. 13.3 Trigeminal Schwannoma. A 58-year-old female with right eye proptosis and vision changes. T1-weighted MRI with gadolinium shows a homogeneously enhancing extra-axial lesion with invasion into the orbit and cavernous sinus involvement on (**a**) axial and (**b**) coronal views. A 66-year-old female with a known history of a left trigeminal schwannoma who underwent surgical resection and radiation presents with worsening left sided facial pain and left facial numbness. (**c**) T2 constructive interference in steady state (CISS) axial view and (**d**) T1-weighted sagittal MRI with gadolinium show a large left sided skull base lesion with involvement of the cavernous sinus, orbital apex, and paranasal sinuses. Patient underwent surgical resection via an expanded endonasal endoscopic approach with neurosurgery, otolaryngology, and ophthalmology

for trigeminal schwannomas presented by Park et al. demonstrates a feasible alternative to microscopic skull base approaches. Another case series of 43 patients shows that 90.7% gross total resection was achieved; however, facial numbness did not improve in most cases [24]. One of the greatest concerns is a postoperative cerebrospinal fluid (CSF) leak, and these approaches require a multilayer reconstruction closure technique. Adjuvant radiation can be considered in patients after surgery or without surgery. In a series of 26 patients, primary or adjuvant gamma-knife radiation therapy has shown favorable risk-to-benefit profile in 72% of patients and tumor shrinkage in 48% of patients [25].

13.5 Sellar/Suprasellar Tumors

Pituitary adenomas make up 10–15% of all intracranial tumors. Pituitary adenomas can have extension into the hypothalamus, laterally into the cavernous sinus, and also toward the orbit. However, orbital invasion is exceedingly rare, with only less than 30 cases reported in the literature [26, 27]. Most of these are functioning adenomas [28, 29]. In the case of orbital invasion, involvement of the orbital apex is ubiquitous, with or without invasion into the superior orbital fissure or optic canal. Presenting ocular symptoms are generally secondary to compression of nerves and ocular structures by the growing tumor, although tissue invasion may also occur. Common symptoms include unilateral retro-orbital pain, proptosis, diplopia, and visual field loss [30]. Other more invasive tumors of the sellar and suprasellar region can include chondrosarcomas, pituitary carcinoma craniopharyngiomas, germ cell tumors, lymphomas, meningiomas, and metastases. Characteristics on MRI can vary depending on the presence of hemorrhage, cystic transformation. Most adenomas show avid homogeneous enhancement with well-defined margins.

Treatment of pituitary adenomas includes a combination of pharmacologic, surgical, and radiation treatments, but transsphenoidal resection is usually the approach of choice. In the case of orbital invasion, surgery should be considered for decompression of ocular structures and adjuvant radiation therapy for any residual. Deterioration of vision or worsening ocular signs and symptoms should prompt surgical evaluation. Endoscopic endonasal approaches provide access for a medial and anterior trajectory, making it ideal for most sellar and suprasellar lesions, but if the tumor extends to the lateral orbit, a combined approach with a lateral craniotomy and orbitotomy may be necessary. In a series of 22 operative cases for patients with adenomas with orbital extension, 7 of these resections were incomplete. Worsening ocular symptoms were also commonly seen postoperatively [27]. After initial mass resection, residual tumor is treated with radiation therapy.

Other lesions of the sellar and suprasellar region include dermoid and epidermoid tumors, which may extend to the orbital apex causing optic nerve compression or invasion via the superior orbital fissure. Dermoid cysts are benign heterotopic inclusion cysts that typically develop along the midline. They can also develop in the cavernous sinus wall or extend into the orbit, and patients may develop ophthalmoplegia (Fig. 13.4). Intracranial epidermoid cysts are typically found in the cerebellopontine angle, but they can also develop in the suprasellar region in 10–15% of cases [31]. Additionally, they can also develop within the orbit, which are less common than dermoid cysts but can have similar features (Fig. 13.5).

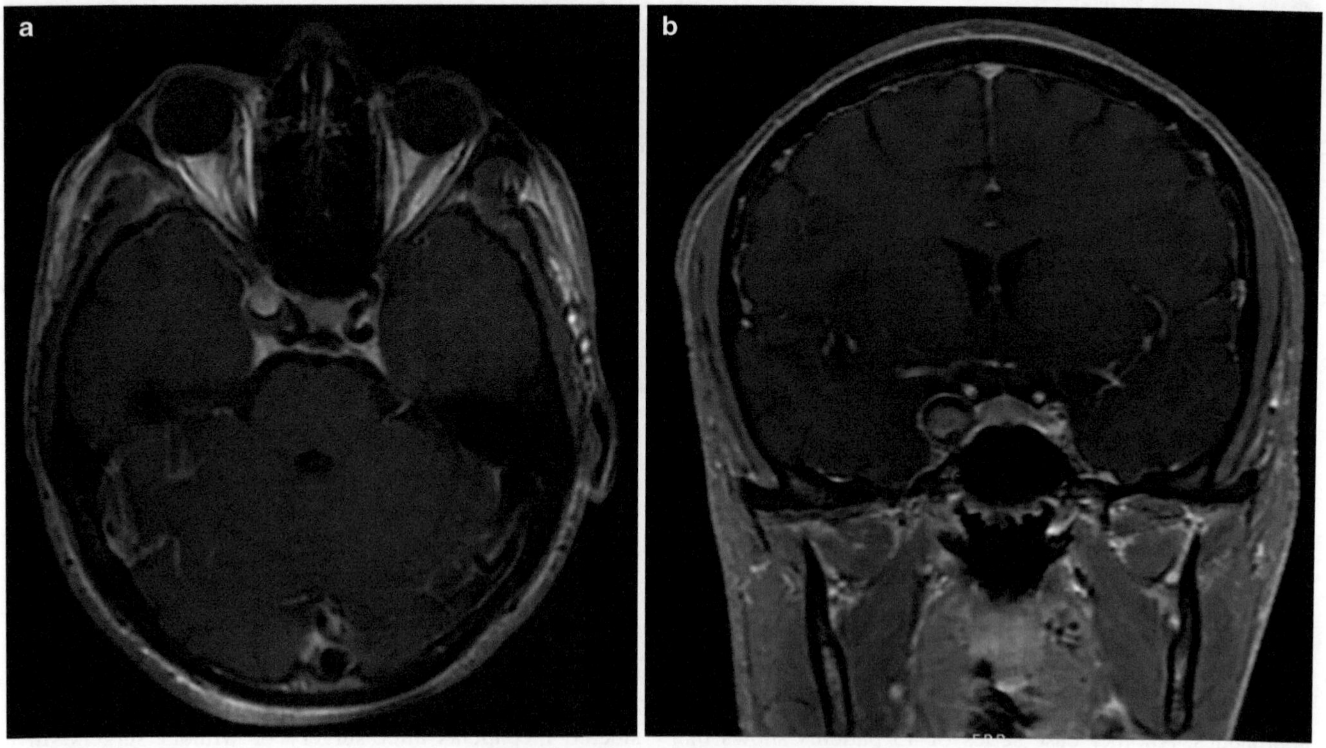

Fig. 13.4 Cavernous sinus dermoid Cyst. A 19-year-old male presenting with right orbital pain, right ptosis and double vision. He was noted to have limited R eye adduction. (**a**) Axial and (**b**) coronal T1-weighted MRI with gadolinium demonstrate a cystic lesion in the right cavernous sinus near the orbital apex. Patient underwent successful resection of this dermoid cyst via an extradural approach to the cavernous sinus

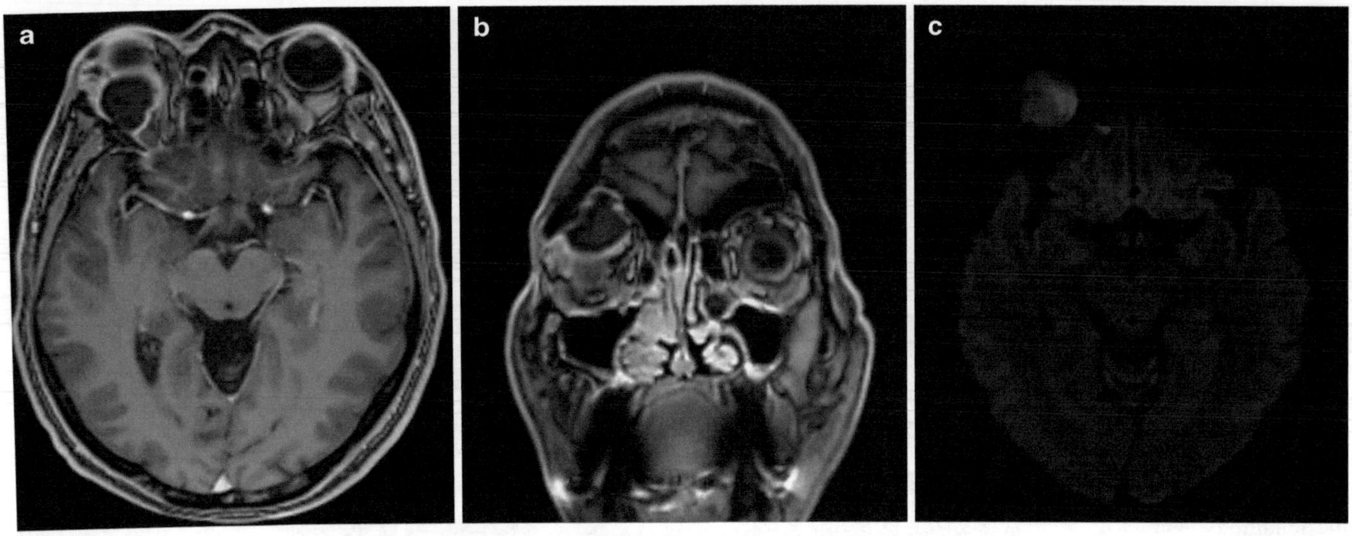

Fig. 13.5 Epidermoid Cyst. A 46-year-old male presenting with complaints of blurry vision and right eye pain for 4 months. Patient also complains of proptosis and diplopia when looking up or to the right. MRI with gadolinium was obtained and demonstrated a 2.5 × 2.2 × 2.4 well-circumscribed ring enhancing, cystic mass in the superior orbit and anterior fossa floor seen on (**a**) axial and (**b**) coronal view. (**c**) The mass also exhibited restricted diffusion on diffusion-weighted imaging

Imaging helps differentiate the two pathologies. A CT scan of dermoid cysts can show fat content in the cyst and demonstrate adjacent osseous changes causing bone remodeling or erosion [32]. On MRI, epidermoid cysts can show some enhancement along the periphery and restriction on diffuse weighted imaging (Fig. 13.5c). The slow growth and location of these tumors allows them to remain asymptomatic until large enough to compress the optic apparatus. Pathologically, both these tumors are lined by keratinizing stratified squamous epithelium. Dermoid cysts contain epidermal content such as hair follicles and sebaceous glands, while epidermoid cysts can contain flaky keratin debris inside the cysts. Treatment involves surgical resection, and complete surgical excision of these cysts is recommended to prevent recurrence. Gross total resection of the cyst and cyst wall can be achieved safely depending on orbital involvement.

13.6 Sinonasal Tumors

Sinonasal neoplasms include a number of different pathologies including squamous cell carcinoma, adenocarcinoma, esthesioneuroblastoma, and sarcomas (discussed later in the chapter) [33]. Epithelial tumors are more common in adults, while sarcomas are more commonly seen in pediatric population. Epithelial tumors arise from the paranasal sinuses and nasal cavity. Specifically, the maxillary, followed by the ethmoid sinuses, is the most common sites. Keratinizing squamous cell carcinomas are the most common, although there is an increase in non-keratinizing squamous cell carcinoma related to human papilloma virus. The incidence of orbital invasion by sinonasal cancers varies with the site of origin and histology. Orbital invasion increases morbidity and mortality and aggressive invasion into the orbital apex gives a T4b grade (Fig. 13.6).

Patients can present with nasal obstruction, or epistaxis, or alternatively, remain asymptomatic until the tumor enlarges. Visual symptoms, including unilateral proptosis and diplopia, occur in 50% of patients as ethmoid or maxillary sinus tumors invade the orbit [34]. There is a grading system for the extent of orbital involvement. Grade I involves erosion or destruction of the medial orbital wall (Fig. 13.6a, b). Grade II is characterized by extraconal invasion of the periorbita (Fig. 13.6d, e), and grade III involves invasion of the medial rectus muscle, optic nerve, ocular bulb, or the skin [35]. On imaging, there is typically a large mass centered in the sinonasal cavity. Though tumor margins can be poorly defined, destruction of the orbital walls is often evident.

Primary treatment for these tumors includes tumor resection through a combination of open and endoscopic endonasal approaches, followed by adjuvant radiation therapy [36]. In the case of extensive invasion and a T4b grade tumor diagnosis with aggressive local extension into the orbital apex, the tumor may be deemed unresectable [37]. Therefore, orbital invasion is a therapeutic challenge and carries a poor prognosis. In all grades of orbital involvement, neither orbital exenteration or preservation has shown to significantly change five-year survival rates [38]. Neoadjuvant induction chemotherapy in T3 and T4 grade disease can help improve outcomes after surgical resection in nonresponders, while induction chemotherapy with radiation alone had better survival rates in responders. Another consideration for treatment of these tumors is reconstruction, especially in the

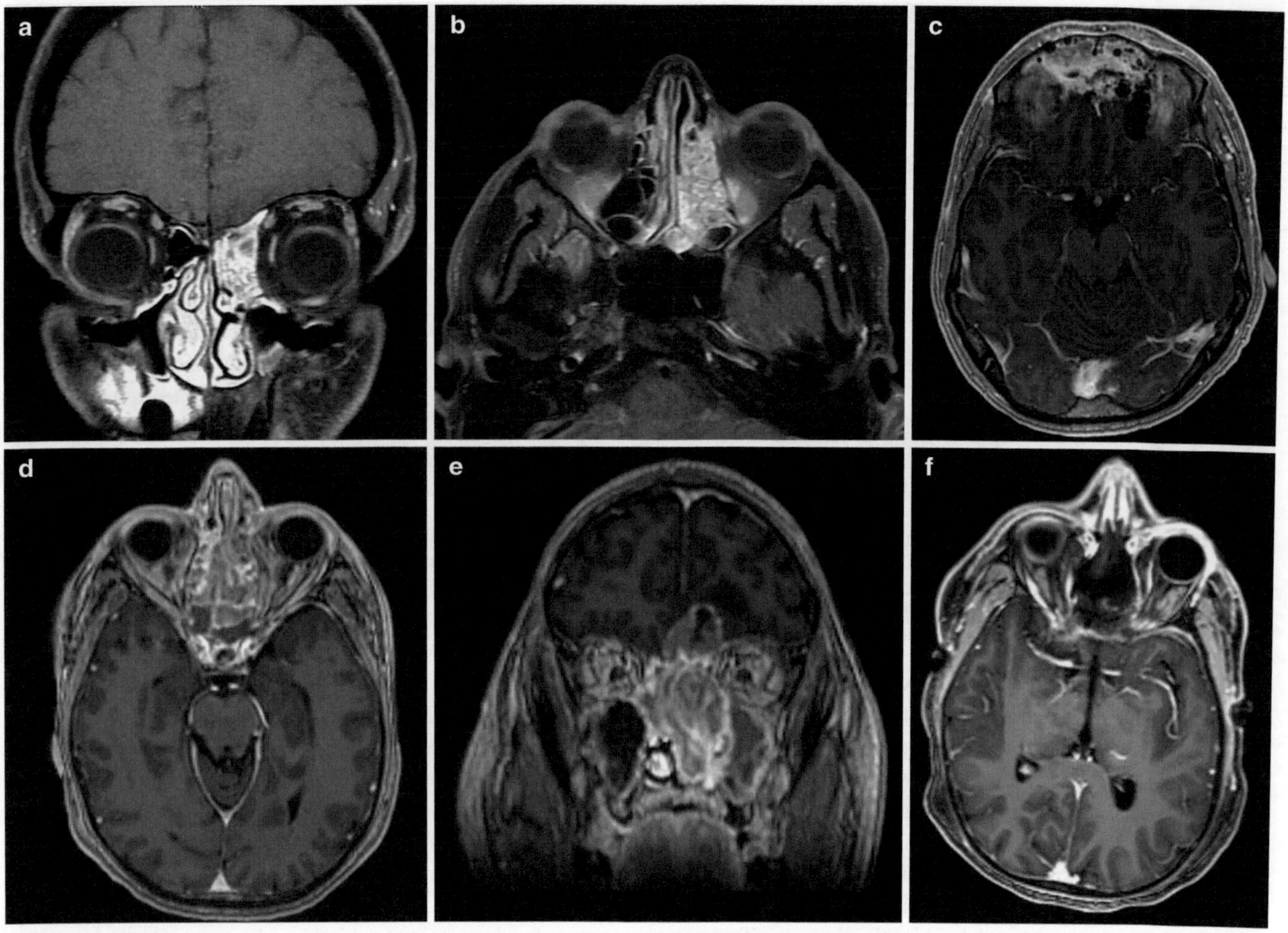

Fig. 13.6 Sinonasal tumors. A 40-year-old male with epistaxis and congestion found to have a sinonasal mass with orbital involvement of the medial orbital wall and periorbita seen on fat suppressed T1-weighted MRI with contrast (**a**) coronal and (**b**) axial views. He underwent a biopsy confirming squamous cell carcinoma and underwent chemotherapy and radiation. Given progression of the tumor, he underwent surgical resection. Later, he developed radiation necrosis and recurrence extending into the medial orbit, skull base and sphenoid (**c**) and required further operations in the form of endoscopic and open skull base debridement. A 43-year-old male with epistaxis presented to medical attention and MRI of the brain with gadolinium demonstrated a large enhancing sinonasal mass that involved the ethmoid, sphenoid, and frontal sinuses with medial orbital involvement on the left (**d**) as well as intracranial extension with vasogenic edema (**e**). This was noted to be esthesioneuroblastoma on biopsy. Patient underwent and expanded endonasal endoscopic approach for surgical resection with good post-operative result (**f**). He then underwent further adjuvant radiation therapy

setting of orbital exenteration. There is also concern for CSF leak in cases where there is intracranial involvement, and prolonged lumbar drainage may be necessary for these cases.

13.7 Cavernous Angiomas

These are typically benign mass lesions made of blood vessels clustered closely together in an abnormal arrangement [39]. They represent the most common intraorbital vascular lesion in adults [40, 41]. According to various sources, they are not classified as tumors but rather vascular malformations and therefore referred to as cavernous hemangioma malformations to make this distinction [42]. Regardless, they represent a large portion of benign orbital lesions and commonly cause ocular symptoms or orbital apex syndrome. In retrospective studies of patients with orbital lesions over a 30-year period, 6–9% were cavernous hemangiomas [42].

The presentation of cavernous angiomas in the orbit, as for all orbital lesions, is directly related to its size and location. There is variation in presentation and timing of progression, but typically, these orbital lesions present with progressive proptosis, often with ptosis, pain, and decreased visual acuity in the affected eye. Most often, lesions are unilateral and solitary; however, there are documented cases of multiple orbital cavernous angiomas, as many as 15 lesions in one orbit [40]. The literature also reveals bilateral cases, although these are exceedingly rare [41].

On imaging, cavernous angiomas are well delineated masses, often but not exclusively intraconal. In one study of orbital cavernous angiomas, 19 out of 23 were intraconal [39]. When bony structures such as the calvarium or skull base are involved, CT shows an osteolytic honeycomb appearance of the affected bone [43]. MRI provides a better depiction of the soft tissues, revealing the lesion's relationship to the extraocular muscles, optic nerve, and extension toward or away from the orbital apex. MRI is instrumental in treatment planning and predicting whether the optic nerve can be preserved. Histopathological analysis reveals distended "caverns" filled with blood [43]. These caverns are large, dilated venous channels contained within a fibrous, well-delineated capsule. Grossly, these lesions are endothelium-lined and blood-filled lesions that are purple, smooth, and encapsulated [40, 41].

Conservative management for cavernous angiomas is a reasonable approach up to the point when they become symptomatic. Treatment for cavernous angiomas of the orbit should take on a multidisciplinary approach. Gross total resection with preservation of the optic apparatus is feasible in some cases if the lesion is well-defined and encapsulated. Recurrence with this treatment modality is uncommon, but patients often experience transient postoperative diplopia [22]. One reported case of orbital cavernous angioma with bony invasion required craniotomy for middle fossa access and an abdominal fat graft [43]. Regardless of the surgical approach, the outcome of resection was largely dependent on size and relationship of the lesion to the optic nerve and the proximity to the apex [42]. For those lesions that are not amenable to resection, multi-session radiosurgery may be a viable option [44]. Kim et al. presented a series of eight patients with greater than 20% tumor shrinkage and improved visual outcomes after radiosurgery [11].

13.8 Lymphangiomas

One of the first cases of orbital lymphangioma was reported by Smith et al. in 1925 regarding a 10-year-old girl who presented with progressive unilateral proptosis. She underwent surgical exploration, and a dark brownish fluid was aspirated from a cystic lesion, with subsequent resolution of her symptoms. Her symptoms recurred 5 years later with ptosis and diplopia. She once again underwent surgical exploration of the orbit and enucleation. On gross pathologic evaluation, cystic cavities with clear gelatinous fluid were reported. Under microscopic evaluation, there was edematous connective tissue, as well as spindle-shaped fibroblasts, and numerous round cells assembled into lymph follicles. Those containing blood were thought to represent lymph spaces in which hemorrhage had occurred. There was also involvement of the optic nerve sheath and extension to episcleral tissues and extraocular muscles. After enucleation, adjunct radiation was performed with small radium implants applied over the socket, brow, and lateral aspect of the orbit [45].

Lymphangioma is a rare, unencapsulated vascular malformation of the lymphatic system. It is common in childhood, especially the first decade of life. They are typically low-flow and have no vascular connection, but they have a clear propensity for recurrent hemorrhage [46]. They account for less than 5% of all orbital tumors but are exceedingly rare in the adult population, with most diagnosed before the age of 10 [47]. The lesion can infiltrate the optic nerve, rendering surgical resection very difficult and making alternative therapies such as systemic steroids and sclerosing agents necessary [48].

MRI shows a solitary cystic lesion with or occasionally without enhancement [49]. The appearance of feeder vessels on MRI would exclude a diagnosis of orbital lymphangioma [48]. Orbital apex lymphangiomas can be confined to a single extraocular muscle or lacrimal gland but often extend far throughout the orbit from globe to apex, making them difficult to resect [50, 51]. On gross examination, orbital lymphangioma appears grayish-red, firm, and lobulated. Dark liquid often escapes from the mass during surgical excision [52]. Goals of treatment typically include preserving visual acuity and extraocular movements. As such, if there is no immediate threat to vision, and low intraocular pressure, conservative measures are taken [48]. Since orbital lymphangiomas are so rare, it is difficult to determine a standard of care. Thus, there remains clinical equipoise regarding the best combination of initial and adjuvant therapies, including mTOR inhibitors [51], sclerotherapy or radiotherapy [48]. Some combination of surgical intervention and sclerotherapy or chemotherapy may be best and should be discussed by a multidisciplinary team to determine what is best for the patient, taking into account size, symptoms, and relationship to the optic nerve and orbital apex.

13.9 Lymphomas

Lymphoma is the most frequently encountered malignant tumor of the orbit, and it typically presents as a primary lesion [2]. Orbital lymphoma represents the most common of the ocular adnexal lymphomas, which include lesions of the orbit, conjunctiva, lacrimal gland, and eyelid in descending order of prevalence. This constellation of non-Hodgkin lymphomas is most commonly seen in females in the fifth to seventh decades of life [53, 54]. According to one report, 70–90% of all orbital lymphomas are primary, and these represent 1% of all non-Hodgkin lymphoma cases. Lymphoma can also invade the orbit from the sinonasal or skull base region [55]. The majority of orbital lymphomas are mucosa-associated lymphoid tissue (MALT), followed by diffuse

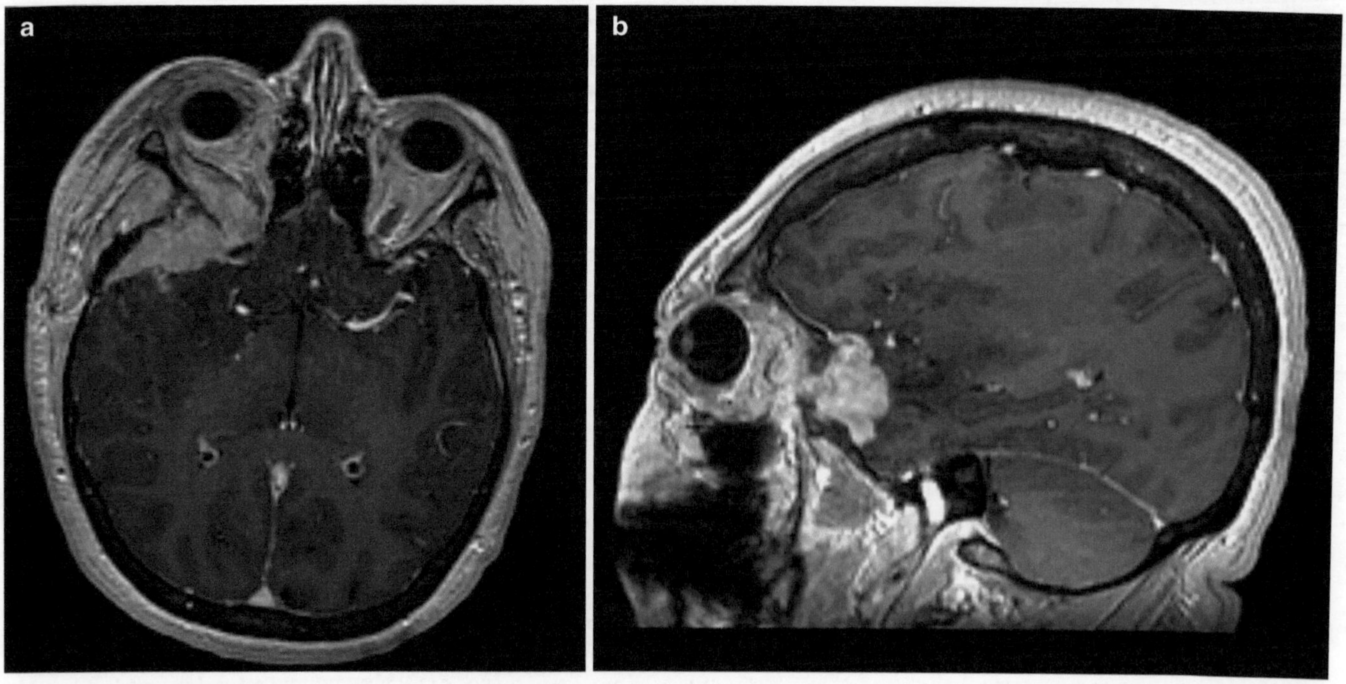

Fig. 13.7 Lymphoma. A 52-year-old female presenting with right sided headache and worsening vision loss over a period of 1 month. She underwent an MRI for evaluation which showed a 3.7 cm × 2.8 cm × 2.8 cm enhancing mass in the right middle cranial fossa with extension into the right cavernous sinus, lateral orbit, and temporalis muscle on (**a**) axial and (**b**) sagittal views shown here. She underwent a biopsy of the mass via right craniotomy and right lateral orbitotomy with neurosurgery and oculoplastics. Pathology identified large B-cell lymphoma. She subsequently underwent radiation therapy and a PET CT which demonstrated no other sites of active disease

large B-cell lymphoma (DLBCL) [54, 56]. Like many other orbital tumors, they present with a palpebral or orbital mass, proptosis, ptosis, decreased visual acuity, or orbital apex syndrome. Frequently located in the superolateral quadrant of the cone, they invade or displace the superior rectus muscle [54]. They can also arise from the skull base and extend to nearby structures including the orbit (Fig. 13.7). However, the location and extent of an orbital lesion on imaging cannot rule out a diagnosis of lymphoma.

Lymphoma is one of the great imitators, and orbital lymphoma is no exception. CT alone can help determine the size and location of the lesion, but MRI is instrumental in depicting the relationship of the lesion to the optic nerve, extraocular muscles, and the presence or absence of intradural extension. It can enhance homogeneously or demonstrate ring enhancement [54]. There are a multitude of histological markers for lymphoma to aid in making the diagnosis, including CD20, CD19, CD45, and Bcl2 [54]. The relative nonspecificity of imaging and the wide array of histological markers available make early surgical biopsy an attractive option in order to diagnose and treat orbital lesions efficiently.

Orbital lymphomas are treated differently from other ocular adnexa, and treatment differs based on presence or absence of systemic disease. Optic nerve involvement in all cases makes gross total resection markedly more difficult and increases the demand for adjuvant therapies. Options for treatment of orbital lymphoma include oral steroids, topical erythromycin, surgical excision, adjuvant radiation, and systemic chemotherapy [54]. Surgery is reserved for tissue diagnosis, debulking, and total resection when safe. Resection is indicated for encapsulated tumors, especially when there is a high risk of recurrence. Endoscopic endonasal approaches are used as well for orbital apex decompression and biopsy, typically for lesions in the inferomedial orbit so as not to interfere with the optic nerve. There remains a lack of consensus on what combination of surgery, radiation, and chemotherapy are best suited for orbital apex lymphoma, but symptoms, prognostic factors, and optic nerve involvement and intradural extension should be taken into account [53].

13.10 Soft Tissue Neoplasms

Orbital rhabdomyosarcoma is the most common primary malignant tumor of the orbit in children and is found in the superior orbit two-thirds of the time, commonly during the first decade of life [57]. The four types of rhabdomyosarcoma are embryonal, alveolar, pleomorphic, and botryoid [58]. Eighty-five percent of these pediatric orbital lesions are of the embryonal variety, and most of the others are alveolar [57]. Other documented orbital soft tissue lesions

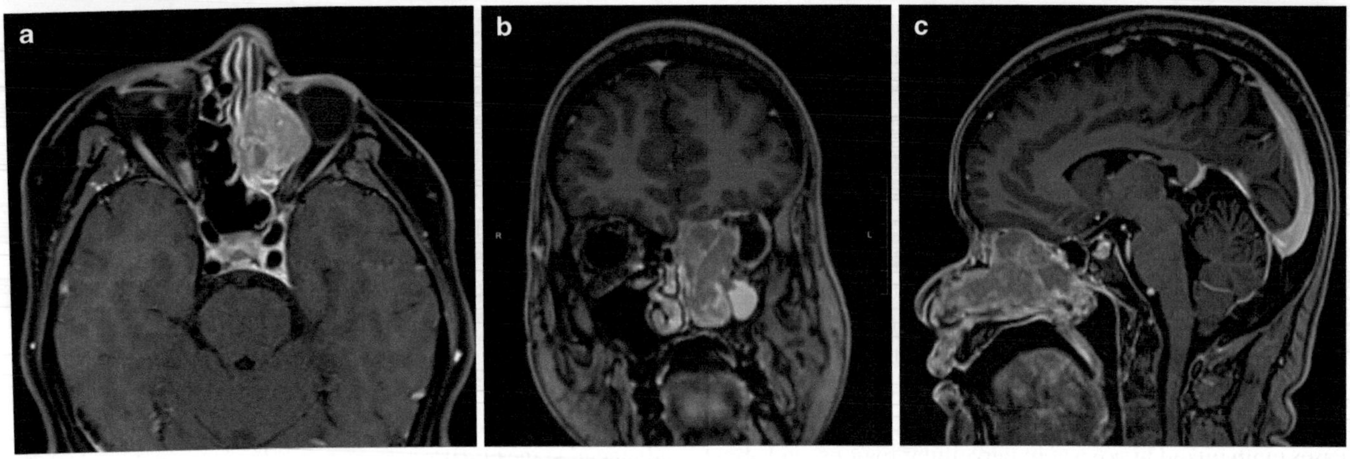

Fig. 13.8 Chondrosarcoma. A 31-year-old female patient with a history of right sided retinoblastoma treated with right eye enucleation and systemic therapy presents with congestion and left sided visual acuity symptoms. MRI revealed a left sinonasal mass with invasion of the left orbit and extension into the anterior skull base seen on (**a**) axial, (**b**) coronal, and (**c**) sagittal views. She underwent surgical resection via expanded endonasal endoscopic approach achieving gross total resection but with some positive margins. She subsequently was treated with adjuvant chemotherapy and proton beam radiation

include leiomyosarcoma, chondrosarcoma, and histiocytic sarcoma, a rare lymphohematopoietic system tumor [20]. Primary orbital leiomyosarcoma represents a malignant smooth muscle tumor, mainly in older women, typically originating in the uterus, GI tract, and vascular tissues [59]. Mesenchymal chondrosarcoma of the orbit is an extremely rare and aggressive cartilage-forming tumor, typically forming in the second to third decade of life, with a female predominance (Fig. 13.8) [60]. Treatment methods for these soft tissue lesions span multiple disciplines, and these lesions often portend a poor prognosis regardless of therapy modality.

CT and MRI help determine what structures are shifted or invaded and the extension of the tumor into bone or dura. On CT, an orbital rhabdomyosarcoma might appear as a well-demarcated inferomedial orbital mass extending to the apex, with no bony erosion, that is homogeneous and isodense to muscle. It can surround orbital structures without displacing them. A heterogeneously enhancing, lobulated orbital mass with multiple cystic areas with calcification on CT would be more consistent with a mesenchymal chondrosarcoma [15]. Orbital rhabdomyosarcomas have been reported to demonstrate restriction on DWI imaging, making this a helpful diagnostic tool [58]. Despite these reported radiology tendencies, tissue biopsy is paramount in the quest for diagnosis. Once a biopsy has been obtained, histological markers aid tremendously in obtaining a definitive diagnosis.

Because these tumors are so rare, a consensus on the best treatment does not exist. Regardless of the type, a combination of surgery, radiation, chemotherapy should be considered for these sarcomas, based on proximity to the optic nerve and staging of the lesion. Surgical approaches range from a simple open biopsy to endoscopic endonasal approaches, to complete resection of the eye and orbital contents for a margin-free resection. A multidisciplinary approach is often the best, with considerations made for tumor size, location, intradural involvement, optic nerve involvement, and comorbidities.

13.11 Solitary Fibrous Tumor

Solitary fibrous tumors (SFTs), previously known as hemangiopericytomas, comprise yet another category of rare orbital apex lesions. These are rare spindle cell tumors, originating from mesenchyme. They typically progress slowly, with a generous blood supply from many feeding arteries. As they mimic meningiomas and neurofibromas, careful workup with history and physical exam, imaging, and histopathological analysis are required to reach an accurate diagnosis [21, 25]. Only 6% of them are found in the head and neck regions, most commonly the sinonasal tract, followed by the orbit, mouth, and salivary glands [61]. There are just under 100 reported cases to date of orbital SFTs [62]. They can present with unilateral painless proptosis, visual disturbance, tearing, ptosis, and restriction of extraocular movements. They can be intraconal or extraconal or involve the lacrimal gland or sinonasal tract. Most are extraconal in the superolateral quadrant of the orbit, but they can exhibit intracranial extension as well as disruption of the optic nerve [7, 63].

CT can help narrow down the diagnosis based on the density of the lesion relative to neighboring structures and can quickly determine the size and extent of the lesion. A CT with contrast of the orbit will show a heterogeneously enhancing extraconal lesion with globe compression, without calcification or bony invasion. SFTs are usually well-defined, isodense to extraocular muscle, enhancing, and normally avoid osseous extension [63, 64]. MRI will show a solid, well-circumscribed mass that does not restrict on DWI [61, 64]. Biopsy may be necessary for accurate diagnosis. Typical SFTs have "patternless architecture" with alternating hypocellular and hypercellular areas separated from each other by thick bands of hyalinized collagen and branching vessels [65]. Once diagnosis is made, all patients require close follow-up since histological evidence of benign or malignant features is an unreliable predictor of clinical outcomes [61, 65].

A study of 17 cases showed vascular proliferation in all cases, with mixed hypo- and hypercellular regions, and about half of the lesions featured a patternless architecture [64]. Histological analysis will usually reveal a mix of coarse and dense spindle cells. However, there are reports of orbital SFTs with very few blood vessels, no perivascular hyalinization, and no regions of alternating density. SFTs of the orbit may stain positively for vimentin, CD34, bcl-2, CD99, STAT6, beta-catenin, progesterone receptor and negatively for CD31, smooth muscle actin, epithelial membrane antigen, WT1, and S100 [61–63, 65]. An absence of S100 helps differentiate from schwannoma. The intra-arterial components will typically have a different staining pattern than the extravascular regions, and the vessels themselves often maintain a staghorn configuration [62, 64].

Treatment of orbital SFTs requires confirmation of diagnosis, but a biopsy without complete resection is dangerous, as it poses a high risk of bleeding. As such, the literature stresses an all-or-nothing strategy, with either complete resection or no surgery. In one study of eight cases of CNS and orbital SFTs, gross total resection was attempted in all orbital cases. In one orbital case, adjuvant radiotherapy was utilized in the treatment plan. Recurrence occurred in two cases [7]. In another study involving 17 cases of orbital SFT, surgical excision was performed in all cases. Seven patients underwent lateral orbitotomy, six had an anterior orbitotomy, three had a transconjunctival approach, and one needed a superomedial orbitotomy. Those treated with chemotherapy had worse outcomes, but there is likely a selection bias inherent in this observation [64]. Distant metastatic disease is extremely rare in SFTs, and the need for systemic chemotherapy would indicate a higher stage of disease burden than those patients only requiring surgical excision [63]. Therefore, it is not surprising that those on chemotherapy would have poorer outcomes than those who are not. Ultimately, complete resection of symptomatic lesions remains the gold standard for these orbital tumors, which rarely metastasize.

13.12 Metastases

Extraocular orbital metastases are rare, accounting for 3–7% of all orbital tumors [66, 67]. Lung cancer makes up 17% of these cases (Fig. 13.9a, b), followed by breast cancer at 14% (Fig. 13.9c, d). More uncommon sources include renal cell (Fig. 13.9e, f), hepatocellular carcinoma, adenoid cystic carcinoma, uterine carcinoma, prostate, and gastric signet ring cell carcinoma [66–73]. One theory explaining the paucity of orbital metastatic disease is the low blood flow to the region. Orbital metastases portend a poor prognosis, as median survival with metastatic disease to the orbit is 15–16 months despite advances in treatments for various primaries at advanced stages [70].

Imaging findings for metastatic disease vary based on the primary tissue and the location of the orbital lesion. Metastatic lesions to the orbit will often show up on MRI as a well-circumscribed, enhancing intraconal mass, with involvement of one or more extraocular muscles, the orbital apex, superior orbital fissure, or occasionally encasing the cavernous sinus [70, 73]. Early biopsy and metastatic workup are imperative in starting an appropriate treatment plan.

Cases of skull base metastases with extension into the orbit include a 62-year-old male with a history of adenocarcinoma of the lung presenting with diplopia. T1-weighted MRI with gadolinium demonstrated a homogenously enhancing mass along the right lateral orbit extending intracranially (Fig. 13.9a, b). Surgical resection was undertaken as a multidisciplinary approach with neurosurgery and ophthalmology, and pathology confirmed metastasis.

Treatment varies widely based on the spread of disease, the patient's goals for their care, the location of the lesion, and involvement of the optic nerve. Typically, surgery and adjuvant radiation represent the mainstay of metastatic treatment, but surgical excision may be too risky close to the optic nerve. Surgical approaches to the orbit for metastatic disease include transorbital, transpalpebral, and endoscopic endonasal approaches in addition to craniotomies. Endoscopic endonasal approaches are best for medial and inferior orbital lesions due to their position relative to the optic nerve and extraocular muscles [71]. Surgical decompression of orbital metastases can serve another purpose in addition to palliation, tissue diagnosis, and relief of mass effect; it can determine the cause of the patient's ocular symptoms and therefore determine whether certain structures have been invaded or simply displaced. In many cases, patients shown to have widespread disease beyond the orbit will opt for palliative measures. However, for those choosing to undergo treatment, there is no consensus on the best method for dealing with orbital metastases.

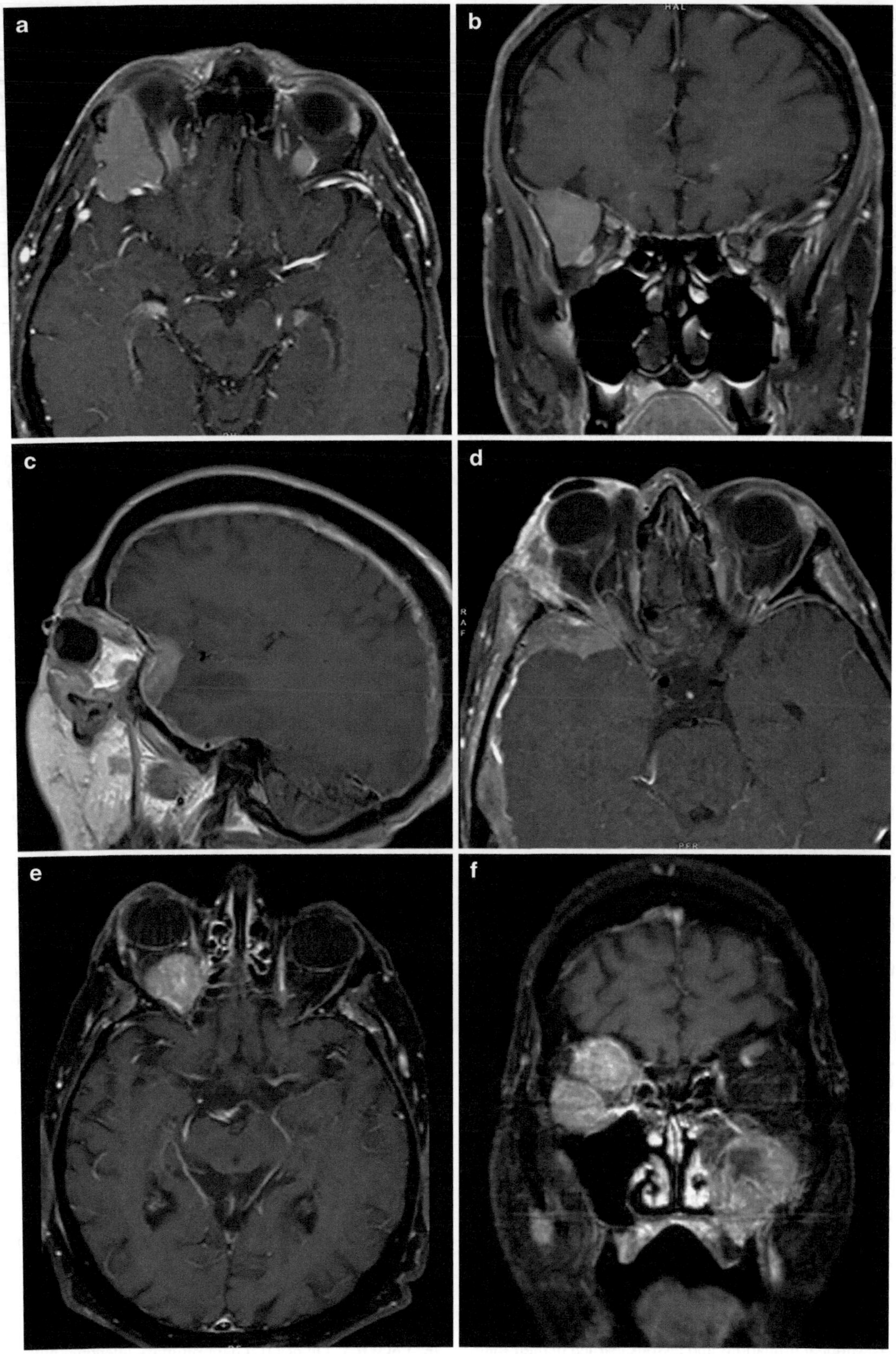

Fig. 13.9 Metastases. A 62-year-old male with a history of adenocarcinoma of the lung presenting with diplopia. (**a**) Axial and (**b**) coronal T1-weighted MRI with gadolinium demonstrated a homogenously enhancing mass along the right lateral orbit extending intracranially. Surgical resection was undertaken as a multidisciplinary approach with neurosurgery and ophthalmology. A 52-year-old female presenting with R orbital pain and blurred vision with a history of invasive ductal carcinoma of the breast. (**c**) Sagittal and (**d**) axial T1-weighted MRI with gadolinium demonstrated a temporal, extra-axial dural based lesion with invasion of the right lateral orbit and involvement of the optic nerve. Patient underwent surgical resection and pathology confirmed metastasis. A 66-year-old male with a history of renal cell carcinoma presenting with proptosis and blurred vision. (**e**) Axial and (**f**) coronal T1-weighted MRI with gadolinium demonstrated a homogenously enhancing mass in the orbit and orbital apex with exophthalmos and compression of neurovascular structures

13.13 Conclusion

Although quite rare, secondary neoplasms of the orbit and orbital apex from the skull base can have devastating consequences if not treated promptly and appropriately. Presentation is fairly constant regardless of the type of tumor and commonly includes proptosis, decreased visual acuity, and restriction of oculomotor movements. Lesions can invade the orbit directly via transosseous route or via foramina. They are typically unilateral but can be bilateral in rare instances. Radiographic appearances can be misleading, but they are important in discerning what structures are involved and whether they are invaded or displaced. Histological markers are instrumental in confirming or ruling out items on the differential diagnosis. These lesions also pose a unique challenge and frequently require multimodal management involving a team approach. Surgical resection is the mainstay of definitive management for most symptomatic lesions, but radiation and chemotherapy play an integral role in more aggressive tumors with a heavier metastatic burden, or those in a precarious location.

References

1. Kannan S, Hasegawa M, Yamada Y, Kawase T, Kato Y. Tumors of the orbit: case report and review of surgical corridors and current options. Asian J Neurosurg. 2019;14(3):678–85. https://doi.org/10.4103/ajns.AJNS_51_19.
2. Jørgensen M, Heegaard S. A review of nasal, paranasal, and skull base tumors invading the orbit. Surv Ophthalmol. 2018;63(3):389–405. https://doi.org/10.1016/j.survophthal.2017.07.001.
3. Gonen L, Nov E, Shimony N, Shofty B, Margalit N. Sphenoorbital meningioma: surgical series and design of an intraoperative management algorithm. Neurosurg Rev. 2018;41(1):291–301. https://doi.org/10.1007/s10143-017-0855-7.
4. Saeed P, Rootman J, Nugent RA, White VA, Mackenzie IR, Koornneef L. Optic nerve sheath meningiomas. Ophthalmology. 2003;110(10):2019–30. https://doi.org/10.1016/S0161-6420(03)00787-5.
5. Kiyofuji S, Casabella AM, Graffeo CS, Perry A, Garrity JA, Link MJ. Sphenoorbital meningioma: a unique skull base tumor. Surgical technique and results. J Neurosurg. 2019;23:1–8. https://doi.org/10.3171/2019.6.JNS191158.
6. Hakuba A, Tanaka K, Suzuki T, Nishimura S. A combined orbitozygomatic infratemporal epidural and subdural approach for lesions involving the entire cavernous sinus. J Neurosurg. 1989;71(5 Pt 1):699–704. https://doi.org/10.3171/jns.1989.71.5.0699.
7. Honeybul S, Neil-Dwyer G, Lang DA, Evans BT, Ellison DW. Sphenoid wing meningioma en plaque: a clinical review. Acta Neurochir (Wien). 2001;143(8):749–757; discussion 758. https://doi.org/10.1007/s007010170028.
8. Shrivastava RK, Sen C, Costantino PD, Rocca RD. Sphenoorbital meningiomas: surgical limitations and lessons learned in their long-term management. J Neurosurg. 2005;103(3):491–7. https://doi.org/10.3171/jns.2005.103.3.0491.
9. Boari N, Gagliardi F, Spina A, Bailo M, Franzin A, Mortini P. Management of spheno-orbital en plaque meningiomas: clinical outcome in a consecutive series of 40 patients. Br J Neurosurg. 2013;27(1):84–90. https://doi.org/10.3109/02688697.2012.709557.
10. Talacchi A, De Carlo A, D'Agostino A, Nocini P. Surgical management of ocular symptoms in spheno-orbital meningiomas. Is orbital reconstruction really necessary? Neurosurg Rev. 2014;37(2):301–9; discussion 309–10. https://doi.org/10.1007/s10143-014-0517-y.
11. Kim BS, Im Y-S, Woo KI, Kim Y-D, Lee J-I. Multisession gamma knife radiosurgery for orbital apex tumors. World Neurosurg. 2015;84(4):1005–13. https://doi.org/10.1016/j.wneu.2015.04.042.
12. Pollack IF, Sekhar LN, Jannetta PJ, Janecka IP. Neurilemomas of the trigeminal nerve. J Neurosurg. 1989;70(5):737–45. https://doi.org/10.3171/jns.1989.70.5.0737.
13. Goel A, Muzumdar D, Raman C. Trigeminal neuroma: analysis of surgical experience with 73 cases. Neurosurgery. 2003;52(4):783–90; discussion 790. https://doi.org/10.1227/01.neu.0000053365.05795.03.
14. Taha JM, Tew JM, van Loveren HR, Keller JT, el-Kalliny M. Comparison of conventional and skull base surgical approaches for the excision of trigeminal neurinomas. J Neurosurg. 1995;82(5):719–25. https://doi.org/10.3171/jns.1995.82.5.0719.
15. Ghosh S, Das D, Varshney R, Nandy S. Orbital extension of trigeminal schwannoma. J Neurosci Rural Pract. 2015;6(1):102–4. https://doi.org/10.4103/0976-3147.143214.
16. Gupta P, Sharma A, Singh J. Solid cystic trigeminal schwannoma with intraorbital extension causing proptosis and vision loss. Asian J Neurosurg. 2016;11(4):456. https://doi.org/10.4103/1793-5482.181142.
17. Masroor FA, Gilde J, Liang J. Vidian nerve schwannoma: a rare skull-base neoplasm presenting with ocular manifestations: a case report and literature review. Perm J. 2018;22:18–021. https://doi.org/10.7812/TPP/18-021.
18. Kapur R, Mafee MF, Lamba R, Edward DP. Orbital schwannoma and neurofibroma: role of imaging. Neuroimaging Clin North Am. 2005;15(1):159–74. https://doi.org/10.1016/j.nic.2005.02.004.
19. Fukaya R, Yoshida K, Ohira T, Kawase T. Trigeminal schwannomas: experience with 57 cases and a review of the literature. Neurosurg Rev. 2010;34(2):159–71. https://doi.org/10.1007/s10143-010-0289-y.
20. Samii M, Migliori MM, Tatagiba M, Babu R. Surgical treatment of trigeminal schwannomas. J Neurosurg. 1995;82(5):711–8. https://doi.org/10.3171/jns.1995.82.5.0711.
21. Shin SS, Gardner PA, Stefko ST, Madhok R, Fernandez-Miranda JC, Snyderman CH. Endoscopic endonasal approach for nonvestibular schwannomas. Neurosurgery. 2011;69(5):1046–1057; discussion 1057. https://doi.org/10.1227/NEU.0b013e3182287bb9.
22. Zoli M, Ratti S, Guaraldi F, et al. Endoscopic endonasal approach to primitive Meckel's cave tumors: a clinical series. Acta Neurochir (Wien). 2018;160(12):2349–61. https://doi.org/10.1007/s00701-018-3708-4.
23. Park HH, Hong SD, Kim YH, et al. Endoscopic transorbital and endonasal approach for trigeminal schwannomas: a retrospective multicenter analysis (KOSEN-005). J Neurosurg. 2020;133(2):467–76. https://doi.org/10.3171/2019.3.JNS19492.
24. Li M, Wang X, Chen G, et al. Trigeminal schwannoma: a single-center experience with 43 cases and review of literature. Br J Neurosurg. 2021;35(1):49–56. https://doi.org/10.1080/02688697.2020.1754334.
25. Sheehan J, Yen CP, Arkha Y, Schlesinger D, Steiner L. Gamma knife surgery for trigeminal schwannoma. J Neurosurg. 2007;106(5):839–45. https://doi.org/10.3171/jns.2007.106.5.839.
26. Levy RA, Quint DJ. Giant pituitary adenoma with unusual orbital and skull base extension. AJR Am J Roentgenol. 1998;170(1):194–6. https://doi.org/10.2214/ajr.170.1.9423631.
27. Naguib MM, Mendoza PR, Jariyakosol S, Grossniklaus HE. Atypical pituitary adenoma with orbital invasion: case report and review

of the literature. Surv Ophthalmol. 2017;62(6):867–74. https://doi.org/10.1016/j.survophthal.2017.01.005.
28. Dhaliwal JS, Seibold LK, Kleinschmidt-Demasters BK, et al. Orbital invasion by ACTH-secreting pituitary adenomas. Ophthalmic Plast Reconstr Surg. 2014;30(2):e28–30. https://doi.org/10.1097/IOP.0b013e31829164cb.
29. Karcioglu ZA, Aden LB, Cruz AAV, Zaslow L, Saloom RJ. Orbital invasion with prolactinoma: a clinical review of four patients. Ophthalmic Plast Reconstr Surg. 2002;18(1):64–71. https://doi.org/10.1097/00002341-200201000-00010.
30. Vaudaux J, Portmann L, Maeder P, Borruat F-X. Orbital invasion by a pituitary macroadenoma without visual loss: case report and review of the literature. Eye (Lond). 2003;17(9):1032–4. https://doi.org/10.1038/sj.eye.6700481.
31. Rehman L, Bokhari I, Siddiqi SU, Bagga V, Hussain MM. Intracranial epidermoid lesions: our experience of 38 cases. Turk Neurosurg. 2017; https://doi.org/10.5137/1019-5149.JTN.21095-17.0.
32. Pushker N, Meel R, Kumar A, Kashyap S, Sen S, Bajaj MS. Orbital and periorbital dermoid/epidermoid cyst: a series of 280 cases and a brief review. Can J Ophthalmol. 2020;55(2):167–71. https://doi.org/10.1016/j.jcjo.2019.08.005.
33. Vahdani K, Rose GE. Ophthalmic presentation and outcomes for malignant sinonasal tumors. Ophthalmic Plast Reconstr Surg. 2021; https://doi.org/10.1097/IOP.0000000000001972.
34. Suárez C, Ferlito A, Lund VJ, et al. Management of the orbit in malignant sinonasal tumors. Head Neck. 2008;30(2):242–50. https://doi.org/10.1002/hed.20736.
35. Iannetti G, Valentini V, Rinna C, Ventucci E, Marianetti TM. Ethmoido-orbital tumors: our experience. J Craniofac Surg. 2005;16(6):1085–91. https://doi.org/10.1097/01.scs.0000164332.81428.ba.
36. Cracchiolo JR, Patel K, Migliacci JC, et al. Factors associated with a primary surgical approach for sinonasal squamous cell carcinoma. J Surg Oncol. 2018;117(4):756–64. https://doi.org/10.1002/jso.24923.
37. Ganly I, Patel SG, Singh B, et al. Craniofacial resection for malignant tumors involving the skull base in the elderly: an international collaborative study. Cancer. 2011;117(3):563–71. https://doi.org/10.1002/cncr.25390.
38. Reyes C, Mason E, Solares CA, Bush C, Carrau R. To preserve or not to preserve the orbit in paranasal sinus neoplasms: a meta-analysis. J Neurol Surg B Skull Base. 2015;76(2):122–8. https://doi.org/10.1055/s-0034-1390403.
39. Akhter AS, El Tecle N, Alexopoulos G, Espinoza G, Coppens J. Intraosseous orbital cavernous hemangioma with frontal extension and dural involvement. Cureus. 2019;11(6):e4823. https://doi.org/10.7759/cureus.4823.
40. Deng C, Hu W. Multiple cavernous hemangiomas in the orbit: a case report and review of the literature. Medicine (Baltimore). 2020;99(29):e20670. https://doi.org/10.1097/MD.0000000000020670.
41. Hentati A, Matar N, Dridi H, Bouali S, Jemel H. Bilateral orbital cavernous hemangioma. Asian J Neurosurg. 2018;13(4):1222–4. https://doi.org/10.4103/ajns.AJNS_96_17.
42. Zhang L, Li X, Tang F, Gan L, Wei X. Diagnostic imaging methods and comparative analysis of orbital cavernous hemangioma. Front Oncol. 2020;10:577452. https://doi.org/10.3389/fonc.2020.577452.
43. Qin X, Akter F, Qin L, et al. Dumbbell shaped craniorbital cavernous hemangioma. BMC Neurol. 2020;20(1):149. https://doi.org/10.1186/s12883-020-01734-z.
44. Young SM, Kim KH, Kim Y-D, et al. Orbital apex venous cavernous malformation with optic neuropathy: treatment with multisession gamma knife radiosurgery. Br J Ophthalmol. 2019;103(10):1453–9. https://doi.org/10.1136/bjophthalmol-2018-312893.
45. Smith ET. A case of lymphangioma of the orbit. Trans Am Ophthalmol Soc. 1925;23:240–6.
46. Patel KC, Kalantzis G, El-Hindy N, Chang BY. Sclerotherapy for orbital lymphangioma - case series and literature review. In Vivo. 2017;31(2):263–6. https://doi.org/10.21873/invivo.11055.
47. Thavara BD, Rajagopalawarrier B, Balakrishnan S, Kidangan GS. A case of adult orbital intraconal lymphangioma. Asian J Neurosurg. 2020;15(1):168–71. https://doi.org/10.4103/ajns.AJNS_282_19.
48. Woo YJ, Kim CY, Sgrignoli B, Yoon JS. Orbital lymphangioma: characteristics and treatment outcomes of 12 cases. Korean J Ophthalmol. 2017;31(3):194–201. https://doi.org/10.3341/kjo.2016.0034.
49. Sen S, Singh P, Bajaj MS, Gaur N. Management of a case of orbital lymphangioma presenting in adulthood with negative-pressure aspiration and bleomycin injection. BMJ Case Rep. 2019;12(6) https://doi.org/10.1136/bcr-2018-227697.
50. Kothari P, Mirani N, Langer PD. Orbital lymphangioma confined to an extraocular muscle. Ophthalmic Plast Reconstr Surg. 2020;36(3):e61–2. https://doi.org/10.1097/IOP.0000000000001572.
51. Lagrèze WA, Joachimsen L, Gross N, Taschner C, Rössler J. Sirolimus-induced regression of a large orbital lymphangioma. Orbit. 2019;38(1):79–80. https://doi.org/10.1080/01676830.2018.1436569.
52. Bagheri A, Amoohashemi N, Salour H, Yazdani S. Lacrimal gland lymphangioma: report of a case and review of literature. Orbit. 2012;31(3):197–9. https://doi.org/10.3109/01676830.2011.648807.
53. Tsen C-L, Lin M-C, Bee Y-S, Chen J-L, Kuo N-W, Sheu S-J. Ocular adnexal lymphoma: five case reports and a literature review. Taiwan J Ophthalmol. 2015;5(2):99–102. https://doi.org/10.1016/j.tjo.2014.05.007.
54. Yuen CA, Pula JH, Mehta M. Primary ocular adnexal extranodal marginal zone mucosa-associated lymphoid tissue (MALT) lymphoma presenting as orbital apex syndrome. Neuroophthalmology. 2017;41(2):94–8. https://doi.org/10.1080/01658107.2016.1263343.
55. Jaiswal AK, Tripathi M, Chandra PS, Sharma MC, Mahapatra AK. An unusual case of primary lymphoma of the skull base extending from cerebellopontine angle to cavernous sinus and orbit. A case report. J Neurosurg Sci. 2000;44(3):145–148; discussion 149.
56. Alkatan HM, Alaraj AM, Al-Ayoubi A. Diffuse large B-cell lymphoma of the orbit: a tertiary eye care center experience in Saudi Arabia. Saudi J Ophthalmol. 2012;26(2):235–9. https://doi.org/10.1016/j.sjopt.2011.09.004.
57. Yazıcı B, Sabur H, Yazıcı Z. Orbital cavitary rhabdomyosarcoma: case report and literature review. Ophthalmic Plast Reconstr Surg. 2014;30(1):e20–2. https://doi.org/10.1097/IOP.0b013e31828de376.
58. Dziedzic TA, Anand VK, Schwartz TH. Endoscopic endonasal approach to the lateral orbital apex: case report. J Neurosurg Pediatr. 2015;16(3):305–8. https://doi.org/10.3171/2015.2.PEDS1575.
59. Chaugule SS, Putambekar A, Gavade S, Deshpande R. Primary orbital leiomyosarcoma in an adult male. Ophthalmic Plast Reconstr Surg. 2019;35(2):e27–9. https://doi.org/10.1097/IOP.0000000000001293.
60. Jakhetiya A, Shukla NK, Muduly D, Kale SS. Extraskeletal orbital mesenchymal chondrosarcoma: surgical approach and mini review. BMJ Case Rep. 2017; https://doi.org/10.1136/bcr-2016-218744.
61. Broggi G, Salvatorelli L, Reibaldi M, et al. Solitary fibrous tumor of the orbital region: report of a case with emphasis on the diagnostic utility of STAT-6. Pathologica. 2020;112(4):195–9. https://doi.org/10.32074/1591-951X-9-20.
62. Mitamura M, Kase S, Suzuki Y, et al. Solitary fibrous tumor of the orbit: a clinicopathologic study of two cases with review of the literature. In Vivo. 2020;34(6):3649–54. https://doi.org/10.21873/invivo.12211.

63. Sayit AT, Elmali M, Gul A, Sullu Y. Solitary fibrous tumor of the orbit: computed tomography and histopathological findings. J Cancer Res Ther. 2019;15(3):719–21. https://doi.org/10.4103/jcrt.JCRT_1194_16.
64. Alkatan HM, Alsalamah AK, Almizel A, et al. Orbital solitary fibrous tumors: a multi-centered histopathological and immunohistochemical analysis with radiological description. Ann Saudi Med. 2020;40(3):227–33. https://doi.org/10.5144/0256-4947.2020.227.
65. Brum M, Nzwalo H, Oliveira E, et al. Solitary fibrous tumors of the orbit and central nervous system: a case series analysis. Asian J Neurosurg. 2018;13(2):336–40. https://doi.org/10.4103/ajns.AJNS_111_16.
66. Crawford L, Sharma S. Orbital apex metastasis from adenoid cystic carcinoma: acute loss of vision and subsequent recovery with the radiation. Cureus. 2017;9(11):e1869. https://doi.org/10.7759/cureus.1869.
67. Hirunwiwatkul P, Tirakunwichcha S, Meesuaypong P, Shuangshoti S. Orbital metastasis of hepatocellular carcinoma. J Neuroophthalmol. 2008;28(1):47–50. https://doi.org/10.1097/WNO.0b013e31816754e7.
68. Kagusa H, Mizobuchi Y, Nakajima K, Fujihara T, Bando Y, Takagi Y. Metastatic tumor to the orbital cavity from a primary carcinoma of the uterine cervix: a case report. J Med Invest. 2019;66(3.4):355–7. https://doi.org/10.2152/jmi.66.355.
69. Kim HJ, Wojno TH, Grossniklaus H. Atypical bilateral orbital metastases of lobular breast carcinoma. Ophthalmic Plast Reconstr Surg. 2012;28(6):e142–3. https://doi.org/10.1097/IOP.0b013e318249d5c0.
70. Pecen PE, Ramey NA, Richard MJ, Bhatti MT. Metastatic pancreatic carcinoma to the orbital apex presenting as a superior divisional third cranial nerve palsy. Clin Ophthalmol. 2012;6:1941–3. https://doi.org/10.2147/OPTH.S30208.
71. Tsuruta Y, Maeda Y, Kitaguchi Y, et al. A case of endonasal endoscopic surgery for intraorbital metastasis of gastric ring cell carcinoma. Ear Nose Throat J. 2020;2020:145561320943372. https://doi.org/10.1177/0145561320943372.
72. Wada K, Tsuda T, Hanada Y, Maeda Y, Mori K, Nishimura H. A rare case of prostate carcinoma metastasis in the orbital apex. Ear Nose Throat J. 2020;2020:145561320973783. https://doi.org/10.1177/0145561320973783.
73. Wadhwani M, Phuljhele S, Kumar R, Shameer A. Cervical carcinoma leading to orbital apex syndrome and blindness. BMJ Case Rep. 2019;12(3):e226587. https://doi.org/10.1136/bcr-2018-226587.

14 Periorbital Bony Diseases

Shuk Wan Joyce Chow

Abstract

Periorbital bony diseases are rare and mostly benign. Most patients present as incidental findings, while others may complain of proptosis or visual impairment. The most common causes are benign osseous tumours such as fibrous dysplasia, meningiomas or osteomas. Malignant neoplasms such as osteosarcomas are very rare. However, tumour-like conditions like Langerhans cell histiocytosis (LCH) may occur in the orbit as a single lesion or part of a multifocal multisystem disease. Orbital LCH usually occurs in children and can be regarded as high-risk lesions for CNS involvement. Other causes in the paediatric age group can be dermoid cysts, craniosynostosis or other congenital conditions, for example, osteopetrosis and craniotubular dysplasias.

Keywords

Periorbital bone disease · Fibrous dysplasia · Intraosseous meningioma · Osteoma · Orbital Langerhans cell histiocytosis · Craniosynostosis · Osteopetrosis · Sclerosing bone disease · Craniotubular dysplasia · Proptosis

14.1 Periorbital Bony Diseases

Diseases of the periorbital bone can be quite rare and are mostly incidental findings unrelated to the initial clinical indications. Benign osseous aetiologies are most frequently found in this region. Among the benign osseous tumours, fibrous dysplasia, meningiomas and osteomas represent the majority of diseases in the orbital bone. Osteosarcomas or other malignant neoplasms are rare. However, these benign lesions may cause debilitating symptoms and compression on optic structures if left untreated.

Tumour-like conditions such as Langerhans cell histiocytosis can also arise in the orbit in patients under 15 years of age. Congenital causes of craniosynostosis with craniofacial abnormalities may affect this region leading to proptosis and hypertelorism, increased risks of astigmatism, strabismus, lateral canthal dystopia, nasolacrimal obstruction and other ocular problems.

14.1.1 Fibrous Dysplasia

Fibrous dysplasia (FD) is a benign, slow growing, non-hereditary condition in which normal bone and marrow is replaced by fibrous tissue and woven bone. Overall incidence of FD is approximately 2.5% of all bone tumours and nearly 7.5% of benign bone neoplasms. The condition is caused by activation of the GNAS gene that results in inhibition of the differentiation and proliferation of bone-formal stromal cells [1].

FD can be either monostotic (80%) or polystostic (20%), or in the rarer form of McCune-Albright syndrome. McCune-Albright syndrome is classically defined by a triad of polyostotic FD (Fig. 14.1), café-au-lait skin patches with irregular borders, and endocrinopathies such as precocious puberty. The vast majority of patients are <30 years old and can present in younger children (<10 years old) in the polyostotic subtype. Ninety percent of patients with polyostotic or McCune-Albright syndrome have craniofacial involvement, whereas the zygomatic-maxillary complex is more affected in the monostotic subtype. Malignant transformation to osteosarcoma or other forms of sarcoma varies from 1% to 4% depending on the subtypes [2].

FD usually behaves as a slow growing mass lesion, but rapid enlargement may occur in some cases, especially young children and pre-pubertal adolescents. The rapid

S. W. J. Chow (✉)
Department of Neurosurgery, Queen Elizabeth Hospital, Hospital Authority, Hong Kong SAR, China
e-mail: csw814@ha.org.hk

T. L. POON et al. (eds.), *Orbital Apex and Periorbital Skull Base Diseases*, https://doi.org/10.1007/978-981-99-2989-4_14

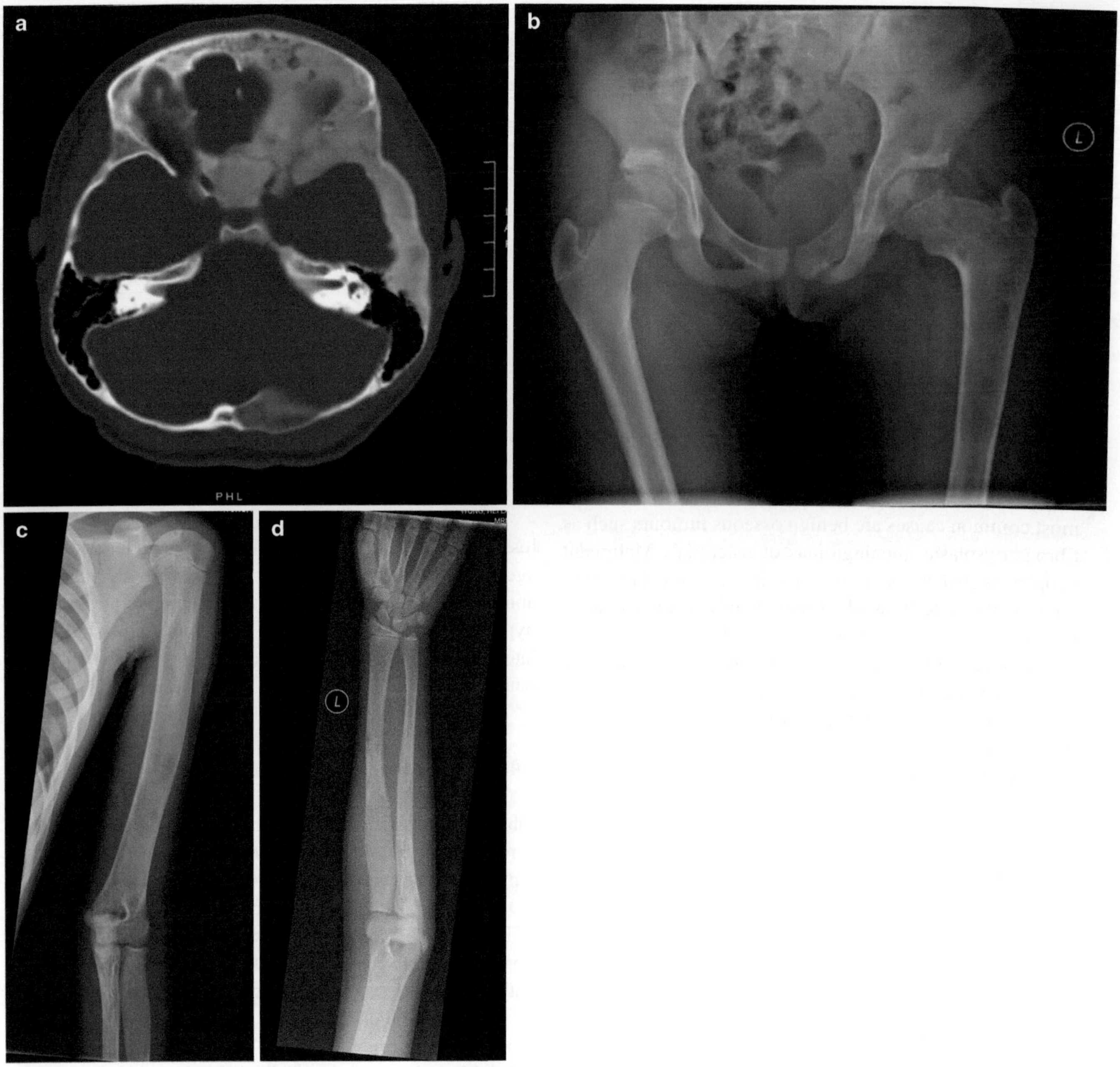

Fig. 14.1 (**a**–**d**) An 11-year-old girl with McCune-Albright syndrome. (**a**) Fibrous dysplasia involving the left fronto-orbital region, the greater and lesser sphenoid wing, anterior clinoid process with optic canal stenosis. Polyostotic involvement of FD. Radiograph showing ground glass appearance in (**b**) left hip and femur, (**c**) left humerus and (**d**) left forearm and metacarpals

growth may compress on vital structures such as the optic nerve, globe, auditory canal or nasal airway causing functional deficits. In non-syndromal cases, the progression may taper off as the patient approaches skeletal maturity. Hence, most patients adopt a conservative approach as there has been no medical therapy that has clearly proven to prevent the progression of FD. Surgical treatments are only reserved for those who have acute or progressive visual impairments or unacceptable cosmetic deformities (Fig. 14.2).

The underlying pathological culprit of visual loss can be due to optic canal stenosis or sometimes cystic degeneration of the tumour, most commonly in the anterior clinoidal process [3]. The diagnosis and extent of FD can be made by CT imaging, which shows an appearance of ground-glass opacity due to the small thin calcified woven trabeculae in fibrous stroma. MRI may not be the best tool to evaluate bony diseases, but it is pertinent in the visualisation of surrounding soft tissue structures, for example the optic nerve for any signals that may suggest compression.

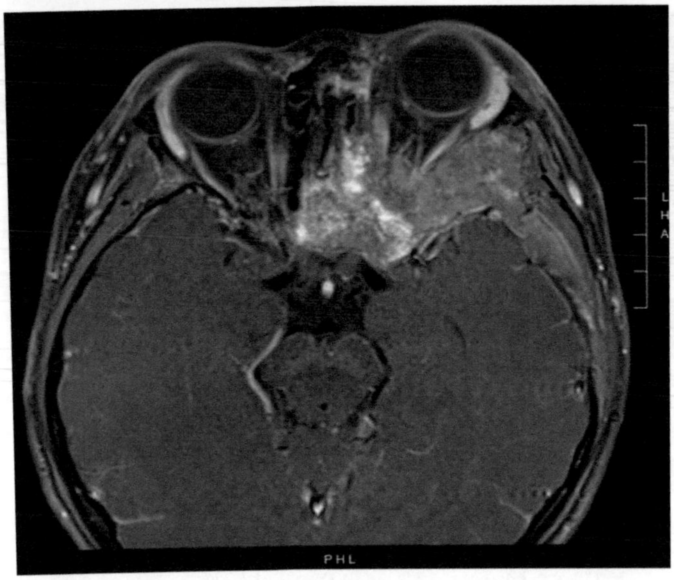

Fig. 14.2 T1-Gd contrast MRI appearance of fibrous dysplasia of frontal and sphenoid bones causing optic canal stenosis and compression onto optic nerve

Resection of the frontal bone complex, along with drilling of the anterior clinoid process and decompression of the optic canal is usually performed for FD involving the orbit. Immediate reconstruction with cranioplasty in the same operation provides excellent cosmetic results. Radical excision resulted in significantly less recurrence (15% vs. 71%) compared to limited reduction burring in previous studies [4].

Visual function can be stabilised or even restored with "timely decompression" in some patients. In a study by Chen et al., they have found that decompression has universally failed in patients who have established blindness of over 1 month. However, the best time for surgery is still controversial as their study only included 13 patients and there has not been large study series that can clearly establish the effect of early decompression from time of visual deterioration. It can only be concluded that patients with progressive or acute visual loss requires early decompression as soon as possible for better outcomes.

Naturally, concerns of the visual function are the most feared complication in fronto-orbital FD surgeries. There has been not one, but a few reported cases of unilateral blindness after surgery in asymptomatic patients [5–7]. As such, many authors proposed that prophylactic transcranial optic canal decompression, with significant associated risks, is still controversial in the current literature.

14.1.2 Meningiomas

Meningiomas are common in adulthood, with a female preponderance and a mean age of onset of 40–50 years old [8]. The en plaque meningiomas (MEP) or intraosseous meningiomas (IOM) comprises 2–9% of all meningiomas and up to 18% of sphenoid wing meningiomas [8]. It was first introduced by Cushing and Eisenhardt in 1938, which described a carpet-like tumour growth associated with significant hyperostosis, most commonly seen in sphenoid ridge with orbital involvement. The most common presenting symptom is proptosis, decrease in vision or even opthalmoplegia. These tumours are often extensive, and complete removal is uncommon; hence, the recurrence rate is higher.

'En plaque' meningiomas differ from the most common 'en masse' meningiomas as it is mainly a bone disease. Most en masse meningiomas may result in hyperostotic reaction of the adjacent skull bone, but MEPs may infiltrate the dura and into bony harversian canals where they continue the neoplastic process intraosseously. Hence, the symptoms of proptosis and visual impairment are more extensive (Fig. 14.3).

There are two important aspects to consider during resection, (1) decompression of the optic nerve and (2) resection of tumour. Most surgeons advocate a frontotemporal craniotomy and removal of tumour in the squamous temporal bone and superolateral orbital wall extradurally. Resection of the anterior clinoid process was also done extradurally if there is tumour involvement. Routine optic canal decompression is recommended by some authors [9, 10] to improve or preserve visual functions of the patients. The dura and intradural component is then excised as far as possible to prevent early recurrence. And the calvarial bony defect is then reconstructed if necessary (Fig. 14.4).

Complete resection is frequently impossible, in a long follow-up period of up to 17 years (mean 4.5 years), 61% of these tumours remain stable, and only 39% were progressive [11]. It is recommended that the surgical aim should be symptomatic relief rather than radical resection. Proptosis generally has a very good outcome after complete resection in reported studies [8]. Visual outcomes may be affected by the duration, extent of compression and severity of visual deficit on presentation. The reported improvement ranges from 27% to 79% due to the heterogeneous data [9, 12, 13].

Recurrence rate may vary depending on the involvement of important vital surrounding structures. Cavernous sinus extension is a main cause of recurrence in many circumstances [14], and some believe that immediate adjuvant

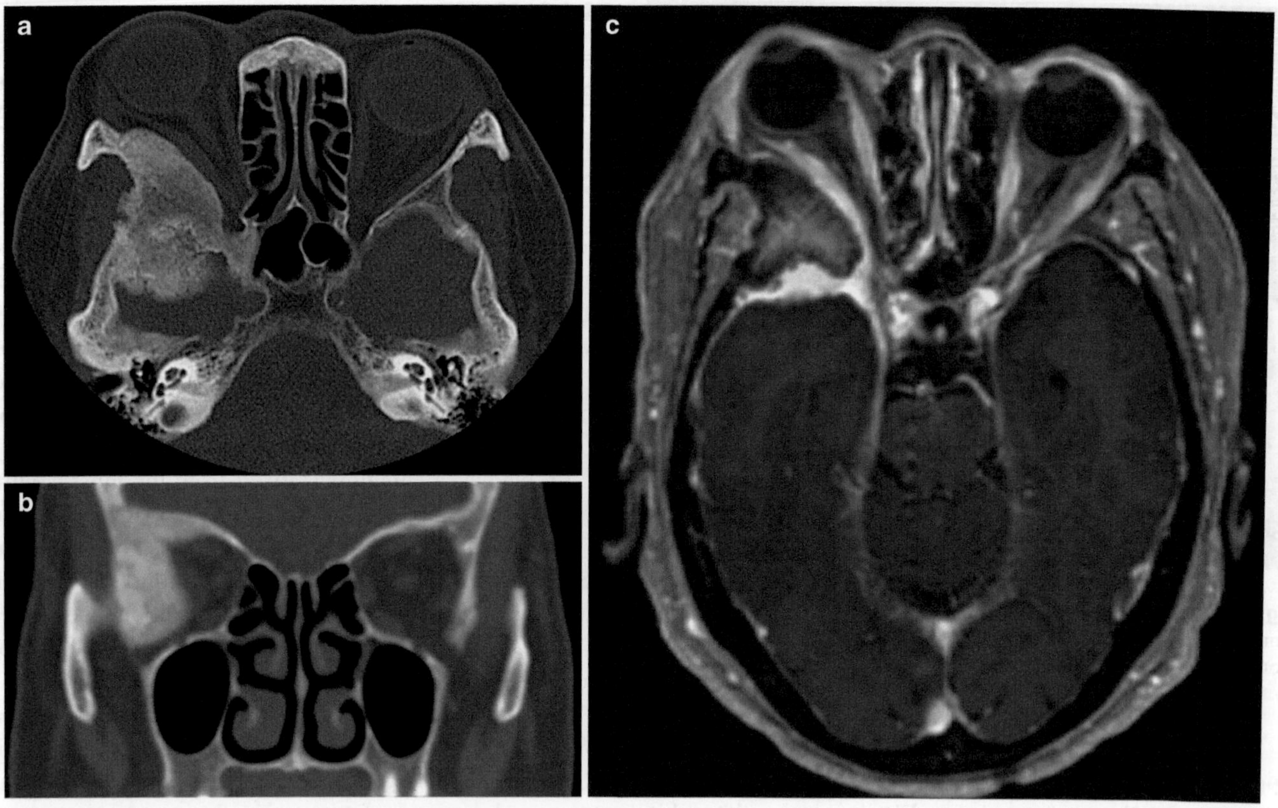

Fig. 14.3 (**a**) Axial and (**b**) coronal CT images of 56-year-old lady with right sphenoid wing intraosseous meningioma causing proptosis and decreased vision. (**c**) T1-Gd contrast MRI images showing large area of dural thickening and enhancement at sphenoid and periorbital region; optic nerve is compressed at orbital apex region

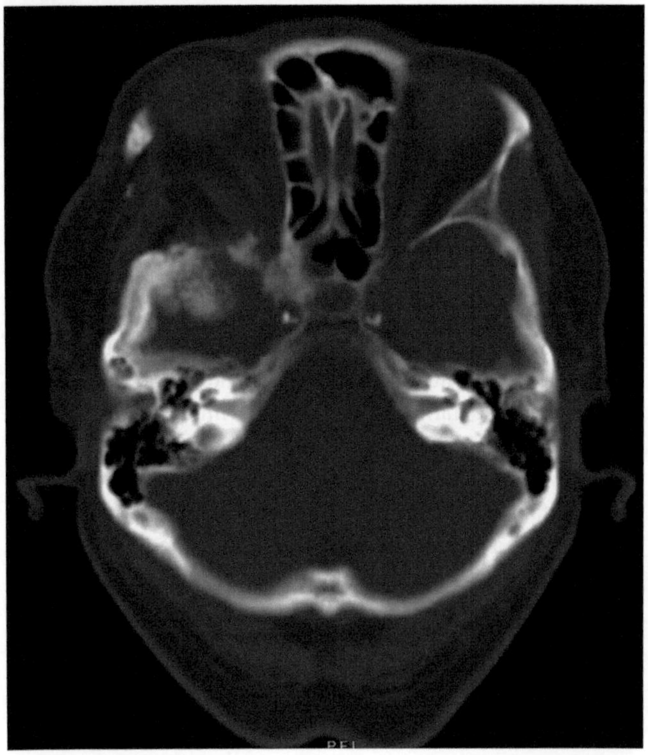

Fig. 14.4 Immediate post-operative CT image after fronto-orbital removal of bone tumour and optic canal decompression with improved proptosis and vision

radiotherapy is necessary for better local control of the disease [14, 15]. Others prefer to defer radiotherapy to those with recurrence or atypical meningiomas. The decision for adjuvant radiotherapy is still a matter of debate.

14.1.3 Osteomas

Osteomas are slow-growing benign bony tumours that are mostly asymptomatic. The overall incidence of skull osteomas is about 0.4% by retrospective analysis of skull radiographs [16], and those arising in the paranasal sinus are even less. The frontal sinus is the most frequently affected region, followed by the ethmoid sinus, maxillary antrum and the sphenoid sinus [16, 17].

Although ongoing debates on a history of childhood trauma causing tumour induction have been repeatedly discussed in the literature, the true pathogenesis of osteomas remains unknown [16, 18]. Notably, multiple osteomas can be associated with Gardner's syndrome, which is characterised by multiple intestinal polyps, desmoid tumours and supranumerary teeth. Given that about half of patients with Gardner's syndrome lack positive family history, some authors even recommend colonoscopy for all patients with osteoma irrespective of age [19].

Osteomas are commonly found as a hard protruding mass at the frontal forehead region with patients complaining of a painless 'bony bump' in the clinic. Rarely, they can grow in the paranasal sinuses causing symptoms of headache, sinonasal obstruction, recurrent sinusitis [20] or sinus abscesses [21]. In the exceptional case, the periorbital region may be affected causing proptosis, impairment of eye mobility and even trigeminal dysaesthesia [16].

These lesions are commonly managed with a 'wait and see' approach, while surgical excision is offered to those with large lesions, for cosmetic reasons, or when symptoms occur. Traditionally, sinonasal osteomas are removed by extranasal approaches with acceptable aesthetic results and shorter operation time. In the recent decade, major improvements have been achieved in endoscopic transanal techniques and are now a valid alternative in many cases [22–25]. Frontal osteomas not extending to a lateral limit passing through the lamina papyracea [22] are typical indications for pure endoscopic approaches. Those that are lateral to this limit may require a combined external-endoscopic technique for complete removal. The recurrence rate after complete resection of this tumour is very rare, and malignant transformation has not been described [20, 26].

14.1.4 Dermoid Cysts

Dermoid cyst is one of the most common orbital lesions encountered in children. They account for 3–9% of orbital tumours [27], usually found at the superolateral orbital margin, near the frontozygomatic suture. It can be superficial or deep, and the deep orbital dermoid cysts usually present later as they lie behind the lacrimal gland. They usually present with a painless solid mass or proptosis, cyst leakage or rupture with or without inflammation that may occur in some cases.

Dermoid cysts are developmental abnormalities or choristoma due to sequestration of ectoderm into underlying mesenchyme along embryonic lines of closure. They are lined by kertanised stratified squamous epithelium with a fibrous wall containing dermal appendages, for example hair follicles, sebaceous and sweat glands. The cyst contents are white sebaceous-like material with cholestrin crystals and hair or oily materials [27, 28].

Superficial dermoid cysts present early at around 1–3 years of age, and they present at birth and may grow slowly. Deep dermoid cysts present later in teenage or adult life with proptosis, and further CT or MRI is required to localise the lesion. Bony erosion may take place due to pressure effect and may occasional involve the underlying dura or even extend intracranially. Treatment is invariably by complete surgical removal without rupture. It is pertinent to evaluate the extent of deep dermoid cysts and approach these lesions with a combined transcranial approach by neurosurgeons and opthalmologists in order to ensure complete removal [29]. In the case of inadvertent rupture, copious irrigation by warm saline is recommended in order to minimise any inflammation in the surrounding area. The bony defect should be curretted clear [30], as remnants of the embryonic epithelium in the surgical cavity can cause recurrence with abscess and fistula formation [31, 32].

14.2 Other Rare Tumours

14.2.1 Langerhans Cell Histiocytosis

Langerhans cell histiocytosis (LCH) is a rare disorder with yearly incidence of four to nine cases per million children younger than 15 years of age [33, 34]. It occurs frequently in the first or second decade of life, with a male predominance. It is characterised by idiopathic inflammatory myeloid neoplasia due to accumulation of clonal histiocytes and granuloma formation with positive immunostaining for CD1a and CD207 (Langerin). There are three main subtypes of LCH: unifocal eosinophilic granuloma, multifocal unisystem disease (Hand-Schuller-Christian syndrome) and multifocal multisystem disease (Letterer-Siwe syndrome).

Isolated eosinophilic granuloma of the orbit accounts for <1% of all orbital tumours [33] but usually occurs in children of 1–5 years old, with the earliest reported case to be 16 months old [33, 35]. These lesions manifest as unilateral eyelid swelling or a palpable mass, with or without proptosis or pain. The superior orbital rim is commonly affected as it still contains bone marrow where the Langerhans cells may proliferate into a tumour mass. These Langerhans cells also produce IL-1 and PGE2 causing disproportionate lytic bone destruction [34–36] and can be reflected as extensive bony destruction in CT images. MRI shows an extraconal isointense T1 and hyperintense T2 mass, which enhances with gadolinium injection. Differential diagnosis of this lytic bone tumour can be dermoid cyst, Ewing's sarcoma or lacrimal gland neoplasms (Fig. 14.5).

The management of LCH is still an ongoing debate as the pathogenesis is still poorly understood [37].There are two polar approaches described in the literature as cases of spontaneous healing with minimal intervention have been reported [36, 38]. Hence, a more 'conservative' approach is advocated by ophthalmologists and orbital surgeons including subtotal curettage with intralesional steroids or low dose focal radiotherapy. However, paediatric oncologists recommend systemic therapy as concerns are raised for the possibility of systemic progression and potential debilitating permanent consequences.

Although involvement of the orbit in LCH can occur in 12–37% of all LCH cases [39–41], 52% of LCH with orbital involvement can have disseminated disease according to the International Histiocyte Society [33]. It is important to refer these patients to paediatric oncologists for extensive evalua-

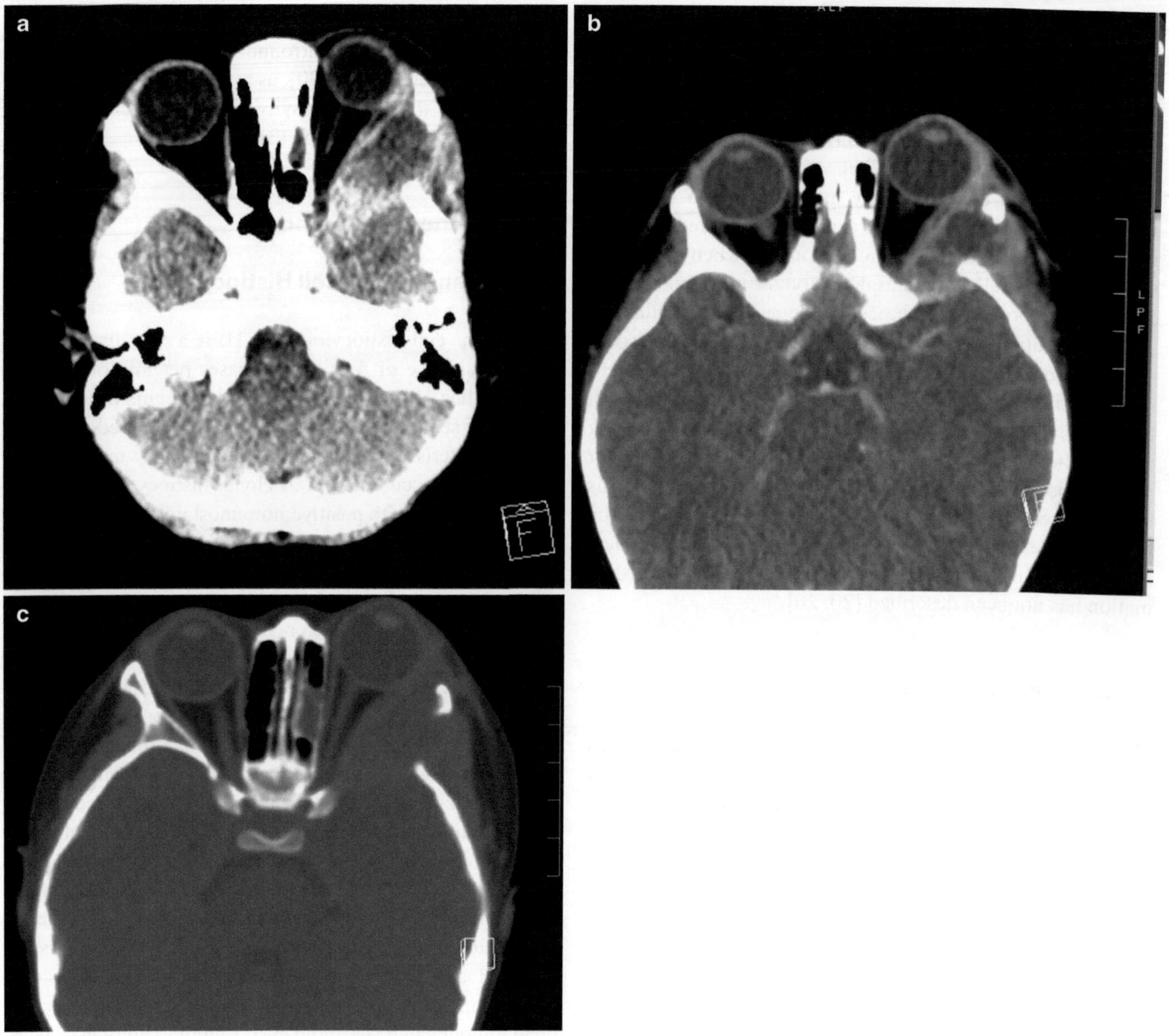

Fig. 14.5 An 8-year-old girl presenting with lateral orbital mass. CT (**a**) plain and (**b**) iodinated-contrast imaging showing lateral orbital mass with heterogeneous contrast enhancement and gross proptosis in left eye with (**c**) lytic bone destruction

tion of systemic involvements. If the disease is solely unifocal and limited to the orbit, the majority of cases can be cured by subtotal curettage and intralesional steroids with low recurrence rates [36, 42]. In case of recurrence or incomplete response, these patients may respond to systemic chemotherapy or additional low dose focal radiotherapy (Fig. 14.6).

In the circumstances where orbital involvement is in the setting of multifocal or multisystemic LCH, it is recommended for these patients to have systemic treatment. These patients have an increased risk of diabetes insidipus and neurodegeneration (CNS-LCH of nongranulomatous type), which may cause inflammation and neuronal loss [43]. Neurodegeneration can occur in the absence of extracranial disease and can lead to refractory or disabling consequences. The presence of unifocal orbital LCH as a risk factor for CNS-related permanent consequences has been implicated, but not substantiated in the current literature [36]. The preventive role of systemic treatment for CNS-LCH lesions or

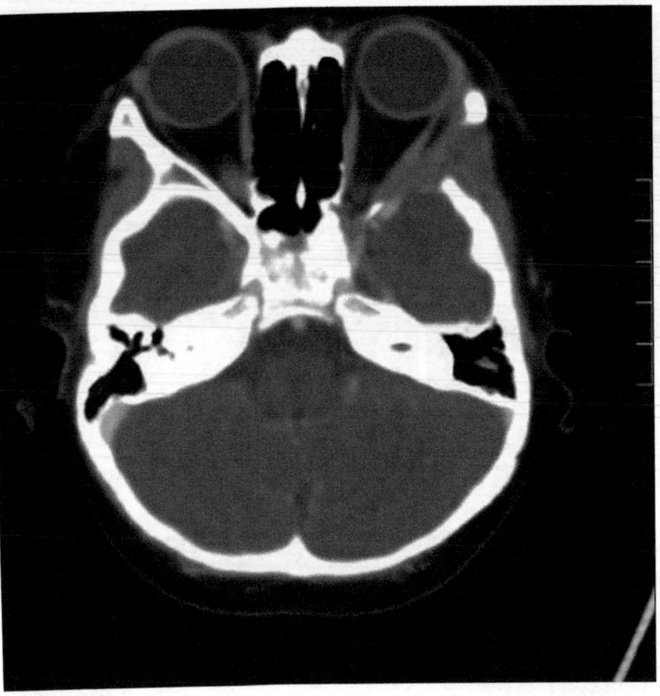

Fig. 14.6 Complete resolution of lesion after a course of systemic chemotherapy

neurodegenerative disease stems from retrospective cohort studies and has been questioned by other authors. The ongoing work by the Histiocyte Society, for example LCH-IV study, may provide the answers in the near future. Meanwhile, the optimal approach is tailored to each individual case by risk stratification through a multidisciplinary approach.

14.3 Congenital Abnormalities

14.3.1 Craniosynostosis

Craniosynostosis is a congenital disorder caused by premature closure of the calvarial sutures, restricting normal growth of bone in both the neuro- and viscero-cranium. This limits the development of the brain and causes deformed skull, midface hypoplasia, and shallow orbits, which leads to clinical symptoms of raised intracranial pressure, obstructive sleep apnoea and proptosis [44].

Majority of the cases are non-syndromal and isolated causing single suture craniosynostosis. However, children with diseases such as Apert, Crouzon or Pfeiffer syndromes typically have multiple suture involvements and require multidisciplinary care at the timing of diagnosis. In many syndromal cases, bilateral premature fusion of coronal sutures leads to restricted growth in the ventral-dorsal direction, compensatory growth occurs in the medial-lateral and the vertical direction according to Virchow's law. This leads to brachycephaly and turricephaly in infants, causing raised intracranial pressure and supraorbital recession [45], which may jeopardise visual functions.

In regard to infants with orbital involvements of anterior skull vault craniosynostosis, most are treated with fronto-orbital advancements at 9–12 months. Early surgery at 3 months of age may be required if symptoms of severely increased intracranial pressure or papilloedema occurs (Fig. 14.7a-d). Surgical methods of anterior advancements have been abounding in the literature, but the mainstay treatment for most brachycephalies and turricephalies is bifrontal remodelling with or without the fronto-orbital bandeau and expansive morcellations depending on their severity. The shallow orbits can be alleviated by the orbital bandeau as demonstrated in a geometrical study, which showed a mean increase of 50.2% in orbital volume after monobloc advancement of the fronto-orbital region [45].

Newer methods such as endoscopic-assisted suturectomies may be utilised in infants of 3–4 months, especially with scaphocephaly, in order to reduce blood loss and shorten operative time. Distraction devices for anterior vault or posterior vault advancements are now also an alternative surgical procedure added to the armamentarium [46, 47]. Despite the need for a second operation for removal of the distraction device, it is a potential procedure when greater degree of advancement is required and is generally recommended to be done at 4–12 years of age [48]. Some also advocate for distraction devices in those patients who had failed multiple corrective surgeries. However, the local infection and CSF leak rates are higher when compared with conventional frontoorbital advancements [47]. Other common complications are operative blood loss, subgaleal haematomas or dural tears, and the mortality rate in craniofacial surgery is very low [49]. Reoperations are common, especially in severe cases that required initial operation at the age of 6 months or below [50].

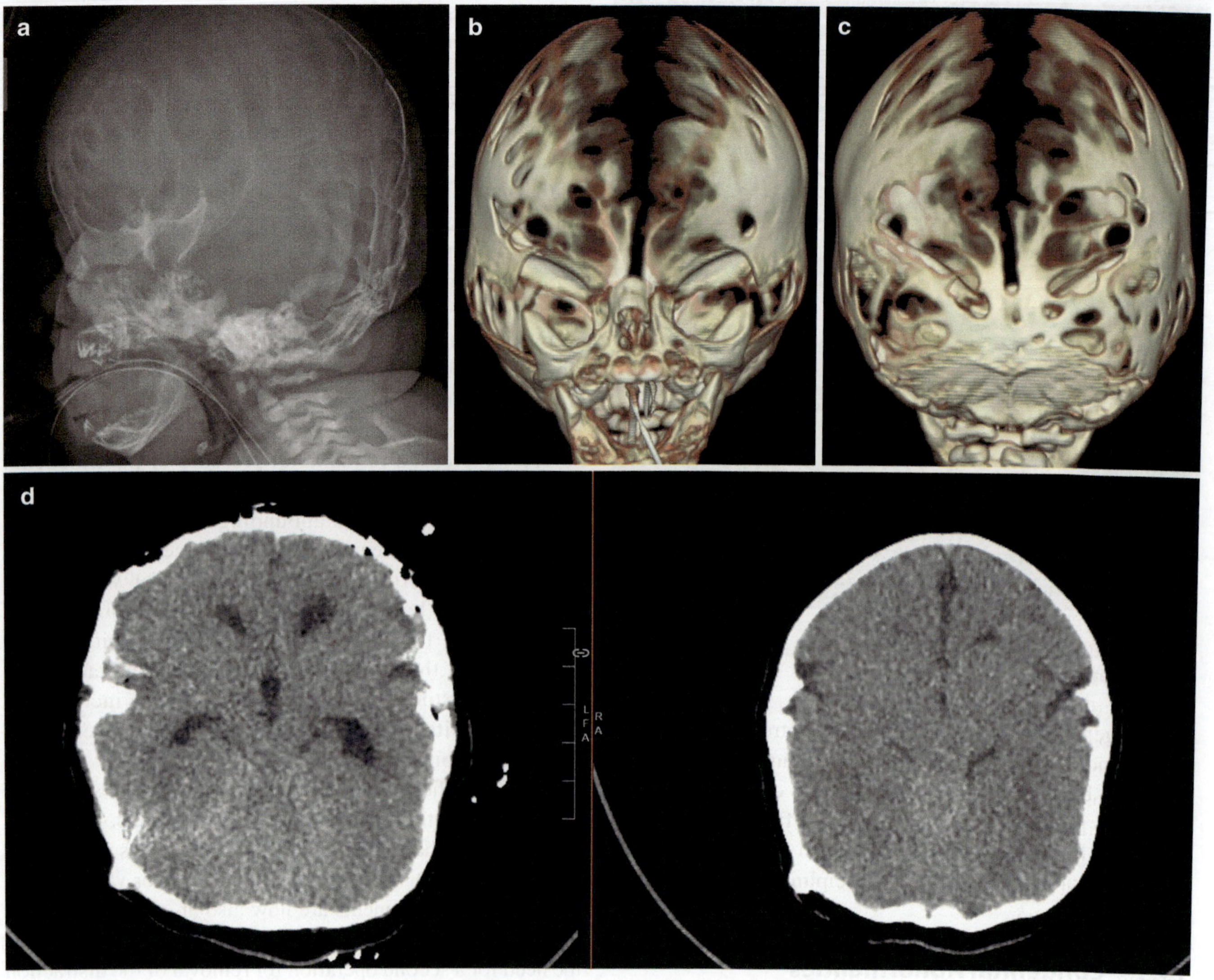

Fig. 14.7 (**a**) Baby girl, with FGFR-related disease, was born with abnormally small head shape at birth. Skull x-ray showed beaten-copper appearance. (**b**) CT reconstruction found severe bilateral coronal, and (**c**) bilateral lambdoid sutures craniosynotosis. (**d**) Early orbitofrontal advancement was done, with prior ventriculo-peritoneal shunt, at 3 months of age to relieve the raised intracranial pressure. The post-operative CT image was shown on the left

14.3.2 Sclerosing Bone Dysplasias [17, 51]

Rare causes of periorbital bony diseases are genetic syndromes of craniofacial hyperostosis. These syndromes have a tendency to present itself during childhood or even infancy, causing severe disfigurement or functional impairment.

14.3.2.1 Osteopetrosis [17, 52, 53]

Osteopetrosis, also termed 'marble bone disease,' is characterised by increased bone density and bone mass resulting in macrocephaly and altered craniofacial features. It is a rare genetic disease that can be inherited in benign autosomal dominant (ADO), intermediate autosomal recessive (ARO) and malignant autosomal recessive forms. The ADO form is more common with an estimated incidence of 1 in 20,000 births, and it presents later in adulthood, and symptoms are milder or even absent. However, the ARO form can occur early in childhood with fractures, short stature, compressive neuropathies (steward), tetanic seizures (steward) and life-threatening pancytopenia.

More than ten genetic mutations have been identified in this heterogeneous condition leading to abnormal osteoclast differentiation and function. Malignant ARO is associated with RANKL gene mutation [52], in which no mature osteoclasts are present. This life-threatening condition occurs in the first few months of life, and the bone is weakened and is predisposed to recurrent fractures and osteomyelitis. The skull base is commonly affected, resulting in an overgrowth of the skull foramina and compressive neuropathies. The optic nerve is most commonly affected [54], subsequently the auditory, trigeminal and lastly the facial nerves.

Diagnosis is mainly clinical and depends on classical radiological features of diffuse sclerosis or tell-tale signs of 'bone-in-bone' appearance, 'rugger-jersey' spine or 'Erlenmeyer flask' deformity. MRI can be used to detect osteomyelitis. Other associated systemic features may help identify the subtype of osteopetrosis.

Unfortunately, no effective medical treatment exists for osteopetrosis. As a neurosurgeon, surgical decompression of the optic nerve can be performed to halt or prevent visual loss. Al-mefty series of six patients underwent supraorbital craniotomies for bilateral optic nerve decompression with no complications. In their paper and thereafter, the key of decompression is to include both sides of the optic nerve, not just unroofing the optic canal [55–57].

14.3.2.2 Craniotubular Dysplasias and Hyperostosis

A group of genetic diseases causes increased bone formation. In craniotubular dysplasias, the cranial and tubular bones are deformed by a defect in bone modelling [51], for example Van Buchem disease. Van Buchem disease, formerly known as hyperostosis corticalis generalisata familiaris, is most prevalent in the Netherlands with less than 50 patients described. Sclerosteosis is similar, usually more severe, and is seen in South Africa with less than 100 cases. Both are autosomal recessive, presents within the first decade of life and is caused by a mutation in the SOST gene, leading to impaired inhibitor feedback mechanism by sclerostin. These patients can have headaches, gigantism, skull base and calvarial hyperostosis causing increased intracranial pressure and cranial nerve entrapments. Decompressive craniectomy is often necessary in the second decade, and the facial and vestibulocochlear nerves are the most commonly affected. Surgical decompression of accessible impaired cranial nerves is advised even in the asymptomatic period in severe cases [58, 59].

In craniotubular hyperostosis, these bones are formed by an active overgrowth of bone tissue. Camurati-Engelmann disease is an autosominal dominant condition in which hyperostosis starts at the diaphysis due to a mutation in the TGFB1 gene. There are only about 200 cases in the literature, and most commonly affects long bones in childhood. Skull base and calvarial involvement occurs in over 50% if cases are severe. Hearing loss is reported to be 19%; optic nerve and facial nerve entrapment can also occur but is less frequent.

Hyperostosis cranialis interna (HCI) is first described by Manni in 1999 [51, 58], with just about 15 cases in the Netherlands so far. It affects the skull base and the calvaria exclusively causing symptoms in childhood. Symptoms are similar to craniotubular diseases leading to raised intracranial pressures or entrapments of cranial nerves. However, the facial appearance is normal as the facial bones and tubular bones are not affected. Hyperostosis frontalis interna (HFI) occurs in 5–12% of the general population that mimics HCI. It is a benign condition, not a disease, of new bone formation in the inner table of the frontal bone that is most commonly found in post-menopausal women. The aetiology is uncertain, yet obesity, diabetes, post-menopausal state and female gender are risk factors for HFI, sparkling debates on hormonal influences on bone growth. It is a common phenomenon in modern populations [60], and the vast majority of cases is asymptomatic.

14.3.2.3 Caffey-Silverman Syndrome [61–63]

Infantile cortical hyperostosis (ICH), also known as Caffey disease, was first reported by Roske in 1930 and then described by Caffey and Silverman in 1945 [62]. It affects the mandible in 70–90% of the cases but can also affect the periorbital bones [64], the clavicle, scapula and rarely parietal bone and ilia.

ICH is autosomal dominant with variable penetrance, associated with a COLIA1 gene mutation. It classically appears as an asymmetrical sudden soft tissue swelling of the face, fever and irritability in the infantile stage and rarely presents beyond the age of 1. The swellings can become hard and fixed to the bone and can also be red and painful [62]. Clinical pictures of periorbital cellulitis [64] associated with anaemia [65] have been reported. Although features can be quite discerning and can mimic that of child abuse, the condition is self-limiting and usually resolves within 2 years of age with no major clinical sequelae.

References

1. Lee JS, Fitzgibbon EJ, Chen YR, Kim HJ, Lustig LR, Akintoye SO, et al. Clinical guidelines for the management of craniofacial fibrous dysplasia. Orphanet J Rare Dis. 2012;7(Suppl 1):1–19.
2. Pack SE, Al Share AA, Quereshy FA, Baur DA. Osteosarcoma of the mandible arising in fibrous dysplasia—a case report. J Oral Maxillofac Surg. 2016;74(11):2229.e1–4. https://www.sciencedirect.com/science/article/pii/S027823911630492X
3. Dumont AS, Boulos PT, Jane JA, Ellegala DB, Newman SA. Cranioorbital fibrous dysplasia: with emphasis on visual impairment and current surgical management. Neurosurg Focus. 2001;10(5):1–8.
4. Denadai R, Raposo-Amaral CA, Marques FF, Ghizoni E, Buzzo CL, Raposo-Amaral CE. Strategies for the optimal individualized surgical management of craniofacial fibrous dysplasia. Ann Plast Surg. 2016;77(2) https://journals.lww.com/annalsplasticsurgery/Fulltext/2016/08000/Strategies_for_the_Optimal_Individualized_Surgical.13.aspx:195.
5. Cutler CM, Lee JS, Butman JA, FitzGibbon EJ, Kelly MH, Brillante BA, et al. Long-term outcome of optic nerve encasement and optic nerve decompression in patients with fibrous dysplasia: risk factors for blindness and safety of observation.

Neurosurgery. 2006;59(5):1011–8. https://doi.org/10.1227/01.NEU.0000254440.02736.E3.
6. Edelstein C, Goldberg RA, Rubino G. Unilateral blindness after ipsilateral prophylactic transcranial optic canal decompression for fibrous dysplasia. Am J Ophthalmol. 1998;126(3):469–71. https://www.sciencedirect.com/science/article/pii/S0002939498001184
7. Chen Y-R, Breidahl A, Chang C-N. Optic nerve decompression in fibrous dysplasia: indications, efficacy, and safety. Plast Reconstr Surg. 1997;99(1):22–30.
8. Samadian M, Sharifi G, Mousavinejad SA, Amin AA, Ebrahimzadeh K, Tavassol HH, et al. Surgical outcomes of sphenoorbital en plaque meningioma: a 10-year experience in 57 consecutive cases. World Neurosurg. 2020;144:e576–81.
9. Mirone G, Chibbaro S, Schiabello L, Tola S, George B. En plaque sphenoid wing meningiomas: recurrence factors and surgical strategy in a series of 71 patients. Oper Neurosurg. 2009;65(Suppl_6):ons100–9. https://doi.org/10.1227/01.NEU.0000345652.19200.D5.
10. Sade B, Lee JH. High incidence of optic canal involvement in clinoidal meningiomas: rationale for aggressive skull base approach. Acta Neurochir (Wien). 2008;150(11):1127–32.
11. Ringel F, Cedzich C, Schramm J. Microsurgical technique and results of a series of 63 spheno-orbital meningiomas. Oper Neurosurg. 2007;60(Suppl_4):ONS-214–22. https://doi.org/10.1227/01.NEU.0000255415.47937.1A.
12. Cristante L. Surgical treatment of meningiomas of the orbit and optic canal: a retrospective study with particular attention to the visual outcome. Acta Neurochir (Wien). 1994;126(1):27–32. https://doi.org/10.1007/BF01476490.
13. Nakamura M, Roser F, Jacobs C, Vorkapic P, Samii M. Medial sphenoid wing meningiomas: clinical outcome and recurrence rate. Neurosurgery. 2006;58(4):626–39. https://doi.org/10.1227/01.NEU.0000197104.78684.5D.
14. Simas N, Farias J. Sphenoid wing en plaque meningiomas: surgical results and recurrence rates. Surg Neurol Int. 2013;4(1):86.
15. Maroon JC, Kennerdell JS, Vidovich DV, Abla A, Sternau L. Recurrent spheno-orbital meningioma. J Neurosurg. 1994;80(2):202–8. https://thejns.org/view/journals/j-neurosurg/80/2/article-p202.xml
16. Friedrich RE. Long-term follow-up control of pedunculated orbital floor osteoma, becoming symptomatic by atypical facial pain. In Vivo (Brooklyn). 2009;23(1):117–22.
17. Van De Voorde N, Mortier GR, Vanhoenacker FM. Fibrous dysplasia, Paget's disease of bone, and other uncommon sclerotic bone lesions of the craniofacial bones. Semin Musculoskelet Radiol. 2020;24(5):570–8.
18. Ma'luf RN, Ghazi NG, Zein WM, Gedeon GA, Hadi UM. Orbital osteoma arising adjacent to a foreign body. Ophthalmic Plast Reconstr Surg. 2003;19(4):327–30.
19. Smud D, Augustin G, Kekez T, Kinda E, Majerovic M, Jelincic Z. Gardner's syndrome: genetic testing and colonoscopy are indicated in adolescents and young adults with cranial osteomas: a case report. World J Gastroenterol. 2007;13(28):3900.
20. Izci Y. Management of the large cranial osteoma: experience with 13 adult patients. Acta Neurochir. 2005;147(11):1151–5.
21. Sahin A, Yildirim N, Cingi E, Atasoy MA. Frontoethmoid sinus osteoma as a cause of subperiosteal orbital abscess. Adv Ther. 2007;24(3):571–4. https://doi.org/10.1007/BF02848779.
22. Turri-Zanoni M, Dallan I, Terranova P, Battaglia P, Karligkiotis A, Bignami M, et al. Frontoethmoidal and intraorbital osteomas. Arch Otolaryngol Neck Surg. 2012;138(5):498.
23. Mulhern M, Kirkpatrick N, Joshi N, Vijh V, Coghlan B, Waterhouse N. Endoscopic removal of periorbital lesions. Orbit. 2002;21(4):263–9.
24. Miman MC, Bayindir T, Akarcay M, Erdem T, Selimoglu E. Endoscopic removal technique of a huge ethmoido-orbital osteoma. J Craniofac Surg. 2009;20(5) https://journals.lww.com/jcraniofacialsurgery/Fulltext/2009/09000/Endoscopic_Removal_Technique_of_a_Huge.22.aspx:1403.
25. Huang Y, Zhu X, Liu Y. Nasal endoscopic surgery for osteoid osteoma of the periorbital skull base: a case report. Lin Chung Er Bi Yan Hou Tou Jing Wai Ke Za Zhi. 2016;30(3):254–5. http://europepmc.org/abstract/MED/27373105
26. Muderris T, Bercin S, Sevil E, Kiris M. Endoscopic removal of a giant ethmoid osteoma with orbital extension. Acta Inform Med. 2012;20(4):266–8. https://pubmed.ncbi.nlm.nih.gov/23378698
27. Ahuja R, Azar NF. Orbital dermoids in children. Semin Ophthalmol. 2006;21(3):207–11.
28. Lane CM, Ehrlich WW, Wright JE. Orbital dermoid cyst. Eye. 1987;1(4):504–11.
29. Gabibov GA, Sokolova ON, Cherekaev VA, Parfenova ND, Khlu S. Dermoid cysts of the orbit spreading into the cranial cavity. Zhurnal Vopr neirokhirurgii Im NN Burdenko. 1989;5:49–51.
30. Vahdani K, Rose GE. Presentation and treatment of deep orbital dermoid cysts. Ophthalmology. 2020;127(9):1276–8.
31. Cavazza S, Laffi GL, Lodi L, Gasparrini E, Tassinari G. Orbital dermoid cyst of childhood: clinical pathologic findings, classification and management. Int Ophthalmol. 2011;31(2):93–7.
32. Wells TS, Harris GJ. Orbital dermoid cyst and sinus tract presenting with acute infection. Ophthalmic Plast Reconstr Surg. 2004;20(6):465–7.
33. Lakatos K, Sterlich K, Pötschger U, Thiem E, Hutter C, Prosch H, et al. Langerhans cell histiocytosis of the orbit: spectrum of clinical and imaging findings. J Pediatr. 2021;230:174–181.e1.
34. Gündüz K, Palamar M, Parmak N, Kuzu I. Eosinophilic granuloma of the orbit: report of two cases. J Am Assoc Pediatr Ophthalmol Strabismus. 2007;11(5):506–8.
35. Yan J, Zhou S, Li Y. Benign orbital tumors with bone destruction in children. PLoS One. 2012;7(2):e32111.
36. Harris GJ, Woo KI, Haik BG, Elner VM. Eosinophilic granuloma of the orbit: a paradox of aggressive destruction responsive to minimal intervention. Trans Am Ophthalmol Soc. 2003;101:93–105.
37. Broadbent V, Gadner H. Current therapy for Langerhans cell histiocytosis. Hematol Oncol Clin North Am. 1998;12(2):327–38.
38. Glover AT, Grove AS. Eosinophilic granuloma of the orbit with spontaneous healing. Ophthalmology. 1987;94(8):1008–12.
39. Erly WK, Carmody RF, Dryden RM. Orbital histiocytosis X. Am J Neuroradiol. 1995;16(6):1258–61.
40. Moore AT, Pritchard J, Taylor DSL. Histiocytosis X: an ophthalmological review. Br J Ophthalmol. 1985;69(1):7–14.
41. Vosoghi H, Rodriguez-Galindo C, Wilson MW. Orbital involvement in Langerhans cell histiocytosis. Ophthalmic Plast Reconstr Surg. 2009;25(6):430–3.
42. Herwig MC, Wojno T, Zhang Q, Grossniklaus HE. Langerhans cell histiocytosis of the orbit: five clinicopathologic cases and review of the literature. Surv Ophthalmol. 2013;58(4):330–40.
43. Grois N, Prayer D, Prosch H, Lassmann H. Neuropathology of CNS disease in Langerhans cell histiocytosis. Brain. 2005;128(4):829–38.
44. Sharma RK. Craniosynostosis. Indian J Plast Surg. 2013;46(1):18–27. https://pubmed.ncbi.nlm.nih.gov/23960302
45. Bender CA, Veneman W, Veenland JF, Mathijssen IMJ, Hop WCJ, Koudstaal MJ, et al. Orbital aspects following monobloc advancement in syndromic craniosynostosis. J Cranio-Maxillofacial Surg. 2013;41(7):e146–53.
46. Meling TR, Due-Tønnessen BJ, Høgevold HE, Skjelbred P, Arctander K. Monobloc distraction osteogenesis in pediatric patients with severe syndromal craniosynostosis. J Craniofac Surg. 2004;15(6) https://journals.lww.com/jcraniofacialsurgery/Fulltext/2004/11000/Monobloc_Distraction_Osteogenesis_in_Pediatric.20.aspx:990.
47. Esparza J, Hinojosa J. Complications in the surgical treatment of craniosynostosis and craniofacial syndromes: apropos of 306 transcranial procedures. Childs Nerv Syst. 2008;24(12):1421–30.

48. Al-Namnam NMN, Hariri F, Rahman ZAA. Distraction osteogenesis in the surgical management of syndromic craniosynostosis: a comprehensive review of published papers. Br J Oral Maxillofac Surg. 2018;56(5):353–66. https://www.sciencedirect.com/science/article/pii/S0266435618300822
49. Dunaway DJ, Britto JA, Abela C, Evans RD, Jeelani NUO. Complications of frontofacial advancement. Childs Nerv Syst. 2012;28(9):1571–6.
50. Wall SA, Goldin JH, Hockley AD, Wake MJC, Poole MD, Briggs M. Fronto-orbital re-operation in craniosynostosis. Br J Plast Surg. 1994;47(3):180–4. https://www.sciencedirect.com/science/article/pii/0007122694900515
51. Manni JJ, Scaf JJ, Huygen PLM, Cruysberg JRM, Verhagen WIM. Hyperostosis cranialis interna. N Engl J Med. 1990;322(7):450–4. https://doi.org/10.1056/NEJM199002153220707.
52. Stark Z, Savarirayan R. Osteopetrosis. Orphanet J Rare Dis. 2009;4(1):1–12.
53. Shapiro F. Osteopetrosis. Current clinical considerations. Clin Orthop Relat Res. 1993;294:34–44. http://europepmc.org/abstract/MED/8358940
54. Mehta M, Pushker N, Sethi S, Bajaj MS, Sharma S, Rajesh R, et al. Oculo–orbital manifestations of osteopetrosis in an Indian patient. Ann Trop Med Parasitol. 2010;104(3):275–81. https://doi.org/10.1179/136485910X12647085215697.
55. Al-Mefty O, Fox JL, Al-Rodhan N, Dew JH. Optic nerve decompression in osteopetrosis. J Neurosurg. 1988;68(1):80–4. https://thejns.org/view/journals/j-neurosurg/68/1/article-p80.xml
56. Hwang J-M, Kim I-O, Wang K-C. Complete visual recovery in osteopetrosis by early optic nerve decompression. Pediatr Neurosurg. 2000;33(6):328–32. https://doi.org/10.1159/000055980.
57. Haines SJ, Erickson DL, Wirtschafter JD. Optic nerve decompression for osteopetrosis in early childhood. Neurosurgery. 1988;23(4):470–5. https://doi.org/10.1227/00006123-198810000-00011.
58. Waterval JJ, van Dongen TM, Stokroos RJ, De Bondt B-J, Chenault MN, Manni JJ. Imaging features and progression of hyperostosis cranialis interna. Am J Neuroradiol. 2012;33(3):453–61. http://www.ajnr.org/content/33/3/453.abstract
59. Waterval JJ, Stokroos RJ, Bauer NJC, De Bondt RBJ, Manni JJ. Phenotypic manifestations and management of hyperostosis cranialis interna, a hereditary bone dysplasia affecting the calvaria and the skull base. Am J Med Genet Part A. 2010;152A(3):547–55. https://doi.org/10.1002/ajmg.a.33205.
60. Hershkovitz I, Greenwald C, Rothschild BM, Latimer B, Dutour O, Jellema LM, et al. Hyperostosis frontalis interna: an anthropological perspective. Am J Phys Anthropol. 1999;109(3):303–25.
61. Kirby K, Wright JE. Infantile cortical hyperostosis (Caffey disease). StatPearls; 2018.
62. Caffey J. Infantile cortical hyperostosis; a review of the clinical and radiographic features. Proc R Soc Med. 1957;50(5):347–54. https://pubmed.ncbi.nlm.nih.gov/13431894
63. Kamoun-Goldrat A, le Merrer M. Infantile cortical hyperostosis (Caffey disease): a review. J Oral Maxillofac Surg. 2008;66(10):2145–50.
64. Rogosin A, Monos T, Shulman H, Shoham A, Lifshitz T. Caffey-Silverman syndrome (infantile cortical hyperostosis) mimicking periorbital cellulitis. J Pediatr Ophthalmol Strabismus. 1999; 36:40.
65. Boyd RD, Shaw DG, Thomas BM. Infantile cortical hyperostosis with lytic lesions in the skull renal cortical necrosis in an infant. Blood Cells. 1970;48(6):57–9.

Traumatic Optic Neuropathy

15

Ka Hing Lok

Abstract

Traumatic optic neuropathy is an important diagnosis in patients with significant face and/or head injuries. It is often associated with unfavorable visual prognosis. Currently, available treatment options, namely, observation, corticosteroids, and surgical measures, are controversial.

Keyword

Traumatic optic neuropathy

15.1 Introduction

Traumatic optic neuropathy (TON) refers to injury to any portions of the optic nerve as a result of trauma. It should be an important entity in every clinician's mind when assessing patients with face and/or head trauma, as the signs could be subtle to pick up.

In order to mitigate the profound visual loss often associated with TON, various treatment options have been studied in the past decades. There is still no clear consensus on the optimal management strategy due to the lack of high-level evidence and the wide spectrum of severity and pattern of optic nerve injury. Therefore, the management should be individualized.

K. H. Lok (✉)
Hong Kong Eye Hospital, Hong Kong SAR, China

Department of Ophthalmology and Visual Sciences, The Chinese University of Hong Kong, Hong Kong SAR, China
e-mail: jerrylkh@cuhk.edu.hk

15.2 Classification

Traumatic optic neuropathy was classically termed direct or indirect based on the primary mechanism of injury [1]. Direct TON is caused by direct disruption of the optic nerve structure by a penetrating object, whereas indirect TON is caused by the force transmitted through the skull from a distant site of impact. The distinction of direct and indirect injuries, however, is not always clear. For example, in the case of blunt trauma with orbital fracture, the optic nerve could be directly lacerated by the bone fragment in a manner similar to what a direct penetrating injury would cause.

TON can also be classified according to the anatomical portion of optic nerve injured. The optic nerve is divided into four parts, namely, the intraocular, intraorbital, canalicular, and intracranial portions. The canalicular portion of the optic nerve is the commonest site affected by TON, as it is within the bony confines of the optic canal, rendering it vulnerable to the force transmitted from a distant site of impact. Optic canal fracture may have a direct effect on this portion of optic nerve.

With relevance to clinical signs, TON can also be classified as either anterior or posterior. The distinction between and anterior and posterior TON lies anatomically at the site of penetration of the central retinal artery/vein into the nerve (i.e., 8–10 mm beyond optic nerve insertion into the globe). Anterior TON could have fundal changes (see below), which are absent in posterior TON.

15.3 Epidemiology

Although the epidemiology of TON varies from region to region, a prospective population-based active surveillance in the United Kingdom estimated the minimum incidence from 2004 to 2006 to be 1.005 per million [2]. Around 80% of the patients were men, with a mean age of around 30, yet a significant proportion (around 20%) were pediatric patients [2,

T. L. POON et al. (eds.), *Orbital Apex and Periorbital Skull Base Diseases*, https://doi.org/10.1007/978-981-99-2989-4_15

3]. Severe trauma such as road traffic accidents, assault, and fall were the leading causes of TON [2, 3], yet apparently, trivial injuries, such as optic nerve massage [4], had been reported to result in TON.

15.4 Clinical Features

The diagnosis of TON is largely clinical, particularly because radiological features were neither specific nor sensitive enough to reflect impairment of optic nerve function [2].

A high index of suspicion should be maintained in order to solicit appropriate input from ophthalmologists. It is expected that patients sustaining significant face and/or head trauma would require immediate attention to stabilize the cardiorespiratory and neurological status. In certain cases, this would lead to a delay in ophthalmological assessment (and thus the diagnosis of TON). In the United Kingdom, only a small proportion of TON patients (7%) presented directly to ophthalmologists, whereas about a quarter of patients had a delay in ophthalmological assessment for 7 days or more [2]. This is more likely to happen to patients with impaired cognitive ability to report visual loss from TON, which could be a relatively common scenario given the significant proportion of TON patients having a history of loss of consciousness (25–45%) [2, 3]. Indeed, since TON has been reported in 0.7–2.5% of head trauma [5, 6], ophthalmological assessment should be considered in every patient with face and/or head trauma.

15.4.1 History

Detailed history should be taken from the patients who can cooperate and from witnesses especially if patients are confused or even comatose. Details about the trauma should be elicited, such as the mechanisms of trauma and the time when it happened. It would be useful to know the past ocular history, history of unconsciousness after the trauma, whether the visual loss is immediate and/or progressive, *etc*.

15.4.2 Physical Examination

Relative afferent pupillary defect (RAPD) is of utmost importance in the diagnosis of TON, as it is always present except for the rare scenario of bilaterally symmetrical involvement. If one pupil failed to be assessed due to an efferent pathway defect (*e.g.,* sluggish pupillary response due to oculomotor nerve palsy or traumatic iritis), reverse RAPD should be looked for. The rationale of reverse RAPD is based on the assumption that the consensual pupillary response is intact and symmetrical, and thus by observing the response of the normal pupil, one can detect if there is an afferent defect in the contralateral side with the swinging-torch test.

Visual acuity should be assessed whenever the patients can cooperate. Commonly, the visual loss is immediate and profound, with 35–40% of patients having no light perception [2, 3]. Only about 10% of patients had a presenting visual acuity of 20/40 or better [2, 3]. A small proportion of patients had delayed visual loss after presentation, and this may signify secondary injury to optic nerve, which might require prompt treatments. Therefore, it is important to serially monitor the visual acuity in patients with TON.

The periorbital region should be examined for the nature and extent of any penetrating injuries. The presence of proptosis, hemorrhagic chemosis, and a tense globe with high intraocular pressure should be assumed to be due to retrobulbar hemorrhage. Ocular examination is important to rule out intraocular causes of visual loss, such as hyphema, lens dislocation, vitreous hemorrhage, *etc*. The presence of a normal red reflex is a useful screening sign for intraocular media pathologies for non-ophthalmologists. The commonest form of TON is posterior indirect TON, in which case the dilated fundal exam would be normal, including a well-perfused optic disc with normal appearance. In the contrary, there would be signs on fundal exam in anterior TON. Optic nerve avulsion would be seen as a ring of hemorrhage (partial or complete depending on the extent of avulsion) or as a deep pit [7, 8]. Injuries to the anterior portion of optic nerve (anterior to the entrance/exit site of the central retinal artery/vein, respectively) would give rise to a picture of central retinal artery and/or vein occlusion. Papilledema (bilateral disc swelling from raised intracranial pressure) could be differentiated from bilateral TON by the absence of RAPD, relative preservation of visual acuity (at least at the initial phase) and (possibly) positive imaging findings, although the distinction is not always clear.

15.4.3 Investigation

Although the diagnosis of TON is clinical, imaging studies are valuable in the assessment of the extent and the exact nature of the injury. Computed tomography (CT) is the preferred imaging of choice for trauma patients since it is fast, gives better details of the bony structure, and is not contraindicated if ferromagnetic foreign body cannot be rule out. It is often not performed for the sole purpose of TON diagnosis, but rather as an overall evaluation of the face and/or head injury. In the context of posterior indirect TON, the presence of optic canal fracture is intuitively the most relevant finding, but it has been suggested that the presence or absence of which does not dictate the visual outcomes [9, 10]. However, CT is still valuable in surgical planning, in detection of orbital/intra-sheath/subperiosteal hematoma/emphysema and compressive bone fragment, which may require treatment, and for prognostication. Blood in the posterior ethmoidal sinuses was presumed to be due to stronger force transmitted to that area (and to the contiguous optic nerve) and thus a higher chance of TON with lower chance of recovery [11, 12].

Optical coherence tomography of the optic nerve head and automated visual field testing are common tools for quantifying the optic nerve function. However, in the acute setting of a retrobulbar insult (as commonly the case for TON), the retinal nerve fiber layer thickness and ganglion cell-inner plexiform complex thickness are expected to remain normal until secondary atrophic changes take place weeks to months later. Both tests would require the patient to be clinically stable, ambulatory, and cooperative, so they may not be practical for some TON patients. Otherwise, a baseline result can be obtained for monitoring as the patients recover.

Visual-evoked potential (VEP) has been investigated as a diagnostic tool in TON [13, 14]. It measures the cortical activity from a visual stimulus, reflecting the integrity of the visual pathway in a waveform. Certainly, there are practical limitations to VEP measurement in the acute setting especially in severely injured patients. The interpretation of waveform requires expertise and caution as there is significant interpersonal variability. Concomitant damage to elsewhere in the visual pathway in the brain would confound the findings [13]. Nevertheless, in certain scenarios, VEP could provide useful information, such as for the diagnosis of bilateral TON in comatose patients (with a handheld device) and for predication of visual potential, which could help in patient triage for intervention. For unilateral TON, the amplitude can be compared with that of the fellow normal eye for prediction of final visual acuity [14]. One series found if the VEP amplitude of 50% or more of that of the normal eye, the visual potential has been reported to be favorable (20/30 or more) [13].

15.5 Management

15.5.1 Observation

Observation is a reasonable management option for TON. Spontaneous recovery of visual acuity could occur in a significant proportion of patients [2, 3, 15, 16]. Even patients without light perception had been reported to have improvement [2, 3, 16–19]. Visual improvement of three lines or more had been reported in 20–57% of indirect TON without any treatment [2, 3].

Nevertheless, the overall visual prognosis of TON had often been poor in a significant proportion of patients (49–65% with final visual acuity of 20/200 or worse, regardless of whether any treatment were given [2, 3]). Some factors had been suggested to adversely affect recovery of vision, including [2, 12]:

- Age of patient (patients less than the age of 40 were more likely to have visual improvement)
- History of loss of consciousness
- History of significant head injury
- History of immediate loss of vision
- Poor initial visual acuity
- Presence of blood in the posterior ethmoidal cells on imaging studies
- Presence of orbital fracture or optic canal fracture
- Failure to respond to steroid after 48 hours of treatment

In the fortunate events of visual recovery, the recovery is often incomplete. The favorable outcomes of observation should be viewed with caution, as it had been suggested that patients with better presenting visual acuity (hence possibly better prognosis for recovery) tended to be observed compared to those with poor visual acuity [2, 9, 20]. In view of these shortcomings, active interventions, namely, systemic corticosteroids and surgical interventions, had been studied.

15.5.2 Systemic Corticosteroids

Corticosteroid treatment is controversial in the management of TON. Proposed benefits of corticosteroids in reducing local edema and secondary inflammatory damages to the optic nerve had led to its use in TON since the early 1980s [21–24]. Various forms and dosage of corticosteroid have been proposed, ranging from: "low-dose" of oral prednisolone (1–2 mg/kg/day) or intravenous dexamethasone; "high-dose" (1,000 mg/day) methylprednisolone; and "megadose" (a bolus of 30 mg/kg methylprednisolone followed by 5.4 mg/kg/hour for 24–48 hours) [2, 3, 9, 20, 22, 24, 25].

Most of the evidence regarding steroid treatment for TON was initially extrapolated from that of another closely related central nervous system structure—the spinal cord. The first National Acute Spinal Cord Injury Studies (NASCIS I) was a multicenter, double-blind, randomized study to evaluate the efficacy of "high-dose" methylprednisolone (1,000 mg bolus and daily thereafter for 10 days) compared with "standard-dose" (100 mg bolus and daily thereafter for 10 days) in 330 patients with acute spinal cord injury [26]. There was no difference in neurological outcomes between the two arms. The lack of effects was attributed to insufficient dosage of methylprednisolone, so a "megadose" approach was investigated in the second NASCIS (NASCIS II), which was a multicenter, double-blind, randomized, placebo-controlled study [27]. Megadose methylprednisolone (a bolus of 30 mg/kg followed by infusion at 5.4 mg/kg/hour for 23 hours) given within

8 hours of injury was found to improve neurologic recovery at 6 months compared to placebo. In the third multicenter, randomized controlled study (NASCIS III), the use of methylprednisolone was further claborated that if the megadose infusion was given for 48 hours instead of 24 hours, some patients (for whom infusion was initiated 3–8 hours after injury) may benefit with better motor recovery [28]. In some ways, this further consolidated the positive effects of steroid.

The efficacy of megadose steroid, however, was questioned by a prospective, randomized, placebo-controlled study conducted in France. In contrast with the findings from NASCIS II, no benefits were demonstrated for megadose steroid in terms of neurologic recovery compared to placebo, yet the steroid group had a higher rate of infectious complications [29].

The debate on whether patients with TON should be treated with megadose steroid (or steroid at all) became more heated after the International Optic Nerve Trauma Study (IONTS) was published. It was an international, multicenter, comparative nonrandomized study to investigate the effects of observation, corticosteroid, and surgical decompression on the visual outcomes in patients with TON. The dosage of corticosteroids used in the trial varied from low dose to megadose, based on the decision of the treating clinicians. Visual improvement was not statistically different among the three groups. In a subgroup analysis, there was no significant difference in the proportion of patients having visual acuity improvement (three lines of more) between the megadose group (41%) and the lower dose group (59%) [3].

In fact, megadose steroid was proven in a subsequent trial to increase mortality in patients with head injury, which is quite invariably associated with TON. The Corticosteroid Randomization After Significant Head Injury (CRASH) trial was a large-scale (including 10,008 adults), multicenter, placebo-controlled study to evaluate the effects of methylprednisolone (2,000 mg methylprednisolone followed by 400 mg/hour for 48 hours) in patients with head injury with Glasgow Coma Scale of 14 or less. The relative risk of death was significantly higher in the steroid group (21% *vs* 18%; $p = 0.0001$) [30, 31]. The study was halted in view of the results, and it became clear that megadose steroid should be avoided in patients with TON.

How about "high-dose" instead of "megadose" steroid? The clinical benefits of lower dose of corticosteroids were mostly described in case reports or small case series. Therefore, they were not designed to scientifically prove the benefits of corticosteroids compared with observation alone. A double-blind, randomized, placebo-controlled study was conducted in Iran comparing the effects of high-dose steroid (250 mg methylprednisolone every 6 hours for 3 days, followed by oral prednisolone at 1 mg/kg/day for 14 days) on TON [32]. Thirty-one patients were included. There was no statistically significant difference between the two groups although the proportion of patients with visual acuity improvement of 0.4 logMAR or more was higher in the steroid group (69%) compared to the placebo group (53%) ($p = 0.38$).

Despite biological plausibility, benefits of corticosteroid are at best uncertain in the treatment of TON. The decision of treatment should be made after weighing benefits against risks. As such, megadose steroid should be avoided. High-dose steroid could be considered on an individualized basis.

15.5.3 Surgical Treatment

There is no standard surgical approach for TON, in part due to the lack of high-level evidence and the heterogeneity in TON nature, severity, timing of diagnosis, *etc*. There are certain scenarios where surgical intervention is deemed appropriate. Optic nerve sheath fenestration can be considered if optic nerve sheath hematoma is detected on neuroimaging [33]. When there is optic nerve dysfunction due to orbital compartment syndrome, such as in the case of retrobulbar hemorrhage, orbital emphysema [34], subperiosteal hematoma [21], orbital decompression should be performed promptly via lateral canthotomy/cantholysis and/or orbitotomy. However, these are relatively uncommon mechanisms of optic nerve damage in most cases of TON.

The commonest form of TON is the posterior indirect type involving the canalicular portion of the optic nerve, with or without optic canal fracture. Therefore, optic canal decompression has been the focus of research and controversy and shall be discussed separately in the following chapter.

References

1. Steinsapir KD, Goldberg RA. Traumatic optic neuropathies. In: Miller NR, Newman NJ, editors. Walsh & Hoyt's clinical neuro-ophthalmology, 6th ed. 2005.
2. Lee V, Ford RL, Xing W, Bunce C, Foot B. Surveillance of traumatic optic neuropathy in the UK. Eye (Lond). 2010;24:240–50.
3. Levin LA, Beck RW, Joseph MP, Seiff S, Kraker R. The treatment of traumatic optic neuropathy: the international optic nerve trauma study. Ophthalmology. 1999;106:1268–77.
4. Borruat FX, Kawasaki A. Optic nerve massaging: an extremely rare cause of self-inflicted blindness. Am J Ophthalmol. 2005;139:715–6.
5. al-Qurainy IA, Stassen LF, Dutton GN, Moos KF, el-Attar A. The characteristics of midfacial fractures and the association with ocular injury: a prospective study. Br J Oral Maxillofac Surg. 1991;29:291–301.
6. Nau HE, Gerhard L, Foerster M, Nahser HC, Reinhardt V, Joka T. Optic nerve trauma: clinical, electrophysiological and histological remarks. Acta Neurochir (Wien). 1987;89:16–27.
7. Tsopelas NV, Arvanitis PG. Avulsion of the optic nerve head after orbital trauma. Arch Ophthalmol. 1998;116:394.
8. Hillman JS, Myska V, Nissim S. Complete avulsion of the optic nerve. A clinical, angiographic, and electrodiagnostic study. Br J Ophthalmol. 1975;59:503–9.

9. Wang BH, Robertson BC, Girotto JA, et al. Traumatic optic neuropathy: a review of 61 patients. Plast Reconstr Surg. 2001;107:1655–64.
10. Tabatabaei SA, Soleimani M, Alizadeh M, et al. Predictive value of visual evoked potentials, relative afferent pupillary defect, and orbital fractures in patients with traumatic optic neuropathy. Clin Ophthalmol. 2011;5:1021–6.
11. Gross CE, DeKock JR, Panje WR, Hershkowitz N, Newman J. Evidence for orbital deformation that may contribute to monocular blindness following minor frontal head trauma. J Neurosurg. 1981;55:963–6.
12. Carta A, Ferrigno L, Salvo M, Bianchi-Marzoli S, Boschi A, Carta F. Visual prognosis after indirect traumatic optic neuropathy. J Neurol Neurosurg Psychiatry. 2003;74:246–8.
13. Holmes MD, Sires BS. Flash visual evoked potentials predict visual outcome in traumatic optic neuropathy. Ophthalmic Plast Reconstr Surg. 2004;20:342–6.
14. Mohammed MA, Mossallam E, Allam IY. The role of the flash visual evoked potential in evaluating visual function in patients with indirect traumatic optic neuropathy. Clin Ophthalmol. 2021;15:1349–55.
15. Yip CC, Chng NW, Au Eong KG, Heng WJ, Lim TH, Lim WK. Low-dose intravenous methylprednisolone or conservative treatment in the management of traumatic optic neuropathy. Eur J Ophthalmol. 2002;12:309–14.
16. Hughes B. Indirect injury of the optic nerves and chiasma. Bull Johns Hopkins Hosp. 1962;111:98–126.
17. Lessell S. Indirect optic nerve trauma. Arch Ophthalmol. 1989;107:382–6.
18. Hooper RS. Orbital complications of head injury. Br J Surg. 1951;39:126–38.
19. Wolin MJ, Lavin PJ. Spontaneous visual recovery from traumatic optic neuropathy after blunt head injury. Am J Ophthalmol. 1990;109:430–5.
20. Cook MW, Levin LA, Joseph MP, Pinczower EF. Traumatic optic neuropathy. A meta-analysis. Arch Otolaryngol Head Neck Surg. 1996;122:389–92.
21. Anderson RL, Panje WR, Gross CE. Optic nerve blindness following blunt forehead trauma. Ophthalmology. 1982;89:445–55.
22. Seiff SR. High dose corticosteroids for treatment of vision loss due to indirect injury to the optic nerve. Ophthalmic Surg. 1990;21:389–95.
23. Fujitani T, Inoue K, Takahashi T, Ikushima K, Asai T. Indirect traumatic optic neuropathy—visual outcome of operative and nonoperative cases. Jpn J Ophthalmol. 1986;30:125–34.
24. Matsuzaki H, Kunita M, Kawai K. Optic nerve damage in head trauma: clinical and experimental studies. Jpn J Ophthalmol. 1982;26:447–61.
25. Spoor TC, Hartel WC, Lensink DB, Wilkinson MJ. Treatment of traumatic optic neuropathy with corticosteroids. Am J Ophthalmol. 1990;110:665–9.
26. Bracken MB, Collins WF, Freeman DF, et al. Efficacy of methylprednisolone in acute spinal cord injury. JAMA. 1984;251:45–52.
27. Bracken MB, Shepard MJ, Collins WF, et al. A randomized, controlled trial of methylprednisolone or naloxone in the treatment of acute spinal-cord injury. Results of the Second National Acute Spinal Cord Injury Study. N Engl J Med. 1990;322:1405–11.
28. Bracken MB, Shepard MJ, Holford TR, et al. Administration of methylprednisolone for 24 or 48 hours or tirilazad mesylate for 48 hours in the treatment of acute spinal cord injury. Results of the third national acute spinal cord injury randomized controlled trial. National Acute Spinal Cord Injury Study. JAMA. 1997;277:1597–604.
29. Pointillart V, Petitjean ME, Wiart L, et al. Pharmacological therapy of spinal cord injury during the acute phase. Spinal Cord. 2000;38:71–6.
30. Edwards P, Arango M, Balica L, et al. Final results of MRC CRASH, a randomised placebo-controlled trial of intravenous corticosteroid in adults with head injury-outcomes at 6 months. Lancet. 2005;365:1957–9.
31. Roberts I, Yates D, Sandercock P, et al. Effect of intravenous corticosteroids on death within 14 days in 10008 adults with clinically significant head injury (MRC CRASH trial): randomised placebo-controlled trial. Lancet. 2004;364:1321–8.
32. Entezari M, Rajavi Z, Sedighi N, Daftarian N, Sanagoo M. High-dose intravenous methylprednisolone in recent traumatic optic neuropathy; a randomized double-masked placebo-controlled clinical trial. Graefes Arch Clin Exp Ophthalmol. 2007;245:1267–71.
33. Mauriello JA, DeLuca J, Krieger A, Schulder M, Frohman L. Management of traumatic optic neuropathy—a study of 23 patients. Br J Ophthalmol. 1992;76:349–52.
34. Jordan DR, White GL Jr, Anderson RL, Thiese SM. Orbital emphysema: a potentially blinding complication following orbital fractures. Ann Emerg Med. 1988;17:853–5.

Part IV

360 Degree of Surgical Approaches

Choices of Approaches

16

Stacey Lam and Hunter Kwok Lai YUEN

Abstract

Orbit is a small area, but there are many surgical approaches to lesions within different parts of the orbit. In this chapter, we will discuss the choice of surgical approaches. We will also discuss visual loss after orbital surgeries, which is the most significant potential complication in orbital surgeries.

Keywords

Orbital surgeries · Surgical approaches · Visual loss

16.1 Choice of Approaches

16.1.1 Background

Orbital apical surgery is particularly challenging due to the narrow anatomic confines of bony walls, limited surgical exposure, and crowding of complex neurovascular structures. Type of approach to the apex depends on the aim of surgery, anatomical location and extent, disease nature, and experience of surgeons.

1. Indication for Surgery
   - Tissue diagnosis (excisional or incisional). Incisional biopsy would need less space, while excisional biopsy would require wider exposure, more dissection, and manipulation.
   - Drainage of abscess.
   - Orbital and optic canal decompression.
   - Orbital and optic canal fractures.
   - Foreign body removal.
2. Anatomical Location. Location of pathology and its relationship to the globe and optic nerve. Besides from the primary indication of surgery, the ultimate goal in orbital surgery is to preserve vision or restore vision, and this is achieved by avoiding manipulation of the optic nerve and its vascular supply. The surgical corridor chosen should therefore not cross the plane of the optic nerve. A useful guideline with various techniques described includes the following:
   - Pathology inferior to the globe is managed inferiorly (transconjunctival, subciliary, infraorbital, or transmaxillary).
   - Pathology medial to globe or optic nerve are managed medially (transconjunctival, endoscopic endonasal, transethmoidal).
   - Pathology lateral to globe or optic nerve are managed laterally (ultradeep lateral wall, frontotemporal craniotomy.
   - Pathology superior to globe are managed superiorly (transfrontal extradural or intradural with removal of orbital root, with combination of sub-brow incision, lid crease incision).
3. Disease Nature
   - Benign versus malignant lesions or metastatic.
   - Circumscribed (e.g., cavernous hemangioma) versus infiltrative lesion (lymphaticovenous malformations). Well encapsulated lesions would be possible to attempt complete removal, while the latter cannot aim complete removal, but can be removed in piecemeal fashion for diagnostic or debulking purpose.
   - More vascular versus less vascular.

S. Lam · H. K. L. YUEN (✉)
Hong Kong Eye Hospital, Hong Kong SAR, China

Department of Ophthalmology and Visual Sciences, The Chinese University of Hong Kong, Hong Kong SAR, China
e-mail: yuenkl1@ha.org.hk

T. L. POON et al. (eds.), *Orbital Apex and Periorbital Skull Base Diseases*, https://doi.org/10.1007/978-981-99-2989-4_16

16.1.2 Clock Model Paradigm

In the past, the traditional approach to the orbital apex used the quadrants to divide the compartment—superotemporal, superomedial, inferomedial, and inferotemporal (Fig. 16.1) [1].

A new method to conceptualize the orbital approach is using the clock model paradigm, which places the right optic nerve at the center of a clock face (Fig. 16.2) [2]. Comprehensive list of approaches and their advantages and disadvantages are listed in Table 16.1 [3–9]. Combination of approaches that involve more than one surgical corridor can be considered in extensive lesions.

16.1.3 Paradigm Shift

The approach to the orbital apex does not differ from that of other regions of the body—to select the approach that allows maximal exposure to attain the aim of the surgery while minimize unwanted structural changes and scarring. This will determine the amount of space the surgeon will need. In recent years, there has been a paradigm shift to less invasive techniques. Reasons for this paradigm shift include advance in technologies in investigation and treatment, increased knowledge in disease and pathology, and increased collaboration amongst surgeons with multidisciplinary approach.

- Imaging: Latest imaging techniques have led to more accurate diagnosis that may not necessitate biopsy in some cases.
- Pathology: Further knowledge on disease pathology has expanded, leading to more options of treatment alternatives. This includes the following:

Orbital decompression: In selected cases where lesions are benign with compressive optic neuropathy, sole orbital decompression without biopsy can be done. Suggested case selection criteria are: benign radiologic features, stable size and characteristics on serial preoperative imaging, no history of malignancy, no rapid clinical decline, biopsy or tumor resection not feasible given tumor size and location [10]. By removing medial bony wall of orbital apex and incising periorbita, it is possible to reverse the compressive optic neuropathy without iatrogenic morbidity associated with lesion removal. However, this method may only provide temporary relief if the lesion regrows and cannot provide histological diagnosis of the lesion [11].

Sclerotherapy: Instead of surgical extensive resection, lymphaticovenous malformations can be managed with percutaneous or endoscopic sclerotherapy, or oral medication such as sirolimus [12, 13].

Gamma knife radiosurgery (GKS): This is a type of stereotactic radiosurgery that administers an accurately focused high dose of radiation. Compared to traditional fractionated radiotherapy that delivers equivalent radiation dose to both lesion and optic nerve, GKS has better spatial accuracy, delivering equivalent dose as fractionated radiotherapy without additional complications to surrounding tissue. Multisession GKS has been found to be able to shrink orbital apex lesions

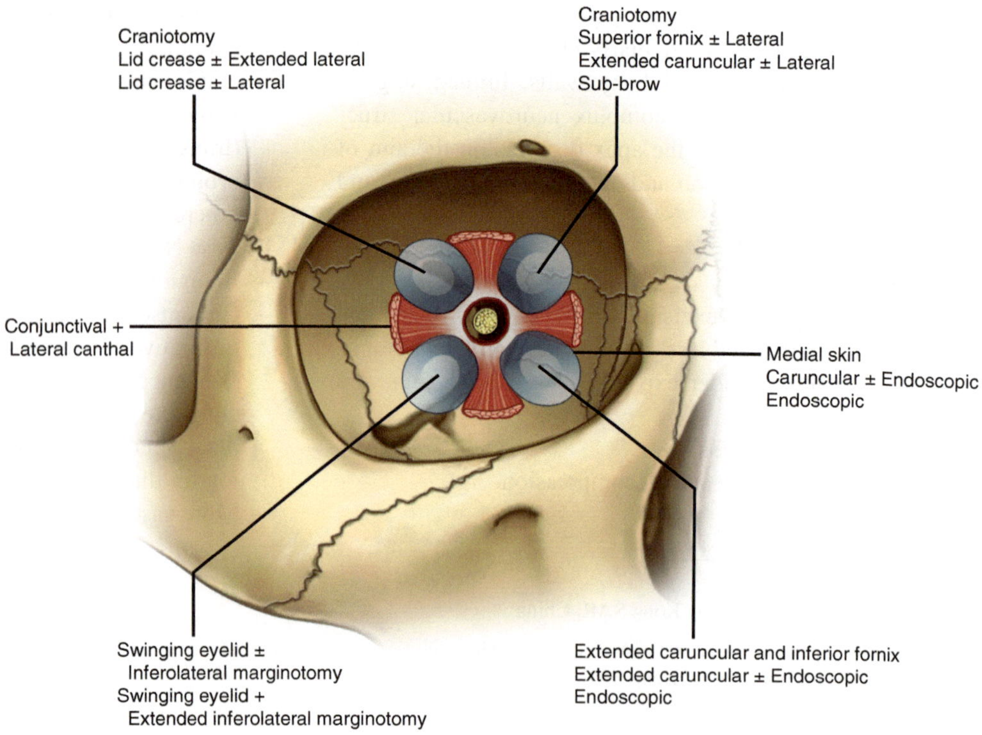

Fig. 16.1 Traditional approach to the orbital apex using quadrant method [1]

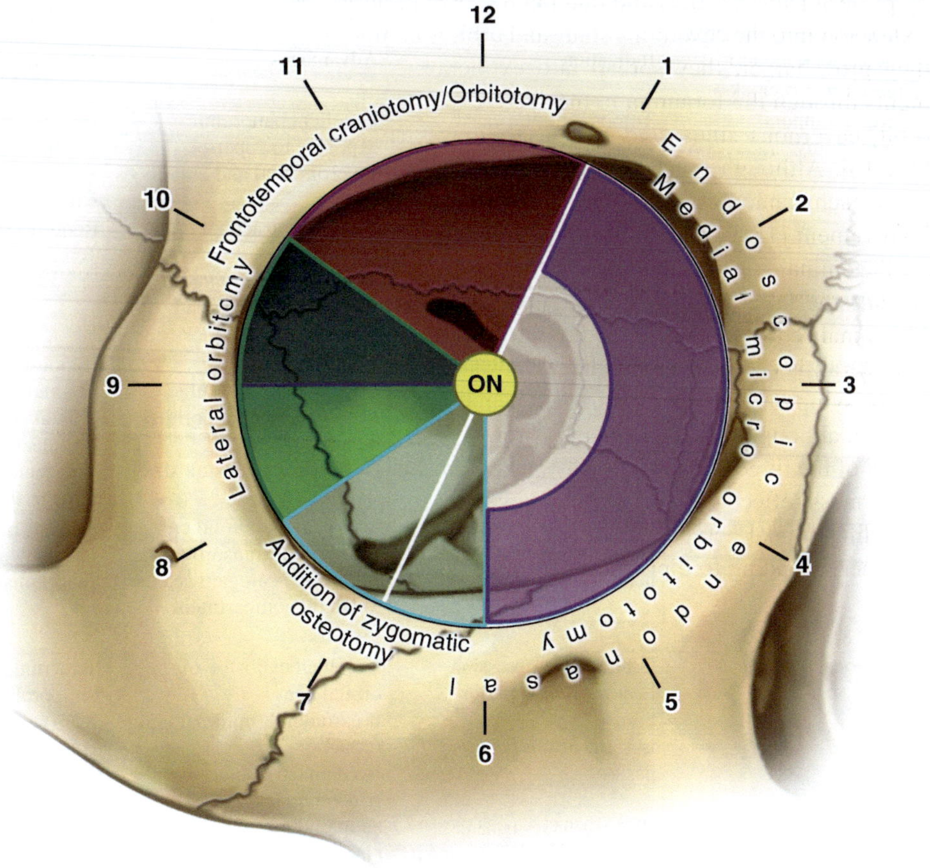

Fig. 16.2 Clock model of the orbit summarizing approaches [2]

such as cavernous hemangiomas, meningiomas, and schwannomas, with improved visual acuity and resolution of visual defect without tumor recurrence [14].

Image-guided radiation therapy: Using advanced computer programs, more accurate delivery of radiation via intensity modulated radiation therapy as nonsurgical options or adjuvant treatment for orbital lesions.

Advances in preoperative radiotherapy, chemotherapy and intra-arterial chemotherapy can reduce tumor size to minimize surgical risk.

- Computer-assisted surgical planning: Technology in computer-aided design (CAD) and computer-aided manufacturing (CAM) computer software to create 3D reconstruction from CT scans. This can aid planning resection and reconstruction, including techniques such as mirroring, segmenting, and repositioning. Mirroring creates a mirror image of the unaffected side, which can be repositioned to abnormal side for reconstruction. These images can be used as models or implants for precise surgical planning.
- Intraoperative navigation: The use of intraoperative image guided orbital surgery has been reported to be precise and safe for complex orbital interventions such as biopsies, apical foreign body removal, tumor removal, fracture reconstruction in crucial areas, abscess drainage, and orbital decompression. For tumor removal, navigation helps in anatomic orientation, target localization, and trajectory information, establishing tumor margins for resection and overall enhanced surgeon's confidence. Additional software can color code the lesion, optic nerve and vessels.
- Innovation in operating microscopes and endoscopy.

Advance in technologies such as three-dimensional (3D) endoscope systems for enhanced depth perception and augmented spatial orientation.

Modern microscopes provide large range of magnification options, stable and bright illumination, and well-designed optics for high resolution. Augmented reality technology has been actively evaluated on the surgical microscope, with additional high-definition (HD) display, image injection techniques, and 3D display.

- Innovation in surgical tools.

Traditional tools for orbital osteotomies include mechanical saw and drills, which include sagittal, oscillating and reciprocating. Complications include ocular laceration, orbital hemorrhage and nerve injury. Piezoelectric ultrasound bone surgery uses 20–30 kHz to cut mineralized tissue selectively, thereby minimiz-

Table 16.1 Clock model of the orbit comparing the different approaches

Approach (using the right orbit as clock model)	Indication	Advantages	Disadvantages
Superior 9–1 o'clock			
Frontotemporal craniotomy	Tumors of optic canal Pathologies extending into cranial cavity Optic nerve glioma Pathologies lateral to optic nerve	Excellent panoramic exposure to superior, superomedial and lateral orbit Ideal for intraconal pathologies Addition of zygomatic osteotomy will extend exposure 6–8 o'clock	Intracranial surgery complications (leakage of cerebrospinal fluid, intracranial injury, meningitis) Bicoronal flap leaves large scar especially in those with receding hairline, risk frontalis palsy Requires brain retraction Temporalis muscle atrophy
Supraorbital	Intraconal and extraconal lesions superior to optic nerve	Minimally invasive Good cosmetic results Minimal brain and orbital manipulation Not limited by lesion size	Hypoesthesia if supraorbital nerve is damaged Limited exposure Frontal sinus contamination Not ideal for posterior lesions Iatrogenic Brown's syndrome and risk of diplopia if damage superior oblique complex
Superior eyelid crease	Intraconal and extraconal lesions superior to optic nerve	Scar is hidden in lid crease Addition of transorbital endoscopy can gain access to lateral compartment	Enophthalmos Narrow window for instrumentation Suboptimal view as orbital fat obscures surgical field
Lateral 8–10 o'clock			
Pterional	Orbital decompression Lesions near superior fissure Lesions near inferior fissure	Excellent exposure of orbital apex If extradural, minimal brain retraction No damage to intraorbital structures, less risk enophthalmos	Intracranial surgery complications Temporalis atrophy Scar (hairline incision and smaller incision behind temporal hairline) Detailed anatomic knowledge essential, smaller surgical field
Lateral orbitotomy	Laterally placed extraconal lesions Orbital apex lesions Intraconal lesions lateral or inferior to optic nerve	Good exposure to orbit Well tolerated Addition of zygomatic osteotomy can increase 6–8 o'clock exposure	Visible but minimal scar Enophthalmos
Medial/inferior 1–6 o'clock			
Transcutaneous (Lynch incision)	Medial and inferior orbit	Excellent exposure	Courses midway between medial canthus and bridge of nose, with risk of medial canthal web formation and visible scarring
Transcutaneous (subciliary)	Medial and inferior orbit	Good exposure to medial and inferior orbit	Lower lid retraction, malposition, scarring
Transconjunctival/ transcaruncle	Medial and inferior orbit	No visible scarring Decreased risk of entropion, given that orbital septum not violated	Poor exposure for orbital apex May need to disinsert medial rectus
Endoscopic endonasal approach (EEA)	Medial aspect of orbital apex Opticocarotid recess Orbital fractures and orbital apical lesions Optic nerve decompression of bony canal in traumatic optic neuropathy Medial wall decompression in thyroid eye disease	Safe and unparalleled visualization of orbit, magnification and illumination Addition of medial maxillectomy can access inferior orbit (4–7 o'clock) No visible scar Low risk of enophthalmos	Endoscopic instrumentation and range of motion are limited compared with ordinary microsurgical instrumentation utilized when working transcranially and with the microscope Limited exposure of orbital apex

ing damage to surrounding soft tissue, improved visualization, optimal bone healing, and reduced surgeon fatigue [15].

New powered instrument such as the microdebrider is an electrically powered device has combined cutting and suction action to excise soft tissue and thin bone. The continuous suction of blood and tissue fragments improves surgeon's visibility, less frequent removal, and reintroduction, minimizing potential for tissue injury and thereby decreasing operative time.

- Hybrid approach. Complex pathologies can be managed with a combination of the above approaches, with more than one surgical corridor by a team of surgeons. transorbital neuroendoscopic surgery (TONES) comprises of a group of endoscopy via access in preseptal plane, precaruncular plane, superior lid crease, lateral retrocanthal approaches [16].

In the following chapters, we will further elaborate the indications, surgical techniques, and possible complications. Even for the same orbital apex lesion, the choice of surgery in the end will depend on surgeon expertise, equipment available, and patient preference.

16.1.4 Vision Loss and Intraoperative Optic Nerve Monitoring

Besides from the specific complications listed in Table 16.1, vision loss is the most dreaded complication after orbital surgery and one that is thoroughly discussed in the informed consent process. Incidence of blindness from orbital surgery varies from 0 to 24% [17, 18]. Risk factors associated with higher risk of vision loss include the following:

Disease Factor

- Location: lesions with optic nerve displacement, optic nerve sheath lesions, closer to orbital apex, in the superomedial vascular quadrant and optic canal invasion [17, 19]. In a series of spheno-orbital meningiomas involving the optic canal, reported major visual loss after surgery was 33% (4 in 12 patients, 1 patient with 20/400 and 3 patients with no light perception) [20]. Higher risk of visual loss in optic canal invasion could be due to damage to small perforating pial vessels that enter the optic nerve while opening optic canal and optic sheath, with optic nerve ischemia [21].
- Nature: vascular lesions such as venous or lymphatic malformations, poorly encapsulated lesions, infiltrative lesions. There is also higher incidence of blindness after orbital tumor excision 4.7% compared to post-traumatic orbital reconstruction and orbital decompression for thyroid orbitopathy 0.15% [22].
- Size: smaller apical lesions with proximity to anterior end of optic canal have higher risk [22].
- Recurrent lesions: scarring from previous surgery resulting in loss of normal anatomic planes renders a more difficult surgery [23].

Patient Factor

- Age: Higher risk in those older than 60 years old. Younger patients are more able to compensate for microvascular deprivation, with greater tissue resilience, associated orbital expansion with chronic expansion, better coagulation profile, less vasculopathic risk factors and vasospasm with better bleeding control than older paitients [24].
- Vision before surgery: longer duration of visual loss before surgery carries worse prognosis due to small vessel compromise, demyelination, and ischemic damage to optic nerve. Visual loss of less than 2 years has a higher rate of visual improvement after surgery [24].

Surgery Factor

- Hypotensive anesthesia, blood loss, and hemodilution could predispose the retina and optic nerve to ischemia [25].
- Surgery: Higher risk in those with orbital floor fracture repair in multiple facial fractures (6.45%), bony decompression of optic canal (15.6%), and intracranial approach to orbital roof (18.2%) [25]. Reason for multiple facial fractures is postulated to be related to underlying traumatic optic neuropathy, optic nerve compression, and more soft tissue edema and less likely to be able to withstand further surgical insult intraoperatively [26].
- Surgical Approach: So far, there is no direct correlation between approach and visual loss. Studies have shown there have been more non-blinding complications such as diplopia and scarring in lateral orbitotomy (35%) compared with anterior orbitotomy (3%) [18]. Incidence in postoperative blindness was similar in lateral, anterior, and coronal approach at 0.5%, 0.4%, and 0.38%, respectively [27].

Mechanism of visual loss includes the following:

- Structural cause: Direct optic nerve injury from mechanical injury, thermal injury secondary to cautery to maintain hemostasis, and vibratory insults from drills during bone removal.
- Vascular cause: Due to anterior ischemic optic neuropathy, posterior ischemic optic neuropathy, central retinal arterial occlusion, or ophthalmic artery occlusion. Arterial vasospasm can be exacerbated by vessel traction, orbital fat traction, vessel compression, surgical sacrifice of vascular structures, direct injury, globe manipulation with transient elevated intraocular pressure, or platelet aggre-

gation following trauma releasing serotonin, which is a potent vasoconstrictor. Delayed ischemia can be related to accumulation of inflammatory mediators and blood that can induce vasospasm [28]. Arterial hypoperfusion can be secondary to blood volume status and multisystem injuries.

– Orbital compartment syndrome: Elevated orbital pressure from bleeding (retrobulbar hemorrhage) or edema, or combination [20].

With the goal being to preserve the visual system, a reliable method to monitor the visual pathway would be ideal. Real-time feedback to the surgeon about the visual pathways can potentially minimize post-operative visual deficits.

For both orbital and cranial surgery, the most straightforward and objective reflection of visual pathway is monitoring the pupil size or shape. A dilated or asymmetric pupil indicates raised intraocular pressure such as in retrobulbar hemorrhage or excessive orbital traction, and, in the unfortunate case, ischemic optic neuropathy. Intermittent pupil dilation can occur when there is manipulation of the ciliary ganglion. Moreover, erroneous pupil measurement can occur when there is significant miosis with opioid anesthesia, dilation due to accidental contact with intranasal vasoconstrictors such as cocaine or adrenaline in endoscopic surgery, and asymmetrical recovery of pupil light reflex after general anesthesia [29]. Hence, intraoperative pupil size and reactivity may not directly correlate with post-operative visual outcome.

In orbital apical surgery, intraoperative neurophysiological monitoring (IONM) with visual evoked potentials (VEP) and electroretinography (ERG) are potential methods to identify injuries to optic nerve. VEP measures the electrical potential resulting from a visual stimulus. The stimulus is applied by light emitting device (LED) placed on the eyes bilaterally, and responses recorded include the cornea, optic chiasm, and occipital lobe. However, literature reports on the use of VEP in intraorbital surgery remain controversial. Studies that support VEP suggested transient abolition of VEP was seen in many circumstances and did not correlate with outcome of surgery, but the absence of previously normal VEP for more than 4 min during surgical manipulation did show a correlation with post-operative visual impairment [30, 31]. Other studies have found VEP to be unstable and unreliable and only feasible in 73% of their patient cohort [32]. Mechanism of optic nerve damage includes optic nerve ischemia, mechanical damage, or a combination of both. It is not known which of these mechanisms are related to VEP changes [33].

ERG is a test to detect an abnormality of the retina. During this test, needle electrode for ERG is inserted in lateral canthus and a reference electrode in the contralateral canthus. To avoid false-negative results in VEP, ERG was introduced to record the response of retina to stimulus. If both VEP and ERG were lost, this indicated displacement of the LED. When VEP is coupled with ERG, predictive power increases from 60 to 100%, but the sensitivity for detecting deterioration is low (47.2%) [34].

The utilization of VEP and ERG can theoretically provide real-time data on any pressure or stretch on the optic nerve during surgical manipulation. However, it is influenced by multiple hemodynamic and physiological parameters such as heart rate, blood pressure, type of anesthesia, the presence of a visual pathway lesion, preoperative severe visual deficit, and cranial surgical manipulation. Its impact therefore remains controversial and is not recommended as routine use of intraoperative monitoring until further evidence is established. Other modalities under investigation includes fiber tracking and diffusion tensor imaging (DTI) in intraoperative magnetic resonance imaging (MRI) with indexes such as fractional anisotropy to test the integrity of visual pathway during surgery [33].

For transcranial approach, global neurophysiologic monitoring including standard somatosensory-evoked potentials (SSEP), electroencephalography (EEG), and transcranial motor-evoked potentials (MEPs) can be used. For orbital approach, no method of neurophysiologic monitoring has been shown to be particularly useful. Therefore, it is important to have careful patient selection, preoperative counseling on risk of visual loss, intraoperative monitoring of pupil size and reactivity, close post-operative monitoring, and urgent management to reverse compressive causes of visual loss.

References

1. Rootman J, Stewart B, Goldberg RA. Orbital surgery: a conceptual approach. 2nd ed. Philadelphia: Lipincott Williams and Wilkins; 1995.
2. Paluzzi A, Gardner PA, Fernandez-Miranda JC, et al. "Round-the-Clock" surgical access to the orbit. J Neurol Surg B Skull Base. 2015;76(1):12–24.
3. Pai SB, Nagarjun MN. A neurosurgical perspective to approaches to the orbit: a cadaveric study. Neurol India. 2017;65(5):1094–101.
4. Kannan S, Hasegawa M, Yamada Y, Kawase T, Kato Y. Tumors of the orbit: case report and review of surgical corridors and current options. Asian J Neurosurg. 2019;14(3):678–85.
5. Abou-Al-Shaar H, Krisht KM, Cohen MA, Abunimer AM, Neil JA, Karsy M, Alzhrani G, Couldwell WT. Cranio-orbital and orbito-cranial approaches to orbital and intracranial disease: eye-opening approaches for neurosurgeons. Front Surg. 2020;7:1.
6. Lee RP, Khalafallah AM, Gami A, Mukherjee D. The lateral orbitotomy approach for intraorbital lesions, vol. 81; 2020. p. 435.
7. Tenzel RR, Miller GR. Orbital blow-out fracture repair, conjunctival approach. Am J Ophthalmol. 1971;71:1141–2.
8. Lynch RC. The technique of a radical frontal sinus operation which has given me the best results. Laryngoscope. 1921;31:1–5.
9. Humphrey CD, Kriet JD. Surgical approaches to the orbit. Otolaryngology. 2008;19:132–9.

10. Kloek CE, Bilyk JR, Pribitkin EA, Rubin PA. Orbital decompression as an alternative management strategy for patients with benign tumors located at the orbital apex. Ophthalmology. 2006;113(7):1214–9.
11. Lund VJ, Rose GE. Endoscopic transnasal orbital decompression for visual failure due to sphenoid wing meningioma. Eye (Lond). 2006;20:1213–9.
12. Cheung SSL, Lam SC, Yuen HKL. Transnasal endoscopic sclerotherapy for orbital apex lymphatic malformation. Ophthalmic Plast Reconstr Surg. 2020;37:S154.
13. Lam SC, Yuen HKL. Medical and sclerosing agents in the treatment of orbital lymphatic malformations: what's new? Curr Opin Ophthalmol. 2019;30(5):380–5.
14. Kim BS, Im YS, Woo KI, Kim YD, Lee JI. Multisession gamma knife radiosurgery for orbital apex tumors. World Neurosurg. 2015;84(4):1005–13.
15. De Castro DK, Fay A, Wladis EJ, Nguyen J, Osaki T, Metson R, Curry W. Self-irrigating piezoelectric device in orbital surgery. Ophthalmic Plast Reconstr Surg. 2013;29(2):118–22.
16. Ramakrishna R, Kim LJ, Bly RA, Moe K, Ferreira M Jr. Transorbital neuroendoscopic surgery for the treatment of skull base lesions. J Clin Neurosci. 2016;24:99–104.
17. Harris GJ, Jakobiec FA. Cavernous hemangioma of the orbit. J Neurosurg. 1979;51:219–28.
18. Purgason PA, Hornblass A. Complications of surgery for orbital tumors. Ophthalmic Plast Reconstr Surg. 1992;8:88–93.
19. Rose GE. The "devil's touch"; visual loss and orbital surgery. A synopsis of the Mustarde Lecture, 2006. Orbit. 2007;26(3):147–58.
20. Cannon PS, Rutherford SA, Richardson PL, et al. The surgical management and outcomes for sphenoid wing meningiomas: a 7-year review of multi-disciplinary practice. Orbit. 2009;28:371–6.
21. Mariniello G, Bonavolontà G, Tranfa F, Maiuri F. Management of the optic canal invasion and visual outcome in spheno-orbital meningiomas. Clin Neurol Neurosurg. 2013;115(9):1615–20.
22. Kansakar P, Sundar G. Vision loss associated with orbital surgery—a major review. Orbit. 2020;39(3):197–208. https://doi.org/10.1080/01676830.2019.1658790.
23. Carlson AP, Stippler M, Myers O. Predictive factors for vision recovery after optic nerve decompression for chronic compressive neuropathy: systematic review and meta-analysis. J Neurol Surg B Skull Base. 2013;74:20–38.
24. Kim TW, Jung S, Jung TY, Kim IY, Kang SS, Kim SH. Prognostic factors of postoperative visual outcomes in tuberculum sellae meningioma. Br J Neurosurg. 2008;22(2):231–4.
25. Lee LA, Roth S, Posner KL, et al. The American Society of Anesthesiologists Postoperative Visual Loss Registry: analysis of 93 spine surgery cases with postoperative visual loss. Anesthesiology. 2006;105:652–9.
26. Jacobs SM, Mcinnis CP, Kapeles M, Chang S. Incidence, risk factors, and management of blindness after orbital surgery. Ophthalmology. 2018;125(7):1100–8.
27. Bonavolontà G. Postoperative blindness following orbital surgery. Orbit. 2005;24(3):195–200.
28. Goepfert CE, Ifune C, Tempelhoff R. Ischemic optic neuropathy: are we any further? Curr Opin Anaesthesiol. 2010;23:582–7.
29. Karkanevatos A, Lancaster JL, Osman I, Swift AC. Pupil size and reaction during functional endoscopic sinus surgery (FESS). Clin Otolaryngol Allied Sci. 2003;28(2):103–7.
30. Harding GF, Bland JD, Smith VH. Visual evoked potential monitoring of optic nerve function during surgery. J Neurol Neurosurg Psychiatry. 1990;53(10):890–5.
31. Susarla SM, Nam AJ, Dorafshar AH. Orbital compartment syndrome leading to visual loss following orbital floor reconstruction. Craniomaxillofac Trauma Reconstr. 2016;9:152–7.
32. Luo Y, Regli L, Bozinov O, Sarnthein J. Clinical utility and limitations of intraoperative monitoring of visual evoked potentials. PLoS One. 2015;10(3):e0120525.
33. Kodama K, Goto T, Sato A, Sakai K, Tanaka Y, Hongo K. Standard and limitation of intraoperative monitoring of the visual evoked potential. Acta Neurochir (Wien). 2010;152:643–8.
34. Metwali H, Kniese K, Fahlbusch R. Literature review intraoperative monitoring of the integrity of the anterior visual pathways: a methodologic review and meta-analysis. World Neurosurg. 2018;110:217–25.

Transcranial Approach to Optic Canal and Orbital Apex

17

Tak Lap POON

Abstract

Neurosurgeons are always often required to approach the optic canal and orbital apex for treatment of various pathologies including neoplastic, vascular, and traumatic in origin. Traditionally and most popularly, this very limited space is approached by transcranial route, of which a wide area of exposure can be achieved. This transcranial route can further be subclassified into extradural approach, intradural approach, and hybrid approach. Development of endoscope-assisted craniotomy with advanced in technology improves the surgical outcome. This chapter is intended to have a comprehensive review of transcranial approach with pros and cons of different subtypes of this surgical approach.

Keywords

Transcranial approach · Optic canal decompression · Anterior clinoidectomy · Meningo-orbital band

17.1 Transcranial Approach to Optic Canal and Orbital Apex

17.1.1 Introduction

Optic canal and orbital apex are very limited anatomical regions connecting the orbit and cranial compartments [1]. Diseases in this region can have presentation including deteriorating visual acuity, visual field deficits, impairment of extraocular movement resulting in diplopia, proptosis, chemosis, cranial nerve palsies related to cavernous sinus, and others.

T. L. POON (✉)
Department of Neurosurgery, Queen Elizabeth Hospital, Hong Kong SAR, China
e-mail: ptl220@ha.org.hk

17.1.2 Indications

Decompression of optic canal and orbital apex is indicated in pathologies causing visual impairment. These causes include neoplasms within optic canal and around periorbital skull base, vascular malformation and other pathologies such as aneurysm, local trauma with or without skull base fracture, bony dysplasia, infection, inflammation, autoimmune, and connective tissue disease [2–4]. Surgical decompression choices include transcranial or endoscopic transnasal transethmoidal approaches [5, 6].

17.1.3 Choices of Transcranial Approaches

Decompression via transcranial route aims to achieve decompression over superior-lateral compartment with respect to optic nerve. Surgical strategy includes unroofing of the optic canal, anterior clinoidectomy, and removal of optic strut (OS) [7]. Removal of anterior clinoid process (ACP) and optic-sheath opening significantly increased the exposure and mobilization of the optic nerve and internal carotid artery (ICA) as well as three- to fourfold expansion of the opticocarotid triangle width [8]. Sofferman in 1981 suggested the following principles of adequate optic nerve decompression [9]:

1. Removal of half the circumference of the osseous canal
2. Removal of bone in a longitudinal dimension to the full extent of the optic canal from 5.5 to 11.5 mm
3. Complete longitudinal incision of the nerve sheath to include the thickened annulus tendinous at the orbital end, that is, annulus of Zinn

Transcranial routes, either via pterional, supraorbital, or orbitozygomatic, are traditionally preferable to most of the neurosurgeons. This approach provides a wide surgical cor-

T. L. POON et al. (eds.), *Orbital Apex and Periorbital Skull Base Diseases*, https://doi.org/10.1007/978-981-99-2989-4_17

ridor but is more invasive and associated with more cosmetic issues compared with other approaches, for example, endoscopic transnasal transethmoidal route [10]. The bony optic canal can be drilled up to 270°, but the inferior and inferomedial floors of the optic canal usually cannot be reached [11–15].

17.1.4 Extradural Approach

Extradural optic canal decompression and anterior clinoidectomy were initially introduced by Vinco Dolenc in 1985 for treatment of aneurysms at cavernous segment of internal carotid artery and traumatic carotid-cavernous fistulas [16, 17]. This approach is often considered as difficult and technique demanding due to the constricted working space and the vulnerability of critical neurovascular anatomical structures [18] (Figs. 17.1 and 17.2).

17.1.4.1 Procedures

The sphenoid ridge is drilled or rougeured flat to the lateral base of the ACP. Dura is stripped off from the floor of the anterior cranial fossa, ACP, and/or the superior orbital fissure (SOF). The orbit can be unroofed and the optic canal can be opened. Another recently favorable way is to open the lateral SOF first, that is, the superior-lateral ACP base and then the inferior greater sphenoid wing portion. The orbitomeningeal artery and vein are then coagulated and divided. Lateral meningo-orbital band (MOB) (or named orbitotemporal periosteal fold or fronto-temporal dural fold) is dissected and cut (Fig. 17.3). Afterward, the optic canal can be unroofed, and the superior-medial connection of the base of ACP can be divided (Fig. 17.4). The final step is the drilling of the OS, either by drilling with a small diamond burr or by using ultrasound bone dissector, and the remaining ACP shell and tip can be disconnected and removed [19–22] (Fig. 17.5).

17.1.4.2 Advantages

1. Extradural space allows a more extensive osteotomy of medial sphenoidal wing and clinoid with protection of intradural neurovascular structures during drilling procedure including optic nerve, ophthalmic artery, and ICA by dura mater as a natural barrier.
2. The approach is less selective and more inclusive.
3. It allows early devascularization in neoplasm case and less traction risk to optic nerve during tumor manipulation.

17.1.4.3 Pearls and Pitfalls

1. Operating surgeon should be aware of clinoid pneumatization and ligament ossification before deciding to complete a clinoidectomy to avoid postoperative cerebrospinal fluid (CSF) leakage [23].
2. Sectioning of lateral MOB for elevation of temporal fossa dura away from lateral wall of the cavernous sinus along the superior orbital fissure (SOF) near the sphenoidal ridge provides an excellent view of the clinoid process.
3. Peeling the temporal dura propria from lateral wall of the cavernous sinus along the length of the ACP may unavoidably cause venous bleeding and/or potential damage to the nerves traveling in the sinus.
4. Drilling should be done with continuous irrigation to avoid thermal injury.
5. Egg-shelling the ACP is a safe method of clinoidectomy.
6. It should be aware that the oculomotor nerve during removal of lower and posterior tip of the clinoid that courses below the ACP.
7. Extradural approach should better be avoided in cases with significant hyperostotic features.
8. En bloc resection of ACP should be avoided.

Dolenc's technique has been refined by minimizing the extent peeling in the lateral wall of the SOF including the limited anterior part of the cavernous sinus. This modified approach is named as trans-Superior Orbital Fissure Approach

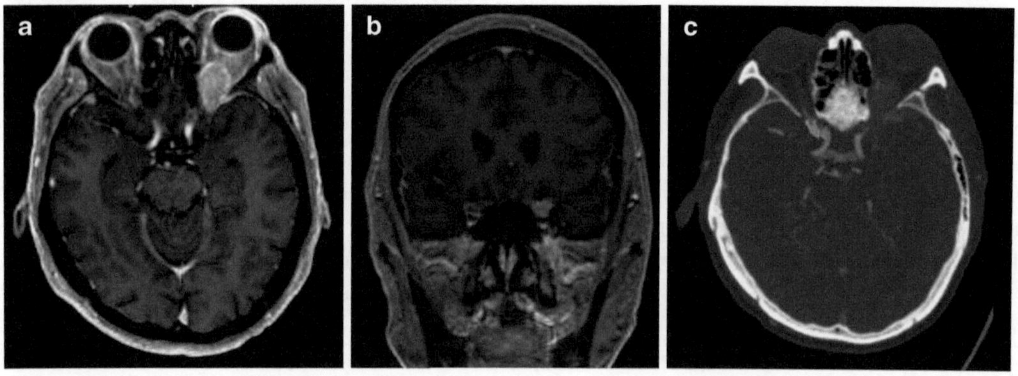

Fig. 17.1 (**a** and **b**) Lymphoma at left orbital apex, and (**c**) post transcranial extradural anterior clinoidectomy and optic canal decompression for partial tumor excision

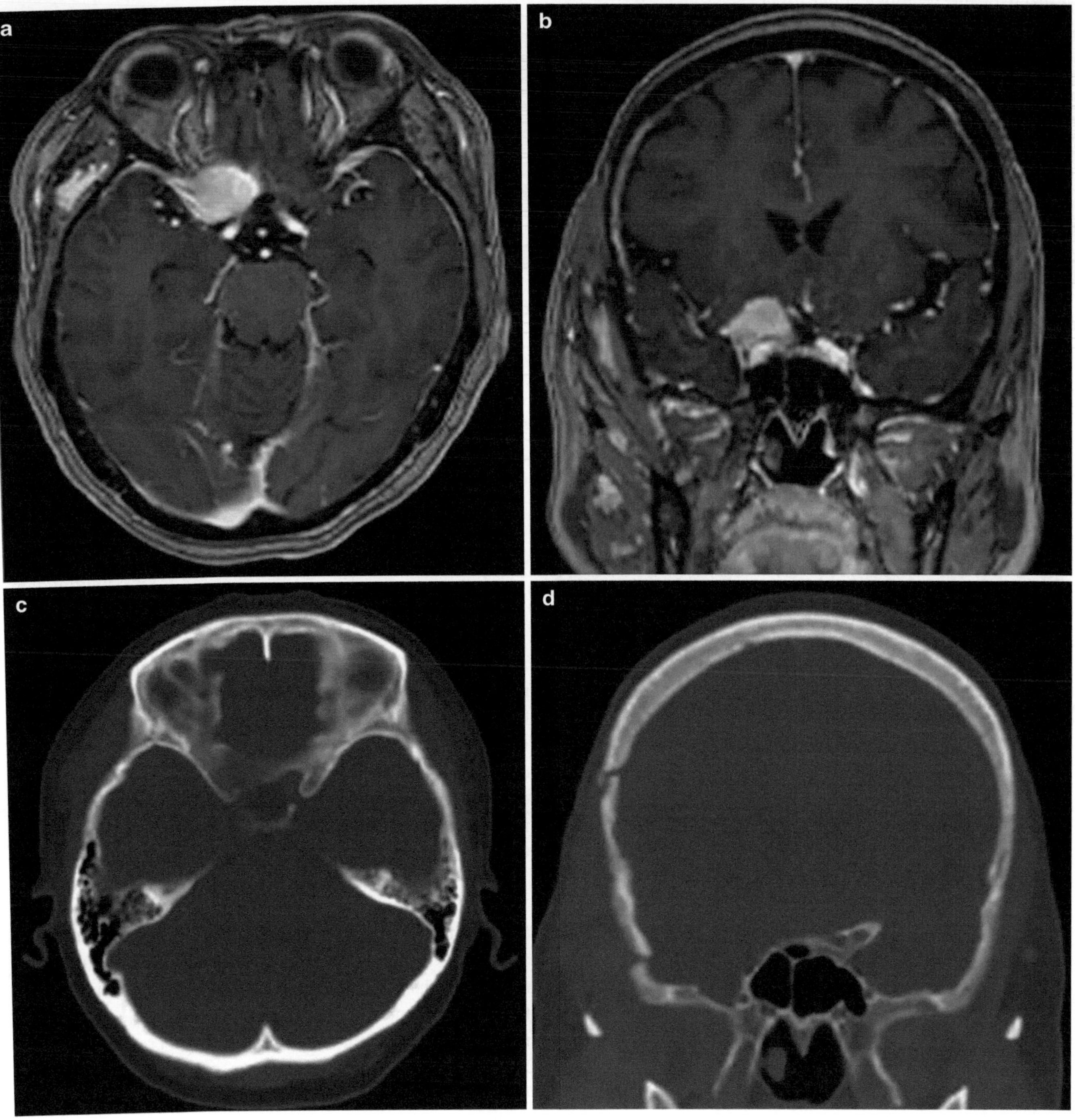

Fig. 17.2 (**a** and **b**) Right clinoidal meningioma, and (**c** and **d**) post transcranial extradural anterior clinoidectomy for tumor excision

[24]. It can provide less invasive but adequate exposure of the ACP and the orifice of the optic canal, resulting in a wider epidural space for safe drilling of the ACP and a wide opening of the optic canal. This approach also allows easy identification of the optic canal after partial removal of the ACP, resulting in fewer surgical complications. Otani et al. applied this approach for emergency optic canal release for traumatic optic neuropathy in eight patients in their series [25].

17.1.5 Intradural Approach

Yasargil et al. in 1977 first described the intradural anterior clinoidectomy by pterional approach for clipping of carotid-ophthalmic aneurysms [26]. Complete splitting of the sylvian fissure additionally improves the working space for identification of the proper anatomy and the pathological lesion.

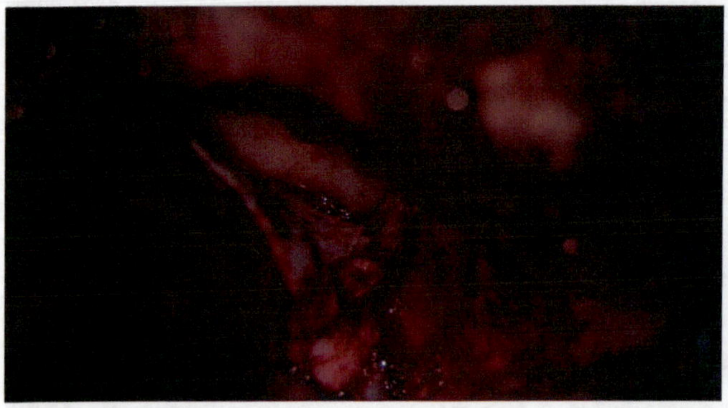

Fig. 17.3 Meningo-orbital band (MOB) is being coagulated and divided

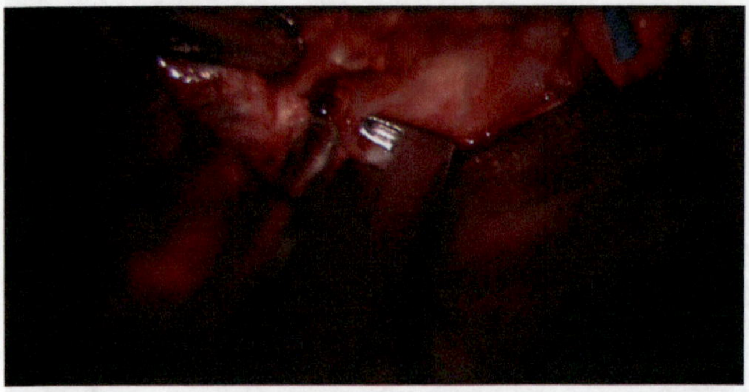

Fig. 17.4 Unroofing of orbital canal

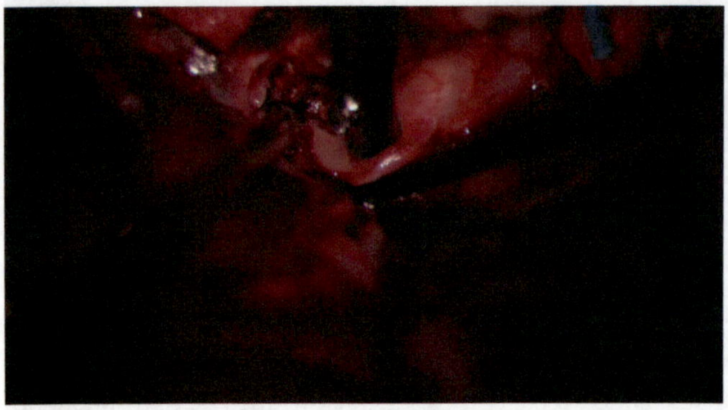

Fig. 17.5 Removal of anterior clinoid process tip

17.1.5.1 Procedures

The intradural clinoidectomy generally begins with a standard pterional craniotomy. The dura over the lesser wing of the sphenoid is stripped and the lesser wing of sphenoid bone is drilled extradurally. Dura is opened and retracted to expose frontal and temporal lobes. Sylvian fissure is dissected widely, and basal cisterns are opened for CSF release and brain relaxation. Dura overlying the optic canal and anterior clinoid is incised. Optic canal and anterior clinoidectomy are performed. The direction is from medial to lateral down to the OS (Fig. 17.6).

17.1.5.2 Advantages

1. Relatively limited osteotomy is required for target lesion.
2. The approach is more selective and more tailor-made.
3. Monitoring of any intraoperative aneurysm rupture during drilling can be achieved.

17.1.5.3 Pearls and Pitfalls

1. This approach is a relatively better choice in cases with highly hyperostotic bone or with ossification of clinoid ligaments.
2. It may be preferable in clipping of aneurysm at clinoidal segment of ICA as bony removal can be tailored based on the pathology with direct visualization on aneurysm sac during manipulations.
3. Egg-shelling the medial clinoid is safe.
4. Copious irrigation is mandatory to avoid thermal injury to optic nerve.
5. Up to one third of patients will have postoperative headache, which are due to subarachnoid accumulation of bone dust.

17.1.6 Hybrid Approach

Ali Tayebi Meybodi et al. in 2019 proposed a two-step hybrid technique called "anterior clinoidectomy using a 2-step hybrid" (ACTH) technique [27]. It combines advantages while avoid shortcomings of individual extradural and intradural approaches. Based on localization of the OS, resection of ACP will be in two steps: the segment anterior to the OS is resected extradurally, while the segment posterior to the OS is resected intradurally.

17.1.6.1 Advantages of the Extradural Phase

Most of the drilling is performed extradurally, and the total amount of intradural drilling is reduced. This greatly minimizes the risk of damage to adjacent neurovascular structures and the amount of bone dust in intradural space, which may prove beneficial in reducing postoperative headache. Furthermore, peeling off the dura propria of the temporal lobe at lateral wall of the cavernous sinus is minimal, potentially reducing venous bleeding and minimizing cranial nerve injury.

17.1.6.2 Advantages of the Intradural Phase

Correct localization and intradural drilling of the OS can be critical, especially in case with unusual origin and course of ophthalmic artery.

The ACTH technique also offers additional advantage over purely extradural approach in ACP with anatomical variations. These include longer whole length of ACP, an interosseous bridge between ACP and posterior clinoid process in about 5% cases, and a carotico-clinoid foramen, that

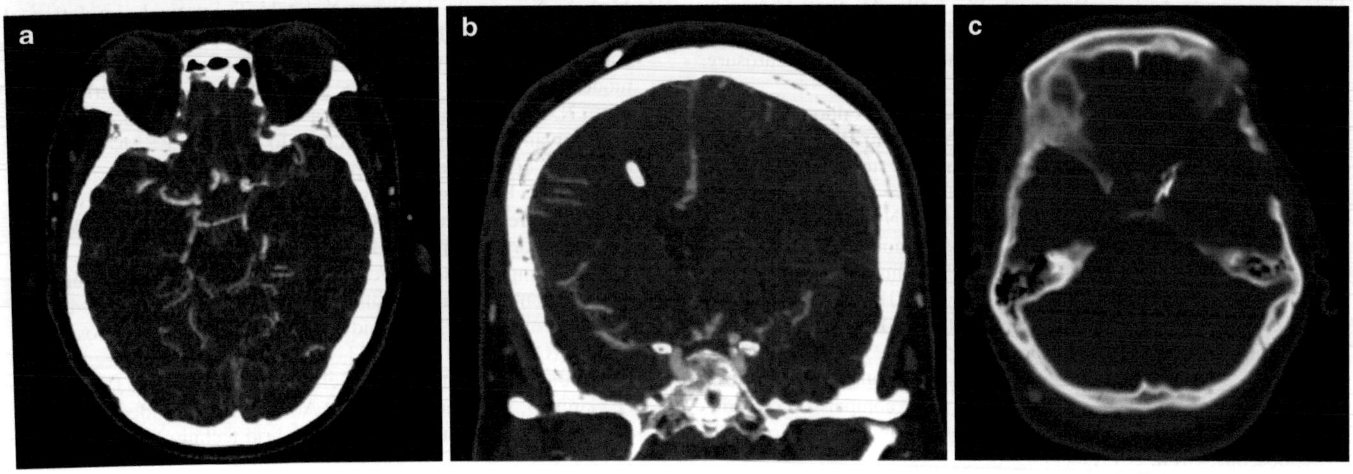

Fig. 17.6 (**a** and **b**) Ruptured left internal carotid artery ophthalmic segment aneurysm, and (**c**) clipping of aneurysm after transcranial intradural anterior clinoidectomy

is, a bony bridge connecting the ACP tip to a middle clinoid process in about 14% cases [28].

17.1.7 Transcranial Extradural Endoscopic Approach

Fuminari Komatsu et al. in 2017 first reported a clinical case of anterior clinoidectomy performed by endoscopy, which was a pathological ACP corroded by a pituitary adenoma [29, 30]. Cai et al. in 2019 reported the first case of extradural anterior clinoidectomy and aneurysm clipping performed using transcranial neuroendoscopic approach [31].

Steps follow the same principles of microscopic extradural anterior clinoidectomy:

1. Osteotomy along medial sphenoid wing to disconnect the lateral connection
2. Osteotomy along the orbital roof to disconnect the anterior and medial connections
3. Drilling within the clinoid to "egg-shell" the bone and disconnect the anteroinferior connection to the OS

Use of endoscope can improve visibility as it provides clear panoramic views of the ACP and its surrounding structures with adequate magnification, and the ACP can be reliably removed without incising the duplication of the dura stretching between the periorbita and temporal fossa dura.

17.1.8 Procedure-Related Complications

Previously described major complications related to optic canal decompression and anterior clinoidectomy include postoperative CSF leak from opening of the sphenoid sinus or ethmoid air cells or pneumatized ACP, damage to optic nerve in terms of visual field deficits (either direct neural damage or ischemia due to ophthalmic artery manipulation), oculomotor palsy and injury to other cranial nerves in SOF, intraoperative aneurysm rupture, profuse bleeding from cavernous sinus during division and retraction of dura fold, and clinoid and cavernous segment of ICA [32, 33].

References

1. Regoli M, Bertelli E. The revised anatomy of the canals connecting the orbit with the cranial cavity. Orbit. 2017;36(2):110–7.
2. Acheson JF. Optic nerve disorders: role of canal and nerve sheath decompression surgery. Eye (Lond). 2004;18:1169–74.
3. Mine S, Yamakami I, Yamaura A, Hanawa K, Ikejiri M, Mizota A, Adachi-Usami E. Outcome of traumatic optic neuropathy. Comparison between surgical and nonsurgical treatment. Acta Neurochir (Wien). 1999;141:27–30.
4. Wohlrab TM, Maas S, de Carpentier JP. Surgical decompression in traumatic optic neuropathy. Acta Ophthalmol Scand. 2002;80:287–93.
5. He Z, Li Q, Yuan J, Zhang X, Gao R, Han Y, Yang W, Shi X, Lan Z. Evaluation of transcranial surgical decompression of the optic canal as a treatment option for traumatic optic neuropathy. Clin Neurol Neurosurg. 2015;134:130–5.
6. Oh HJ, Yeo DG, Hwang SC. Surgical treatment for traumatic optic neuropathy. Korean J Neurotrauma. 2018;14(2):55–60.
7. Norris JH, Norris JS, Akinwunmi J, Malhotra R. Optic canal decompression with dural sheath release; a combined orbito-cranial approach to preserving sight from tumours invading the optic canal. Orbit. 2012;31(1):34–43.
8. Natori Y, Rhoton JRAL. Transcranial approach to the orbit: microsurgical anatomy. J Neurosurg. 1994;81:78–86.
9. Sofferman RA. Sphenoethmoid approach to the optic nerve. Laryngoscope. 1981;91:184–96.
10. Abou-Al-Shaar H, Krisht KM, Cohen MA, Abunimer AM, Neil JA, Karsy M, Alzhrani G, Couldwell WT. Cranio-orbital and orbitocranial approaches to orbital and intracranial disease: eye-opening approaches for neurosurgeons. Front Surg. 2020;7:1.

11. Di Somma A, Andaluz N, Gogela SL, Keller JT, Prats-Galino A, Cappabianca P. Surgical freedom evaluation during optic nerve decompression: laboratory investigation. World Neurosurg. 2017;101:227–35.
12. Filho PMMM, Prevedello DM, Prevedello LM, Filho LFD, Fiore ME, Dolci RL, Buohliqah L, Otto BA, Carrau RL. Optic canal decompression: comparison of 2 surgical techniques. World Neurosurg. 2017;104:745–51.
13. Gogela SL, Zimmer LA, Keller JT, Andaluz N. Refining operative strategies for optic nerve decompression: a morphometric analysis of transcranial and endoscopic endonasal techniques using clinical parameters. Oper Neurosurg (Hagerstown). 2018;14(3):295.
14. Onofrey CB, Tse DT, Johnson TE, Neff AG, Dubovy S, Buck BE, Casiano R. Ophthal Plast Reconstr Surg. 2007;23(4):261–6.
15. Roth J, Fraser J, Singh A, Bernardo A, Anand VK, Schwartz TH. Surgical approaches to the orbital apex: comparison of endoscopic endonasal and transcranial approaches using a novel 3D endoscope. Orbit. 2011;30(1):43–8.
16. Dolenc VV. Direct microsurgical repair of intracavernous vascular lesions. J Neurosurg. 1983;58:824–31.
17. Dolenc VV. A combined epi- and subdural direct approach to carotid-ophthalmic artery aneurysms. J Neurosurg. 1985;62:667–72.
18. Yasargil MG, Gasser JC, Hodosh RM, Rankin TV. Carotid-ophthalmic aneurysms: direct microsurgical approach. Surg Neurol. 1977;8(3):155–65.
19. Froelich SC, Abdel Aziz KM, Levine NB, Theodosopoulos PV, Van Loveren HR, Keller JT. Refinement of the extradural anterior clinoidectomy: surgical anatomy of the orbitotemporal perioteal fold. Neurosurgery. 2007;61(ONS Suppl 2):ons179–86.
20. Kim JS, Lee SI, Jeon KD, Choi BS. The pterional approach and extradural anterior clinoidectomy to clip paraclinoid aneurysms. J Cerebrovasc Endovasc Neurosurg. 2013;15(3):260–6.
21. Lehmberg J, Krieg SM, Meyer B. Anterior clinoidectomy. Acta Neurochir (Wien). 2014;156:415–9.
22. Mishra S, Leao B, Rosio DM. Extradural anterior clinoidectomy: technical nuances from a learner's perspective. Asian J Neurosurg. 2017;12(2):189–93.
23. Mikami T, Minamida Y, Koyanagi I, Baba T, Houkin K. Anatomical variations in pneumatization of the anterior clinoid process. J Neurosurg. 2007;106:170–4.
24. Mori K, Yamamoto T, Nakao Y, Esaki T. Surgical simulation of extradural anterior clinoidectomy through the trans-superior orbital fissure approach using a dissectable three-dimensional skull base model with artificial cavernous sinus. Skull Base. 2010;20:229–36.
25. Otani N, Wada K, Fujii K, Toyooka T, Kumagai K, Ueno H, Tomura S, Tomiyama A, Nakao Y, Yamamoto T, Mori K. Usefulness of extradural optic nerve decompression via trans-superior orbital fissure approach for treatment of traumatic optic nerve injury: surgical procedures and techniques from experience with 8 consecutive patients. World Neurosurg. 2016;90:357–63.
26. Yang Y, Wang H, Shao Y, Wei Z, Zhu S, Wang J. Extradural anterior clinoidectomy as an alternative approach for optic nerve decompression: anatomic study and clinical experience. Neurosurgery. 2006;59(ONS Suppl 4):ons253–62.
27. Meybodi AT, Lawton MT, Yousef S, Guo X, Sanchez JJG, Tabani H, Garcia S, Burkhardt JK, Benet A. Anterior clinoidectomy using an extradural and intradural 2-step hybrid technique. J Neurosurg. 2019;130:238–47.
28. Kulwin C, Tubbs RS, Cohen-Gadol AA. Anterior clinoidectomy: description of an alternative hybrid method and a review of the current techniques with an emphasis on complication avoidance. Surg Neurol Int. 2011;2:140.
29. Komatsu F, Komatsu M, Inoue T, Tschabitscher M. Endoscopic extradural anterior clinoidectomy via supraorbital keyhole: a cadaveric study. Neurosurgery. 2011;68(ONS Suppl 2):ons334–8.
30. Komatsu F, Imai M, Shigematsu H, Aoki R, Oda S, Shimoda M, Matsumae M. Endoscopic extradural supraorbital approach to the temporal pole and adjacent area: technical note. J Neurosurg. 2018;128:1873–9.
31. Cai Q, Guo Q, Zhang W, Ji B, Chen Z, Chen Q. Extradural anterior clinoidectomy and aneurysm clipping using transcranial neuroendoscopic approach. Medicine. 2019;98:17.
32. Lehmberg J, Krieg SM, Mueller B, Meyer B. Impact of anterior clinoidectomy on visual function after resection of meningiomas in and around the optic canal. Acta Neurochir. 2013;155:1293–9.
33. Romani R, Elsharkawy A, Laakso A, Kangasniemi M, Hernesniemi J. Complications of anterior clinoidectomy through lateral supraorbital approach. World Neurosurg. 2012;77(5/6):699–703.

Transcranial Approach to Cavernous Sinus and Middle Cranial Fossa

18

King Fai Kevin Cheng and Wai Man Lui

Abstract

Despite the advances in skull base techniques, lesions involving cavernous sinus and deeper part of the middle cranial fossa still pose a challenge to neurosurgeons. Even with the advancement of endoscopic instruments, these lesions cannot be completely resected via endoscopic approach and require open surgery. Transcranial approach to this region can be combined with others depending on necessity, for example, anterior clinoidectomy, splitting the lateral wall of cavernous sinus, cutting of tentorium, and anterior petrosectomy. To choose the best approach, we have to ascertain thorough understanding of the involved anatomical structures, clinical symptoms and signs, tumors' nature, and patients' expectation. Here, we would like to focus on a standard transcranial approach to the cavernous sinus via the middle cranial fossa approach, its variation to expand the operative corridor to suit different pathology, the technical nuances, and how to avoid major complications.

Keywords

Cavernous sinus · Middle cranial fossa · Trans-zygomatic approach · Anterior clinoidectomy · Kawase approach · Glasscock triangle · Fukushima bypass

18.1 Introduction

Despite the advances in skull base techniques, lesions involving the cavernous sinus or petroclival region still pose a challenge to neurosurgeons. The route from the lateral skull base is still the most widely adopted approach to this region, and when combined with anterior clinoidectomy, opening of tentorium, anterior petrosectomy, it can lead us to different windows of attack visualizing from anterior to posterior the superior orbital fissure (SOF), optic canal (OC), cavernous sinus (CS), Meckel's cave, and internal auditory canal (IAC) in treating majority of skull base pathologies, which includes the medial sphenoidal ridge meningioma with or without orbital or optic canal extension, anterior clinoidal meningioma, cavernous sinus lesion be it a meningioma or hemangioma etc., or cranial nerves Schwannoma, for example, a dumbbell-shaped trigeminal schwannoma, or the notorious petroclival meningioma. Other than tumor, some vascular pathology is also amenable by this approach including anterior inferior cerebellar artery aneurysm, dural arterio-venous fistula involving the medial cerebellopontine angle, or even for cerebral bypass surgery the famous Fukushima bypass.

More recently, within the last decade, endonasal endoscopic approaches to the cavernous sinus region have been developed as an alternative to an open craniotomy. The current trend in anterior and middle cranial base surgery is to incorporate these strategies as a minimally invasive alternative. Here, we will focus on the transcranial techniques in detail.

18.2 Goals of Surgery

The ideal goal of surgery is complete resection of the tumor without causing additional deficits to the patient. Neurosurgeons must weigh the increased morbidity produced by aggressive surgery against the natural history of residual tumor particularly in older patients. The best treatment strategy for each patient involves various considerations. These include prognostic factors, applicability of other options such as radiosurgery, and consequences of the outcome on the patient's quality of life. For example, it is extremely difficult to achieve total excision of a petroclival

K. F. K. Cheng (✉) · W. M. Lui
Division of Neurosurgery, Department of Surgery, Queen Mary Hospital, Li Ka Shing Faculty of Medicine, The University of Hong Kong, Hong Kong SAR, China
e-mail: ckf414@ha.org.hk

T. L. POON et al. (eds.), *Orbital Apex and Periorbital Skull Base Diseases*, https://doi.org/10.1007/978-981-99-2989-4_18

meningioma, including excision of its dural attachment, its dural tail, and the involved bone. Therefore, our primary goal is brain stem decompression to restore clinical function with either total or subtotal excision. For tumors with neurovascular invasion, we prefer performing an excision of the tumor that leaves the parts infiltrating the neurovascular structures undisturbed, rather than attempting total excision of the tumor, which may leave the patient with a major neurologic deficit. Devascularization of the residual capsule of a skull base lesion may result in limited growth for a long period.

The surgeon must constantly weigh the benefits of complete resection, the risk of morbidity by injury to vital structures, and the natural history of potentially residual tumor. To keep morbidity to a minimum, other alternative to surgery includes safe debulking and stereotactic radiosurgery.

18.3 Preoperative Neuroradiologic Evaluation

Thorough evaluation of preoperative neuroimaging studies is of utmost importance in the management of skull base lesion. The tumor size, consistency, vascularity, location, and extension of dural attachment; tumor-brain stem interface; degree of brain stem displacement displacement of the vertebrobasilar arterial system; and tumor extension into the cavernous sinus or internal auditory canal are all important details to look into before operation.

Computed tomography (CT) of brain is valuable in evaluating the anatomy of the temporal bone, the degree of pneumatization of the mastoid bone, anatomy of the anterior clinoid, the relationship of the petrous apex and ICA, the cochlear, and its relation to the jugular bulb. Magnetic resonance imaging (MRI) T1-weighted images (Fig. 18.1) delineates the tumor and its relationships to the surrounding structures. MRI T2-weighted images are useful for assessment of the arachnoid cleavage plane, brain stem edema, and infiltration. Flow voids on MRI T2-weighted images can reveal the location of major vertebrobasilar vessels and its vascularity. The absence of a definite arachnoid cleavage plane between the tumor and the brain stem may represent pial infiltration and can make resection extremely challenging. This is one of the main obstacles preventing safe total resection of skull base tumor.

Understanding the venous anatomy can reduce related complications during middle fossa dissection [1]. CT Venogram or MR Venogram can illustrate the temporal venous drainage pattern [2], size of the vein of Labbe, which is very important before consideration of peeling of lateral of cavernous sinus and tentorial cutting. Cerebral angiography is sometimes helpful in showing the tumors' blood supply for example the meningohypophyseal trunk of the internal carotid artery, the posterior branch of the middle meningeal artery, the clival artery from the carotid siphon, and the petrosal branches of the meningeal arteries. Angiography can be used for preoperative tumor embolization to reduce surgical blood loss.

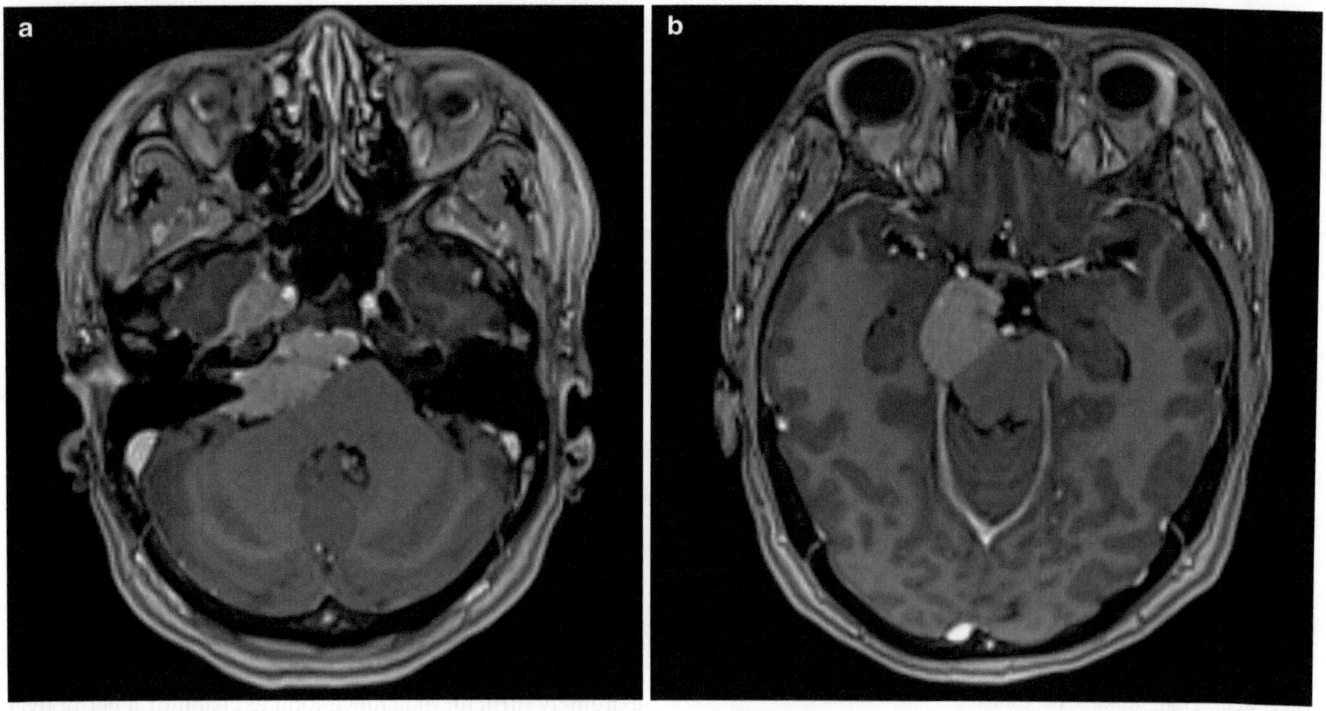

Fig. 18.1 (a) Tumor involving IAC and Meckel's cave. (b) Tumor involving suprasellar part encasing PCA. (c) Tumor crossing midline, compressing brainstem and displaced the vertebrobasilar artery. (d) Postoperative MRI at 3 months showing the anterior petrosectomy window with good decompression of brainstem achieved, thin sheet of dural tail left in the clival dura

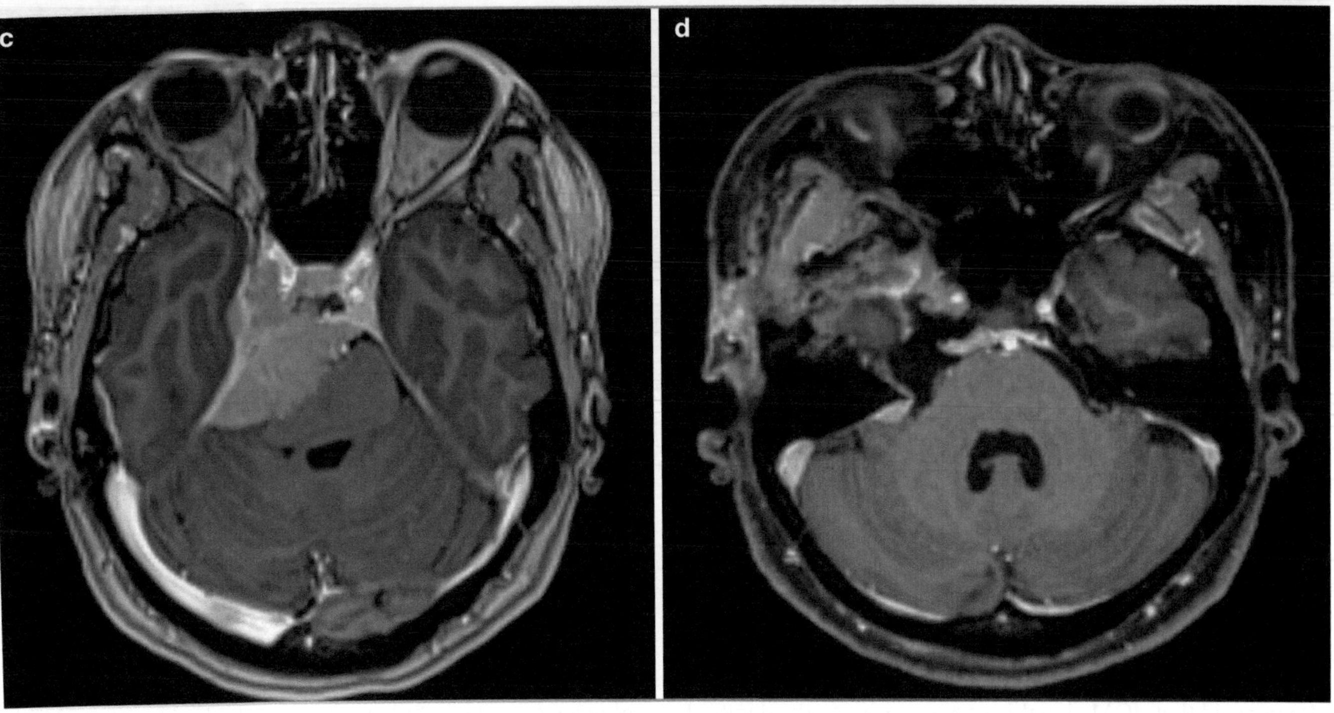

Fig. 18.1 (continued)

18.4 Surgical Procedures

18.4.1 Patient Position and Skin Flap Design

Under general anesthesia, the patient is positioned supine with the head fixed by headpins and the head holder, elevated above the level of the heart to improve venous drainage, extended, and rotated 60° to the opposite side to bring the malar eminence to the highest point of the operative field. Depending on the location of pathology, rotation of more than 60° is advised if anterior petrosectomy and tentorial opening is planned. A curvilinear frontotemporal incision begins at the superior border of the zygomatic arch (Fig. 18.2a), close to the tragal cartilage and anterior to the superficial temporal artery (STA). STA can be preserved if sizable as an arterial donor in case of anticipated cerebral revascularization procedure; otherwise, it can be ligated and cut to gain more access to zygomatic arch. The incision then proceeds posteriorly above the ear pinna, and this aims to gain more exposure to the subtemporal space for later tentorial exposure [3], before curving anterior-superiorly to the frontal region behind the hairline. Interfascial dissection [4] is applied to preserve the frontotemporal branch of the facial nerve. At the same time, a long vascularized pericranium (Fig. 18.2c) together with superficial temporalis fascia can be harvested and based inferior-posteriorly for dural repair and wound closure. Leaving a muscle cuff on the superior temporal line for later suturing aids better cosmetic result.

18.4.2 Anesthetic Considerations

The goals of modern neuroanesthesia are to provide a stable hemodynamic condition, maintain cerebral perfusion pressure, allow optimum intraoperative monitoring, and leave no residual anesthetic effects to facilitate the postoperative assessment of patient's neurologic condition. For complex skull base surgery, brain relaxation can be provided by the use of Mannitol and Furosemide or Hypertonic Saline. Muscle relaxation is not utilized because of cranial nerve and motor tract monitoring.

18.4.3 Intraoperative Neurophysiologic Monitoring

Intraoperative neurophysiologic monitoring (IOM) has been utilized to minimize neurologic morbidity from operative manipulations. Intraoperative monitoring facilitates safe tumor resection with cranial nerve preservation especially when dealing with large tumor involving cranial nerves. Somatosensory-evoked potentials (SSEPs) and motor-evoked potentials (MEPs) are particularly important to detect hemispheric ischemia or major vascular territory injury. And facial MEP and brain stem auditory-evoked potentials (BAEPs) are very sensitive and accurate when detecting CN VII and VIII function when the lesion involves internal auditory canal. Electroencephalography (EEG) is generally used

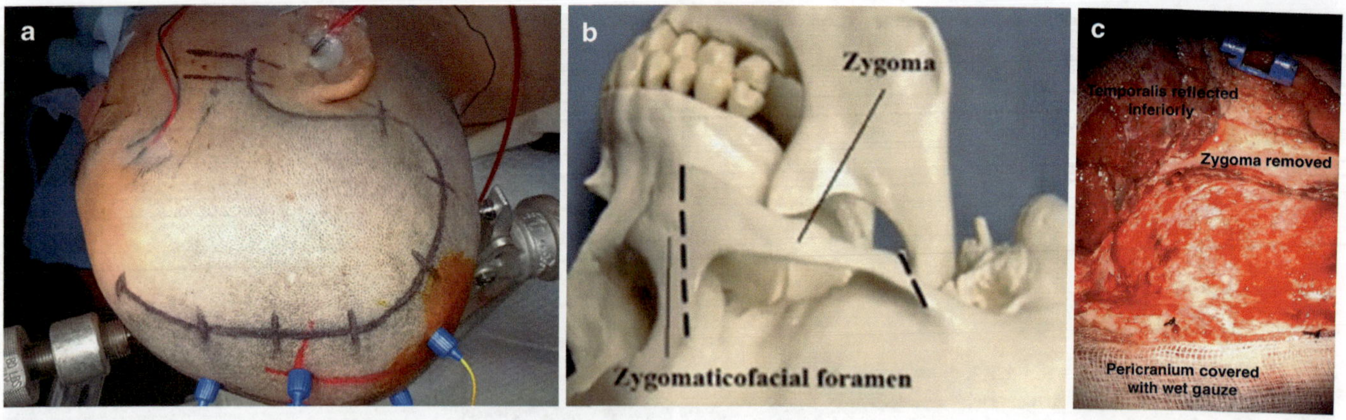

Fig. 18.2 (**a**) Scalp incision with posterior extension at temporal base (**b**) excision of zygoma, (**c**) inferior reflection of temporalis flap with the preparation of pericranial flap

to monitor burst suppression in case of bypass surgery. Specific cranial nerves III to VII and IX to XII are performed by recording electromyogram activity from the appropriately innervated muscles via an intraoperative stimulation probe. Having said that, IOM signal is very sensitive to the depth of anesthesia and the use of muscle relaxants, and experienced neurophysiologist for accurate signal interpretation is as important as having IOM machine in place.

18.4.4 Craniotomy

The craniotomy is a standard pterional craniotomy with temporal extension. Transzygomatic approach [5] is suited where expanded access to the middle fossa is necessary, two beveled cuts are made by electric saw at the anterior and posterior ends of the zygomatic arch, and the anterior cut is made parallel to the lateral orbital rim, beginning at the frontozygomatic suture, leaving as little bone overhanging the frontozygomatic recess as possible (Fig. 18.2b); the posterior cut is made roughly parallel to the surface of the temporal squama through the root of the temporal zygomatic process and avoid invasion of the temporomandibular joint. This step helps to achieve inferior reflection of the temporalis muscle. In order to further minimize temporal retraction in dominant hemisphere, we prefer to remove the zygoma when the pathology is over the left side. We strongly recommend to place the temporal burr hole flush with the floor of the middle fossa, and this can minimize excessive bone loss. Exposed mastoid air cells must be bone waxed. The sphenoid wing is then drilled from its lateral to medial extension until the anterior clinoid process (ACP) is reached. This exposes the meningo-orbital artery, which is coagulated and cut. During this step, the posterior third of the lateral and superior orbital wall is removed, preserving the peri-orbita. This mini-lateral orbidotomy helps the clear identification of plane separating the dura propria and lateral wall of cavernous sinus.

18.4.5 Cerebrospinal Fluid Drainage (CSF) Via External Ventricular Drainage (EVD)

External ventricular drainage is placed occasionally for several purposes: one is for sure to relax the brain and minimize the chance of brain retraction injury especially on the dominant side. Second it serves as an intracranial pressure (ICP) sensor when intubation overnight is anticipated after a long surgery. Thirdly to keep the CSF drainage for few days can help minimize the formation of pseudomeningocele and better wound healing. Lumbar drain may serve similar purpose, but in case of large intracranial lesion, lumbar drainage may post the harm of brain coning. And the caring of lumbar drain is relatively difficult and prone to dislodgement or blockage.

18.4.6 Epidural Dissection of the Lateral Wall of the Cavernous Sinus

The meningo-orbital artery is a point where the dissection plane between the dura propria of the temporal lobe and the lateral wall of the cavernous sinus starts, and cranial nerves (CNs) III and IV and V1 and V2 nerves are identified. Peeling starts at the lateral edge of superior orbital fissure, usually the bony prominence of anterior clinoid process is a safe point to guide the cutting. Once the dural propria is elevated, the thin layer covering the cranial nerves can be observed under high power magnification. The peeling should be smooth and feel like "peeling the skin of an orange" and continue laterally toward the V1 and V2 branches [6], between which is a common area for bleeding that can be controlled by fibrin glue injection. The middle sphenoid ridge is a good landmark between V2 and V3, extra care must be taken not to damage the temporal dura, or it has to be repaired before starting the temporal epidural dissection; otherwise, during the process of temporal elevation, the temporal brain tissue may herniate through the dural defect leading to temporal lobe injury.

Middle fossa dural elevation begins posteriorly and laterally, over the petrous ridge, and continues antero-medially to the foramen ovale. The middle meningeal artery and surrounding venous plexus are coagulated and divided near the artery's exit from the foramen spinosum, a piece of bone wax is used to cover the foramen spinosum. The greater superficial petrosal nerve (GSPN) lies in the major petrosal groove of the middle fossa floor and is covered by a thin layer of periosteum, dura is elevated in posterior to anterior manner to avoid traction on the GSPN, which may result in facial nerve compromise. The next key landmark is to expose the arcuate eminence. The entire length of the IAC is exposed.

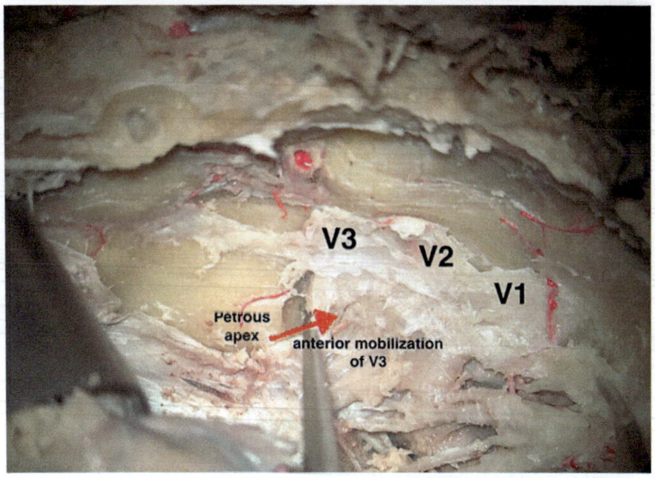

Fig. 18.3 Anterior mobilization of V3 enlarges the windows for drilling of petrous apex (RED arrow)

18.4.7 Removal of Anterior Clinoid Process

After peeling the lateral wall of the CS, the ACP removal can be performed. It is helpful to first locate the exit point of the nerve from the optic canal, and it is easier especially when lateral orbidotomy has been performed. Drilling should be directed over the superior and lateral aspects of the optic canal first with copious irrigation, which does not extend medially over the optic nerve to prevent risks of entering the spheno-ethmoidal air cells with subsequent CSF rhinorrhea. If the sinus is opened, it must be carefully packed with either muscle or fat. The anterior clinoid process is next removed on the lateral side of the optic canal. Optimal technique is critical because the anterior clinoid process is surrounded by the optic nerve, ICA, and contents of the superior orbital fissure. The ACP is gradually hollowed out with the diamond drill, thinned to the point at which the sides can be lightly fractured and dissected free from the dura. The very tip of the anterior clinoid is usually removed with the aid of small clinoid ronguer, with the small curved tip we can gently twisted free after careful dural dissection. Some venous bleeding may counter as it is the opening to the anterior cavernous sinus compartment [7], which could easily be controlled by some Surgicel or fibrin glue material.

18.4.8 Removal of Petrous Apex

It is also called anterior transpetrosal or Kawase approach [8], and it is a narrow corridor providing limited access to the postero-inferior triangle and region surrounding the porus trigeminus. The major obstacle hindering drilling of petrous apex [9] is the trigeminal nerve; hence, adequate subtemporal extradural peeling together with anterior migration of V3 segment is the key for adequate anterior petrosectomy. To identify the rhomboid shaped Kawase triangle [8], it is crucial to identify firstly the GSPN on the lateral side, the arcuate eminence on the posterior side, then the petrous ridge on the medial side, and finally the V3 segment after anterior migration (Fig. 18.3) as described above [10]. One point to add is that the petrous ridge harbors the superior petrosal sinus, and excessive tentorial split may venture into sinus causing venous bleeding, coring out of the petrous apex followed by early identification of petrous ICA to avoid inadvertent injury. After that, the pre- and post-meatal triangle bone should be drilled to achieve 270-degree exposure of IAC [11]. Care must be taken not to injure the cochlear and superior semicircular canal, which may result in permanent hearing loss. The concept of petrous apex drilling is similar to anterior clinoidectomy, with the principle of coring out followed by circumferential dissection, and the lower limit for anterior petrosectomy is reaching the posterior fossa dura and the inferior petroal sinus, while the anterior limit is reaching the clival bone and Dorello's canal. Adequate petrosectomy is the key to extend the operative window when the tumor or dural tail extends across the midline at clival dura.

18.4.9 Skull Base Triangle

Among the many triangles in the cavernous sinus region [6], there are several that are more clinically important. First is the anterior triangle, which is exposed after anterior clinoidectomy; it helps us to identify the C3 carotid segment that enters this space by piercing the carotico-oculomotor membrane. It is useful for identifying the clinoid ICA segment.

Lateral triangle is also called Parkinson triangle, and it is a very narrow space in normal individual, but for true cavernous sinus tumor, this window is enlarged as the trochlear nerve is pushed upward.

Glasscock described the posterolateral triangle, and it helps to define the horizontal intrapetrous carotid artery, which is important in case of bypass surgery.

Kawase first described this posteromedial triangle [12], and this volume of bone that can be removed to make a window in the petrous apex to the posterior fossa. If this triangle is drilled, the anterior brain stem [13] and root of the trigeminal nerve can be reached without encountering neural or vascular structures in the bone.

Pre- and post-meatal triangle is used to help defining the location of the cochlea from the middle fossa angle of view. In order to achieve 270° of IAC exposure, the bone over these two triangles has to be drilled out.

18.4.10 Dura Opening and Tentorial Cut

With the bone dissection complete, we use multiple tack-up sutures on the dura over the temporal lobe to maintain the surgical field. The dura is opened at the porus trigeminus above the superior petrosal sinus. This incision is carried laterally as far as the arcuate eminence and exposes the superior surface of the tentorium. A parallel incision is then made inferior to the superior petrosal sinus [14]. The superior petrosal sinus is either coagulated or ligated and divided at its medial aspect [15]. The temporal lobe is retracted more superiorly under protection (Fig. 18.4a). The tentorium can be cut after identifying the CN 4 and go posterior to its dural entrance [16]. The trigeminal root is also liberated from its dural attachment at the porus trigeminus; with this maneuver, a corridor to the posterior cavernous sinus and the entrance of CN VI into Dorello's canal can be traced.

In situation where the tumor involves anterior cavernous sinus or extend to the parasellar region [17], another dural cut from the ACP tip, the durotomy extends toward the frontal side, joining the temporal dural cut. In the intradural part, the Sylvian fissures can be split at the proximal end, hence mobilizing the ICA and CN II by cutting the distal dural ring and the falciform ligament, achieving a half-and-half Hakuba approach.

18.4.11 Tumor Resection

Once the exposure is completed and well prepared, the time needed for tumor resection is usually shorter. For tumor involving the Meckel's cave [18], during the splitting of cavernous sinus wall, tumor might already be seen inside, and usually, there is a nice plane separating majority of the V3 nerve rootlets with CSF released from the Gasserian ganglion.

For tumor where the attachment is mostly over the tentorium, early cutting of the involved tentorium makes the whole procedure easier, find the posterior limit of tumor by elevating the temporal lobe gently above the tentorium, early detachment, and devascularization from the tentorial blood supply, and the remaining part usually has a good arachnoid layer separating from the cerebellar superior surface, brain stem surface, and the cranial nerves. Early opening of posterior fossa dura from the tentorium downward toward IPS to find the lower edge and tumor can be sucked easily by suction and ultrasonic aspirator, at the end the CN 6 at the cisternal segment can be identified.

Biggest challenge is still the petroclival meningioma where the dural attachment might cross to the midline to the contralateral side with extensive brainstem compression.

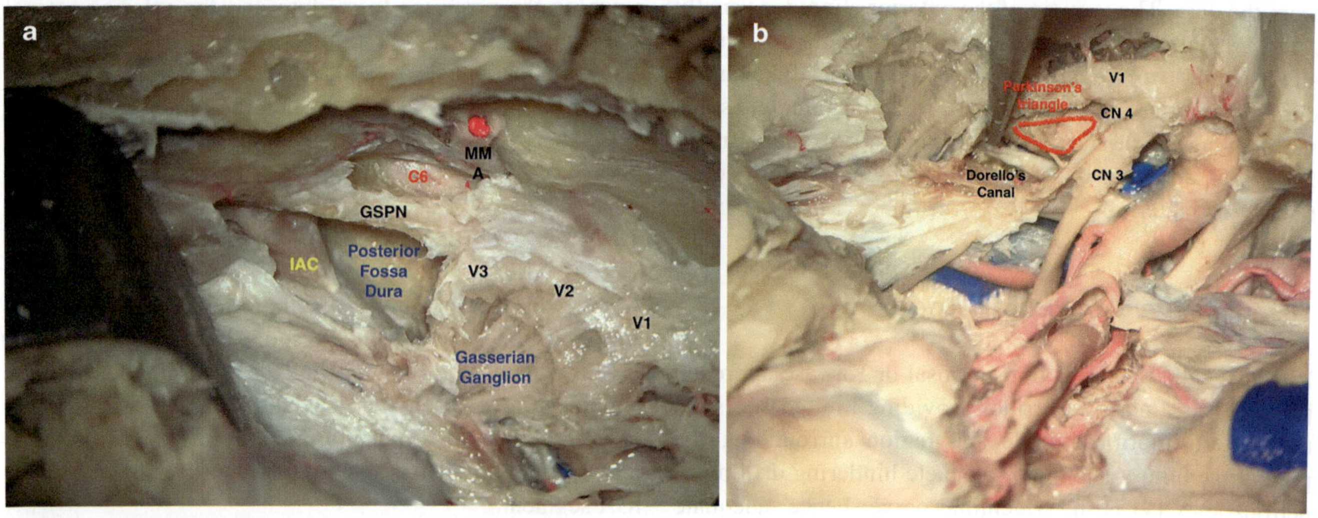

Fig. 18.4 (**a**) Dural opening includes temporal base, posterior fossa dura and medial tentorial cut with ligation of superior petroasal sinus. (**b**) Free mobilization of CN 5 with working window between CN 4 and CN 6

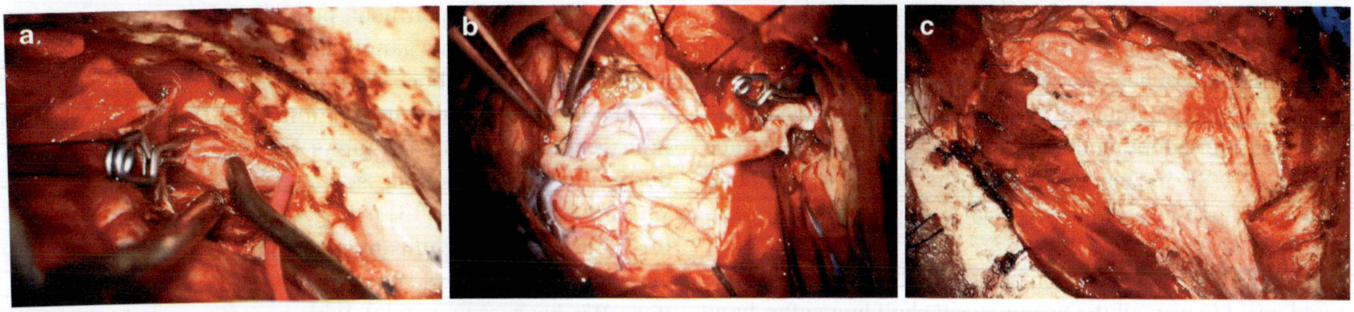

Fig. 18.5 (**a**) Intrapetrous exposure with proximal control by inflated balloon and distal control by a curved aneurysm clip. (**b**) Petrous ICA and supraclinoid ICA Bypass for Cavernous ICA mycotic aneurysm. (**c**) Pericranium with superficial temporalis fascia for dural closure

The CN 5 needs to be mobilized and retracted inferiorly, while the remaining tentorial sleeve together with the CN 4 is also gently retracted superiorly. The window between the CN 4 and CN 5 provides an angle of attack for clival lesion (Fig. 18.4b), the only cranial nerves in between is the CN 6 entering the Dorello's canal, as long as the drilling of petrous apex is adequate, line of vision could be in parallel to the clival angle. Dural attachment of meningioma can be removed safely in that case. As mentioned before, in case of pial invasion, dissection of tumor from brain stem surface may create damage to tiny pontine perforator, and it is not recommended. Adequate brain stem decompression is not a bad choice compared to brain stem injury.

In case the tumor has involved parasellar region [19], it is wise to open the fronto-temporal dura and early identification of ICA and CN 3 via Sylvian fissure opening. The CN 3 is easily identified before entering the oculomotor triangle [14] at the fronto-temporal side rather than from below the tentorium. Again, the tumor extending to the parasellar region is usually removable by gentle suction with preservation of arachnoid plane.

After gross total tumor excision, hemostasis in general can be achieved by gentle packing and seldom required aggressive bipolar coagulation.

18.4.12 Wound Closure

The dura is closed by running suture over the temporal side, and the dural defect at the skull base is repaired with the harvested pericranial flap, anchoring over the dural remnant at the peri-orbita, lateral wall of cavernous sinus, and posterior fossa dura. It is further reinforced with artificial dura, fat graft, and fibrin glues in a sandwich fashion (Fig. 18.5c). The bone flap is placed back and augmented by bone cement. The temporalis muscle is sutured back to the muscle cuff left on the bone flap, and the fractured zygoma is secured in place with screws and plates. Exudrain is placed for free drainage 1–2 days. The skin flap is then closed in standard fashion.

18.4.13 Skull Base Carotid Bypass Procedures

The GSPN in most of the case has to be sectioned and reflected lateral for exposure needs. The carotid is exposed in the posterolateral triangle from V3 to the tensor tympani muscle (Fig. 18.5a). To expose the intracavernous carotid artery [20], it is necessary to open the outer cavernous membrane between the trigeminal ganglion and the posterolateral fibrous ring surrounding the carotid's entrance to the cavernous sinus at the foramen lacerum.

For bypass surgery in this area, one of the biggest challenge after adequate exposure is to achieve proximal and distal control. First of all, we have to anticipate the extra length of the aneurysm clip, and to achieve maximal clipping force, the tips of the aneurysm clip after closing will be hitting on the bone, which means extra bone drilling deeper than the carotid artery has to be done in order to accommodate the tips of aneurysm clips. The petrous ICA has a quite robust connective tissue wall protection and is not as fragile as intradural ICA; this will give us some confidence in doing bone drilling near petrous ICA. We would suggest to use two curved clip to slide into the vertical petrous carotid segment and the intracavernous segment (Fig. 18.5b). Another option for achieving proximal control is by endovascular means using balloon inflation, of course that would involve an extra endovascular procedure.

18.5 Outcomes and Complications

After all skull base tumor is a challenging entity even for experienced neurosurgeons, the chance of having complication is high in general, be it reversible or permanent [21]. That is why always set the goal of surgery and remember not to create additional neurological problem to the patients.

It is difficult to compare the recurrence and regrowth rates in the published series due to variation in the follow-up duration and the definition of the degree of resection. Recurrence rate depends on location, cavernous sinus involvement, brainstem infiltration, grade of resection, and histopathologic result. In general, for meningioma over petroclival region, the recurrence rate ranges from 0 to 42%.

Brain retraction injury over temporal lobe was not uncommon, but after adopting the use of transzygomatic route and release of CSF by inserting EVD, the degree of temporal edema is much less. Anticonvulsant for covering perioperative period is recommended.

CSF leakage is another challenge, and the first thing we could avoid is wax all the pneumatized skull bone after bone drilling, second is to prepare a long pericranium and fascia pedicle during wound opening, and thirdly together with the use of fat graft and dural substitute in a sandwich fashion, CSF leakage can be prevented. In the early postoperative period, we do see pseudomeningocele formation, but as long as it is not under tension, not leaking and clinically the patient is aseptic, it might improve spontaneously within few weeks. If infection is suspected, we can perform lumbar drainage or even direct tapping of pseudomeningocele for fluid culture.

Cranial nerves palsies are one of the biggest determining factor if the surgery is successful or not [22]. Third nerve palsy is uncommon for petroclival region, but if it could happen during peeling of cavernous sinus, coagulation of bleeding on the lateral wall of CS, or at the cisternal segment when some tumor extended to the oculomotor cistern [14]. Third nerve palsy would cause complete ptosis and significant diplopia, and the end result is very disabling and should always be cautious when near the course of third nerve. Trochlear nerve is the thinnest cranial nerves, and its long course including the portion entering the tentorium makes it vulnerable for petroclival lesion. Most of the time, the CN 4 can be preserved during tentorial cutting; however, at the point where it enters the tentorium and adherent to the main tumor bulk, it is very easy to have it damaged. Fortunately, the deficit and impact on daily life for a patient with CN 4 palsy is relatively less than other cranial nerves.

Facial numbness is another common complaint, it could be due to the tumor direct invasion to the Gasserian ganglion, but I could also be due to the opening of porus trigeminus and mobilization of the trigeminal complex during dissection. At the most medial part of the CN 5, you can identify the Dorello's canal. The abducens nerve travels from the lower brain stem up and makes a sharp turn into the Dorello's canal; in case of petroclival tumor crossing the midline, the dissection or coagulation of the dural tail attachment makes CN 6 vulnerable.

From this approach, mostly, the petroclival lesion pushes the CN 7/8 complex postero-inferiorly, majority of cases we might not actually see the CN 7/8 complex even after tumor excision, but careful dissection is also recommended when removing the portion of tumor at the posterior fossa, because it might be adherent to the CN 7/8 nerve or its blood supply from anterior inferior cerebellar artery. Another reason in case of hearing impairment postoperatively is the direct injury to the geniculate ganglion or cochlear during temporal dural dissection and bone drilling.

The most dreadful complication includes major vascular injury especially when the tumor invades the pial layer, and during tumor dissection, some tiny branches from the verterobasilar system [13] may get avulsed accidentally, and this could cause significant arterial bleeding and difficult hemostasis in a narrow space in the middle of tumor dissection. We have seen patient with posterior cerebral artery injury at the level of ambient cistern causing PCA infarct, another patient with bleeding from an avulsed parapontine artery, both patients ended up in major neurological disability.

Another concern in long term is cosmetic, and the temporal hollow secondary to bone drilling and temporalis atrophy is quite disfiguring especially for young ladies. We would suggest the use of bone cement to fill the pterion part to alleviate the cosmetic concern and psychological burden.

18.6 Discussion

There are many skull base approaches, but how to choose the best one depends on many factors. Patient's chief complaint is the first thing into consideration, for example, for facial numbness or neuropathic pain secondary to trigeminal nerve compression, the aim of surgery is to adequately decompress the Meckel's cave. On the other hand, if the clinical picture is due to long tract sign secondary to brain stem compression, then the goal of surgery is to achieve brainstem compression. As stated above, detailed neuroradiological evaluation of the tumor characteristics could avoid many potential complication, in particular pay attention to the tumor epicenter, and any involvement of optic canal, cavernous sinus, Meckel's cave, posterior fossa, and IAC will all make your strategy a bit different.

In our series, for skull base lesion over dominant hemisphere, we prefer the removal of zygoma to enhance temporal base exposure and insertion, of external ventricular drainage can further minimize the chance of temporal retraction injury. One thing important is the temporal venous drainage pattern [1] rarely, but it does happen the whole temporal venous [2] drainage is heavily dependent on the spheno-parietal sinus, and this group of patients has high chance of venous infarction if the venous plexus is jeopardized during peeling of cavernous sinus wall.

The knowledge of skull base triangles become useful when we start the elevation of dural propria, careful gentle splitting of the two layers, anticipation of venous channel, and control with gentle packing or fibrin glue keep the operative clean. Identify the key skull base triangles and protect the important cranial nerves, and after judicious temporal elevation, the bone drilling of anterior clinoid process and petrous apex is straightforward, avoiding cracking the ACP or PA in big piece; rather, we should hollow out the core and dissect it from the attaching dura to avoid injury to the underlying neurovascular structures.

Dural opening and tentorial cut are the final key steps for the whole middle cranial fossa exposure; from our experience, the dural opening can be classified into the temporal side above the superior petrosal sinus; the posterior fossa side below the superior petrosal sinus and in between the two is the tentorial splitting. The aim is to elevate the temporal lobe, make a wide cut of tentorium behind the CN 4 tentorial entrance, and mobilize the CN 5 to create a wide window between CN 4/5 in tackling the petroclival region.

Tumor removal is mostly done by gentle suction and preservation of existing intact arachnoid layer as much as possible; those adherent tumor over brain stem should be left behind for fear of permanent neurological damage.

18.7 Conclusions

There is nothing more gratifying than the successful removal of a complex skull base lesion with a subsequent perfect functional recovery for a neurosurgeon. The goal of surgical resection should be avoidance of permanent neurological dysfunction with maximum tumor removal. The art is simultaneously aggressive and judicious. Detailed studying of the pre-operative images to know your enemy, good rapport with the patient and family with full understanding of the treatment goal, and endless hours of practice to excel your operative skills are all necessary to make a good skull base neurosurgeon. Incomplete excision is not necessarily a failure, and for some tumors, brain stem decompression after subtotal resection is the most appropriate course of action. Residual tumors can be successfully followed or treated with other means. As the old saying goes, your patients give you experience, and they are your best teacher. Train hard, being caring, and empathic to your patients will drive you a better skull base neurosurgeon.

References

1. Guppy KH, Origitano TC, Reichman OH, Segal S. Venous drainage of the inferolateral temporal lobe in relationship to transtemporal/transtentorial approaches to the cranial base. Neurosurgery. 1997;41:615–20.
2. Hayashi N, Sato H, Tsuboi Y, Nagai S, Kuwayama N, Endo S. Consequences of preoperative evaluation of patterns of drainage of the cavernous sinus in patients treated using anterior transpetrosal approach. Neurol Med Chir (Tokyo). 2010;50:373–7.
3. Transzygomatic extended middle fossa approach for upper petroclival skull base lesions Neurosurgical Focus. 2008;25(6). https://doi.org/E5-10.3171/FOC.2008.25.12.E5.
4. Yasargil MG, Reichman MV, Kubik S. Preservation of the frontotemporal branch of the facial nerve using the interfascial temporalis flap for pterional craniotomy. Technical article. J Neurosurg. 1987;67:463–6.
5. Yoshida K, Kawase T. Zygomatic transpetrosal approach for Dumbbell-shaped parasellar and posterior fossa chordoma. Oper Tech Neurosurg. 2002;5(June):104–7.
6. Kawase T, van Loveren H, Keller JT, Tew JM. Meningeal architecture of the cavernous sinus: clinical and surgical implications. Neurosurgery. 1996;39:527–34.
7. Dolenc VV. A combined epi- and subdural direct approach to carotid-ophthalmic artery aneurysm. J Neurosurg. 1985;62:667–72.
8. Aziz KM, Tew JM Jr, Chicoine MR. The Kawase approach to retrosellar and upper clival basilar aneurysm. Neurosurgery. 1999;44:1225–36.
9. Altieri R, Zenga F. Detailed anatomy knowledge: first step to approach petroclival meningiomas through the petrous apex. Anatomy lab experience and surgical series. Neurosurg Rev. 2017;40:231–9.
10. Yasuda A, Campero A, Martins C, Rhoton AL, de Oliveira E, Ribas GC. Microsurgical anatomy and approaches to the cavernous sinus. Neurosurgery 2008;62(6):SHC1240–63: https://doi.org/10.1227/01.NEU.0000333790.90972.59.
11. Aoyagi M, Ohno K. Combined extradural subtemporal and anterior transpetrosal approach to tumours located in the interpeduncular fossa and the upper clivus. Acta Neurochir (Wien). 2013;155:1401–7.
12. Tripathi M, Srivastav V. Quantitative analysis of the Kawase versus the modified Dolenc-Kawase approach for middle cranial fossa lesions with variable anteroposterior extension. J Neurosurg. 2015;123:14–22.
13. Krist AF, Kadri PA. Surgical clipping of complex basilar apex aneurysms: a strategy for successful outcome using the pretemporal transzygomatic transcavernous approach. Neurosurgery. 2005;56(2 Suppl):261–73.
14. Kawase T, Shiobara R, Toya S. Anterior transpetrosal-transtentorial approach for sphenopetroclival meningiomas: surgical method and results in 10 patients. Neurosurgery. 1991;28:869–76.
15. Hafez A, Nader R. Preservation of the superior petrosal sinus during the petrosal approach: technical note. J Neurosurg. 2011;114:1294.
16. Kusumi M, Friedman AH, Fujii K. Tentorial detachment technique in the combined petrosal approach for petroclival meningioma. J Neurosurg. 2012;116:566–73.
17. Krisht AF. Transcavernous approach to diseases of the anterior upper third of the posterior fossa. Neurosurg Focus. 2005;19(2):E2.
18. Liao C-H, Chen M-H. Pretemporal trans-Meckel's cave transtentorial approach for large petroclival meningiomas. Neurosurg Focus. 2018;44(4):E10.
19. Kobayashi M, Yoshida K, Kawase T. Inter-dural approach to parasellar tumours. Acta Neurochir (Wien). 2010;152:279–85.
20. Liu JK, Fukushima T, Sameshima T, Al-Mefty O, Couldwell WT. Increasing exposure of the petrous internal carotid artery for revascularization using the transzygomatic extended middle fossa approach: a cadaveric morphometric study. Neurosurgery. 2006;59:ONS309–18.
21. Siindou M, Wydh E, Jouanneau E, Nebbal M, Lieutaud T. Long-term follow-up of meningiomas of the cavernous sinus after surgical treatment alone. J Neurosurg. 2007;107:937–44.
22. Couldwell WT, Kan P, Liu JK, Apfelbaum RI. Decompression of cavernous sinus meningioma for preservation and improvement of cranial nerve function. Technical note. J Neurosurg. 2006;105:148–52.

Infratemporal Fossa and Orbital Apex

19

Kentaro Watanabe

Abstract

This chapter discusses the surgical treatment of diseases in the orbit, middle temporal fossa, cavernous sinus, and infratemporal fossa from an anatomical perspective, focusing on the superior orbital fissure and the orbital apex. The orbital apex is the area where the nerves enter the orbit converge and is adjacent to and connected to the cavernous sinus.

Based on anatomical evidence, this chapter shows how to safely approach this complex area, which includes the oculomotor nerve, trochlear nerve, trigeminal nerve, optic nerve, superior and inferior ophthalmic vein, and ophthalmic artery running from the cavernous sinus to the orbit. Variations in surgical reach were considered based on microanatomy, and their application to clinical cases was demonstrated. In addition, the safe removal of the middle cranial bone allows for an expanded approach to diseases that span both the cavernous sinus and the orbit.

Keywords

Orbital apex lesion · Transcranial approach · Orbital and cavernous sinus diseases · Infratemporal fossa

This chapter consists of four parts.

1. Surgical Anatomy
2. Types and manifestations of different pathologies
3. Approaches
4. Illustrative Case presentations

K. Watanabe (✉)
Department of Neurosurgery, Tokyo Jikei University School of Medicine, Tokyo, Japan
e-mail: k_wtnb0623@jikei.ac.jp

In the treatment of orbital apex, visual function is a special area that requires great attention because the visual function, eye movement, and cosmetic aspects are directly related to life. It requires an understanding of nerves, arteries, veins, muscles, and bone structures. It is very important to understand the microanatomy and choose a rational surgical method to remove the lesion and plan the treatment based on the tumor origin and microanatomy. The surgical timing is also delicate, and patients are often very discouraged by the loss of visual function, even if the loss of vision is after they already have a visual deficit before the treatment.

In addition, the utmost meticulousness is required during surgery because the optic nerve is a very weak part of the body, and even the slightest stimulation can cause loss of visual function. The release of the optic canal requires special training as it requires the removal of bone with a drill.

19.1 Surgical Anatomy of Orbit

The orbital function and microanatomy are complicated and sensitive because of the optic nerve fragility and the possibility of affection of binocular vision. These anatomical structures are related to the optic nerve and eye movements and visual functions. Visual function directly impacts our quality of life. The anatomy and structure of the orbit must be fully understood through cadaveric dissection training before surgery.

The most complex and concentrated structure is the orbital apex. The optic canal and the superior orbital fissure (SOF) cross and join into the orbital cavity. The optic nerve and ophthalmic artery run in the optic tract, and the cranial nerve (CN) III, IV, V, VI, and superior ophthalmic veins (SOV) run in the SOF. Within the orbital apex, there is a unique structure, the Annulus of Zinn, which is an integration in the fibrous ligaments of all straight ("recti") extraocular muscles.

T. L. POON et al. (eds.), *Orbital Apex and Periorbital Skull Base Diseases*, https://doi.org/10.1007/978-981-99-2989-4_19

Annulus of Zinn

Anterior to the optic canal and the medial aspect of the SOF, the periorbita thickens, creating the tendinous attachments of the four rectus muscles, the levator palpebrae superioris, and the superior oblique muscle, forming a tendinous ring known as the annulus of Zinn.

Periorbita

The periorbita, also playing the role of orbital periosteum, covers the orbital bone. This thin membrane of dense connective tissue membrane serves as an attachment site for muscles, tendons, and ligaments, a support structure for the blood supply to the orbital bones, and its preservation is important for the protection of orbital structures during surgery. Below it, the orbital cavity is filled with fat, which protects as a cushion the complex nerve and vascular structures. Once the periorbita is damaged even a little, orbital fat will tend to protrude. Thus, by protecting the periorbita integrity, it will be possible to prevent the protrusion of orbital contents.

19.1.1 Intraconal and Extraconal Structure

Within the common orbital compartment made by the orbital wall and the periorbita, there is another smaller compartment produced by the extraocular muscles attached posteriorly to the Zinn's ring and their fascias, having the shape of a conus (Fig. 19.1a). This partition of two compartments, one inside the other, allows the division of the pyramidal internal orbital space into two compartments, both reaching the orbital (pyramid's) apex as follows:

1. Intraconal compartment
2. Extraconal compartment

In each of these compartments can be found the following important structures:

Intraconal Area

Supero-medial foramen: optic nerve and ophthalmic artery

Superolateral foramen: superior and inferior branches of the oculomotor nerve, nasochiliary nerve, and abducens nerve

Extraconal Area

Superior part (entry from superior orbital fissure): lacrimal nerve, frontal nerve, trochlear nerve, superior orbital vein

Inferior part (entry from the inferior orbital fissure): inferior ophthalmic vein, infraorbital nerve, zygomatic nerve, infraorbital artery and vein, ganglionic branch from pterygopalatine ganglion

The osseous orbital apex is formed by the superior orbital fissure (SOF) and the optic canal. The optic canal is in the superomedial corner of the orbital apex, and its contents include the optic nerve and the ophthalmic artery. The optic nerve is separated from the SOF by an osseous structure called the optic strut.

The trochlear and frontal nerves locate outside the annulus of Zinn. The SOF is lateral to the optic canal.

The lateral portion of the SOF contains the trochlear, lacrimal, and frontal nerves, together with the superior orbital vein (SOV). Superior and medial to the SOF, the

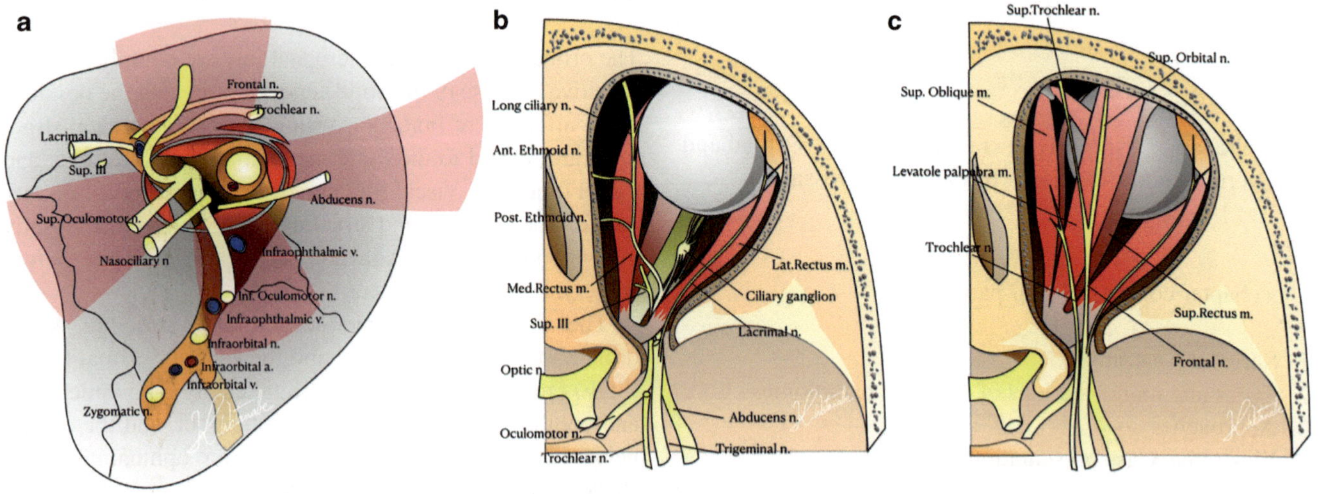

Fig. 19.1 An illustration of the orbit. (**a**) Anterior view of the right orbital apex showing the distribution of nerves as they enter through the superior orbital fissure and optic canal. This view also shows the annulus of Zinn, the fibrous ring formed by the common origin of the four rectus muscles. (**b**) Superior view of the orbit without the orbital roof. The optic nerve, the ciliary nerve, oculomotor nerve (superior and inferior branch), and abducens nerve run through the annulus of Zinn. (**c**) The frontal nerve, lacrimal nerve, and trochlear nerve run the outside of the annulus of Zinn

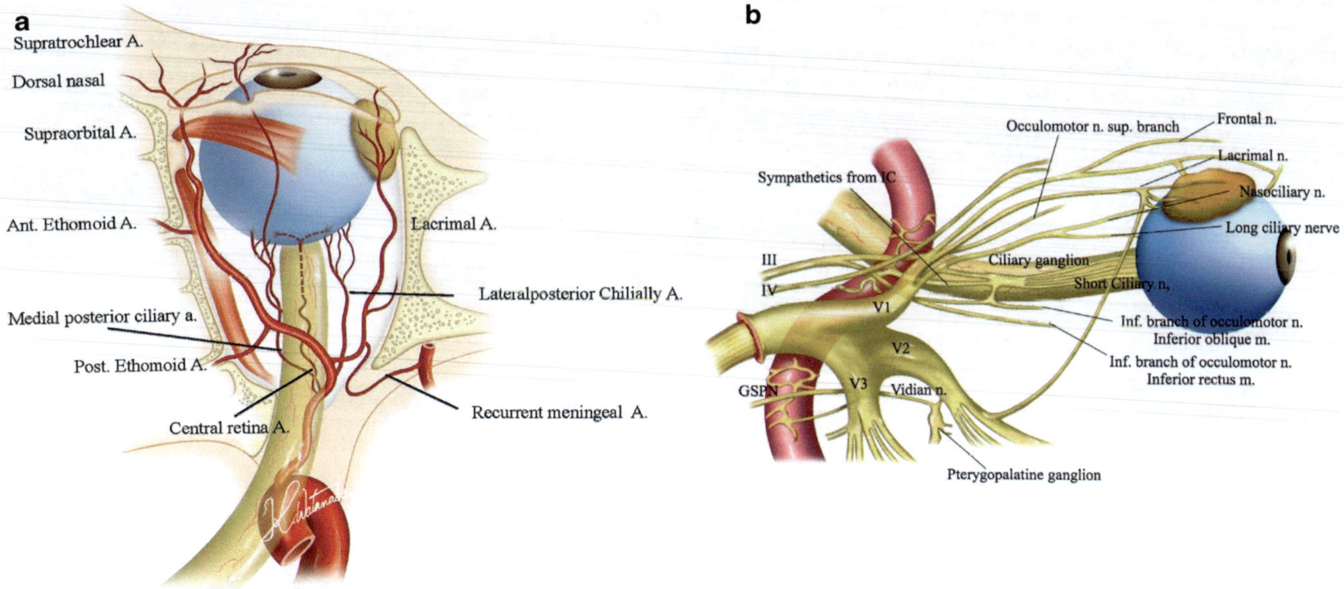

Fig. 19.2 Orbital arteries and nerves. (**a**) An illustration of arteries of the orbit. The central retina artery is the most important artery in the orbit. (**b**) An illustration of the orbital nerve connection. The inferior branch of the oculomotor nerve, the ciliary nerve from the trigeminal nerve and the sympathetic nerve are connected in the ciliary ganglion

annulus of Zinn contains the optic nerve and ophthalmic artery exiting from the optic foramen. The medial portion of the SOF contains the oculomotor, abducens, and the nasociliary nerves, the superior ophthalmic vein, and they are enclosed in the annulus of Zinn, the tendinous ring attaching four of the six extraocular muscles. The oculomotor nerve further anterior divides into two, the superior and inferior branches before entering the annulus of Zinn. After passing the annulus, two branches go to each muscle that they innervate (Fig. 19.1b, c).

There is a small ganglion in the orbit, which is the ciliary ganglion (Fig. 19.2b). A fine ramification from the inferior branch of the oculomotor nerve, a small branch from the ciliary nerve of the CN V, and a sympathetic branch supply the ciliary ganglion.

All V1 and V2 divisions of the trigeminal nerve, oculomotor, and trochlear nerves pass through the lateral wall of the cavernous sinus. CN VI passes through the sinus between the ICA and the lateral wall. The ICA and neighboring sympathetic fibers pass through the medial portion of the sinus. The greater petrosal nerve, which is the specialized sensory branch of the facial nerve, and the deep petrosal nerve, which is the sympathetic branch from the ICA, join to give the origin of the vidian nerve (Fig. 19.2b).

19.1.2 Arteries

The most important artery—the central retinal artery—is a small branch of the ophthalmic artery. This artery emerges on the eye fundus at the papilla after traveling with the optic nerve in the dural sheath. It provides arterial supply to the inner surface of the eye bulb wall. This artery supplies blood to the nerve fibers of the optic nerve, and when occluded, there will be a complete loss of vision, even though the fovea is not affected (Fig. 19.2a). Since this blood vessel originates from the ophthalmic artery near the orbital apex, great care must be taken when performing orbital apex surgery.

The other vessel to be considered in orbital apex surgery is the lacrimal artery. This vessel has an anastomosis with the anterior branch of the MMA and the inferior lateral trunk (ILT), so its relationship as a tumor-feeding vessel needs to be considered in meningioma surgery. The ethmoidal arteries also need to be cared for during transnasal endoscopic surgery.

19.1.3 Anterior Infratemporal Fossa and Lateral Orbital Wall

The infratemporal fossa can be exposed by an extradural approach. After temporal dura is exposed and retracted, it is penetrated between its periosteal and meningeal layers to reach the lateral wall of cavernous sinus. Next is removed the lateral wall of the orbit and periorbita exposed. The first branch of the trigeminal nerve that enters the SOF and the second entering the foramen rotundum (FR) are identified. SOF and FR walls and surrounding osseous structure have to be removed to have exposed the periorbital surface to the pterygopalatine fossa [1].

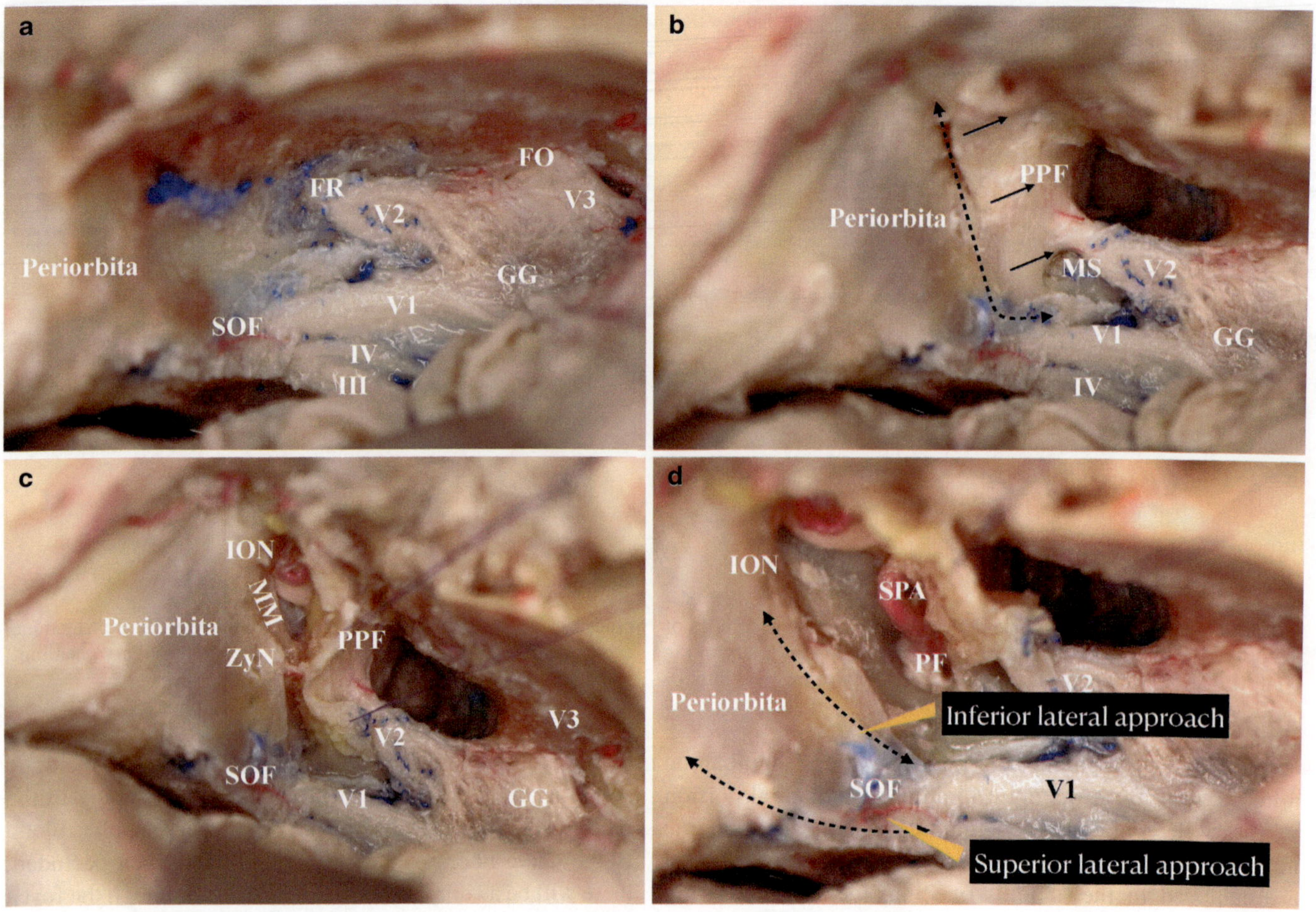

Fig. 19.3 Infratemporal fossa exposure and access route to the orbital apex. *IV* Trochlear nerve, *III* oculomotor nerve, *FO* foramen ovale, *FR* foramen rotundum, *FS* foramen spinosum, *GG* gasserian ganglion, *PPF* pterygopalatine fossa, *PF* pterygopalatine foramen, *SPA* sphenopalatine artery, *ION* inferior orbital nerve, *MS* maxillary strut, *SOF* superior orbital fissure, *V2* second branch of the trigeminal nerve, *V3* third branch of the trigeminal nerve, *VN* vidian nerve, *ZyN* zygomatic nerve. (**a**) The infratemporal fossa exposure in cadaveric dissection. The lateral wall of cavernous sinus is exposed. The orbital roof and lateral wall is removed and the foramen rotundum is unroofed toward the pterygopalatine fossa. (**b**) The pterygopalatine fossa is exposed. An incision is made between the orbit and pterygopalatine fossa. (**c**) Part of the pterygopalatine fossa is sectioned to allow the mobilization of the maxillary nerve together with the pterygopalatine fossa. (**d**) There are two corridors to access in the orbit. Inferior lateral approach and superior lateral approach are the safe entry zone to the orbital apex. *FO* foramen ovale, *FR* foramen rotundum, *SOF* superior orbital fissure, *IV* trcholar nerve, *III* oculomotor nerve, *ICA* internal carotid artery, *GG* Gasserian ganglion, *MS* maxillary strut, *PPF* pterygopalatine fossa, *SS* sphenoid sinus, *V1* ophthalmic nerve, *V2* maxillary nerve, *V3* mandibular nerve, *ZyN* zygomatico temporal nerve

After the trigeminal nerve peripheral V2 root was exposed, beyond it to the periorbita, there is a fat tissue pad containing the pterygopalatine ganglion in the so-called ptergopalatine fossa (PPF). There is a fine fiber structure between the PPF and periorbita called the Muller's muscle, and it can be incised. After cutting the zygomatic nerve (ZyN), the inferior border of the orbit can be exposed. Then, it is possible to access to the inferior parts of the orbital cavity and maxillary sinus and sphenoid sinus by moving the second branch of the trigeminal nerve posteriorly (Fig. 19.3a–d).

The anatomical view of the anterior infratemporal fossa. (a) The view of the lateral cavernous sinus wall. The trigeminal nerve is exposed, and the superior orbital fissure, foramen rotundum, and foramen ovale are shown. (b) Between the periorbita and the pterygopalatine fossa (PPF) is placed the incision line to expose the inferior aspect of the orbit. (c) The V2 is retracted posteriorly. The zygomatic nerve (ZyN) can be seen between the PPF and periorbita. (d) The two dotted lines are the incision lines to enter the orbital apex.

19.1.4 Symptoms and Syndromes

Syndromes associated with orbital apex include the Rochon-Duvigneaud syndrome (orbital apex syndrome) [2], Jacod syndrome (superior orbital fissure syndrome) [3], and cavernous sinus syndrome (cavernous sinus syndrome) [4]. However, with proper anatomical knowledge, it will be easy to understand the structural and functional effects of the different locations of lesions.

(a) Orbital apex syndrome
(b) Superior orbital fissure syndrome
(c) Cavernous sinus syndrome

These syndromes are reported as syndromes because of the concentration of nerves and blood vessels in the orbital apex, which the symptoms complex and specific. Because of the concentration of nerves and blood vessels in the orbital apex region, it is sometimes difficult to determine the origin of tumor development using MRI alone. Clinical diagnosis is also important to determine whether the tumor is intraconal or extraconal in origin. By considering the relationship between bones, ligaments, and nerves and the mechanism of tumor development, we can understand the symptoms.

19.2 Disease

Although there are some rare diseases, there are not so many tumors that we encounter as neurosurgeons [5].

In this chapter, some of the most common diseases are presented. In cases of benign tumors, if function is still present, the goal is to perform surgery that preserves function as much as possible. Opposite, for tumors that are benign but cannot be removed without functional deterioration, surgery will have a role when the patient has completely lost visual function. This needs to be discussed in depth, as it depends on the patient's perspective on function.

In the case of malignant tumors, the procedure of removal is completely different. If we aim for radical surgery, we need to consider the removal of the orbital area with an extent of removal to the cavernous sinus and the anterior part of the middle skull base with adequate tumor margin, even with the loss of function and anatomical structure.

Neoplasm, Inflammatory Disease, and Trauma

- Meningioma
- Spheno-orbital meningioma
- Optic sheath meningioma
- Schwannoma
- Orbital cavernous hemangioma
- Malignancy
- Metastasis
- Dermoid, epidermoid
- Fibrous dysplasia
- Lymphoma
- Lacrimal gland tumor

19.3 Approaches

1. Transcranial: for an intra-orbital lesion
   Frontotemporal approach
   Superior lateral approach
   Inferior lateral approach
   Medial approach
2. Transcranial: for an intra- and extra-orbital lesion
   Orbital and infratemporal fossa exposure
3. Endoscopic: orbital lesion
   Endoscopic: transnasal-trans-sphenoidal-trans-maxillary-trans-ethmoid approach

1. Transcranial Approach to the Orbit
   (a) Superolateral approach
   In case of a tumor located in area A (Fig. 19.4a), the approach is between the levator palpebrea muscle and the lateral rectus muscle. Trochlear and frontal nerves (V1) run medially, and lacrimal nerve runs laterally from V1 as showed in figure. After dissection of these structures, the orbital cavity can be entered. In case the tumor is in the SOF, care should be taken not to damage these nerves. Most fragile is the oculomotor nerve.
   (b) Inferior lateral approach
   In case of the tumor is located in the area C (Fig. 19.4a), it is possible to use the corridor between the lateral rectus and inferior rectus muscles. When the anterior infratemporal fossa is sufficiently exposed, the inferior border of the lateral rectus muscle can be identified. This approach is useful if the tumor is on the lateral inferior border; however, in practice, this approach is rarely used. In case of otolaryngological diseases such as maxillary sinus malignant pathology, the surgeon should be aware of the specific anatomical landmarks.
   (c) Medial approach
   The medial approach is inevitably difficult as an approach due to the limited access (Fig. 19.4b). At the orbital apex, the medial approach is the least structured route for access to the optic nerve. In case of sacrificing the optic nerve, such as in optic glioma cases, proximal optic nerve ligation can be performed in this approach. The annulus of Zinn can be opened between the superior rectus muscle and superior oblique muscle. Only the trochlear nerve should be divided before access to the orbital apex.
2. Transcranial Intra and Extraorbital Lesion
   Diseases of the lateral orbital wall and periorbital region often progress to the anterior infratemporal fossa. In case

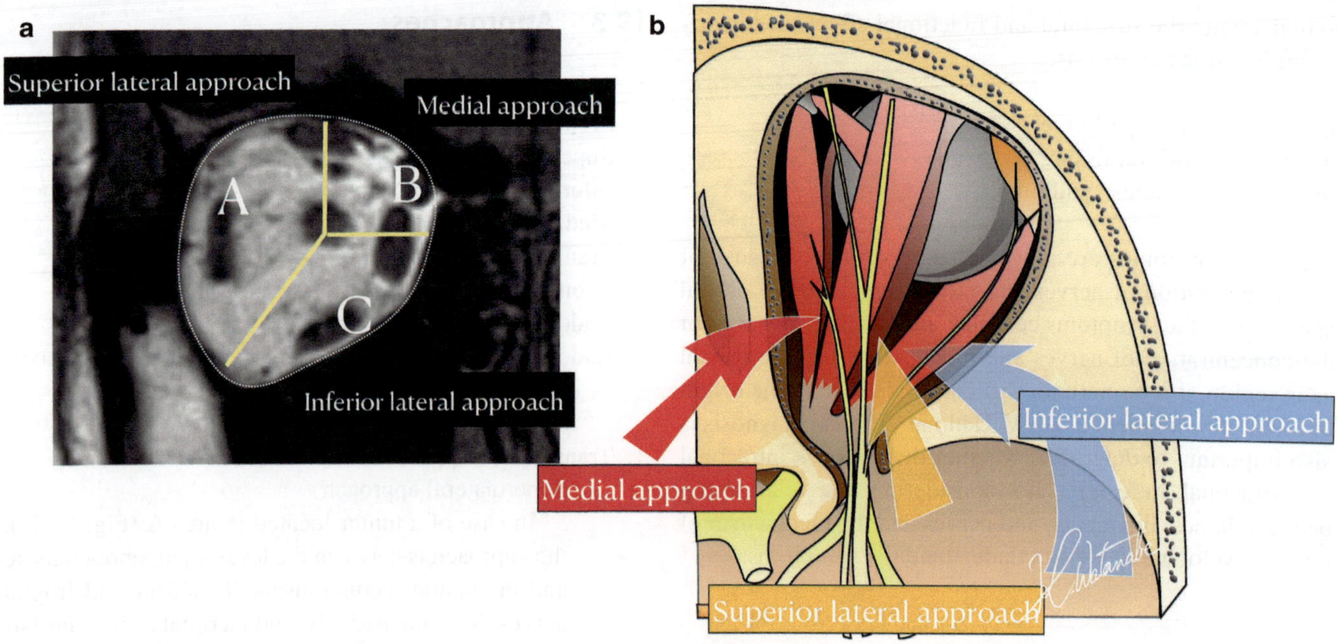

Fig. 19.4 Three approaches to the orbital lesion. (**a**) Three areas of the orbital lesion. Area A is able to approached via superior lateral approach. Area B is able to approach via medial approach. Area C is able to approach via infra lateral approach. (**b**) The schema of the three approach corridors

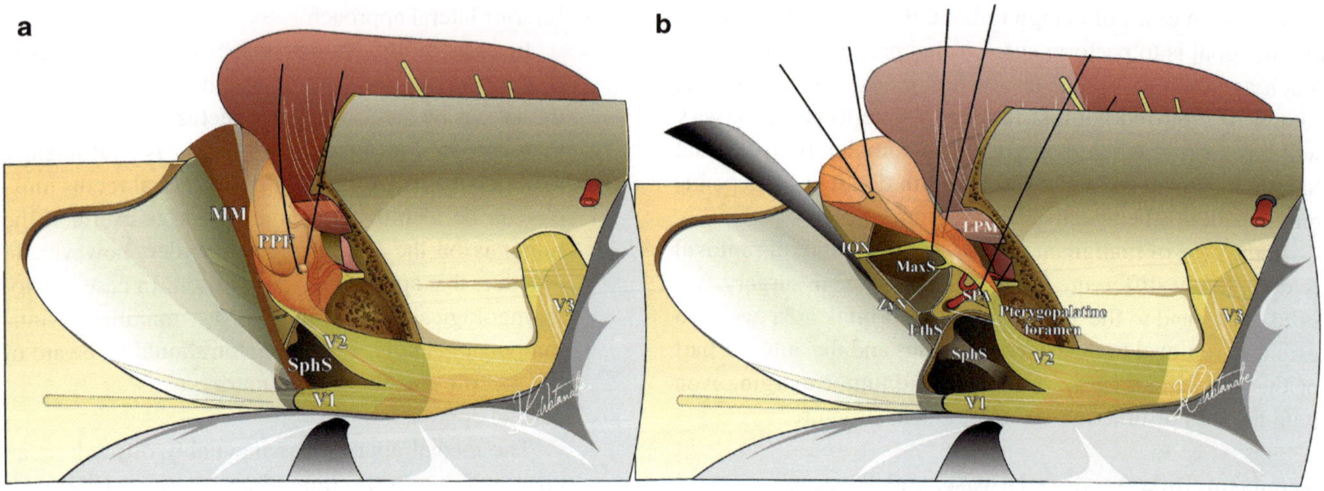

Fig. 19.5 Orbital and infratemporal fossa exposure. *ION* inferior orbital nerve, *LPM* inferior head of lateral pterygoid muscle, *MM* Muller muscle, *MPM* medial pterygoid muscle, *MaxS* maxillary sinus, *PPF* pterygopalatine fossa, *SphS* sphenoid sinus, *V1* ophthalmic nerve, *V2* maxillary nerve, *V3* mandibular branch, *ZyN* zygomatic nerve. (**a**) The schema of the anterior infra temporal fossa exposure. Pterygopalatine fossa is translocated laterally and the sphenoid sinus is opened between the V1 and V2. (**b**) TheV2 branch is translocated laterally and exposing the maxillary sinus, ethmoid sinus and sphenoid sinus through the V1 and V2 corridor

the tumor extends to the orbit and cavernous sinus and/or pterygopalatine fossa, the extradural transcranial infratemporal fossa approach is appropriate (Fig. 19.5a and b). Furthermore, sphenoid sinus, maxillary sinus, and ethmoid sinus are also accessible by extradural approach. This is a very useful approach in otolaryngology and is the region providing access to the middle cranial fossa through the sinuses.

(d) Endoscopic Transnasal Approach

The nasal endoscopic technique also allows a less invasive approach to the orbit. The inferior wall of the orbit and the orbital apex is accessible through the ethmoid, sphenoid, and maxillary sinuses. By opening the paranasal sinuses, the medial or inferior orbital walls can be reached, and optic canal decompression can be performed [6].

19.4 Clinical Cases

19.4.1 Sphenoorbital Meningioma

Sphenoid or spheno-orbital meningiomas are supplied by the MMA, lacrimal artery, recurrent meningeal artery, and ILT. If the meningioma is fed by anastomotic vessels of the MMA and the lacrimal artery through a recurrent meningeal artery or a lacrimal meningeal artery, there is a possibility for the orbital wall and roof to be thickened.

If the recurrent meningeal artery is the feeding vessel, the anterior clinoid process may also be thickened in continuity with the thickening of the orbital wall. In cases of severe bony hyperplasia of the orbital wall, it should be noted that the periorbita within the orbit may also be tumorigenic (Fig. 19.6a–d).

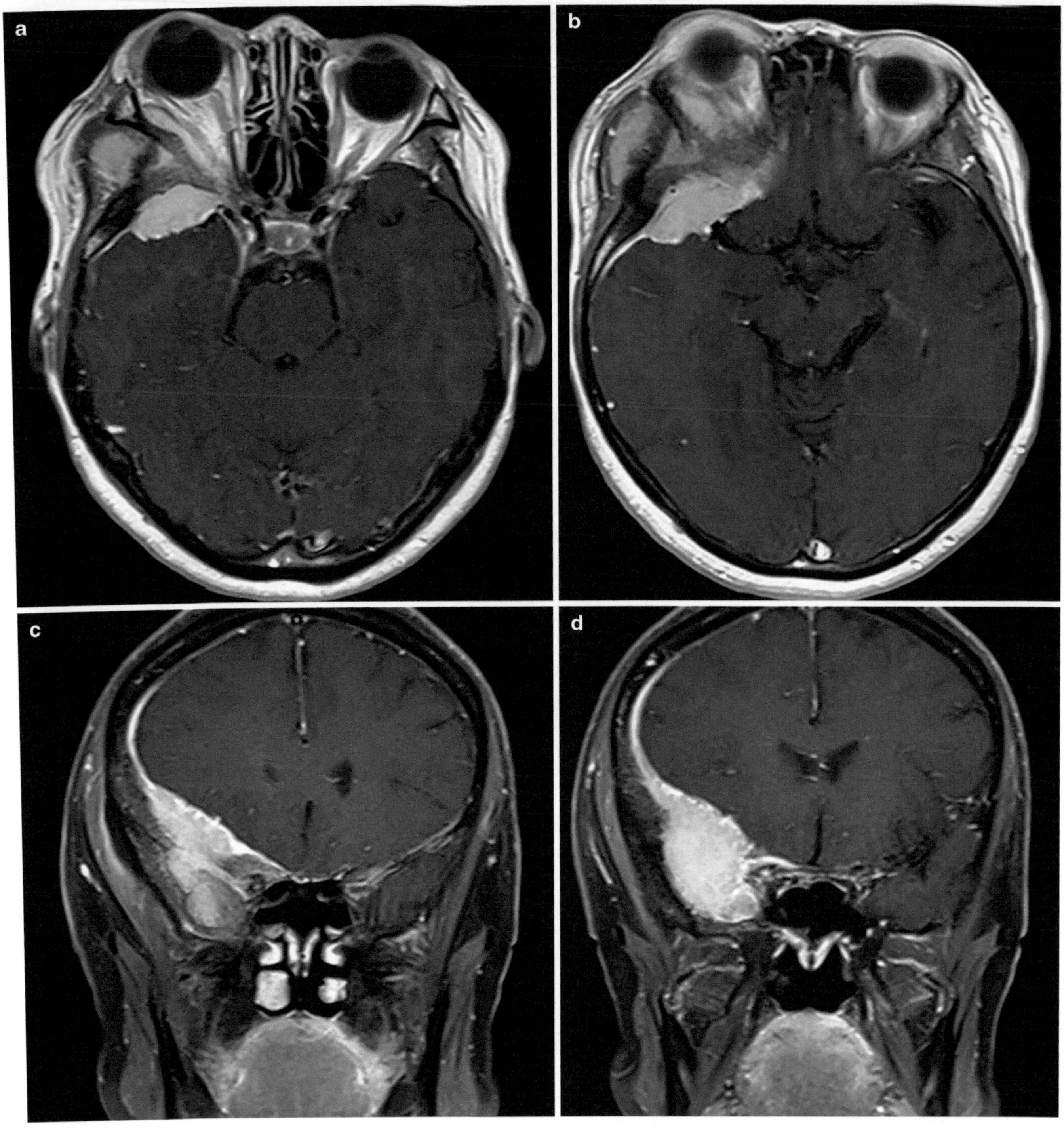

Fig. 19.6 MRI image of sphenoorbital meningioma clinical case. (**a**, **b**) Gadolinium enhanced MRI axial image show the enhanced mass lesion in the right sphenoid wing. The tumor invaded in the lateral and superior wall of the orbit, temporal and frontal dura mater, and medial aspect of temporal muscle. (**c**, **d**) Gadolinium enhanced MRI coronal image shows the mass lesion invades in the sphenoid wing

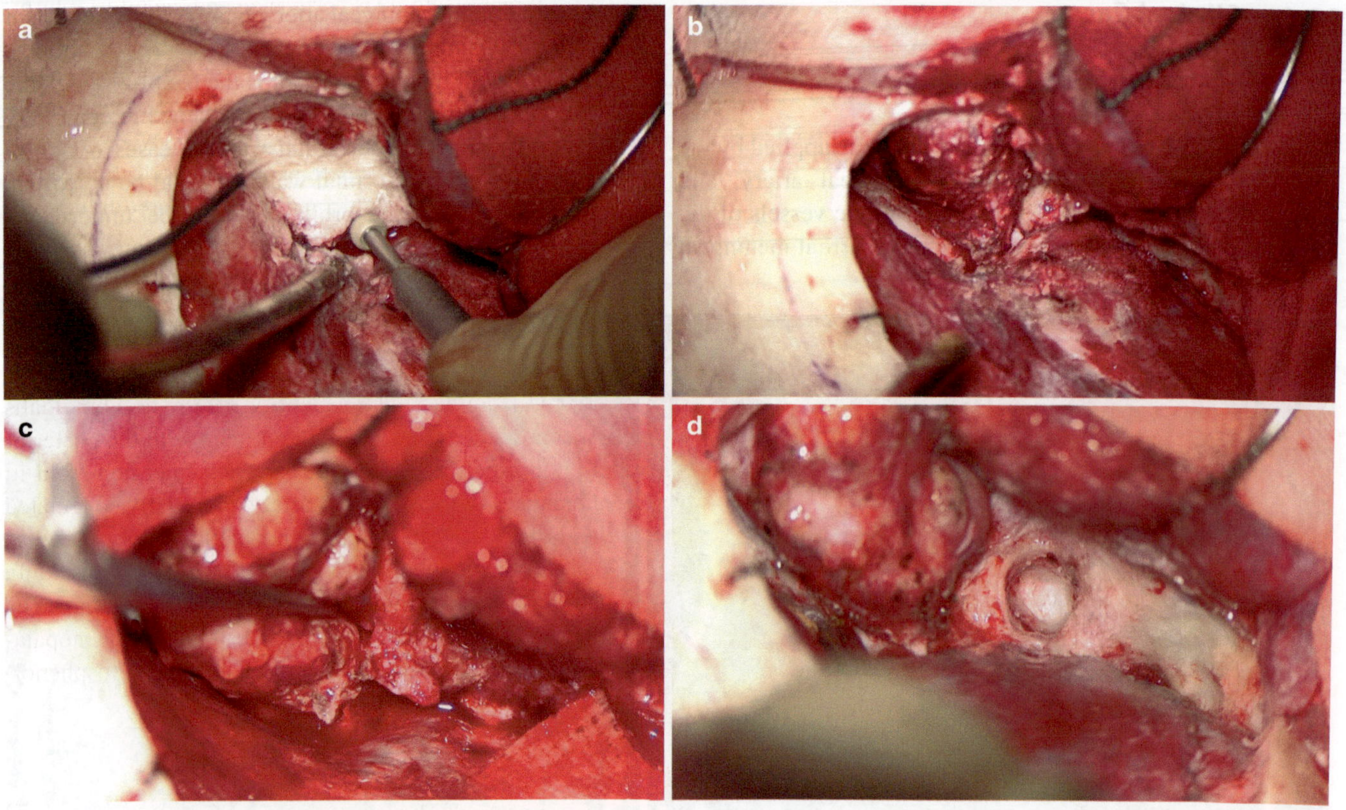

Fig. 19.7 Intraoperative image of sphenoorbital meningioma clinical case. (**a**) Removal of the thickened orbital roof. (**b**) Exposing the invaded meningioma on the periorbita. (**c**) After removing the periorbital meningioma. (**d**) Removal of the anterior infratemporal fossa bone. The peripheral branches of the trigeminal nerve are exposed

Periorbital meningiomas should be removed well with the periorbita until exposing fat; otherwise, recurrence rate would be high. The ligamentous tissue of the Annuls of Zinn has not been observed to be the origin of meningiomas; thus, it is not necessary to cut the ligament to release it. However, if the tumor invades into the optic canal with optic nerve compression, the optic canal needs a bony decompression followed by dural incision over the nerve (Fig. 19.7a–d).

19.5 Schwannoma

Orbital schwannoma is often located in the superior or medial superior aspect of the orbit. Orbital schwannomas most commonly arise from the supraorbital or supratrochlear branch of the trigeminal nerve [7]. In schwannomas presenting with orbital pain, exophthalmos, and visual deficit, surgical treatment is indicated.

There are two surgical options: transnasal endoscopic or transcranial open tumor removals. Orbital apex tumors that affect the optic nerve need removal, even if they are small. The choice of surgical approach depends on tumor location. For tumors located in the medial parts of the orbit, the transnasal endoscopic approach can be recommended. When the tumor locates in the superior parts of the orbit, the extradural fronto-temporal transcranial approach is appropriate. Since schwannomas rarely arise from motor nerves responsible for eye movements, the safe way to remove a tumor is to perform internal decompression of the tumor. Because the surrounding fine nerves, such as the ciliary nerve may be involved, great care must be taken during surgery at its entry to the orbit.

19.6 Orbital Cavernous Hemangioma

Cavernous hemangiomas are the most common vascular lesions of the orbit in adults and account for 5–7% of all orbital tumors. Nowadays, stereotactic radiosurgery (SRS) might be effective and safe.

In cases where they are symptomatic, or growth of the lesion is demonstrated on follow-up imaging, surgical

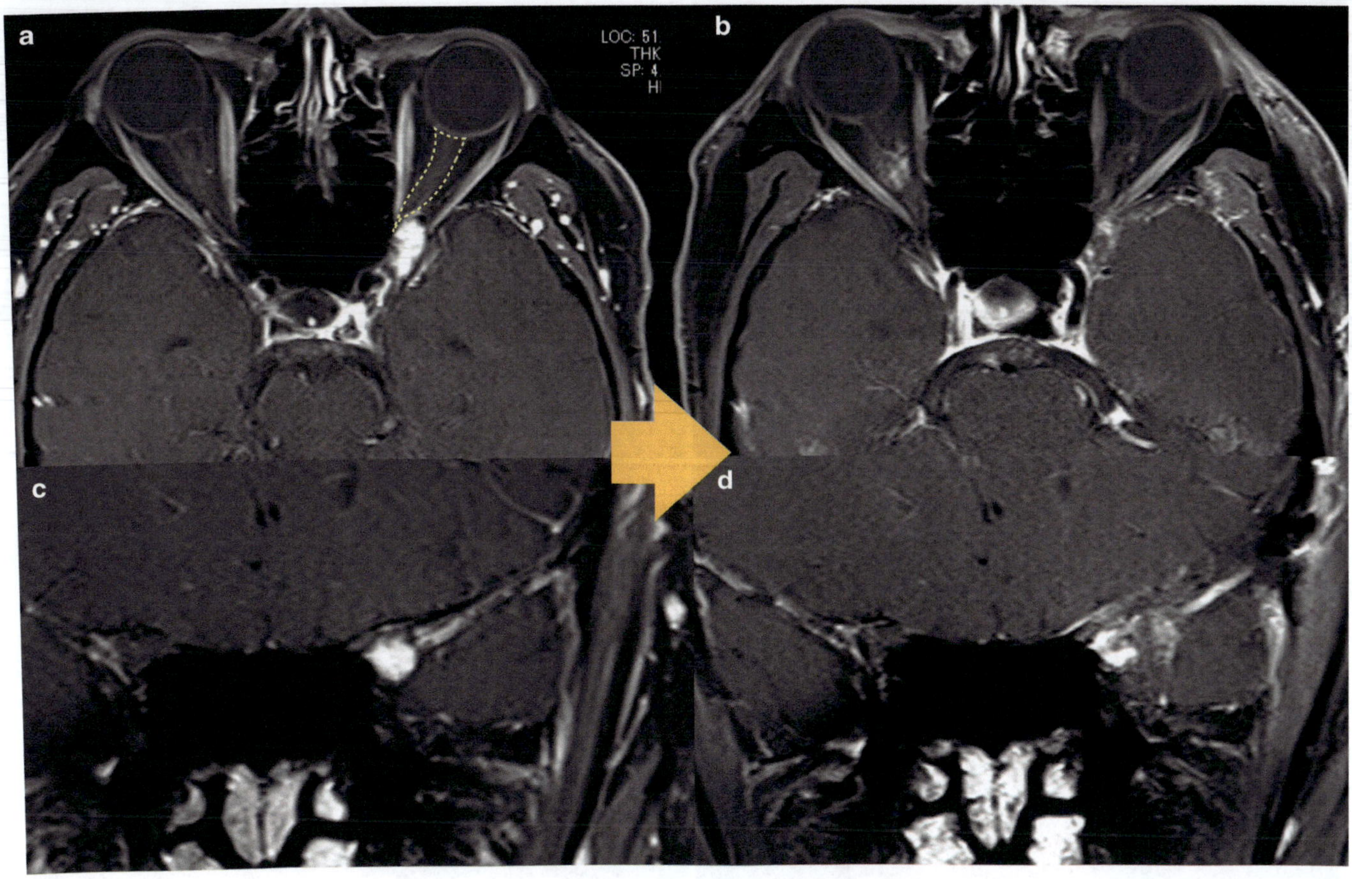

Fig. 19.8 Clinical case of cavernous hemangioma in the superior orbital fissure. (**a**, **c**) Preoperative MRI image. MRI shows that the enhanced small mass lesion on the orbital apex. The optic nerve is pushed medially by the tumor. (**b**, **d**) Postoperative MRI image. MRI shows the tumor is removed and small residual tumor is seen in the superior orbital fissure

removal is required (Fig. 19.8a–d). Intraorbital cavernous hemangiomas have relatively clear margins, with a fine fibrous tissue layer adhering to the surface of the hemangioma where small blood vessels penetrate and adhere to the surrounding structures (Fig. 19.9a–d). If this vascular supply is coagulated and detached, the tumor can be removed as a single mass. Unlike the case of schwannoma, the tumor can be removed at the plane external to the capsule. Since the orbital cavity is filled with fat, it is important to avoid unnecessary fat manipulation and remove just the cavernous hemangioma itself. Once the fat protrudes, it will continue further and further out, so adequate precaution is needed. As an extracapsular removal, constant attention to the surrounding neural and vascular structures should be given. However, in the rare case when the hemangioma is intraconal in the orbital apex and the lesion is surrounded by nerves, extracapsular removal may not be possible. Therefore, the purpose of surgical procedure will be to obtain a pathological diagnosis and decompression of the optic nerve by debulking, also considering the SRS an effective and safe additional option.

SRT remains one of the alternative treatments for orbital cavernous hemangioma [8, 9].

If the tumor is in the inferior part of the orbit, the transnasal endoscopic resection can be useful. The intraconal space can be accessed between the inferior and medial rectus muscles. In the past, when the tumor was located infero-medially, it was difficult to reach the lesion from the lateral side by open surgery, and a contralateral approach was also advocated. Since the development of nasal endoscopic surgery and the improvement of surgical techniques, the approach to the medial inferior orbit has become much easier.

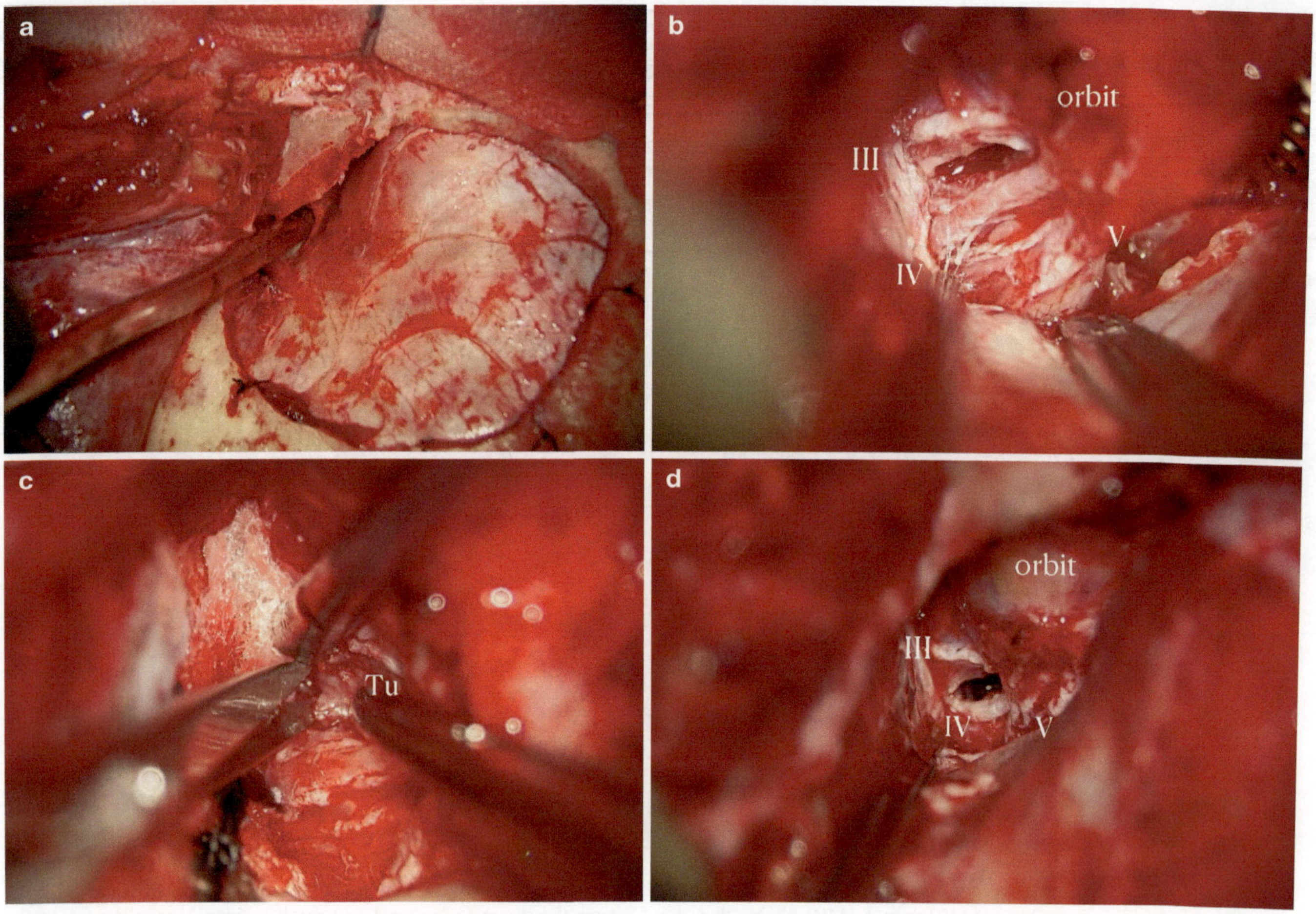

Fig. 19.9 Intraoperative image of the superior orbital fissure cavernous malformation. (**a**) Frontotemporal craniotomy is performed. (**b**) Orbit and superior orbital fissure are exposed and the small corridor between the oculomotor and trochlear nerve. (**c**) Small piece of a tumor is seen between the oculomotor and trochlear nerve. (**d**) The tumor is removed without damaging the nerves

19.7 Optic Nerve Sheath Meningioma (ONSM)

ONSMs consist of proliferations of meningothelial cells, which are thought to originate from the arachnoid villi of the arachnoid layer. Optic sheath meningioma is more difficult to remove because the tumor grows in the orbit along and in direct contact with the optic nerve.

If the tumor is small but localized to the orbital apex and compresses the optic nerve, causing visual field disturbance or vision loss, surgery is required to open the optic canal and biopsy by taking only a portion of the tumor. There are three management options for ONSM: follow-up, surgical removal, and radiation therapy. However, due to the nature of the tumor and the characteristics of the optic nerve function, a cure by surgical treatment means a loss of optic nerve function. ONSM is a benign tumor, but due to its relationship to optic nerve function, it can only be completely removed under certain conditions, and complete removal is difficult and unpredictable. Because the tumor is benign, it is unacceptable for patients to sacrifice their vision. Surgical treatment is only recommended when a definitive tissue diagnosis is made and for complete removal of the tumor when the patient eye is completely blind.

The results of stereotactic radiotherapy are acceptable [10] and in some cases can be expected to reduce or control tumor size and even improve visual function. In the situation where the tumor is in the orbital apex and the optic nerve function is decreasing, it is desirable to release the pressure on the optic nerve by performing optic nerve canal decompression to prevent the optic nerve function from decreasing due to temporary tumor growth after radiosurgery [11, 12].

19.8 Conclusion

Orbital lesions are directly related to the visual and ocular functions and have a great impact on patient's life, requiring very well planned, indicated, and understood by the patient treatment. The anatomical complexity of the lesion requires a rational and often combined treatment strategy. Surgical treatment is based on the detailed anatomy of the intraorbital and apical portions of the orbit.

The relationship of the orbital apex to the orbit, anterior infratemporal fossa, and paranasal sinuses is very important. This is an area where there is a wide range of surgical options, and a thorough knowledge of both transcranial and nasal endoscopic approaches is required.

References

1. Oyama K, Watanabe K, Hanakita S, Champagne PO, Passeri T, Voormolen EH, Bernat AL, Penet N, Fukushima T, Froelich S. The orbitopterygoid corridor as a deep keyhole for endoscopic access to the paranasal sinuses and clivus. J Neurosurg. 2020;134(5):1480–9. https://doi.org/10.3171/2020.3.JNS2022. PMID: 32534497.
2. Lenzi GL, Fieschi C. Superior orbital fissure syndrome. Review of 130 cases. Eur Neurol. 1977;16(1–6):23–30. https://doi.org/10.1159/000114876. PMID: 210020.
3. Badakere A, Patil-Chhablani P. Orbital apex syndrome: a review. Eye Brain. 2019;11:63–72. https://doi.org/10.2147/EB.S180190. PMID: 31849556; PMCID: PMC6913296.
4. Fernandez S, Godino O, Martinez-Yelamos S, et al. Cavernous sinus syndrome: a series of 126 patients. Medicine (Baltimore). 2007;86:278–81.
5. Ohtsuka K, Hashimoto M, Suzuki Y. A review of 244 orbital tumors in Japanese patients during a 21-year period: origins and locations. Jpn J Ophthalmol. 2005;49(1):49–55. https://doi.org/10.1007/s10384-004-0147-y. PMID: 15692775.
6. Chen L, White WL, Xu B, Tian X. Transnasal transsphenoid approach: a minimally invasive approach for removal of cavernous haemangiomas located at inferomedial part of orbital apex. Clin Exp Ophthalmol. 2010;38(5):439–43. https://doi.org/10.1111/j.1442-9071.2010.02274.x. PMID: 20649613.
7. Sweeney AR, Gupta D, Keene CD, Cimino PJ, Chambers CB, Chang SH, Hanna E. Orbital peripheral nerve sheath tumors. Surv Ophthalmol. 2017;62(1):43–57. https://doi.org/10.1016/j.survophthal.2016.08.002. Epub 2016 Aug 26. PMID: 27570221.
8. Sasaki Y, Miyazaki S, Fukushima T. Multisession CyberKnife radiosurgery for orbital cavernous hemangiomas. Cureus. 2021;13(1):e12711. https://doi.org/10.7759/cureus.12711. PMID: 33614316; PMCID: PMC7883522.
9. Lee CC, Sheehan JP, Kano H, Akpinar B, Martinez-Alvarez R, Martinez-Moreno N, Guo WY, Lunsford LD, Liu KD. Gamma knife radiosurgery for hemangioma of the cavernous sinus. J Neurosurg. 2017;126(5):1498–505. https://doi.org/10.3171/2016.4.JNS152097. Epub 2016 Jun 24. PMID: 27341049.
10. Arvold ND, Lessell S, Bussiere M, Beaudette K, Rizzo JF, Loeffler JS, Shih HA. Visual outcome and tumor control after conformal radiotherapy for patients with optic nerve sheath meningioma. Int J Radiat Oncol Biol Phys. 2009;75(4):1166–72. https://doi.org/10.1016/j.ijrobp.2008.12.056. Epub 2009 May 4. PMID: 19406585.
11. Parker RT, Ovens CA, Fraser CL, Samarawickrama C. Optic nerve sheath meningiomas: prevalence, impact, and management strategies. Eye Brain. 2018;10:85–99. https://doi.org/10.2147/EB.S144345. PMID: 30498385; PMCID: PMC6207092.
12. Bloch O, Sun M, Kaur G, Barani IJ, Parsa AT. Fractionated radiotherapy for optic nerve sheath meningiomas. J Clin Neurosci. 2012;19(9):1210–5. https://doi.org/10.1016/j.jocn.2012.02.010. Epub 2012 Jun 22. PMID: 22727747.

Endoscopic Endonasal Approach to Optic Canal and Orbital Apex

20

Karen Kar Wun Chan, Christine Chi Ying Lam, and Kelvin Kam Lung Chong

Abstract

In this chapter, we highlight the essential perioperative preparations, anatomical landmarks, and step-by-step surgical techniques for endoscopic endonasal approach to lesions in the optic canal and orbital apex.

Keywords

Endoscopic endonasal · Optic canal · Orbital apex · Navigation-guided · Surgical techniques · Endoscopic landmarks

20.1 Introduction

Optic canal and orbital apex lesions are difficult to approach surgically due to the conglomeration of critical structures confined in the anterior skull base. While lesions are usually benign, they may cause significant morbidities including visual loss, ptosis, diplopia, exposure keratopathy, proptosis, and facial deformities. Surgeries may also induce iatrogenic injuries to neural (cranial nerves II, III, IV, V, VI, parasympathetic and sympathetic innervation), vascular (ophthalmic artery and veins), muscular (extraocular muscles), and other adnexal and periocular (lacrimal gland, lacrimal drainage, and eyelid) structures.

The three borders of the orbital apex can be reached by lateral (transcutaneous, transforniceal, or transtemporal), medial (transcutaneous, transcaruncular, or transethmoidal), and superior (transcutaneous, transconjunctival, or transcranial) orbitotomy. Endoscopic transethmoidal approach utilizes fiberoptic scopes through natural orifices avoiding periocular incisions. Importantly, this is among the more popular "extraorbital" (the others are transtemporal and transcranial) approaches to minimize intraoperative orbital retraction and iatrogenic compressive damage to the globe and the apical structures. Operative view is enhanced by fiberoptic illumination and magnification, and allows real-time capturing as high-definition or even three-dimensional videos. Orbital fat herniation into the surgical field should be minimized before periosteal incision. On the other hand, pre-existing nasal pathologies including deviated nasal septum may need to be managed, possibly in the same operation. In appropriately selected lesions (medial, inferior, or inferomedial based), patients and surgical teams, endoscopic approach to the orbital apex offers a less traumatic alternative to the classic transorbital approach.

The intricate anatomies limit surgical trajectories and direct visualization of critical structures (e.g., skull base, optic nerve, carotid, and ophthalmic artery). Dedicated instruments including endoscopic video setup is required, while navigation system and sinus surgery instruments (either powered or cold steel) are optional. A steep learning curve is expected for surgeons without prior endoscopic experience (e.g., endoscopic lacrimal surgeries), while postoperative endoscopy follow-up is essential.

Endoscopic orbital surgeries are primarily performed through paranasal sinuses to access to the medial orbit (transethmoidal), inferior orbit (transmaxillary), and optic nerve (transethmoidal or trans-sphenoidal), or through the subperiosteal space to reach all quadrants of the orbit during endoscope-assisted orbitotomies/ endoscopic transorbital (ETO) approach or transorbital neuroendoscopic surgery (TONES). Applications are wide and have been covered elsewhere in the book.

K. K. W. Chan · C. C. Y. Lam
Department of Ophthalmology and Visual Sciences, Prince of Wales Hospital, Hong Kong SAR, China

K. K. L. Chong (✉)
Department of Ophthalmology and Visual Sciences, Prince of Wales Hospital, Hong Kong SAR, China

Department of Ophthalmology and Visual Sciences, The Chinese University of Hong Kong, Hong Kong SAR, China
e-mail: chongkamlung@cuhk.edu.hk

T. L. POON et al. (eds.), *Orbital Apex and Periorbital Skull Base Diseases*, https://doi.org/10.1007/978-981-99-2989-4_20

Surgery to the orbital apex may be indicated for decompression, incisional or excisional biopsy, or removal of foreign bodies. These may be combined with lateral (transcutaneous) or inferolateral (transantral, transconjunctival, transcutaneous) bone and/ or fat removal to augment the amount of proptosis reduction in thyroid-associated orbitopathy or other conditions. Traumatic optic neuropathy (TON) and idiopathic intracranial hypertension (IIH) are indications for optic canal decompression with or without optic nerve sheath fenestration.

20.2 Pertinent Surgical Anatomy

The optic canal is formed by the two struts of the lesser wing of the sphenoid bone. It contains the optic nerve and the ophthalmic artery. This canal is approximately 10 mm long and 4–5 mm wide. It is thinner and wider proximally and thicker and narrower distally. At this point, the dura mater and the periosteal layer of the optic canal fuse to form the periorbita. Typically, the ophthalmic artery lies inferolateral to the optic nerve, but a more medial trajectory is possible and hence should be considered during decompression. The central retinal artery leaves the ophthalmic artery 10 mm behind the globe. As seen from below, the optic canal is in direct contact with the lateral sphenoid recess and the most posterior ethmoidal cells. Among these cells are sphenoethmoidal Onodi cells, which may directly cover the optic canal and must be opened to expose the optic nerve [1].

The orbital apex is the area between the orbit and intracranial space. The lesser wing of the sphenoid bone forms the roof of the apex, the ethmoidal sinus forms the medial wall, the greater wing of the sphenoid forms the lateral wall, and the orbital process of the palatine bone forms the floor. The optic canal is bordered by the sphenoid bone, superiorly by the lesser wing, inferolaterally by the optic strut, and medially by the sphenoid body. The superior orbital fissure is inferolateral to the optic canal separated by the optic strut and bordered by the lesser wing of the sphenoid superiorly and medially, by the greater wing of the sphenoid bone laterally and the orbital process of the palatine bone inferiorly [2].

The anterior skull base receives significant blood supply from the anterior (AEA) and posterior ethmoidal arteries (PEA). They arise from the ophthalmic artery in the medial third of the orbit and range in between 0.5 and 1 mm in diameter [3]. The anatomy of the ethmoidal arteries is of concern to surgeons performing endoscopic sinus surgery, as injury to these arteries may cause uncontrolled intraorbital hemorrhage and vision loss. These arteries enter the anterior and posterior ethmoidal canals and leave the canals to enter the anterior cranial fossa at the anterior and posterior ends of the lateral edge of the cribriform plate. They mark important landmarks of the skull base by forming the superior surgical limit at the frontoethmoidal junction. The "24-12-6" rule of thumb is proposed for the distance from the anterior lacrimal crest to the anterior ethmoidal foramen (24 mm), from the anterior to posterior foramina (12 mm), and from the posterior foramina to the optic canal (6 mm) to estimate the locations of the AEA and PEA [4].

20.3 Surgical Technique

20.3.1 Perioperative Preparation

A detailed ophthalmological assessment should include thorough documentation of visual acuity, visual fields, relative afferent pupillary defect, optic nerve head appearance, color vision, exophthalmometry, eyelid position, presence of diplopia, and limitations and pain on extraocular muscle movements. A thorough preoperative endoscopic nasal examination looking for nasal septal deviation, nasal polyps, and signs of chronic rhinosinusitis is required to identify conditions, which may require co-management with rhinologists. If needed, 2–3 days' course of Rhinocort Aqua 64 mcg/ actuation nasal spray (McNeil Products, United Kingdom) and Otrivin nasal drops (GlaxoSmithKline, United Kingdom) are prescribed to decongest the nasal mucosa.

Preoperative orbital imaging including computed tomography (CT) and magnetic resonance imaging (MRI) of the orbits is complementary in apical surgeries. CT orbits are a valuable tool for evaluation of detailed bony anatomy. Preoperative knowledge of the height of the skull base, location of cribriform plate, depth of olfactory fossa (based on Keros classification), and anatomical variations permit safe surgical access and guide setting up of the navigation system. MRI is superior at delineating soft tissue layers and provides useful information including degree of inflammation, vascularity, and cellularity (from perfusion and diffusion-weighted imaging). It also details the relationship of surrounding neurovascular structures including the globe, optic nerve, cranial nerves, extraocular muscles, cavernous sinus, and intracranial structures. Decision for the need of preoperative embolisation or sclerotherapy should be determined to achieve optimal intraoperative hemostasis and completion of excision.

Finally, surgical precision is assisted by the use of image-guided navigation system based on preoperative CT and/ or MRI images to track and visualize the surgical procedure in real-time in relation to the preoperative imaging in two- or three-dimensional modes. Appropriate instrumentations, including long-handled endo-diathermy, cryoprobe, microscissors, and functional endoscopic sinus surgery set, should be available.

20.4 Step-by-Step Surgical Technique

20.4.1 Preparation and Anesthesia

Surgery is typically performed under general anesthesia. With the patient in supine position, patient's head should be elevated to decrease venous congestion, and neck slightly extended. Nasal packing with ribbon gauzes or neurosurgical cottonoid soaked in 5% cocaine, 1:10,000 adrenaline, 0.05% oxymetazoline, and/ or topical tranexamic acid is placed under the middle meatus to decongest and vasoconstrict the nasal mucosa. The middle turbinate is medialized, fractured, or a limited middle turbinectomy can be performed to improve middle meatal access. Optional limited conjunctival periotomy is performed to isolate and sling any rectus extraocular muscle with 4-0 silk sutures.

20.4.2 Uncinectomy and Ethmoidectomy

Ethmoidectomy widens the surgical corridor to the ventrolateral skull base [3]. The extent of ethmoidectomy (partial or complete) can be guided by intraoperative navigation system to ensure targeted removal of lesion. Ethmoidectomy begins with an uncinectomy, performed using Stammberger or swinging door techniques. The anterior, middle, and posterior ethmoidal air cells are then sequentially removed with cold steel (e.g., Blaksley forceps) or powered (e.g., microdebrider) instruments. The nasofrontal opening must be preserved while removing the Agger Nasi air cells. As mentioned, the anterior and posterior ethmoidal vessels are useful landmarks of the superior surgical limit at the frontoethmoidal suture.

After ethmoidectomy, the sphenoid sinus entry and lamina papyracea will be evident. The lamina can be punctured with a seeker probe or periosteal elevator, while the bone fragments can be removed with Blaksley or Takahashi forceps. Depending on the extent of decompression required and the size and location of the lesion, the lamina can be removed in part or in whole up to the sphenoethmoidal junction including the posterior part of the ethmoidomaxillary strut and the orbital process of the palatine bone especially for apical decompression (Fig. 20.1a). At this stage, the periorbita should preferably be kept intact to prevent fat prolapse into the surgical field. The skull base is recognized by the characteristic granular surface of the fovea ethmoidalis and increased bone thickness (Fig. 20.1b). Maxillary antrostomy should be done to prevent occlusion of sinus drainage by prolapsing orbital tissues, which may lead to postoperative sinusitis (Fig. 20.1c).

20.4.3 Endoscopic Transethmoidal Approach to Orbital Apex Lesions

Following adequate removal of lamina papyracea, the periorbita is incised as guided by location and size of lesion using a sickle knife, a bent 18-gauge needle on a tuberculin syringe, or a crescent knife. Lesions are gently dissected from surrounding intra- or extraconal fat with a blunt-tipped instrument, for example, a seeker probe or transphenoidal dissector. Extraconal lesions are readily visible after periorbita incision. Intraconal lesions are accessed following retraction of medial, superior, and/or inferior rectus muscles either endonasally or conjunctivally with/ without muscle detachment. Orbital fat will come into view and retracted using wet neurosurgical cottonoids. Fat removal should be limited using a manual suction punch under direct visualization in a controlled manner. Image-guidance can be useful for small lesions. Once the lesion is identified, blunt and limited sharp dissection begins from distal to proximal. Incisional biopsy can be performed should the representative part of the lesion is exposed, confirmed with the navigation images. Gentle, intermittent, and controlled traction by sutures, forceps, or cryoprobe is performed while monitoring pupillary changes. Any feeding vessel may be cauterized before delivering the entire lesion into the nasal cavity. If complete excision is deemed impossible, for example, an infiltrative lesion or sustained mydriasis, debulking followed by an orbital apex and/or optic canal decompression can be an alternative.

A four-hands, binarial transeptal approach may be adopted after a posterior nasal septectomy to allow access from contralateral nare to accommodate multiple instrumentations.

20.4.4 Optic Canal Decompression: Transethmoidal or Trans-Sphenoidal Approach

The medial aspect of the optic canal can be decompressed endoscopically through the ethmoid or sphenoid sinus. During transethmoidal approach, complete ethmoidectomy is performed as described above until sphenoid sinus entry is reached. Alternatively, during transsphenoidal approach, the superior turbinate is removed to expose the sphenoid sinus ostium, with or without a posterior bony septoplasty. Once the sphenoid sinus is reached, anterior sphenoidotomy is performed to expose the optic canal, internal carotid artery, and medial and lateral opticocarotid recesses (Fig. 20.2a and b). These landmarks should be confirmed with navigation system before the following steps (Fig. 20.2c and d).

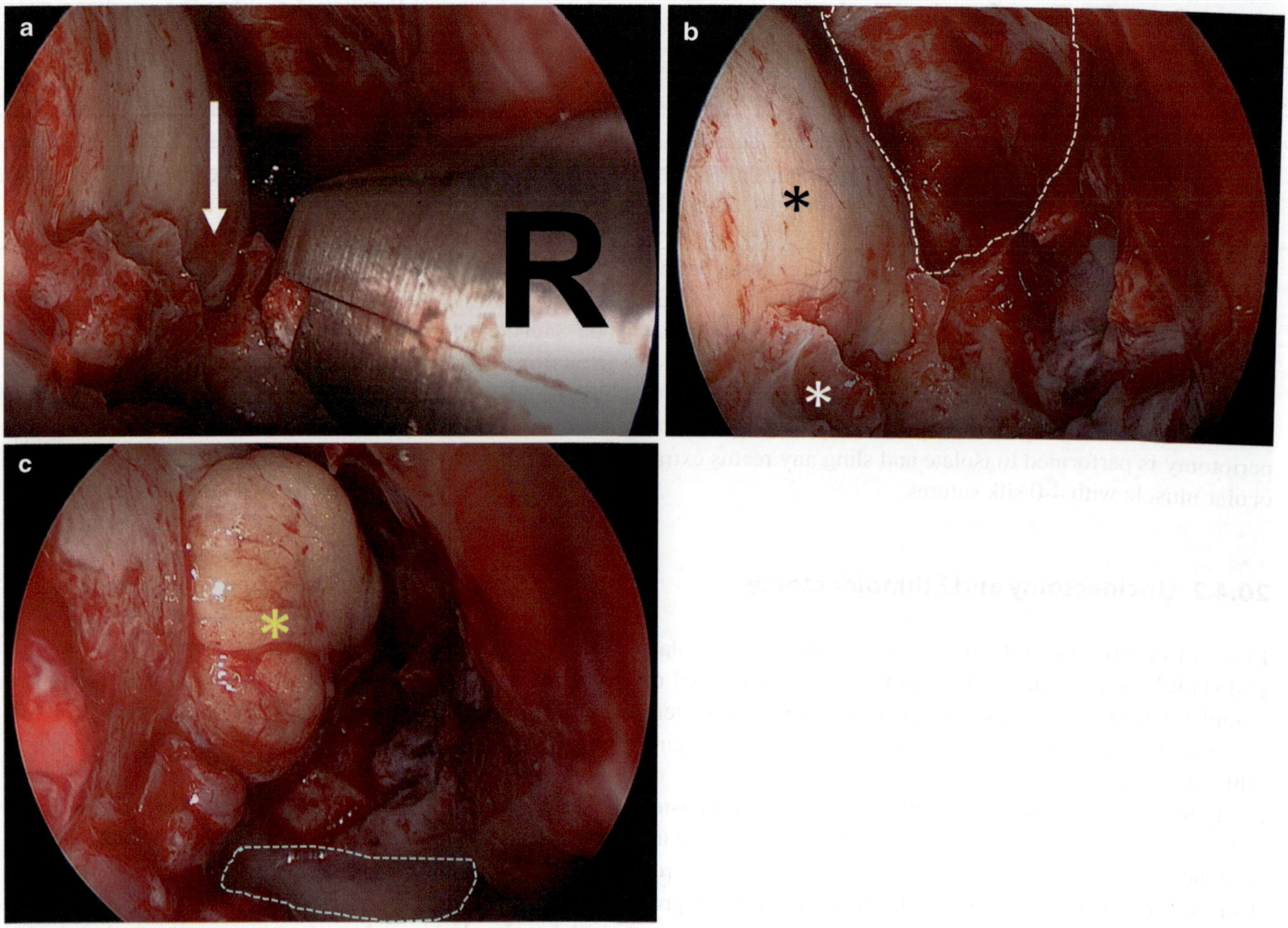

Fig. 20.1 (**a**) Endoscopic view (right side). Following complete ethmoidectomy and removal of lamina papyracea demonstrating removal of the posterior ethmoidomaxillary strut (white arrow) and later posterior orbital floor and the orbital process of the palatine bone with rongeur (R) to achieve maximum apical decompression. (**b**) Endoscopic view (right side). Identification of surgical landmarks including fovea ethmoidalis (white dotted lines), medial periorbita (black asterisk), and a preserved anterior ethmoidomaxillary strut (white star). (**c**) Endoscopic view (right side). Incision of the retrobulbar part of the periorbita exposing orbital fat (yellow asterisk). Note the enlarged maxillary antrum to avoid postoperative sinus occlusion (blue dotted line)

A long-handled diamond burr is used to drill over a segment of the bony optic canal, typically the middle section, with constant irrigation to prevent heat damage to the underlying optic nerve. Once the canal bone becomes eggshell thin, a periosteal elevator is used to peel off the remaining bone away from the optic nerve and sheath. Pulsations of the optic nerve signal good decompression are achieved. The rest of the bony canal from the apex toward the chiasm can be removed by drilling or with a 1-mm sphenoid rongeur mechanically. The optic nerve sheath should be examined for any hematoma, particularly when there is associated canal fracture. If indicated, the optic nerve sheath and annulus of Zinn are incised with a sickle knife, crescent knife, or bent 18-gauge needle, to expose the underlying pia matter. Incisions should be shallow, as the superomedial quadrant of the cone is where damage to the inferiorly positioned ophthalmic artery may occur.

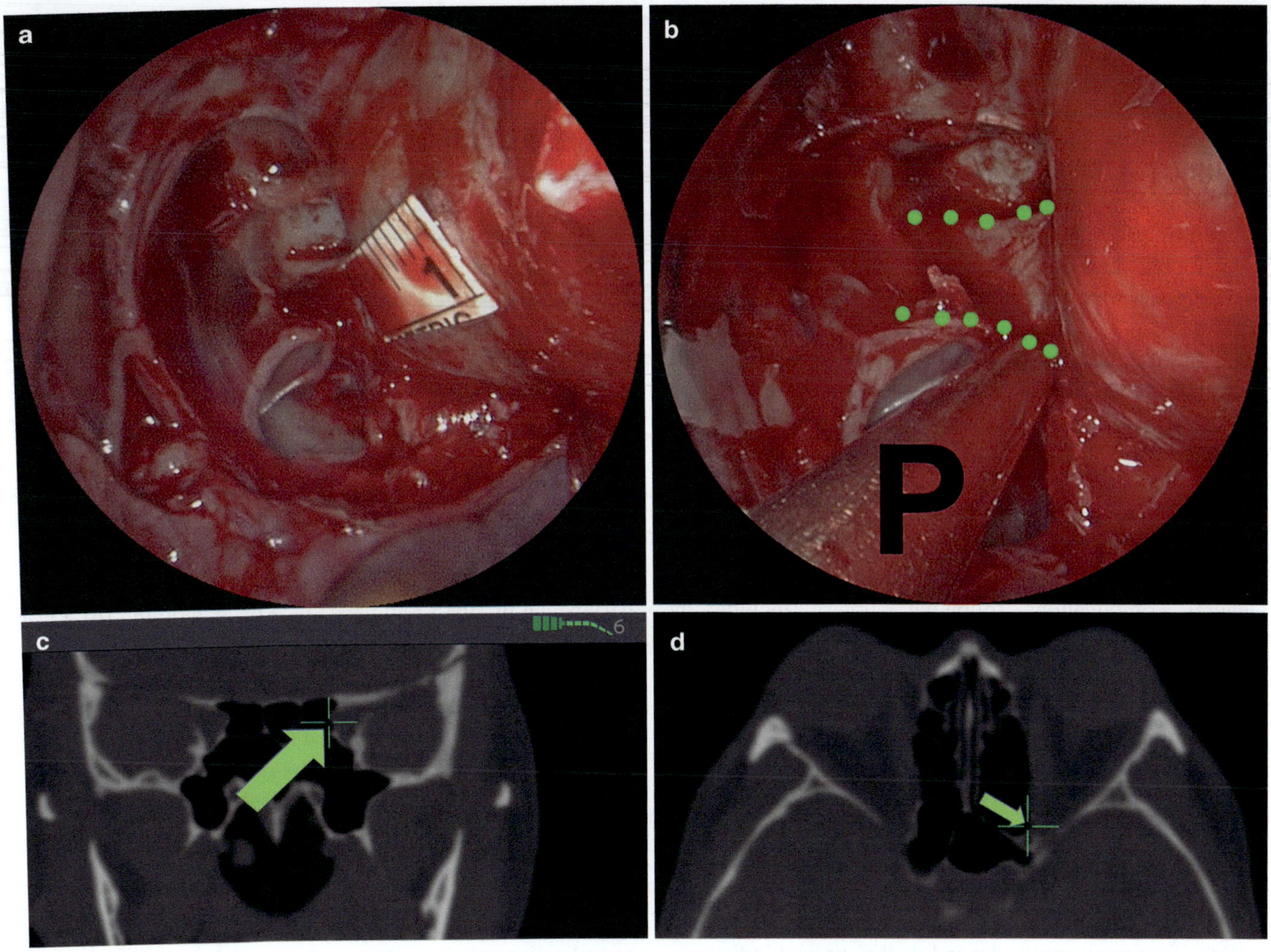

Fig. 20.2 (**a**) Endoscopic view (left side). After left ethmoidectomy and anterior sphenoidotomy. (**b**) Endoscopic view (left side). The medial aspect of the optic canal (green dotted line). Pointer is identified (P) (**c** and **d**) Navigation panel showing location of navigation pointer from (**b**) (green cross) over at the optic canal opening on coronal (**c**) and axial (**d**) computerized tomography images

20.5 Surgical Pearls

Pupil size should be monitored throughout the surgery either manually or by a pupillometer. Traction, irritation, or vascular compromise to the optic nerve may lead to pupil dilatation, while vasoconstricting or anesthetic agents applied locally after periorbita is opened may cause sectoral mydriasis. Traction should be released immediately and surgery resumed after pupil achieves a small and round state.

Hemostasis is achieved intraoperatively with the 6Ps: pressure (nasal packing), physical (cold saline irrigation), pharmacological (topical vasoconstrictants), position (head-up), procedural (cautery), and patience (of the operating surgeons). To limit the use of cauterization in the orbital apex, the use of topical agent (e.g., tranexamic acid)-soaked cottonoids (neuropatty) may displace a broad area of fat while achieving hemostasis to facilitate dissection. Monopolar cautery and vasoconstrictor (e.g., adrenaline) should be avoided around the orbital apex. Small pieces of Surgicel (absorbable hemostat, oxidized cellulose polymer) is useful over sinus mucosa, and bone wax over bleeding bone edges may be left at the end of the surgery if necessary. Nasal packing with absorbable (e.g., nasopore, gelfoam) or nonabsorbable (ribbon-gauze, merocel) materials can be placed at conclusion of operation to avoid adhesions between the septum and the middle turbinate.

20.6 Postoperative Management

Preliminary visual and pupillary assessment should be performed in the recovery room after anesthesia is reversed. A short course of intravenous steroid may enhance decongestion and relieve any pre-existing and postoperative optic neuropathy. Patients should be nursed 30 degrees inclined with frequent cold compress to the forehead. Hot food, drinks, and nose-blowing should be avoided during the first week postoperatively. Nasal steroidal sprays, steroid-antibiotic eyedrops, and systemic antibiotics are prescribed based on the surgeon's discretion.

Upon postoperative endoscopic examination, if nasal tamponades were placed, they should preferably be moistened before removal. Electrocautery, silver nitrate, or repacking can be used under endoscopic monitoring when active mucosal bleeding is present. Following removal of nasal packs, patients are instructed to perform nasal douching to remove crusts and hasten mucosal healing. Endoscopic toileting around the maxillary antrum is performed to prevent postoperative sinusitis. Adjunctive postoperative endoscopic manipulation including periosteal release or intraorbital steroidal injection can be performed before mucosa is healed.

20.7 Complications

General complications following surgery include the following:

- Bleeding ranging from epistaxis and periorbital hematoma, to retrobulbar hemorrhage
- Infection of sinus, orbit, or meninges
- Nasolacrimal duct injury
- Cerebrospinal fluid leakage and rhinorrhea
- Direct and indirect (ischemia) injury to optic nerve with reduced vision or blindness

Specific complications depend on the surgical indication. New-onset or worsening of existing diplopia following orbital apex decompression may be due to displacement, entrapment, and/ or injuries to extraocular muscles, cranial nerve palsies, and fat adhesion syndrome. Removal of intraconal fat to improve visualization may inadvertently traumatize branches of the ophthalmic artery and branches of the third cranial nerve. Compared to extraconal lesions, intraconal lesions are associated with greater incidence of incomplete removal and postoperative morbidities including new-onset diplopia and enophthalmos [5]. Carotid artery injury may lead to stroke and shock while ethmoidal vessels retrobulbar hemorrhage.

It is prudent to have access to suitable endonasal equipment to reduce complications. High speed bone drilling with a coarse diamond burr is useful as heat created may facilitate hemostasis. The Sonopet Ultrasonic Aspirator (Stryker, USA) provides fine bone emulsification while protecting soft tissues and avoiding collateral damage. Three-dimensional video endoscopic system enhances depth perception and skull-base appreciation especially in distorted anatomies or for less experienced surgeons. Bipolar cautery and cryoprobes of appropriate length and angulation (Bayonet) facilitate endonasal hemostasis and lesion removal.

20.8 Surgical Outcomes: Scientific Evidence

The first descriptions of endonasal approaches to orbital surgery began in 1990s and have since been evolving [6]. Over the years, only limited case series from high-volume institutions were published in the literature, and as such, evidence of efficacy of the surgical approach is limited by small sample sizes and lack of randomized controlled trials.

Orbital cavernous hemangioma (OCH) is the most common benign orbital space-occupying lesions in adults. Due to its well-circumscribed and compressible nature, it is a classic indication for endoscopic endonasal removal. Table 20.1 shows case series reporting outcomes following surgery. Although visual loss is a potentially devastating complication of the surgery, it was only reported in one series, including 77.8% (14/18) who had improved or stable vision, while 22.2% (4/18) had dropped vision postoperatively [12]. Transient, new diplopia was common, though the majority does not result in permanent morbidity. Incomplete resection was reported and may be due to proximity to optic nerve to avoid risk of optic neuropathy from vasospasm or undue traction during dissection [10]. Enophthalmos was infrequently recorded and may warrant subsequent orbital reconstruction. A global multicenter clinical study in 2015 revealed that 21.7% patients had enoph-

Table 20.1 Outcomes of orbital cavernous hemangioma resection following endoscopic endonasal surgery

Author	Year[a]	No. of patients	M:F	Location IC:EC	Incomplete excision	Visual loss	Transient diplopia	Permanent diplopia	Enophthalmos
Muscatello et al. [7]	2012	3	1:2	3:0	0	0	1 (33.3)	0	0
Castelnuovo et al. [8]	2012	16	10:6	9:7	0	0	3 (18.9)	2 (12.5)	1 (6.25)
Netuka et al. [9]	2013	3	0:3	2:1	0	0	0	0	0
Chhabra et al. [10]	2014	5	3:2	5:0	1 (20)	0	5 (100)	1 (20)	2 (40)
Bleier et al. [5]	2015	23	10:13	16:7	6 (26.1)	0	9 (39.1)	1 (4.35)	21.7
Ma et al. [11]	2019	23	10:13	16:7	7 (30.4)	0	8 (34.7)	0	0
Li et al. [12]	2021	18	7:11	18:0	6.7	4 (22.2)	0	0	0

F female; *IC:EC* intraconal: extraconal, *M* male, *No.* number; numbers are expressed in percentages within brackets
[a] Year published

Table 20.2 Outcomes of idiopathic intracranial hypertension following optic canal decompression with or without optic nerve sheath fenestration

Author	Year[a]	No. of patients	M:F	Visual improvement	Visual Deterioration	Papilloedema improvement	Headache improvement	VF improvement	CSF leak
Sencer et al. [13]	2014	10	1:9	7 (70)	1 (10)	7 (78)	4/7 (57.1)	8 (80)	0 (0)
Yildirim et al. [14]	2015	2	0:2	2 (100)	0 (0)	NS	1 (50)	2 (100)	0 (0)
Tarrats et al. [15]	2017	34	5:29	29 (85.3)	0 (0)	27 (81.4)	27 (81.8)	32 (93.8)	0 (0)
Goksu et al. [16]	2021	9	2:7	7 (78)	0 (0)	6 (66.7)	6 (66.7)	5/8 (62.5)	0 (0)
Wadikhaye et al. [17]	2021	21	2:19	19 (90.5)	0 (0)	19 (90.5)	14 (66.7)	17 (81.0)	0 (0)

Numbers are expressed in percentages within brackets
CSF cerebrospinal fluid, *F* female, *M* male, *No.* number, *NS* not specified, *VF* visual field
[a] Year published

Table 20.3 Outcomes of traumatic optic neuropathy following optic canal decompression

Author	Year[a]	No. of patients	M:F	Visual improvement	Visual loss	CSF rhinorrhea	Need for further surgery
Berhouma et al. [1]	2014	11	3:8	6 (54)	0 (0)	0 (0)	4 (36.4)
He et al. [18]	2016	11	8:3	5 (45.5)	0	2 (18.2)	0
Yu et al. [19]	2016	96	86:10	45 (46.9)	0 (0)	4 (4.17)	0
Yu et al. [20]	2018	62	53:9	34 (54.8)	2 (3.23)	3 (4.84)	0

Numbers are expressed in percentages within brackets
CSF cerebrospinal fluid, *F* female, *M* male, *No.* number
[a] Year published

thalmos and 26.1% patients with worsened diplopia after endoscopic endonasal resection of OCH [5]. Current data suggests that endoscopic removal of intraconal cavernous hemangiomas is feasible and safe.

Outcomes of idiopathic intracranial hypertension (IIH) following optic canal decompression with or without optic nerve sheath fenestration is included in Table 20.2, while Table 20.3 shows outcomes of TON following optic canal decompression. Without conclusive evidence from randomized controlled trials evaluating the natural course and optimum management of IIH or TON, the current management is tailored according to the stage of presentation.

References

1. Berhouma M, et al. Endoscopic endonasal optic nerve and orbital apex decompression for nontraumatic optic neuropathy: surgical nuances and review of the literature. Neurosurg Focus. 2014;37(4):E19.
2. Engin Ö, et al. A systematic review of the surgical anatomy of the orbital apex. Surg Radiol Anat. 2021;43(2):169–78.
3. Cecchini G. Anterior and posterior ethmoidal artery ligation in anterior skull base meningiomas: a review on microsurgical approaches. World Neurosurg. 2015;84(4):1161–5.
4. Necmettin Pamir M, Rudolf Fahlbusch PMB. Meningiomas. In: Meningeal anatomy, vol. 2. Saunders; 2010.
5. Bleier BS, et al. Endoscopic endonasal orbital cavernous hemangioma resection: global experience in techniques and outcomes. Int Forum Allergy Rhinol. 2016;6(2):156–61.
6. Curragh DS, Halliday L, Selva D. Endonasal approach to orbital pathology. Ophthalmic Plast Reconstr Surg. 2018;34(5):422–7.
7. Muscatello L, et al. Transnasal endoscopic surgery for selected orbital cavernous hemangiomas: our preliminary experience. Head Neck. 2013;35(7):E218–20.
8. Castelnuovo P, et al. Endoscopic transnasal intraorbital surgery: our experience with 16 cases. Eur Arch Otorhinolaryngol. 2012;269(8):1929–35.
9. Netuka D, et al. Endoscopic endonasal resection of medial orbital lesions with intraoperative MRI. Acta Neurochir (Wien). 2013;155(3):455–61.
10. Chhabra N, et al. Endoscopic resection of orbital hemangiomas. Int Forum Allergy Rhinol. 2014;4(3):251–5.
11. Ma J, et al. Transnasal endoscopic resection of orbital cavernous hemangiomas: our experience with 23 cases. Int Forum Allergy Rhinol. 2019;9(11):1374–80.
12. Li C, et al. Retrospective case analysis of transnasal endoscopic resection of benign orbital apex tumors: some thoughts on transnasal endoscopic surgery. J Ophthalmol. 2021;2021:6691203.
13. Sencer A, et al. Unilateral endoscopic optic nerve decompression for idiopathic intracranial hypertension: a series of 10 patients. World Neurosurg. 2014;82(5):745–50.
14. Yildirim AE, et al. Endoscopic endonasal optic nerve decompression in a patient with pseudotumor cerebri. J Craniofac Surg. 2015;26(1):240–2.
15. Tarrats L, et al. Outcomes of endoscopic optic nerve decompression in patients with idiopathic intracranial hypertension. Int Forum Allergy Rhinol. 2017;7(6):615–23.
16. Goksu E, et al. Endoscopic bilateral optic nerve decompression for treatment of idiopathic intracranial hypertension. Brain Sci. 2021;11(3):324.
17. Wadikhaye R, Alugolu R, Mudumba VS. A 270-degree decompression of optic nerve in refractory idiopathic intracranial hypertension using an ultrasonic aspirator—a prospective institutional study. Neurol India. 2021;69(1):49–55.
18. He ZH, et al. Endoscopic decompression of the optic canal for traumatic optic neuropathy. Chin J Traumatol. 2016;19(6):330–2.
19. Yu B, et al. The outcome of endoscopic transethmosphenoid optic canal decompression for indirect traumatic optic neuropathy with no-light-perception. J Ophthalmol. 2016;2016:6492858.
20. Yu B, et al. Outcome of endoscopic trans-ethmosphenoid optic canal decompression for indirect traumatic optic neuropathy in children. BMC Ophthalmol. 2018;18(1):152.

21 Endoscopic Endonasal Approach to Cavernous Sinus and Middle Cranial Fossa

Arianna Fava, Paolo di Russo, Thibault Passeri, Lorenzo Giammattei, and Sébastien Froelich

Abstract

Cavernous sinus surgery has evolved in the last decades moving toward less invasive approaches to reduce postoperative morbidities. Endoscopic endonasal techniques have been a revolution in skull base surgery providing a natural and direct line of sight to deep-seated skull base lesions such as the cavernous sinus, complementing the standard transcranial approaches. In this chapter, endoscopic anatomy, patient selection and contraindications, and surgical technique among clinical cases are provided.

Keywords

Cavernous sinus · Middle cranial fossa · Petrous apex · Meckel's cave · EEA · Endoscopic endonasal techniques · Chondrosarcomas · Chordomas · ICA

21.1 Introduction

Treatment for skull base tumors involving the cavernous sinus (CS) and middle fossa has significantly evolved during the last decades. After pioneer surgery performed by Parkinson [1] to treat vascular lesions within the parasellar compartment, several transcranial approaches such as the frontotemporal, orbitozygomatic epidural [2], and the middle fossa approaches have been described to access the CS using the so-called "Kawase," "Hakuba," or "Dolenc" techniques [3–5]. Transcranial approaches, through a lateral-to-medial trajectory, have provided optimal surgical results for tumors along the sphenoid ridges, for lesions of the lateral wall of CS or the resection of the extracavernous temporal, petroclival, supra-cavernous, and suprasellar portions of CS tumors. Contrariwise, in case of intra-cavernous tumors, the transcranial routes are less favorable because of higher risk of cranial nerve deficits and the high rate of morbidity [6, 7]. Moreover, as reported by Larson et al., in the case of CS meningiomas, the evidence of cranial nerve infiltration suggests that total removal inside the CS may be futile and provide no oncological advantage with a high morbidity [6].

For Meckel's, petrous apex and petroclival tumors, the subtemporal approach through Kawase triangle has been shown to provide favorable results for meckel's cave and petrous bone tumors as well as for the resection of the petroclival part of cavernous tumors or petroclival lesions, such as for meningiomas, trigeminal schwannoma, or chondrosarcomas. However, drawbacks of such approach are the soft tissue trauma, the retraction of the temporal lobe, the venous issues, and the risk to damage the inner ear during bone drilling.

In the last decades, the development of endoscopic endonasal techniques has changed the surgical strategies offering new options in term of surgical approach. The natural opening through the nose and the medial-to-lateral trajectory allow access to tumors originating medial to the internal carotid artery (ICA) with invasion of the CS without crossing the cranial nerves decreasing the surgical morbidity. In the same manner, petrous apex tumors can be reach from an endoscopic endonasal approach (EEA) medial or inferomedial to the posterior ascending segment of the cavernous ICA avoiding soft tissue trauma, bone drilling, or extended transcranial approaches [8–12]. In particular, angled endoscopes

A. Fava (✉)
Laboratory of Experimental and Skull Base Neurosurgery, Department of Neurosurgery, Lariboisière Hospital, Paris, France

P. di Russo
Department of Neurosurgery, Lariboisière Hospital, Assistance publique—Hôpitaux de Paris, Paris, France

T. Passeri · L. Giammattei · S. Froelich
Laboratory of Experimental and Skull Base Neurosurgery, Department of Neurosurgery, Lariboisière Hospital, Paris, France

University of Paris Diderot, Paris, France
e-mail: thibault.passeri@curie.fr; sebastien.froelich@aphp.fr

T. L. POON et al. (eds.), *Orbital Apex and Periorbital Skull Base Diseases*, https://doi.org/10.1007/978-981-99-2989-4_21

and dedicated instruments, together with the improvement of endonasal techniques, have helped to push the limits of this corridor.

21.2 Indications and Advantages

Nowadays, endoscopic endonasal techniques have an essential role in the armamentarium of a skull base surgeon who has to decide for a specific patient and pathology, which is the best approach strategy between endoscopic endonasal or transcranial or the combination of both. In general, the EEA represents a suitable choice for:

(a) Pituitary tumors invading CS, such as pituitary adenomas. As a contrary to cavernous meningiomas, the cranial nerves into the CS are most often surrounded by a preserved arachnoid sheath, which offer a protection for the CNs and lower the risk of oculomotor dysfunction (Fig. 21.1c).
(b) Extradural tumors, such as chordomas and chondrosarcomas, extending from the midline or from the petroclival junction to the CS and middle fossa. Chordoma are most often medial and soft and intra-cavernous extension usually pushes the cranial nerves laterally. However, preserving the sixth CN, which is the most frequently impaired cranial nerve and often surrounded by the tumor, remains one of the main challenges. Chondrosarcomas are usually often more lateral, more fibrous, and sometimes highly calcified, being thus more challenging to remove than chordomas.
(c) Cholesterol granulomas of the petrous apex. Most of the cholesterol granuloma cysts bulge in the clival depression of the sphenoid sinus, thus accessible medial or infero-medial to the paraclival ICA.
(d) Trigeminal schwannomas. Tumors located into Meckel's cave are accessible through the quadrangular space or through extensions into infratemporal fossa or sphenopalatine fossa. Even if EEA is a valuable and straightforward option to access trigeminal schwannomas, it remains difficult to predict their consistency as well as the location of the cranial nerves, trigeminal divisions, and ganglion around the tumor.
(e) CS hemangiomas. The vast majority are located between the ICA, medial to the lesion, and the cranial nerves pushed laterally, which make them quite suitable for an EEA. There is most often a single and direct feeder from the intra-cavernous ICA. Once the feeder is controlled along the medial aspect of the tumor lateral to the ICA, the tumor is usually significantly devascularized.
(f) Rare nonadenomatous sellar and parasellar diseases (metastasis, esthesioneuroblastomas).

A fundamental criterion for the choice of the approach is the consistency of the tumor. Soft and suckable lesions are more suitable for an EEA. According to the suspected diagnosis, tumor behavior, its consistency, and its relationship with the ICA and cranial nerves, the goal of EEA varies from maximal resection for oncological purpose, decompression for intra-cavernous tumors causing cranial nerves' deficits, and biopsy in the case of a holocavernous tumor spreading (Fig. 21.1).

Obviously, for each case, patient's characteristics, surgical objectives, anatomical relationships, and variations must be taken into consideration, as described below.

Potential advantages in favor of an EEA to CS and middle fossa include avoidance of soft tissue trauma and craniotomy, a direct trajectory with minimal manipulation of the cranial nerves if the lesion is medial to them and avoidance of brain retraction, which may offer better cosmetic result,

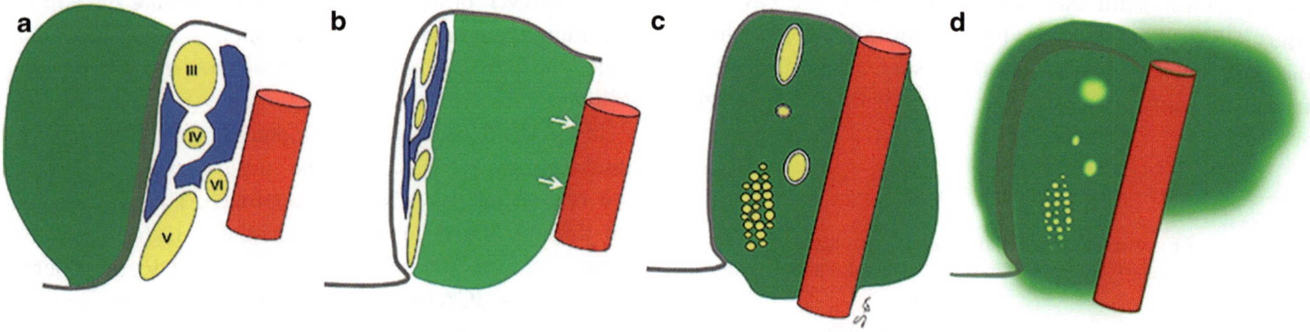

Fig. 21.1 Schematic representation of the various relationship between the tumor and the cavernous sinus. (**a**) Meningioma of the lateral wall of CS: open transcranial approaches are recommended because of the direct access to the tumor without handling with neurovascular structures within the CS. (**b**) Tumor within the CS displacing the ICA laterally and compressing the cranial nerves (chordomas and chondrosarcomas): EEA is a valuable option for maximal safe resection. (**c**) Intra-cavernous tumors surrounding the ICA and cranial nerves but without infiltration of the nerves: in case of soft tumor, EEA may offer a significant tumor reduction, while the nerves remain protected by their arachnoid sheath (pituitary adenomas). (**d**) Holocavernous tumors with cranial nerves infiltration (meningiomas): EEA could be an option for decompression and/or biopsy only

less morbidity, and depending on the lesion and its extension, faster recovery, and shorter hospital stay.

21.3 Contraindications

The perfect approach does not exist, and each surgical corridor carries advantages and drawbacks.

21.3.1 Patient's Characteristics

Previous endonasal surgeries or radiation therapies are important factors to consider before choosing the EEA, particularly in case of intradural pathologies. Previous surgical procedures could modify the usual anatomical landmarks and make the tumor dissection more difficult because of adherences and the skull base reconstruction more challenging. Surgeons must be particularly careful in case of previous radiation therapy, in which the ICA can be more fragile increasing the risk of injuries. Moreover, higher BMI increases the intracranial pressure with a higher risk of postoperative CSF leak.

21.3.2 Anatomy

Considering CS tumors, the exact origin and the pattern of growth are essential factors to consider for the choice of the approach. Tumors originating from the lateral wall of CS or tumors infiltrating the CS from lateral to medial should not be treated using an EEA because of the necessity to work between cranial nerves and the ICA with an associated increased risk of injury. Moreover, ICA encasement remains one of the limitations for EEA.

Tumors of the anterior aspect of the middle fossa extending into the CS, pterygopalatine fossa (PPF), or infratemporal fossa, such as meningiomas and chondrosarcomas, may be considered [13]. However, pro and cons should be carefully considered and balanced with other options such as endoscopic-assisted transcranial techniques or combined strategies.

21.4 Diagnosis and Preoperative Workup

According to the nature and the pattern of growth of the tumor, different clinical presentations can occur. In case of chordomas and chondrosarcomas, with clival and sphenopetroclival epicenters, the posterior aspect of the CS is usually infiltrated first, and diplopia caused by abducens nerve paresis is the most common presenting sign, followed by headache [11, 14–17]. When tumors invade the CS, infiltrating or stretching the nerves, ophtalmoplegia and proptosis can occur. Considering the proximity to the optic nerve, pituitary gland and stalk, visual field impairment, and pituitary dysfunction can also occur [7, 10, 11, 15, 18–22]. Moreover, trigeminal nerve dysfunction can be present with facial numbness or facial pain, particularly in case of middle fossa and Meckel's cave tumors.

CT scan is the first exam to perform to obtain important information about skull base and nasal anatomy, the degree of pneumatization, bone erosion or hyperostosis, and tumor calcifications. MRI study helps to establish a diagnosis and generates high spatial resolution images that allow the visualization of cranial nerves, dura mater, and vessels and to clarify their involvement by adjacent pathology, becoming paramount to define the surgical strategy [23]. T2-weighted images may identify a dural defect through which the tumor extent intradurally, reveal intradural portions, and provide information about the consistency of the tumor (not always completely reliable) [24]. Sequences such as constructive interference in steady-state (CISS) or fast imaging employing steady-state acquisition with phase cycling (FIESTA) are useful to study the cranial nerves trajectory (Fig. 21.2).

CT angiography is recommended to study important vessels, especially the ICA.

In case of total ICA encasement, an angiography with a balloon test occlusion (BTO) may be performed [20], and ICA occlusion may be considered preoperatively in case of high risk of vascular injury (infiltrative lesion, malignancy, previous surgery, previous radiation, highly calcified lesion). In case of vascular tumors, preoperative embolization should also be considered.

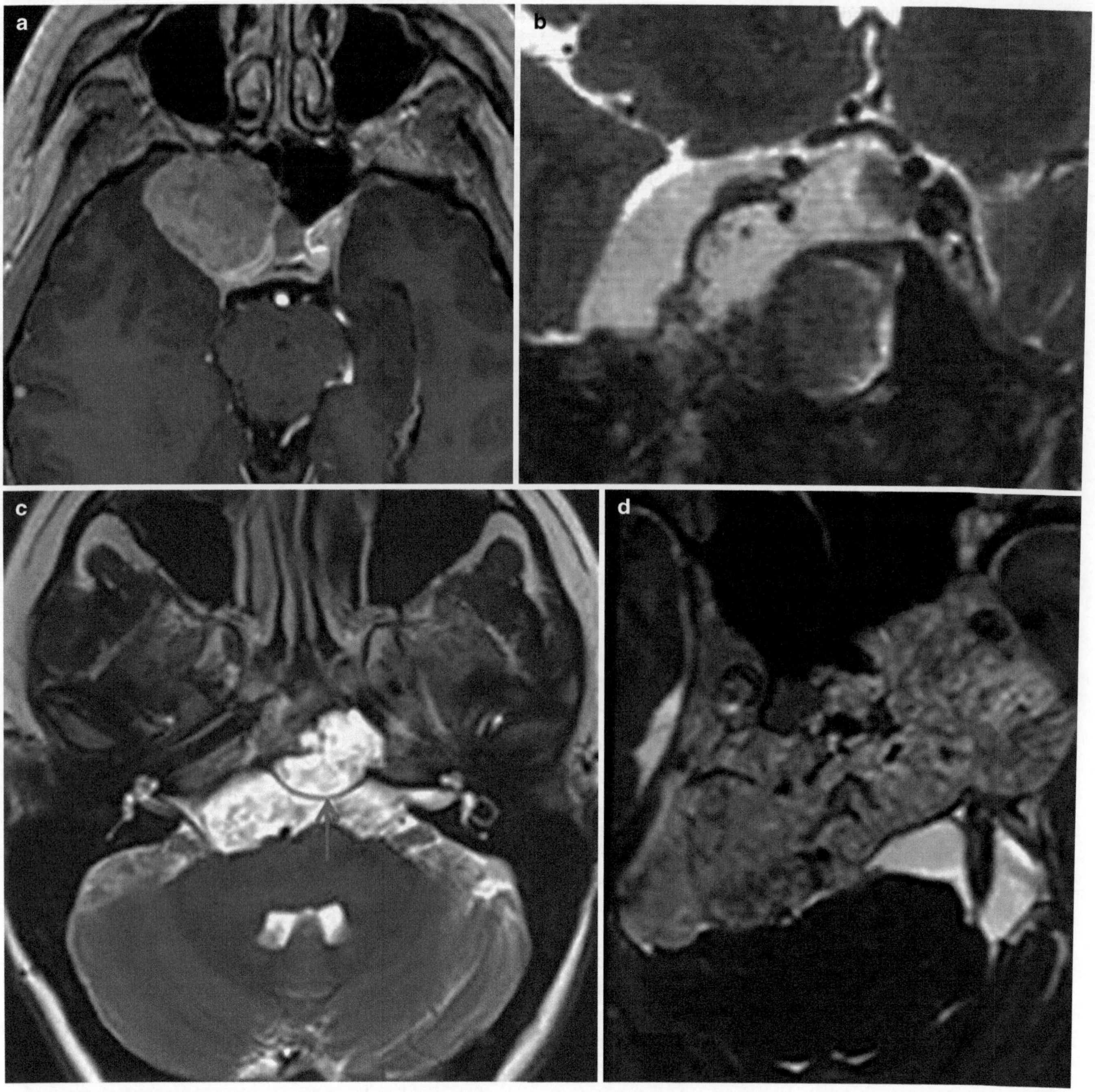

Fig. 21.2 MRI findings to define the best surgical strategy. (**a**) T1-weighted images with gadolinium showing a right trigeminal schwannoma compressing the ICA medially. (**b**) T2-weighted MRI images that highlight the lateral wall of cavernous sinus, which creates a clear demarcation between the extra- and intra-cavernous parts of a cavernous meningiomas. (**c**) T2-weighted MRI image showing a hyperintense intra- and extra-dural chordoma (red arrow: dura mater), suggesting a soft and suckable consistency. (**d**) FIESTA sequence showing the cisternal segment of trigeminal nerve

21.5 Surgery

21.5.1 Instrumentation and Preparation

The patient is placed in the supine position, and the head is fixed in a Mayfield head holder with the head slightly flexed and turned toward the surgeon with slight rotation and lateral inclination. To reduce the venous congestion, the thorax is elevated. The nasal mucosa is decongested with cottonoids soaked with epinephrine. The nasal cavity is cleaned with povidone-iodine solution and the abdomen prepared for the fat harvesting. Reverse Trendenlenbourg position should be anticipated and tested before the surgery in case of profuse venous bleeding from the cavernous sinus or basilar plexuses.

Intraoperative micro-Doppler is used to check the ICA, particularly in case of tumor encasement and second surgeries. Neuronavigation and cranial nerves monitoring are prepared.

In our experience, using the chopstick technique [25], angled endoscopes and instruments and malleable rotating suction are key to perform an EEA taking advantage from a wider visualization field and a higher degree of freedom. 0° endoscope is rarely used. With this technique, the surgeon holds in the same nondominant hand, the endoscope and a rotative malleable suction and in the other hand, a working instrument: rongeur, dissector, scissor, etc. It allows a single surgeon to control all the instruments and to work in an extremely small corridor preserving the normal anatomy and avoiding sword conflict. In fact, a one-nostril approach is most often used to reduce soft tissue trauma and morbidities, and the soft endonasal structures (nostril, inferior turbinate, middle turbinate, etc.) serve as a buttress for the endoscope (Fig. 21.3). Thus, the endoscope rests on the thumb being only supported and not hold with strength, allowing other fingers to control the rotative and malleable suction. One of the main advantages is the ability to have the tip of the endoscope very close to the tip of the working instruments, with limited sword conflict.

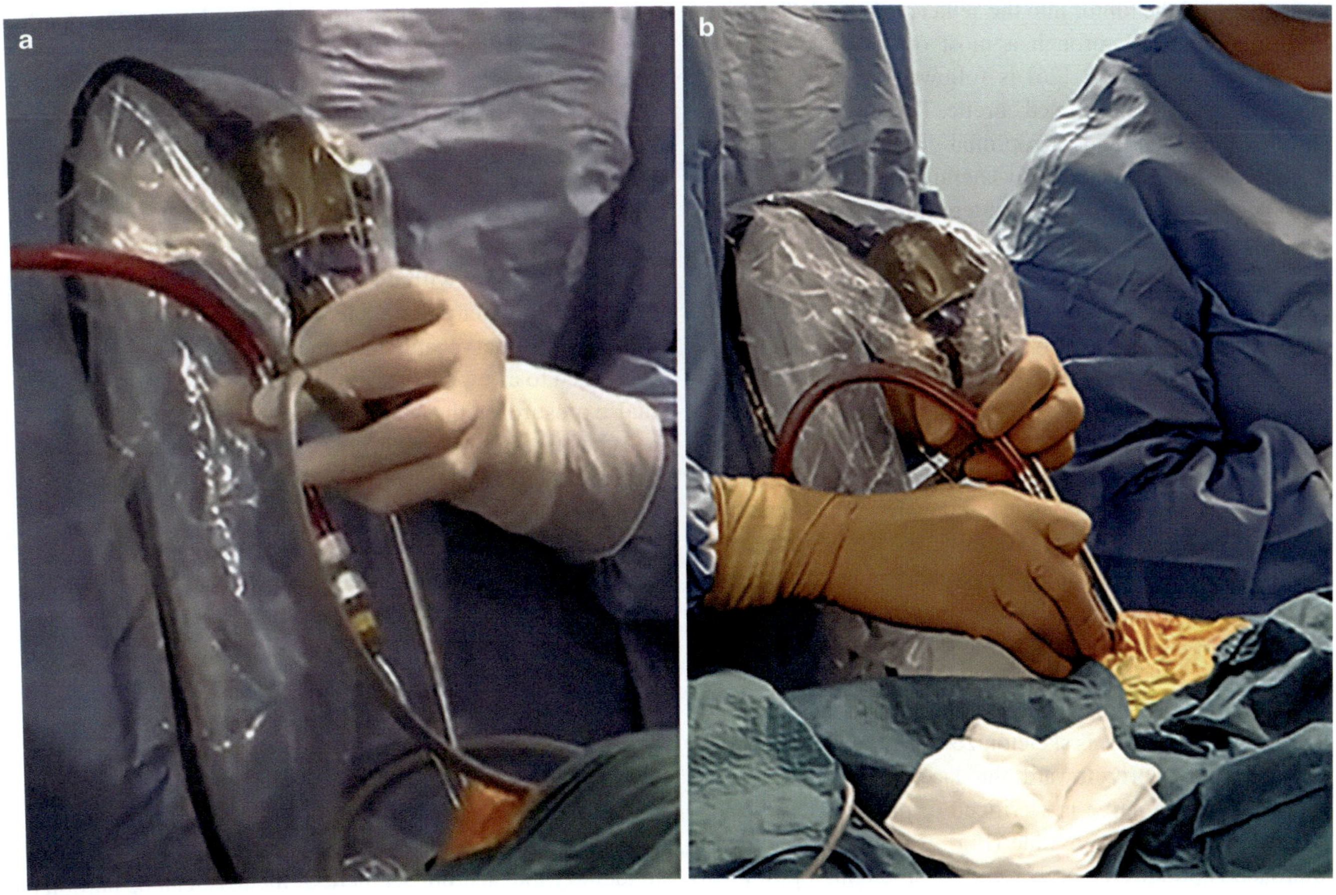

Fig. 21.3 Chopstick's technique. (**a**) The endoscope and the suction can be held in the nondominant hand of the surgeon like chopsticks. A simple rolling motion of the fingers on the rotative shaft with the unused thumb and index allows access to a wide surface of the surgical field with the bended extremity of the malleable suction. (**b**) Surgical example of the technique

21.6 EEA to Cavernous Sinus

The cavernous sinus can be access through a midline or a lateral approach, according to the location of the tumor into the CS and its relationship with the cavernous ICA.

The midline endoscopic transsphenoidal approach is suitable for tumors involving the medial and the posterosuperior compartments of the CS, such as in case of invasive pituitary adenomas or chordomas extending into the CS. Figure 21.4 shows a clinical case of an invasive pituitary adenoma. After the standard transsphenoidal approach to the sella, the floor of the sella and the anterior bony wall of CS (lateral wall of the sphenoid sinus) is removed either with a small kerrison rongeur or a pure diamond drill and the anterior ascending segment of the ICA is exposed. Care is taken to preserve the periosteum intact to avoid venous bleeding and carotid injury. Because of the 2D view and loss of depth perception, it is therefore mandatory, for this step, to have a close look to the tip of the kerrison rongeur, which is one of the advantages provided by the chopstick technique, as there is very limited sword conflict. The periosteum of the sella turcica is then open and the tumor into the sella is removed. The tumor infiltrating the CS through a most often weak or absent medial wall of the CS [26] is followed and resected with malleable suction and angled curette. The angled endoscopes and instruments provide an optimal visualization and working angle during the medial-to-lateral dissection.

When tumors involve the anteroinferior and the lateral compartments of the CS, a more lateral approach should be preferred. After a wide sphenoidotomy, as described above, the transpterygoid approach can be performed starting with the ipsilateral uncinectomy and maxillary antrostomy. To create the corridor, the sphenopalatine artery must be sacrificed. Thus, the nasoseptal flap (NSF) for skull base reconstruction is prepared on the contralateral side. The posterior wall of maxillary sinus is removed preserving the periosteum, which covers the contents of the pterygopalatine fossa (PPF). The PPF is mobilized laterally, and the vidian nerve is identified exiting from the vidian (pterygoid) canal before reaching the sphenopalatine ganglion into the PPF. This nerve represents a reliable landmark for identifying the position of the anterior genu and lacerum segment of the ICA. The vidian canal, situated into the superomedial part of the pterygoid process, is skeletonized, and the vidian nerve is followed posteriorly toward the lacerum segment of the ICA. The vidian nerve is sacrificed or preserved and transposed laterally when possible (Fig. 21.5). If a mononostril approach is preferred, another more challenging option is to harvest the NSF on the same side, which require the section of the vidian nerve in order to mobilize the sphenopalatine artery together with the entire PPF and to store the NSF in the ipsilateral maxillary sinus.

The vidian nerve is often fragile, and the risk of injury is high with the consequence of an ipsilateral dry eye. For this reason, in case of preoperative trigeminal V1 branch impairment or high risk of impairment with tumor resection, (i.e., by tumor) and associated reduction or loss of corneal sensation, it is recommended to avoid the sacrifice of the vidian nerve, which would increase the risk of corneal ulcers. V2 and its branch, the infraorbital nerve, are identified. The bone over the cavernous ICA is now surgically accessible via the lateral sphenoid recess. Depending on the pathology, the ICA can be skeletonized using pure diamond drill to avoid injuries. The micro-doppler is used to identify the ICA behind the periostal layer. The doppler is particularly useful when bony landmarks are missing in case of redo surgery or in case of limited pneumatization of the sphenoid sinus. Finally, the transpterygoid approach allows access to the quadrangular area bordered by the orbital apex antero-superiorly, the opticocarotid recess postero-superiorly, the prominence of V2 antero-inferiorly, and paraclival carotid prominence postero-inferiorly (Fig. 21.6).

If additional inferior exposure is needed during the transpterygoid approach, PPF can be skeletonized and completely transposed laterally en bloc with the preservation of the neurovascular structures within it. The medial wall of PPF, formed by the orbital process and the perpendicular plate of the palatine bone, is removed. Inferiorly, the bone of the greater palatine canal is drilled to freed completely the greater palatine nerve and the descending palatine artery, guaranteeing an adequate lateral mobilization of the PPF without injuries. Superiorly, the vidian nerve is identified and skeletonized, as described above. Finally, the PPF with vidian nerve, descending palatine artery, and greater palatine nerve are transposed laterally en bloc. Vidian nerve and palatine nerve sometimes can be sacrificed to allow further mobilization of the PPF and optimal exposure of the anterior aspect of the pterygoid process. After mobilization, the lateral pterygoid plate is exposed to access the medial aspect of the infratemporal fossa (Figs. 21.5 and 21.6).

However, the transpterygopalatine approach and the endonasal maneuvers required to expose the PPF also carry a risk of morbidity related to the extended approach and resection of normal structures in the nasal cavity. Thus, an oblique line of sight using a contralateral mononostril approach is a more conservative option that, together with the use of angled endoscope, can also provide an adequate exposure of the lateral sphenoid recess of the sphenoid through the rostrum of the sphenoid without a need for a transpterygoid approach. The vidian canal, which is an important landmark to identify the lacerum segment of the ICA, can be unroofed without a need to expose the PPF. The NSF if needed is harvested on the same side of the approach and stored during the surgery in the nasopharynx.

A careful analysis of the penumatisation prior surgery is mandatory to take advantage of it and to avoid useless maneuver.

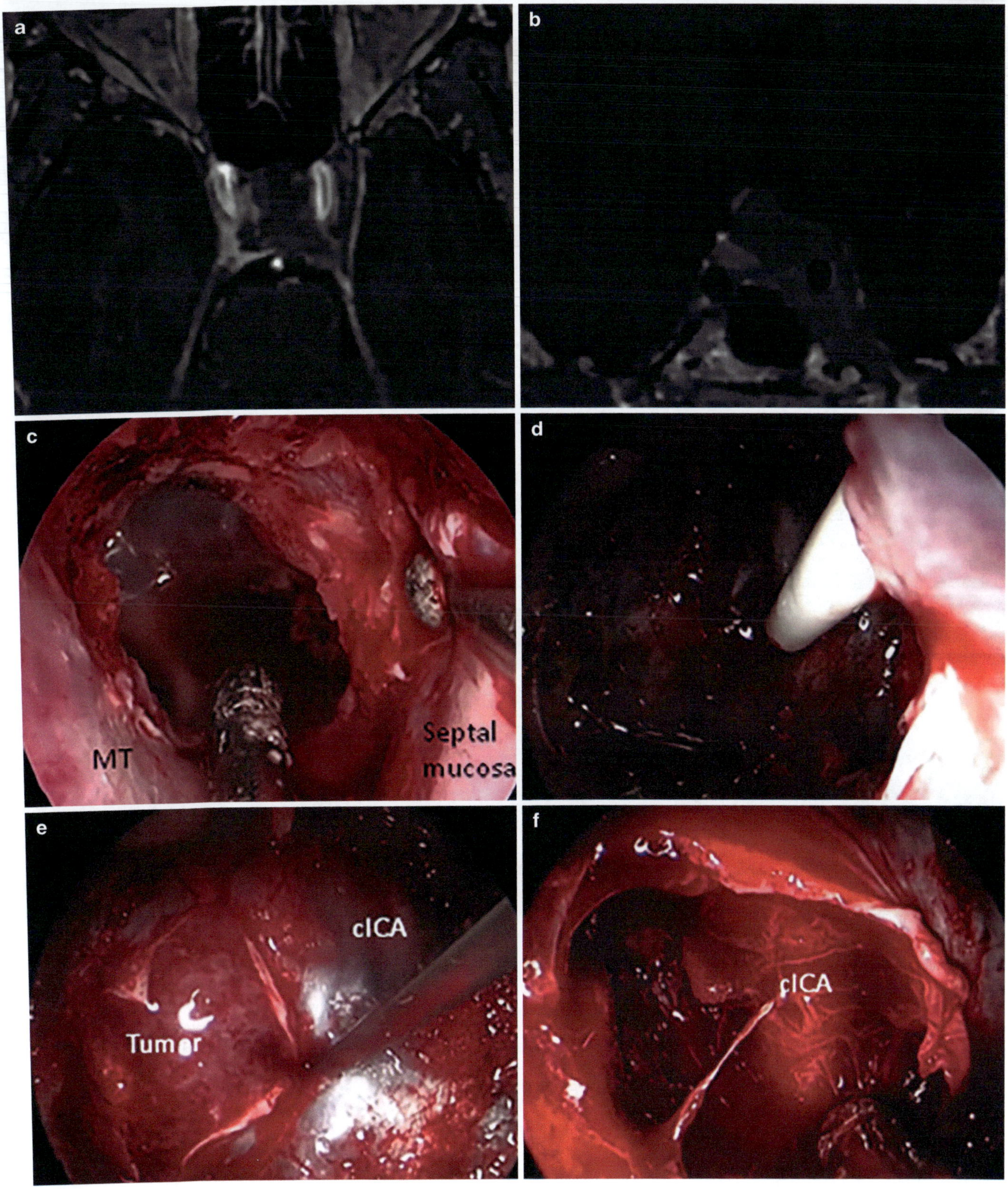

Fig. 21.4 (**a**, **b**) Enhanced T1-weighted MRI images showing a pituitary adenoma invading the left cavernous sinus. (**c**) Standard one-nostril (right side) transsphenoidal approach after drilling the sphenoid rostrum. (**d**) Exposure of the sella and cavernous ICA after drilling the posterior wall of sphenoid sinus. Micro-doppler is used to confirm the position of the left ICA. (**e**) Midline opening of the sellar periosteum with exposure of the tumor. (**f**) Tumor removal from the left CS, around the cavernous ICA with angled-endoscope and curved suction. *MT* middle turbinate, *cICA* cavernous segment of ICA

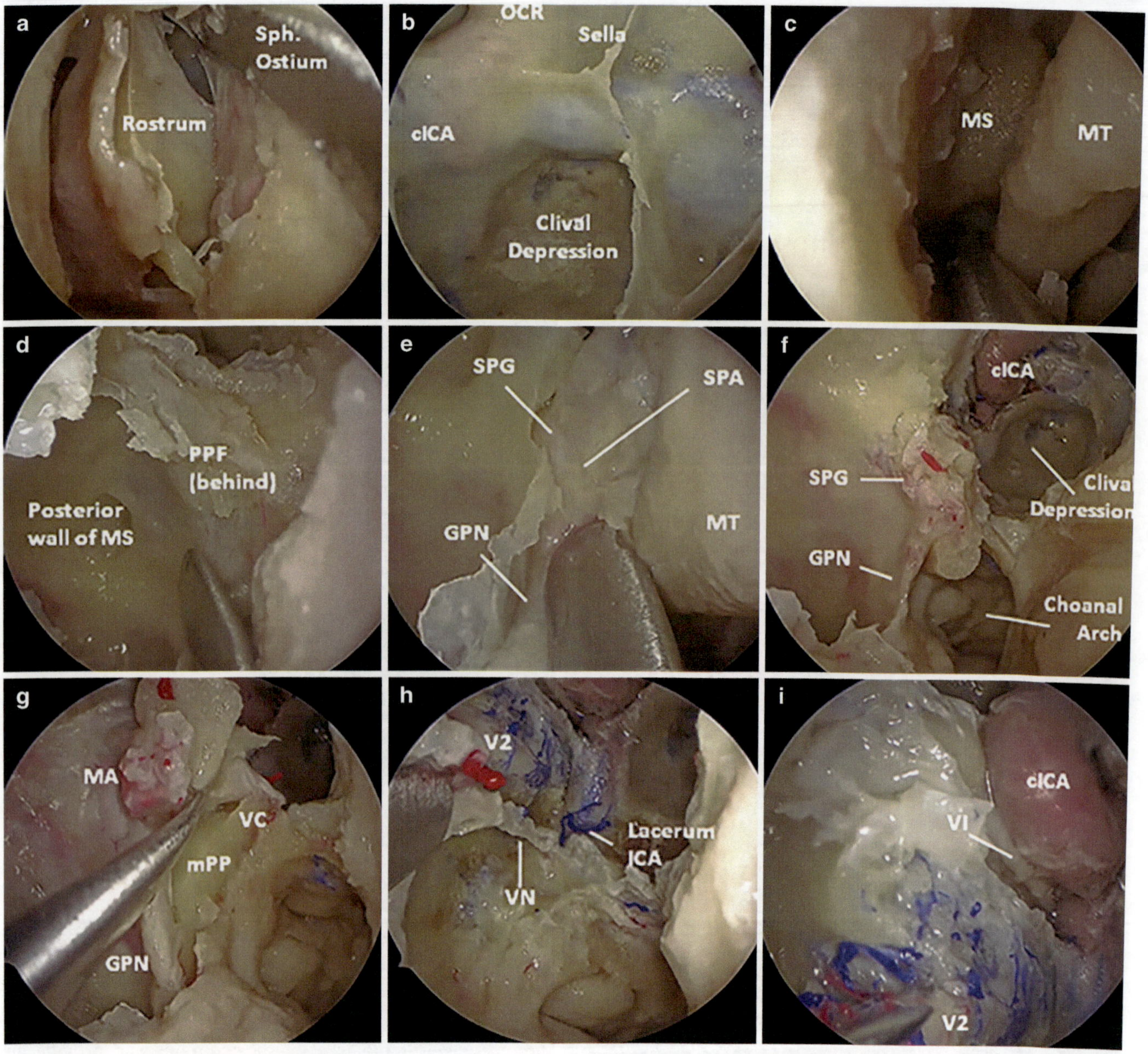

Fig. 21.5 Step-by-step cadaveric dissection of EEA for the anteroinferior and lateral compartments of cavernous sinus. (**a**) Rostral mucosa incision and rostrum exposure. (**b**) Posterior wall of the sphenoid sinus after SS opening. (**c**) Lateralization of middle turbinate with exposure of the medial wall of MS. (**d**) MS with identification of PPF behind the posterior wall of MS. (**e**) Identification of SPG and SPA medially and GPN inferiorly. (**f, g**) Skeletonization of the PPF with its lateralization identifying the medial PP and the VC. (**h**) Drilling of the medial PP with skeletonization of the VN identifying lacerum segment of the ICA. (**i**) Exposure of the anteroinferior and lateral compartments ofCS. *MS* maxillary sinus, *PPF* pterygopalatine fossa, *SPG* sphenopalatine ganglion, *SPA* sphenopalatine artery, *GPN* greater palatine nerve, *mPP* medial pterygoid plate, *VC* vidian canal, *VN* vidian nerve

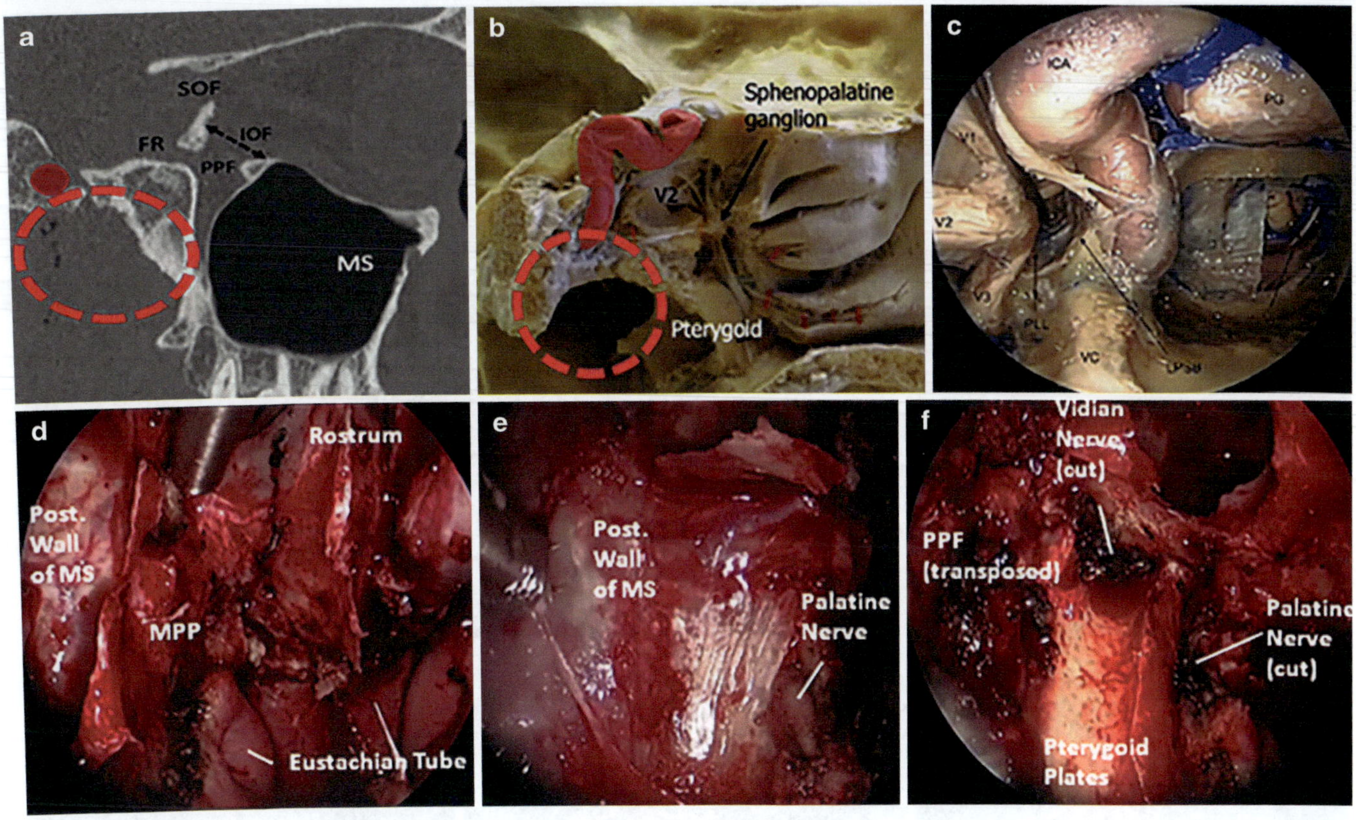

Fig. 21.6 Representation of the PPF in a sagittal CT scan (**a**) and in a cadaveric specimen (**b**). (**c**) Cadaveric dissection showing the quadrangular area to access the inferior and lateral portion of the CS and petrous apex. (**d**–**f**) Transpterygoid approach with lateralization of the PPF after vidian and palatine nerve section exposing the anterior aspect of the pterygoid process. *MS* Maxillary sinus, *MPP* medial pterygoid plate, *PG* pituitary gland, *VC* vidian canal

21.7 EEA to Middle Fossa

21.7.1 Medial Petrous Apex

The infrapetrous approach is ideal for extradural lesions centered on petrous apex such as cholesterol granulomas and cholesteatomas. The key points of the approach are the exposure of the lacerum segment of the ICA and the lateral mobilization of the posterior ascending of the ICA to access the underlying petrous bone. Firstly, a wide sphenoidectomy is performed, and then the sphenoid floor is drilled. A posterior maxillary antrostomy is performed, and the PPF is exposed. The vidian canal is identified and unroofed leading to the lacerum segment of the ICA as its petrous portion turns vertical. Depending on the medial extension of the lesion, it may be needed, in order to access it, to drill the bone lateral to the ICA in order to be able to mobilize it laterally. Once the ICA is slightly displaced laterally, the underlying lesion into the petrous apex can be exposed (Figs. 21.7 and 21.8).

As described above, 45°- or 75°-angled endoscopes, malleable rotating aspirators and angled instruments can be used in order to access and remove the lesion reducing the extension of the approach, the need for paraclival ICA mobilization and the related risks of vascular injury (Fig. 21.9).

Moreover, the contralateral nostril approach as described above also provides a more adequate line of sight for the petrous apex.

Similarly, a recent study [27] has described the contralateral transmaxillary (CTM) corridor to extend the lateral trajectory and improve access for petrous apex tumors while reducing the morbidity associated with manipulation of the paraclival ICA.

21.7.2 Middle Fossa

To access the middle fossa, the transpterygoid approach is performed, as described previously in case of lesions of lateral compartment of CS. Once the PPF contents are lateralized, V2 and FR are identified. FR is then drilled and opened. Then, moving posteriorly and inferiorly through the pterygoid wedge, the foramen ovale (FO) is identified and V3 exposed. The anterolateral triangle between V2 and V3 is drilled to expose the temporal fossa dura.

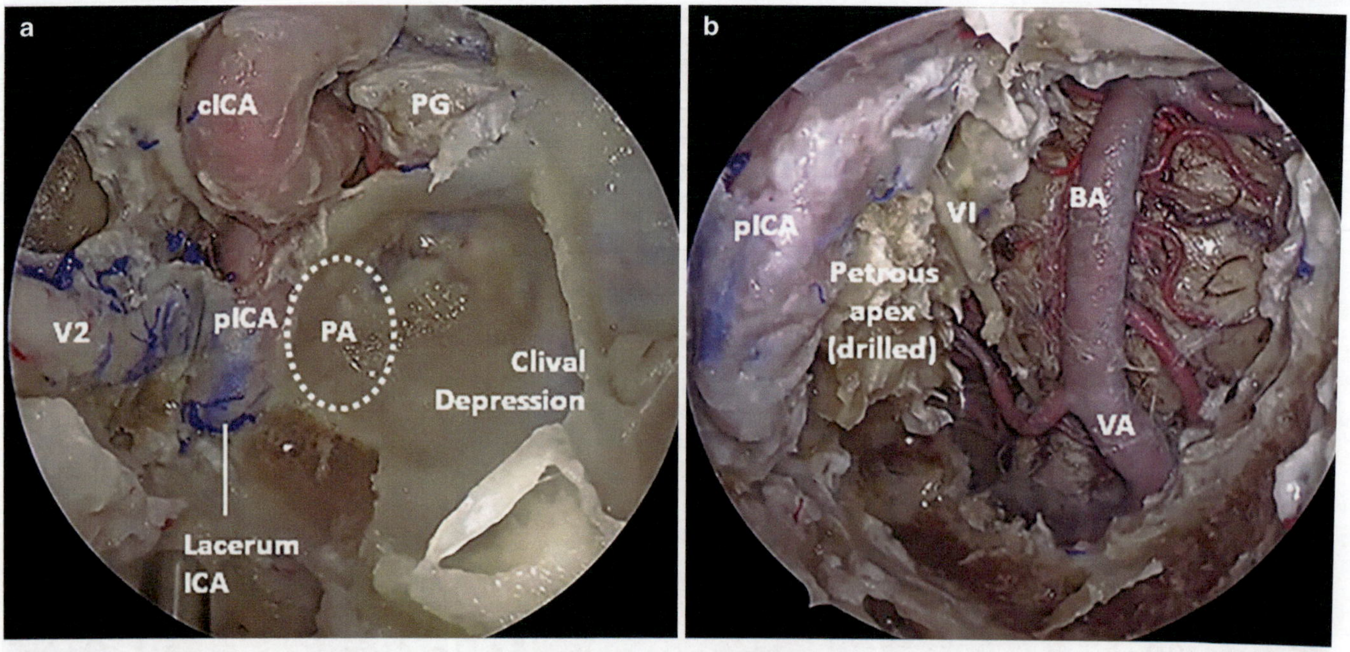

Fig. 21.7 Cadaveric dissection showing (**a**) the corridor to access the petrous apex after a transpterygoid approach and (**b**) the relationship between intra- and extra-dural compartment after ICA lateralization, petrous apex drilling and dura opening. *cICA* cavernous ICA, *pICA* paraclival ICA, *PG* pituitary gland, *PA* petrous apex, *BA* basilar artery, *VA* vertebral artery

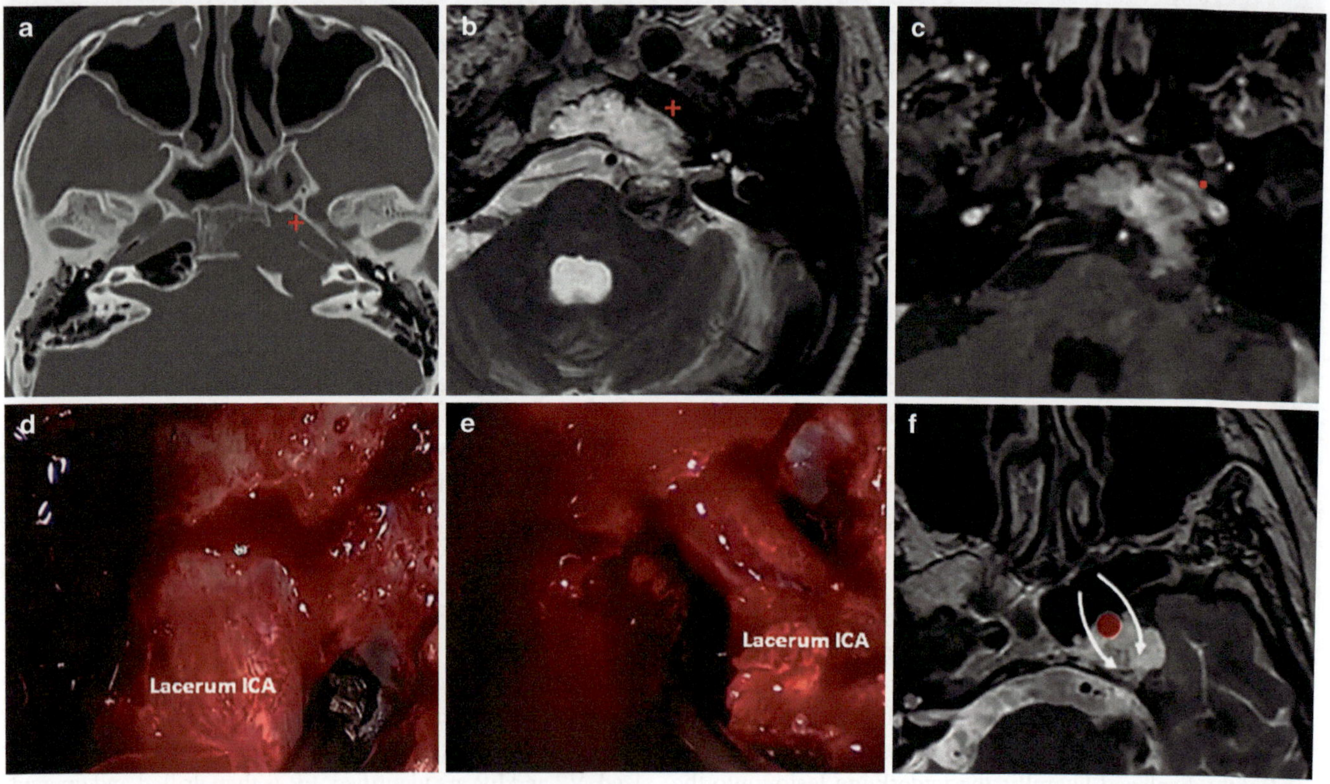

Fig. 21.8 (**a–c**) Axial CT scan, T2-weighted, and enhanced T1-weighted MRI images showing a left-side petrous apex chondrosarcoma extending from the petrous apex to the jugular foramen behind the petrous (red cross) and lacerum (red dot) segment of ICA. (**d–f**) A transpterygoid approach was performed with the mobilization of the ICA working on both side of the artery as illustrated in the axial MRI (**f**) (white arrows, red point: ICA)

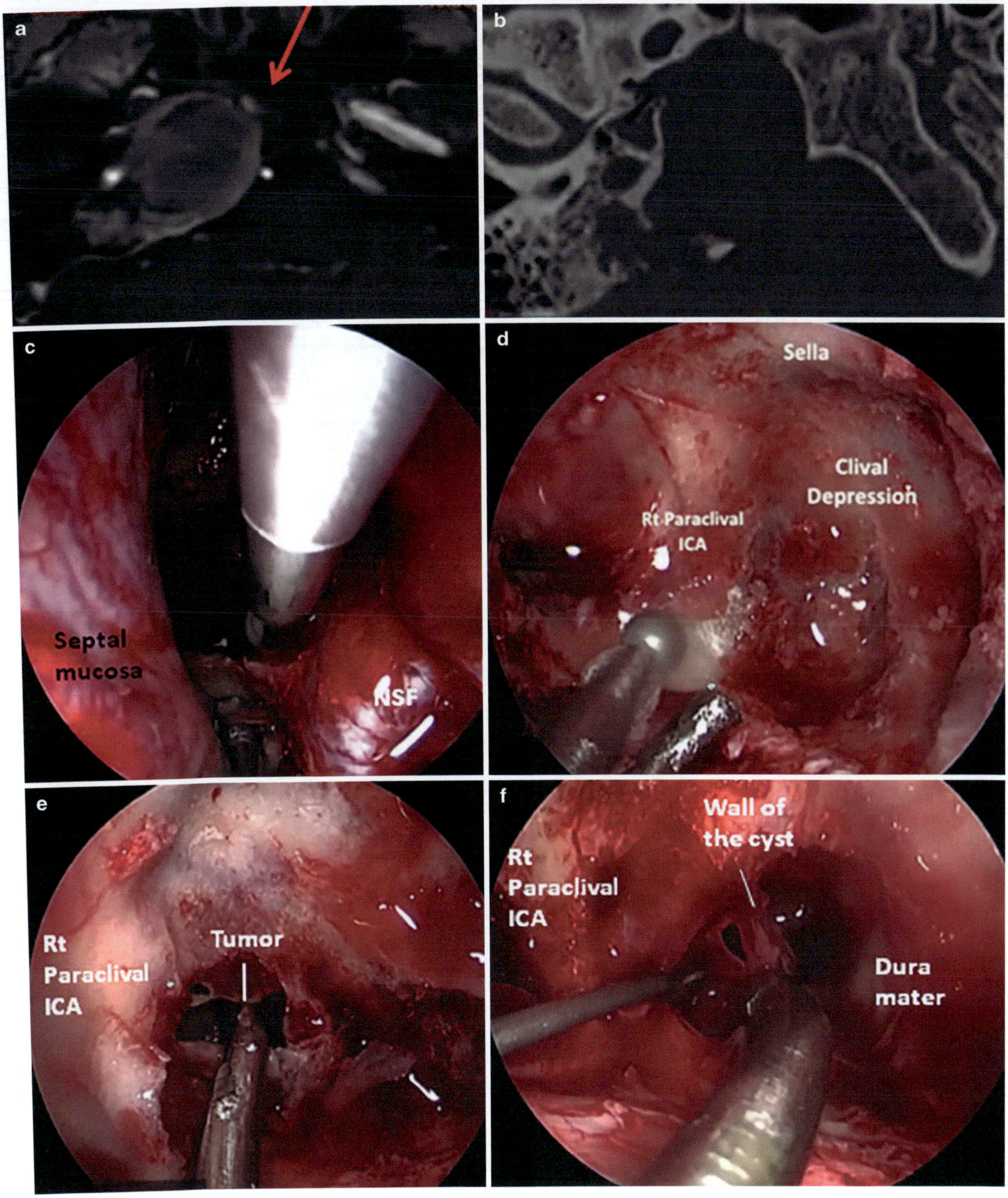

Fig. 21.9 (**a**, **b**) Axial MRI image and CT scan showing a right-side cholesterol granuloma of petrous apex. A contralateral one-nostril approach was performed (red arrow) from the left to the right side in order to have a better angle of attack for the petrous apex without a need for paraclival ICA lateralization. (**c**) Drilling of the sphenoidal rostrum after preparation of the NSF. (**d**) left-to-right view with an angled endoscope exposing the bone covering the right paraclival ICA and the sella. (**e**) Drilling of the bone corresponding to the petrous apex, medial and posterior to the paraclival ICA and lateral to the clival depression. (**f**) Tumor debulking and removal of the cyst wall using the chopstick techniques and angled instruments

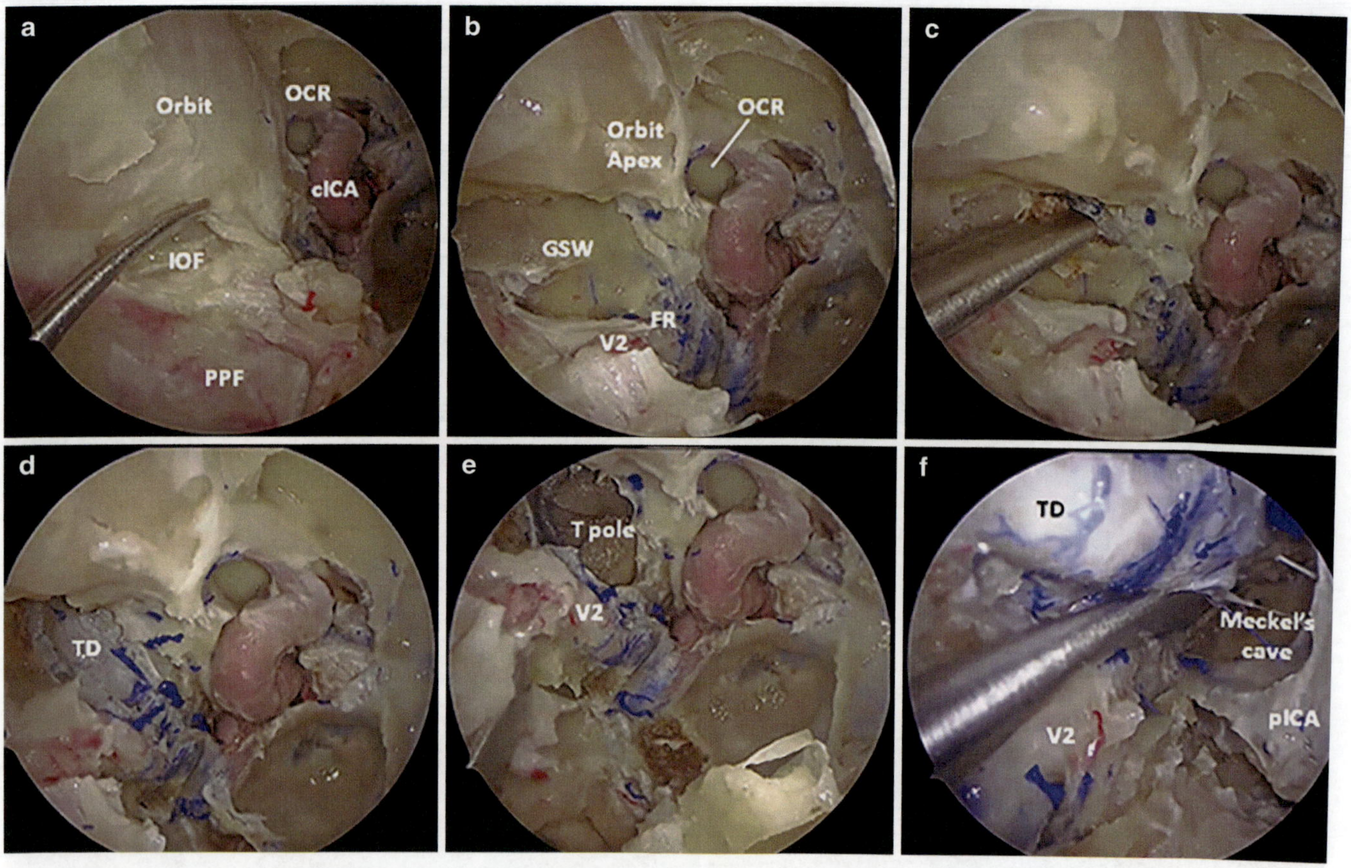

Fig. 21.10 Cadaveric dissection showing middle fossa and Meckel's cave exposure. (**a**) Identification of the PPF and orbit (after the removal of the lamina papyracea) separated by the IOF. (**b**) Identification of V2 into FR following the infraorbital nerve into the PPF and exposure of the GSW. (**c**–**f**) Exposure of the temporal dura and Meckel's cave after GSW removal. *OCR* opticocarotid recess, *IOF* inferior orbital fissure, *FR* foramen rotondum, *TD* temporal dura, *T pole* temporal pole

Recently, our group [13] has described an endoscopic endonasal technique to expose the antero-medial temporal fossa and the lateral wall of CS, by approaching these regions more laterally through a corridor between the orbital apex, and the superior orbital fissure (SOF) superiorly and V2 inferiorly. This technique is a lateral extension of the EEA to the CS, wherein the greater wing of sphenoid and temporal fossa dura are exposed through the inferior orbital fissure. The surgical steps are as follow: partial anterior ethmoidectomy and posterior ethmoidectomy to expose the lamina papyracea, antrostomy to expose the posterior wall of the maxillary sinus, removal of the lamina papyracea and the posterior wall of the maxillary sinus to expose the orbit and PPF, opening of the SOF and FR unroofing, drilling of the maxillary strut (between V1 and V2), resection of the orbital muscle of Muller, exposure and resection of the greater wing of sphenoid, peeling of the outer layer of the lateral wall of the CS, and opening of the dura matter.

Frequently, middle fossa tumors displace the trigeminal nerve superiorly and laterally allowing for a direct corridor. Dural opening is performed below the abducens nerve and laterally to the ICA. Tumor removal can continue with a posterior and lateral trajectory through the Meckel's cave, the petrous bone, and into the posterior fossa as required (Figs. 21.10 and 21.11).

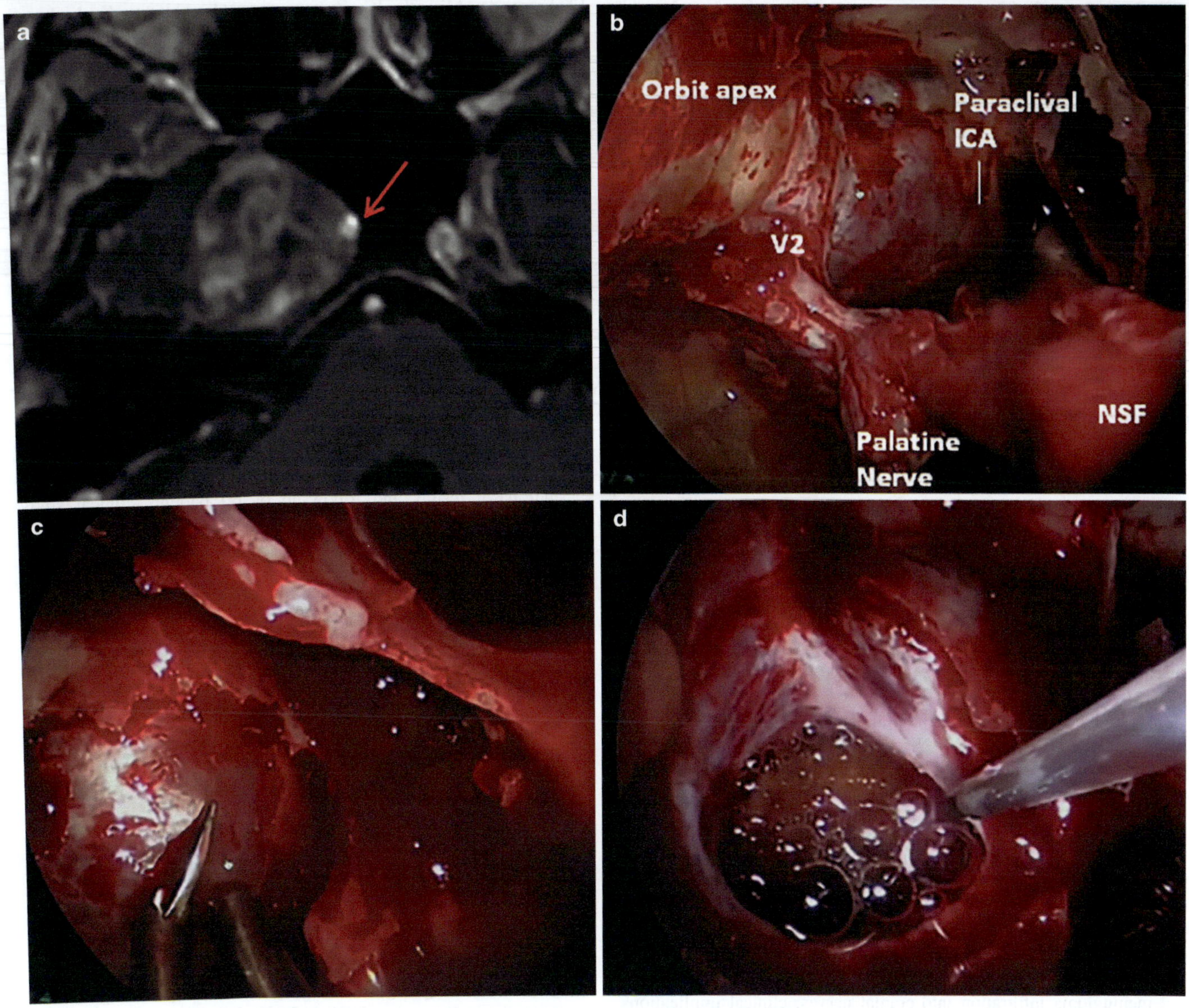

Fig. 21.11 (**a**) MRI image showing a right-side trigeminal schwannoma bulging into the sphenoid sinus and displacing the paraclival ICA. (**b**, **c**) Preparation of the NSF. Removal of the posterior wall of maxillary sinus and identification of PPF, V2 and orbital apex. The paraclival ICA is identified with the micro-doppler, and the periosteum is incised to enter and remove the tumor. (**d**) Closure with fat graft and fibrin glue

21.8 Closure

In case of tumors showing a large dural invasion and intradural component, the risk of CSF leak increases significantly and even more in case of recurrent tumor. Several reconstruction techniques have been described [9] such as the nasoseptal flap (NSF) [28], multilayer vascularized technique [29], Gasket Seal technique [30], and temporo-parietal fascia flap [31]. Recently, the 3F (Fat, Flap, Flash) technique [32] have demonstrated that not only an accurate closure is essential to reduce CSF leak but also an early control of the intracranial pressure with fast patient mobilization. Nevertheless, effective dural reconstruction remains the main issue for EEA, and postoperative CSF leak represents a serious risk for the patient.

Recently, our group [33] have described a new reconstruction strategy, applying to EEAs, the initial and final steps of transcranial approaches: skin opening and closure. The key concept is to consider the mucosa of the rostrum as a main barrier to close, similar to the skin in transcranial approaches, which is closed at the end of surgery. The mucosa of the rostrum can be incised in different fashion to expose the bone and open the sphenoid sinus, and it can be then sutured at the end of the procedure, after cranialization of the SS, as the physiological barrier to prevent CSF leak.

21.9 Conclusions

In the last decade, the refinement and the advances in endoscopic endonasal instrumentation and techniques have pushed the limits of endoscopic skull base surgery moving from medial transphenoidal approaches to more lateral, inferior, and posterior corridors. The decision for the best surgical approach should take into consideration multiple factors: patient characteristics, goal of the surgery, localization and consistency of the lesion, and relationship with critical neurovascular structures. The medial-to-lateral corridor created with endoscopic endonasal approaches has changed the surgical indications, making sometimes feasible tumor resection within "holy" compartments like cavernous sinus with a reduced morbidity. Confidence with angled scopes (30°, 45°, and 70°) and flexible and rotating instruments is fundamental to tailor the approach to laterally located lesions and reduce the surgical footprint.

References

1. Parkinson D. A surgical approach to the cavernous portion of the carotid artery. Anatomical studies and case report. J Neurosurg. 1965;23(5):474–83.
2. Dolenc VV. Transcranial epidural approach to pituitary tumors extending beyond the sella. Neurosurgery. 1997;41(3):542–52.
3. Kawase T, Shiobara R, Toya S. Anterior transpetrosal-transtentorial approach for sphenopetroclival meningiomas: surgical method and results in 10 patients. Neurosurgery. 1991;28(6):866–9.
4. Hakuba A, Tanaka K, Suzuki T, Nishimura S. A combined orbitozygomatic infratemporal epidural and subdural approach for lesions involving the entire cavernous sinus. J Neurosurg. 1989;71(5 Pt 1):699–704.
5. Dolenc V. Direct microsurgical repair of intracavernous vascular lesions. J Neurosurg. 1983;58(6):824–31.
6. Larson JJ, van Loveren HR, Balko MG, Tew JMJ. Evidence of meningioma infiltration into cranial nerves: clinical implications for cavernous sinus meningiomas. J Neurosurg. 1995;83(4):596–9.
7. Pamir MN, Kilic T, Özek MM, Özduman K, Türe U. Non-meningeal tumours of the cavernous sinus: a surgical analysis. J Clin Neurosci. 2006;13(6):626–35.
8. Fraser JF, Nyquist GG, Moore N, Anand VK, Schwartz TH. Endoscopic endonasal transclival resection of chordomas: operative technique, clinical outcome, and review of the literature—clinical article. J Neurosurg. 2010;112(5):1061–9.
9. Wang EW, Zanation AM, Gardner PA, Schwartz TH, Eloy JA, Adappa ND, et al. ICAR: endoscopic skull-base surgery. Int Forum Allergy Rhinol. 2019;9(S3):S145–365.
10. Patrona A, Patel KS, Bander ED, Mehta A, Tsiouris AJ, Anand VK, et al. Endoscopic endonasal surgery for nonadenomatous, non-meningeal pathology involving the cavernous sinus. J Neurosurg. 2017;126(3):880–8.
11. Koutourousiou M, Vaz Guimaraes Filho F, Fernandez-Miranda JC, Wang EW, Stefko ST, Snyderman CH, et al. Endoscopic endonasal surgery for tumors of the cavernous sinus: a series of 234 patients. World Neurosurg [Internet]. 2017;103:713–732. https://doi.org/10.1016/j.wneu.2017.04.096.
12. Fernandez-Miranda JC, Zwagerman NT, Abhinav K, Lieber S, Wang EW, Snyderman CH, et al. Cavernous sinus compartments from the endoscopic endonasal approach: anatomical considerations and surgical relevance to adenoma surgery. J Neurosurg. 2018;129(2):430–41.
13. Hanakita S, Chang W-C, Watanabe K, Ronconi D, Labidi M, Park H-H, et al. Endoscopic endonasal approach to the anteromedial temporal fossa and mobilization of the lateral wall of the cavernous sinus through the inferior orbital fissure and V1-V2 corridor: an anatomic study and clinical considerations. World Neurosurg. 2018;116:e169–78.
14. George B, Bresson D, Herman P, Froelich S. Chordomas: a review. Neurosurg Clin N Am. 2015;26(3):437–52.
15. Arnold H, Herrmann HD. Skull base chordoma with cavernous sinus involvement. partial or radical tumour-removal? Acta Neurochir (Wien). 1986;51:48–51.
16. Almefty K, Pravdenkova S, Colli BO, Al-Mefty O, Gokden M. Chordoma and chondrosarcoma: similar, but quite different, skull base tumors. Cancer. 2007;110(11):2467–77.
17. Gay E, Sekhar LN, Rubinstein E, Wright DC, Sen C, Janecka IP, Snyderman CH. Chordomas and chondrosarcomas of the cranial base: results and follow-up of 60 patients clinical study. Neurosurgery. 1997.
18. Al-Mefty O. Chordoma. Acta Neurochir (Wien). 2017;159(10):1869–71.
19. Goel A, Muzumdar DP, Nitta J. Surgery on lesions involving cavernous sinus. J Clin Neurosci. 2001;4:71–7.
20. Lanzino G, Sekhar LN, Hirsch WL, Sen CN, Pomonis S, Snyderman CH. Chordomas and chondrosarcomas involving the cavernous sinus: review of surgical treatment and outcome in 31 patients. Surg Neurol. 1993;40(5):359–71.
21. Wanebo JE, Bristol RE, Porter RR, Coons SW, Spetzler RF. Management of cranial base chondrosarcomas. Neurosurgery. 2006;58(2):249–54.
22. Zada G. Atlas of sellar and parasellar lesions. 2016.
23. Zamora C, Castillo M. Sellar and parasellar imaging. Neurosurgery. 2017;80(1):17–38.
24. Yao A, Pain M, Balchandani P, Shrivastava RK. Can MRI predict meningioma consistency?: a correlation with tumor pathology and systematic review. Neurosurg Rev. 2018;41(3):745–53.
25. Labidi M, Watanabe K, Hanakita S, Park HH, Bouazza S, Bernat AL, et al. The chopsticks technique for endoscopic endonasal surgery—improving surgical efficiency and reducing the surgical footprint. World Neurosurg. 2018;117:208–20.
26. Kehrli P, Ali M, Reis M, Maillot C, Dujovny M, Ausman J, et al. Anatomy and embryology of the lateral sellar compartment (cavernous sinus) medial wall Anatomy and embryology of the lateral sellar compartment (cavernous sinus) medial wall. 2017;6412(February).
27. Patel CR, Wang EW, Fernandez-Miranda JC, Gardner PA, Snyderman CH. Contralateral transmaxillary corridor: an augmented endoscopic approach to the petrous apex. J Neurosurg. 2018;129(1):211–9.
28. Kassam AB, Thomas A, Carrau RL, Snyderman CH, Vescan A, Prevedello D, et al. Endoscopic reconstruction of the cranial base using a pedicled nasoseptal flap. Neurosurgery. 2008;63(1 Suppl 1):ONS44–52; discussion ONS52-3.
29. Simal-Julián JA, Miranda-Lloret P, de San Román Mena LP, Sanromán-Álvarez P, García-Piñero A, Sanchis-Martín R, et al. Impact of multilayer vascularized reconstruction after skull base endoscopic endonasal approaches. J Neurol Surg B Skull Base. 2020;81(2):128–35.
30. Garcia-Navarro V, Anand VK, Schwartz TH. Gasket seal closure for extended endonasal endoscopic skull base surgery: efficacy in a large case series. World Neurosurg. 2013;80(5):563–8.

31. Thomas R, Girishan S, Chacko AG. Endoscopic transmaxillary transposition of temporalis flap for recurrent cerebrospinal fluid leak closure. J Neurol Surg B Skull Base. 2016;77(6): 445–8.
32. Cavallo LM, Solari D, Somma T, Cappabianca P. The 3F (fat, flap, and flash) technique for skull base reconstruction after endoscopic endonasal suprasellar approach. World Neurosurg. 2019;126:439–46.
33. di Russo P, Fava A, Giammattei L, Passeri T, Okano A, Abbritti R, et al. The rostral mucosa: the door to open and close for targeted endoscopic endonasal approaches to the clivus. Oper Neurosurg (Hagerstown). 2021;21(3):150–9.

Endoscopic Endonasal Approach to the Infratemporal Fossa

22

Stefan Lieber and Sébastien Froelich

Abstract

The infratemporal and pterygopalatine fossae are anatomically and functionally linked and highly significant for skull base surgery and other specialties including otolaryngology, ophthalmology, maxillofacial surgery, and radiation oncology due to their central location and their extensive connections with neighboring skull base regions. Endoscopic surgery is rendered possible by advanced endoscopic instrumentation, dependable strategies for closure and reconstruction, and an intimate knowledge of the surgical anatomy; this holds particularly true for the complex anatomical contents of the pterygopalatine and infratemporal fossae. Four figures have been included in this chapter with the aim to provide a review of the relevant anatomy, to identify reliable surgical landmarks, and to illustrate the surgical steps of the expanded endoscopic endonasal transpterygoid-transmaxillary approach to the pterygopalatine and infratemporal fossae (Figs. 22.1, 22.2, 22.3, and 22.4).

Keywords

Endoscopic endonasal approach · Transpterygoid approach · Transmaxillary approach · Infratemporal fossa · Pterygopalatine fossa · Skull base · Coronal plane · Maxillary artery · Sphenopalatine artery · Medial maxillectomy · Transantral approach · Trigeminal schwannoma · Juvenile angiofibroma · Sinonasal carcinoma

S. Lieber (✉) · S. Froelich
Department of Neurosurgery, Lariboisière Hospital, University of Paris, Paris, France
e-mail: Stefan.Lieber@aphp.fr

22.1 Introduction

The infratemporal fossa (ITF) is a deep-seated, retromaxillary space that contains the pterygoid muscles, the maxillary artery with its branches, the mandibular division of the trigeminal nerve with its branches, the otic ganglion, and the pterygoid venous plexus [1–8]. It is bounded by the lateral pterygoid plate medially, the posterolateral surface of the maxillary sinus anteriorly, the infratemporal crest laterally, and the mandibular fossa posterolaterally. The roof of the infratemporal fossa is formed by the greater wing of the sphenoid bone, posteromedially it is separated from the post-styloid compartment of the parapharyngeal space by the stylopharyngeal and sphenopharyngeal fasciae; the plane of these fasciae largely corresponds to the petrosphenoidal fissure.

Functionally and anatomically, the infratemporal fossa is closely linked to the pterygopalatine fossa (PPF), a small space in the shape of an inverted quadrangular pyramid, which is located at the angle of the inferior orbital and pterygomaxillary fissures. The pterygopalatine fossa accommodates terminal branches of the maxillary artery, the Vidian nerve, the maxillary division of the trigeminal nerve, and the pterygopalatine ganglion. The pterygopalatine fossa represents a critical crossroad of the skull base as it communicates with the orbit (via the orbital apex and the posteromedial segment of the inferior orbital fissure), the nasal cavity (via the sphenopalatine foramen), the middle cranial fossa (via the foramen rotundum, and the Vidian canal), the nasopharynx (via the palatosphenoidal canal), and the oropharynx (via the greater and lesser pterygopalatine canals). It is in continuum with the infratemporal fossa through the pterygomaxillary fissure which in turn communicates with the orbit (via the anteromedial segment of the inferior orbital fissure), the middle cranial fossa (via the foramen ovale, spinosum, and venosum Vesalii), and the parapharyngeal space [9–17]. Pathological processes and neoplasms can arise primarily or extend into the infratemporal fossa from these adjacent

T. L. POON et al. (eds.), *Orbital Apex and Periorbital Skull Base Diseases*, https://doi.org/10.1007/978-981-99-2989-4_22

regions and include vascular tumors such as juvenile nasopharyngeal angiofibroma and hemangiopericytoma, meningioma with extracranial extension, schwannoma originating primarily from the extracranial portion of the mandibular nerve, lymphoproliferative disorders, and sinonasal carcinoma [18–20].

Numerous surgical corridors to the infratemporal fossa have been described, among them the anterior transmaxillary approach (Le Fort I and II osteotomies with a sublabial or facial incision), the transmandibular approach (requiring a facial degloving), the transcranial extension of the fronto-temporo-orbito-zygomatic approach (through the anterolateral triangle and the middle cranial fossa floor), and the lateral transtemporal approaches (Fisch type A-C) [21–28]. While a comprehensive review of all these approaches is beyond the scope of this chapter, some are discussed elsewhere in this volume (Chap. 22: transcranial approaches, and Chap. 25: endoscopic transorbital approaches).

This chapter addresses the endoscopic endonasal approach to the pterygopalatine and infratemporal fossae. Expanded endoscopic approaches (EEA) have become an important part in the armamentarium of skull base surgeons and can be classified into approach modules in the sagittal plane (cranio-caudal) and coronal plane (medio-lateral).

Extended endoscopic approaches to the paramedian skull base, including the transpterygoid-transmaxillary approach to the PPF and ITF, are approaches of minimal access but rarely of minimally invasiveness [6, 19]. However, they avoid the cosmetic and (at least partially) the functional morbidity associated with more traditional open approaches, shorten postoperative recovery time, and thereby accelerate transition to adjuvant radiotherapy. EEAs provide a well-illuminated, magnified, and multiangled view for safe and effective manipulation of tissues in a deep-seated region, and thereby maximize the probability of complete resection.

The expanded transpterygoid-transmaxillary approach entails the following steps:

- Exposure of the maxillary sinus
- Identification of the sphenopalatine artery
- Removal of the posterior wall of the maxillary sinus
- Removal of the perpendicular plate and the pyramidal process of the palatine bone
- Exposure of the periosteum wrapping the content of the pterygopalatine fossa
- Identification of the Vidian and maxillary nerve
- Identification of vascular structures (branches of the maxillary artery)
- Transposition or removal of the contents of the pterygopalatine fossa
- Removal of the pterygoid base with transposition or transection of the Vidian nerve
- Closure and reconstruction

22.2 Principles of Approach Selection, Modifications, and Limitations

Although the initial steps are similar, each surgical target requires slight modification to the endoscopic endonasal transpterygoid-transmaxillary approach for access to the PPT and ITF. These modifications largely depend on the topography, morphology, and anticipated pathology of the targeted lesion, the patient's individual anatomy and preexisting loss of function, and the skull base surgeon's preference and experience.

For resection of malignant tumors, adequate surgical exposure should not be compromised by efforts to limit the invasiveness of the approach or by concerns for subsequent loss of sinonasal function since insufficient maneuverability, and loss of visualization and control over tumor margins invariably hampers oncologic integrity of the resection [18–20].

The addition of a posterior septectomy has various advantages: first, it is the prerequisite for a binostril, 2-surgeon, 4-hand technique. Second, it permits the elevation of a nasoseptal flap on the contralateral side for later reconstruction since the vascular pedicle on the ipsilateral side is usually sacrificed during the approach. Third, it greatly improves angulation and therefore lateral reach. Access lateral to the infraorbital nerve is possible with a maxillary antrostomy, modified medial maxillectomy, or total maxillectomy in 63.3% of cases; this is improved to 97.6% when a posterior transseptal approach is used [18].

While the PPF can be reached by limited endoscopic approaches such as the medial transpalatine approach (for the medial aspect of the PPF) or a middle meatal transantral approach (for a more lateral exposure where the infraorbital nerve is the first landmark to be identified), lateral access to the ITF usually requires at least an inferior turbinectomy and a modified medial maxillectomy. The lateral pterygoid plate is considered the lateral boundary accessible via a purely endonasal approach, further lateral and posterior reach is limited by the nasal osseous pyramid and the nasolacrimal canal.

In addition to the use of angled endoscopes and instruments, the exposure of the posterior and posterolateral wall of the maxillary sinus and laterally toward the ITF can be maximized by the following approach modules:

- The addition of a posterior septectomy (as detailed above)
- Using a total rather than a modified medial maxillectomy, where the maxillary sinus is entered anterior to the nasolacrimal duct
- The addition of an endoscopic anterior maxillotomy (Denker's procedure), where the entire medial buttress is removed without the need for a separate sublabial incision

- The addition of a prelacrimal approach, which usually permits to preserve function of the nasolacrimal duct without the need for further reconstruction
- The addition of a Caldwell-Luc approach, an anterior transmaxillary approach through the canine fossa with a sublabial incision (providing direct lateral access and permitting removal of anteriorly based lesions in the maxillary sinus)
- The combination of some of these approach adjuncts, e.g., access via a contralateral transmaxillary corridor

Major challenges of the endoscopic endonasal transpterygoid-transmaxillary approach remain the technical difficulty in controlling hemorrhage from the abundant and highly variable vasculature and the limitation in reaching the lateral aspect of the infratemporal fossa.

22.3 Surgical Comorbidity

Nasal crusting, impaired sense of olfaction, empty nose syndrome, and bad smell are well-established sequelae of endoscopic endonasal surgery. The transpterygoid-transmaxillary approach and removal of lesions in the PPF and ITF invariably result in sacrifice of functional tissues, and the following postoperative comorbidities are to be expected for this type of surgery; patients need to be counseled accordingly. Sacrifice of the Vidian nerve results in xerophthalmia, which carries the risk of corneal dysfunction, especially in conjunction with functional loss of the ophthalmic branch of the trigeminal nerve. Transection of the descending palatine nerves results in a variety of sensory dysfunctions of the palate (hypoesthesia, anesthesia, or deafferentation pain). Surgical manipulation within the masticator space with partial resection of the lateral and medial pterygoid muscles leads to immediate postoperative muscle swelling or permanent trismus. Facial numbness, oroantral fistulas, recurrent sinusitis, and devitalized teeth can result from the medial access to the maxillary sinus; dacryocystitis can develop due to the disruption of the nasolacrimal duct. Complications related to the Caldwell-Luc approach and Denker's endoscopic maxillotomy include injury to the anterior superior alveolar nerve, the canine roots, and facial deformity. The latter is due to the loss of lateral support of the alar cartilage to the pyriform aperture when the medial buttress is removed during an endoscopic anterior maxillotomy (Denker's procedure).

22.4 Surgical Setup

Following the administration of preoperative antibiotics, and disinfection and decongestion of the nasal cavity, the patient's head is secured in a Mayfield head holder. For EEA, we usually position the patient in a slight reverse Trendelenburg with the head elevated to 15° to decrease central venous pressure and to aid hemostasis. An MRI- and CT-based neuronavigation system is referenced, for lesions originating in the orbit, PPF and ITF fat suppressed T1 post-contrast MRI sequences are useful due to the high content of fat in these regions. Neuromonitoring for the relevant cranial nerves is installed.

If the harvest of autologous tissue for reconstruction or obliteration of a resection cavity is anticipated (e.g., abdominal fat, fascia lata, temporoparietal flap), the respective surgical sites are prepared accordingly. We use angled endoscopes (30° and 45°) for all skull base procedures including the nasal stage because of the dynamic multidirectional visualization and the minimization of interference between instruments and the endoscope.

22.5 Nasal Stage, Access to the Maxillary Sinus, Considerations for Reconstruction (Figs. 22.1 and 22.2)

Expansive lesions often invade, distort, or obliterate normal anatomy that usually guides endoscopic surgery. Following stable anatomic landmarks and establishing the boundaries of the lesion are key principles to ensure safe surgery. In the nasal cavity, nasal floor, posterior choana, Eustachian tube orifice, and nasal crest can aid in orientation [29].

The nasal stage of the endoscopic transpterygoid-transmaxillary approach begins with an uncinectomy, a wide maxillary antrostomy and a sphenoethmoidectomy until the medial wall of the maxillary sinus and its transition into the medial orbital wall (lamina papyracea) is reached. A modified medial maxillectomy is performed and the inferior turbinate resected; its mucosa can be used for a free flap reconstruction. Similarly, a flap from the nasal floor can be harvested and reflected medially. A posterior septectomy is added and the ethmoid's perpendicular plate saved for reconstruction. If a nasoseptal flap is to be harvested, this can be done on the contralateral side and the flap stored in the oropharynx [30–32]. The medial maxillary wall is resected posteriorly to the level of the greater palatine canal and anteriorly to the level of the nasolacrimal duct; the maxillectomy should be flush with the nasal floor to ensure free movement of instruments. The mucosa is elevated from the orbital process of the palatine bone to identify the crista ethmoidalis and to expose the sphenopalatine foramen with the posterior septal and posterior lateral nasal arteries emerging from it; these branches of the maxillary artery are usually coagulated for hemostatic control. The sphenopalatine artery provides 90% of the blood supply to the nasal cavity and commonly branches before exiting the sphenopalatine foramen. Its branches can serve as landmarks to identify the sphenopalatine foramen (toward the PPF), as well as the palatosphenoidal and Vidian canals [33–36].

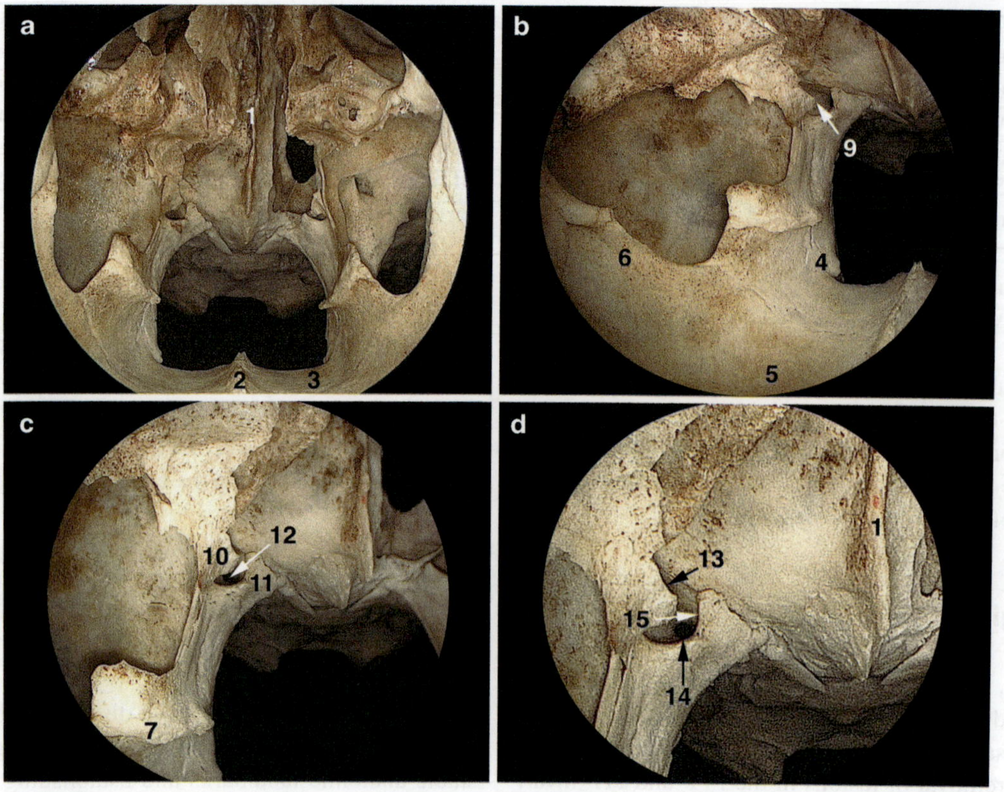

Fig. 22.1 Osteology, endoscopic endonasal approach to the pterygopalatine and infratemporal fossae. Dry skull specimen. Bilateral maxillary antrostomies and a nasal septectomy have been conducted, on the left side supplemented by a sphenoidotomy and removal of the maxillary sinus' posterior wall. (**a**) The osseous nasal septum consists of the perpendicular plate of the ethmoid bone and the vomer, it inserts at the sphenoidal rostrum (1) and the nasal crest (2). The horizontal plates of each palatine bone (3) merge in the midline to form the posterior part of the hard palate and the nasal crest. (**b**) (view toward the right) The pyramidal process of the palatine bone (4) accommodates the pterygopalatine canal and the greater palatine foramen. The palatine processes of the maxillary bone (5) represent the anterior part of the hard palate. The perpendicular plate of the palatine bone connects anteriorly with the rough surface of the maxillary bone to form the maxillary sinus' medial wall (6); its conchal crest (7) serves as the attachment for the inferior turbinate. (**c**) (zoomed detail of **b**) The middle turbinate belongs to the ethmoid bone, yet the most posterior aspect of its basal lamella blends into the ethmoidal crest of the palatine bone (8) which terminates just anteroinferior to the sphenopalatine foramen (9). (**d**) (zoomed detail of **c**) The anatomy of the palatine bone is central to the understanding of endoscopic endonasal approaches in the coronal plane. Superolaterally, the orbital process (10) attaches to the orbital surface of the maxillary bone, superomedially, the sphenoidal process (11) attaches to the base of the medial pterygoid plate. The orbital and sphenoidal processes are separated by the sphenopalatine notch, which becomes the sphenopalatine foramen when covered by the sphenoid bone superiorly. A shallow recess in the anterior surface of the base of the pterygoid process represents the posterior wall of the pterygopalatine fossa (12) and contains the orifices of the foramen rotundum (13, view obstructed by the orbital process) superolaterally, the Vidian/pterygoid canal (14) posteriorly, and the palatosphenoidal canal (15, view obstructed by the sphenoidal process) medially. The anterior wall of the pterygopalatine fossa is formed by the maxillary bone. (**e**) (view toward the left) The maxillary sinus' posterior wall (16) has been removed to expose the pterygopalatine fossa medially and the infratemporal fossa (17) laterally. (**f**) (more medial view when compared with **e**) The foramen rotundum (13) connects the middle cranial fossa with the pterygopalatine fossa; it opens into its superolateral aspect. The infraorbital canal in the roof of the maxillary sinus is often dehiscent and joins the posteromedial aspect of the inferior orbital fissure. It accommodates the infraorbital nerve (orbitomaxillary segment of the maxillary nerve), which courses posteromedially to enter the pterygopalatine fossa (see also Figs. 22.3 and 22.4. (**g**) (lateral extracranial view onto the left side, posterior wall of the maxillary sinus removed) at the junction of the perpendicular and horizontal plates, the pyramidal process of the palatine bone attaches to the maxillary bone (19) anteriorly and to the oblique inferior margins of the lateral pterygoid plate (20) posterolaterally; the pterygomaxillary fissure (18) lies superior. The pterygoid process of the sphenoid bone connects superiorly to the body and greater wing; it consists of the base and the medial and lateral pterygoid plates. The infratemporal fossa is bounded by the lateral pterygoid plate medially, the posterolateral surface of the maxillary sinus anteromedially, the infratemporal crest (21) laterally, and the mandibular fossa (22) posterolaterally. (**h**) (extracranial view from below, left side) The greater wing of the sphenoid bone (23) forms the roof of the infratemporal fossa, whereas the squamous part of the temporal bone (24) overlies the poststyloid compartment of the parapharyngeal space. In the pterygoid fossa, the depression between the medial and lateral (20) pterygoid plates, an inconstant foramen venosum Vesalii (25) can be found, more posterolaterally and anterior to the petrosphenoidal fissure (26), foramen ovale (27) and foramen spinosum (28) are located

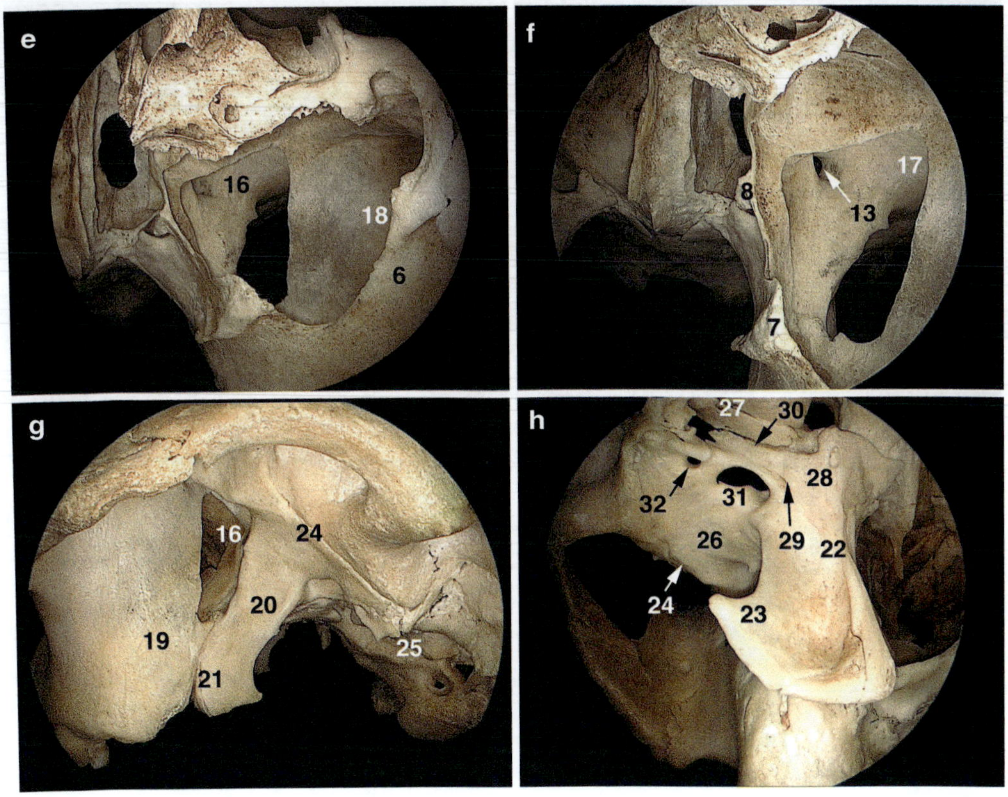

Fig. 22.1 (continued)

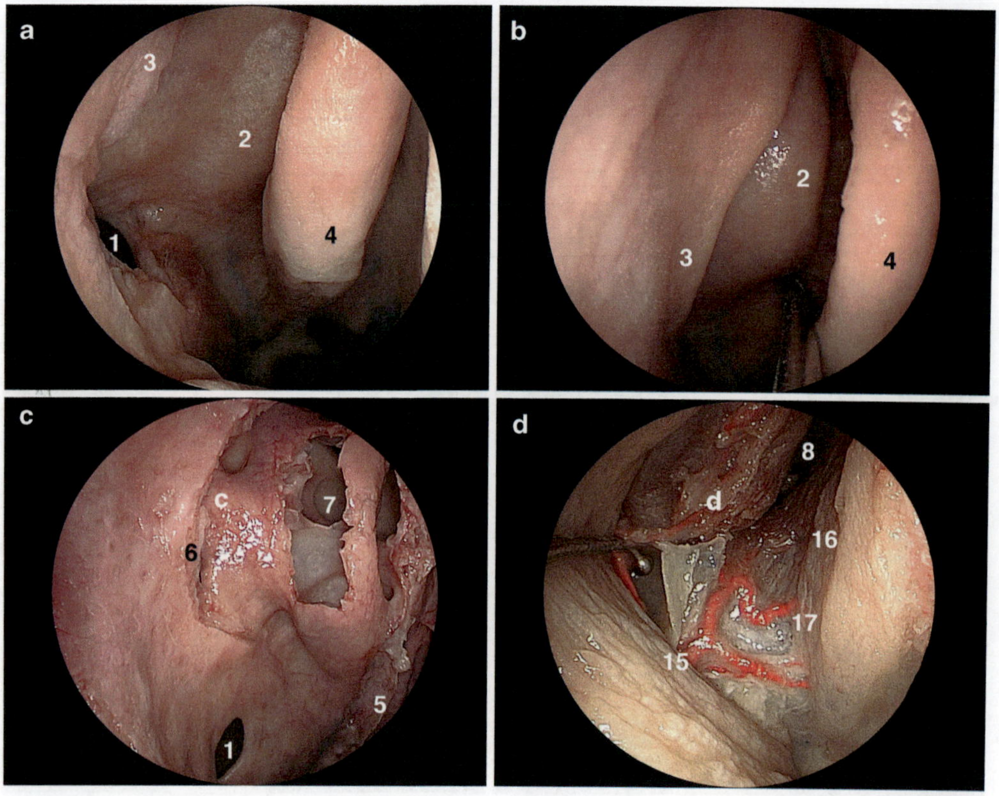

Fig. 22.2 Nasal stage, terminal branches of the maxillary and sphenopalatine arteries. Color-injected, fixed specimen. (**a–f**) right side, (**g, h**) left side. (**a**) The maxillary ostium (1) is located inferior to the bulla ethmoidalis (2) and is partially covered by the inferior aspect of the uncinate process (3). (**b**) The middle turbinate (4) is medialized to expose the medial wall of the maxillary sinus and the afore mentioned structures. (**c**) View after middle turbinectomy (5 showing the residual of its basal lamella), uncinectomy (6), and partial ethmoidectomy (7). (**d**) The sphenoidal ostium (8) opens into the sphenoethmoidal recess (9). The sphenopalatine artery represents a terminal branch of the pterygopalatine segment of maxillary artery, it divides into the posterior lateral nasal artery and the posterior septal artery within the pterygopalatine fossa, both branches exit into the nasal cavity via the sphenopalatine foramen. The posterior septal artery (10) courses on the anterior wall of the sphenoid sinus (11) between the sphenoidal ostium and the choana to reach the posterior aspect of the nasal septum; it usually divides into a superior and inferior branch. The inferior turbinate is supplied by a branch of the posterior lateral nasal artery (12). (**e**) The mucosa overlying the ethmoidal crest (13) has been elevated to expose the sphenopalatine foramen and the posterior lateral nasal and the posterior septal arteries emerging from the pterygopalatine fossa (14). (**f**) The terminal segment of the pterygopalatine segment of maxillary artery (16) bifurcates into the sphenopalatine artery (17) and the descending palatine arteries (18). The sphenopalatine artery then branches into the posterior lateral nasal artery (12) and the posterior septal artery (10). Direct branches can often be identified such as the artery of the foramen rotundum (19), the Vidian artery, or the palatosphenoidal arteries; they emerge variably from the pterygopalatine segment of maxillary artery. (**g, h**) If a nasoseptal flap (20) is to be harvested, this is usually done on the contralateral side since its vascular pedicle consisting of the inferior and superior posterior septal arteries (10), would be sacrificed during the surgical approach to the pterygopalatine fossa. The harvested flap can be stored in the nasopharynx (21) or the contralateral maxillary antrum

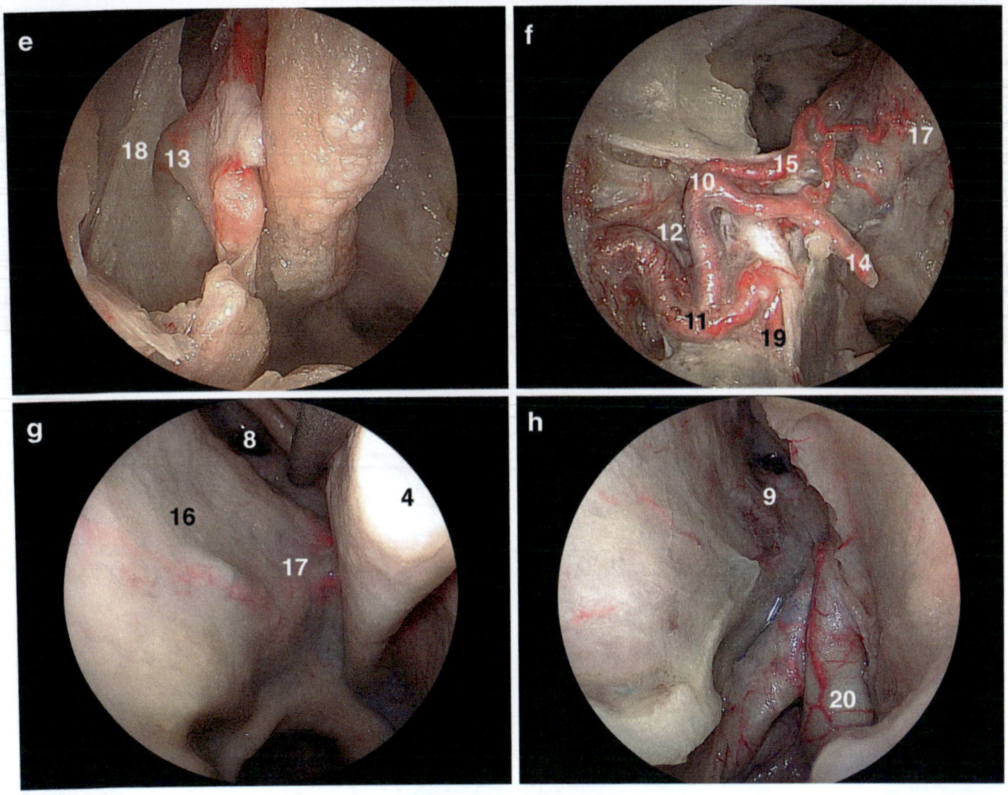

Fig. 22.2 (continued)

22.6 Pterygopalatine Fossa (Figs. 22.1, 22.2, and 22.3)

Drilling continues through the perpendicular plate of the palatine bone, the descending greater and lesser palatine nerves and their artery usually need to be transected for transposition of the PPF contents. The medial pterygoid plate and muscle lie just posterior. The sphenopalatine foramen is largely formed by the orbital and sphenoidal processes of the palatine bone, these can be reduced to expose the pterygopalatine fossa in a medial to lateral direction. The fibrous tissues encountered superolaterally correspond to the Mueller muscle, which is a vestigial muscle surrounded by a thin periosteal sheath that covers the posteromedial segment of the inferior orbital fissure and separates the pterygopalatine fossa from the orbit; manipulation should be minimized to not disrupt postganglionic fibers coursing into the orbit [37, 38]. Once the mucosa is elevated off the maxillary sinus, the infraorbital artery and nerve are readily visualized coursing anterosuperior toward the floor of the orbit. Further resection of the posterior wall of the maxilla exposes the periosteum of the pterygopalatine and infratemporal fossae [39].

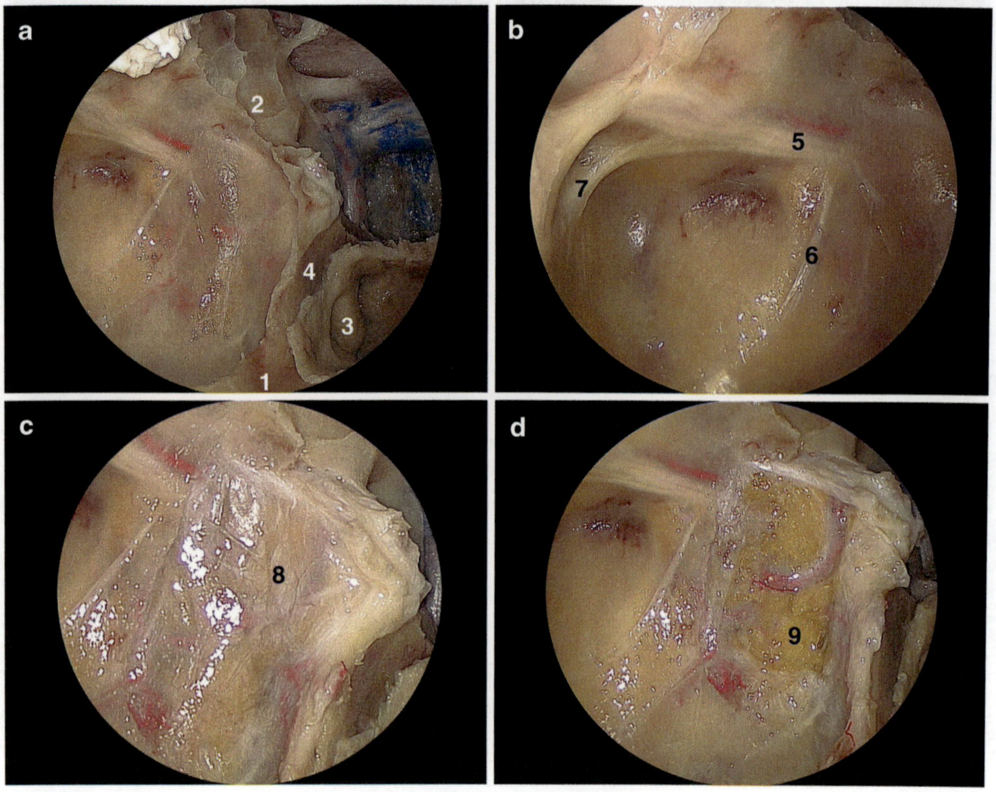

Fig. 22.3 Pterygopalatine and infratemporal fossae I. Color-injected, fixed specimen. Stepwise exposure, right side. (**a**) View following removal of the maxillary sinus' medial wall (medial maxillectomy), from the level of the hard palate (1) inferiorly to the lamina papyracea (2) superiorly. The torus tubarius (3), the nasopharyngeal ostium of the Eustachian tube, is located posterior to the perpendicular plate of the palatine bone (4). (**b**) Removal of the mucosa reveals the infraorbital nerve and artery (5). The orbitomaxillary segment of the infraorbital nerve gives off the middle superior (6) and the anterior superior alveolar nerves (7) which descend on the maxillary tuberosity. (**c**) Removal of the thin maxillary sinus' posterior wall exposes the subjacent periosteum (8). (**d**) Incision of the periosteum reveals a fat pad (9) that overlies the pterygopalatine and infratemporal fossae. Within this fat pad, the pterygopalatine fossa is organized in two distinct compartments: a superficial vascular compartment and a deep neural compartment. (**e, f**) Lateral dissection exposes contents of the pterygopalatine and infratemporal fossae. The junction of the infraorbital canal (10) and the maxillary sinus' posterior wall is just medial to the vertical fibers of the temporalis muscle (11); this point can be used as a landmark to divide the infratemporal fossa and the pterygopalatine fossa from the endoscopic perspective. The pterygopalatine ganglion consists of an assortment of parasympathetic, sympathetic, and somatosensory nerve fibers that regulate secretomotor functions to and provide sensation from various structures including lacrimal glands, and mucous membranes of the oropharynx, nasopharynx, nasal cavity, and the oral cavity. Pterygopalatine segment of the maxillary nerve (12), infraorbital nerve and artery (5), greater and lesser palatine nerves and artery (13), and middle superior alveolar nerve (6). (**g**) Detail of the posterior aspect of the pterygopalatine fossa. The maxillary nerve enters superolaterally via the foramen rotundum (14), while the Vidian nerve enters posteriorly via the Vidian/pterygoid canal (15). The pneumatized lateral recess of the sphenoid sinus (16) belongs to the pterygoid bone. Mueller's muscle (17) covers the inferior orbital fissure and serves as a landmark between orbit and pterygopalatine fossa. The zygomatic nerve (18) courses into Muller's muscle, essentially dividing it into a superior and an inferior part. (**h**) Detail of the perpendicular plate (4) and the descending greater and lesser palatine nerves (13). For details on the pterygopalatine segment of the maxillary artery see Fig. 22.2

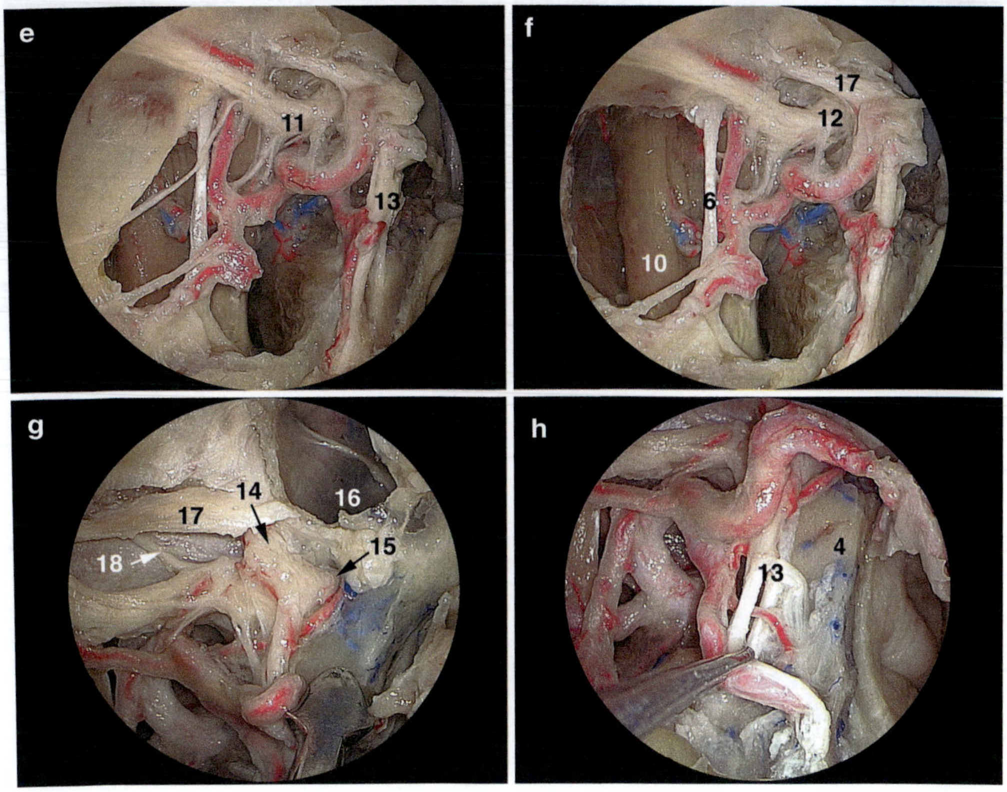

Fig. 22.3 (continued)

The contents of the pterygopalatine fossa are organized in two distinct compartments: gentle dissection of the fat at first exposes the superficial vascular compartment. The vascular compartment contains the pterygopalatine segment of the maxillary artery which traverses the PPF in a characteristic corkscrew loop (coursing anteriorly, medially, then superiorly); its branches are usually encountered prior to the main artery [40]. The neural compartment lies deeper, its most important structures are the pterygopalatine ganglion, the maxillary and infraorbital branches of the trigeminal nerve, the Vidian nerve, and the greater and lesser descending palatine nerves. Three obliquely oriented foramina are consistently found on the posterior aspect of the pterygopalatine fossa: superolaterally the foramen rotundum, medially the Vidian canal, and inferomedially the palatosphenoidal canal [41]. The Vidian nerve is formed by the union of the greater superficial petrosal and the deep petrosal nerves. It is readily identified at the inferolateral aspect of the sphenoid sinus floor at the junction of the sphenoid body and the pterygoid process. The Vidian canal and the fibrous tissues of the pterygosphenoidal fissure serve as excellent surgical guides to identify the lacerum segment of the internal carotid artery if the approach is taken more posteriorly [42, 43]. The transposition of the pterygopalatine fossa contents with preservation of a mobilized Vidian nerve is generally feasible after transection of the greater and lesser descending palatine nerves, in malignant tumors or for extended exposure its sacrifice is necessary.

22.7 Infratemporal Fossa (Figs. 22.1, 22.3, and 22.4)

The pterygoid plates can be followed to their base and attachment to the middle cranial fossa. During the endonasal endoscopic transpterygoid-transmaxillary approach, the medial pterygoid muscle can be recognized by fibers coursing in the vertical plane, complete drilling of the perpendicular plate of the palatine bone and the lateral pterygoid plate is required for its exposure. Its two heads descend in a posterior and lateral direction to insert at the medial surface of the ramus and angle of the mandible. The lateral pterygoid muscle, which occupies most of the superior aspect of the ITF, equally consists of two heads: the superior head originates on the infratemporal surface and crest of the greater wing of the sphenoid bone, just posterolaterally of the inferior orbital fissure, its lower head originates from the lateral surface of the lateral pterygoid plate [44]. Both course posterolaterally, their fibers directed in the horizontal plane. The lateral pterygoid plate is the most useful landmark for the location of the

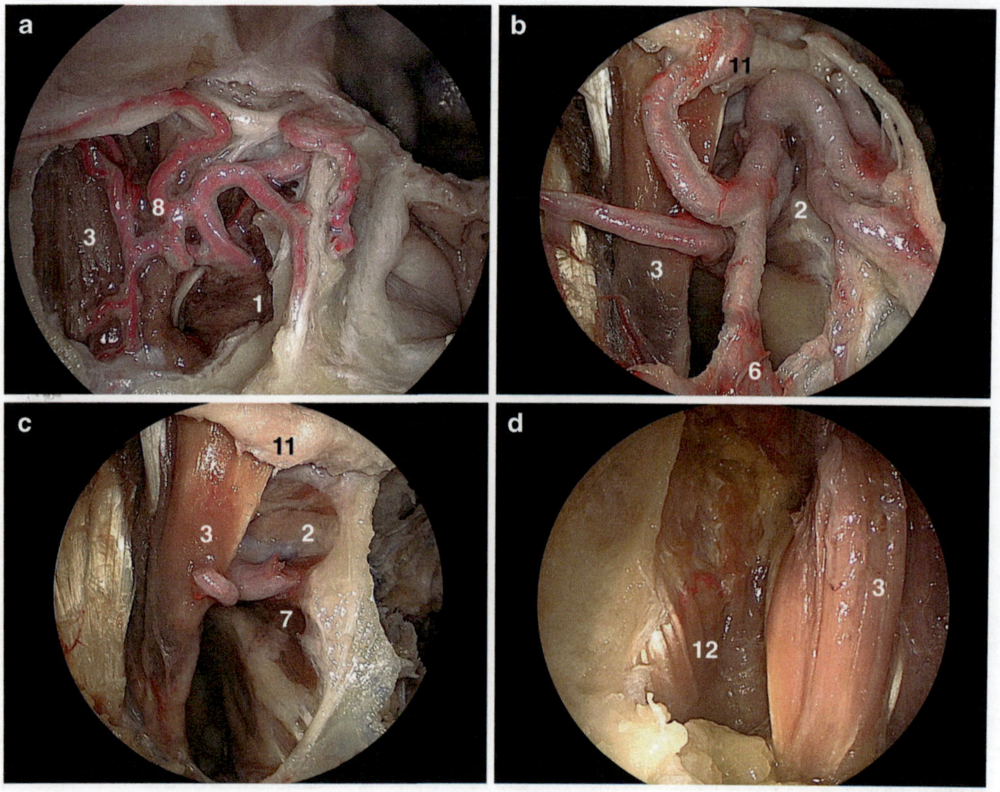

Fig. 22.4 Pterygopalatine and infratemporal fossae II. Color-injected, fixed specimen. Stepwise exposure, right side. (**a**) The infratemporal fossa is largely occupied by the medial and lateral (1) pterygoid muscles; its lateral boundary is formed by the inner fascia of the temporal muscle (2) which inserts at the infratemporal crest. (**b**) The maxillary artery (3) arises from the external carotid artery and courses anteromedially to enter the infratemporal fossa via an orifice formed by the condylar process of the mandible (4) and the sphenomandibular ligament. There are three named segments to the maxillary artery: mandibular, pterygoid, and pterygopalatine. The mandibular segment spans from the external carotid artery to the lateral aspect of the lateral pterygoid muscle; five branches originate: the deep auricular, anterior tympanic, middle (5) and accessory meningeal, and inferior alveolar arteries. The pterygoid segment continues to the pterygomaxillary fissure; it gives rise to a variable number of muscular branches: the anterior and posterior deep temporal, masseteric, buccal, and pterygoid arteries (see Figs. 22.2 and 22.3 for a description of the pterygopalatine segment). (**c**) The lateral pterygoid muscle consists of two heads: the superior head (1 sup) originates on the infratemporal surface and crest of the greater wing of the sphenoid bone, just posterolateral of the inferior orbital fissure, whereas the lower head (1 inf) originates from the lateral surface of the lateral pterygoid plate. Both course in a posterolateral direction, their fibers directed in the horizontal plane, to inserts at the temporomandibular joint (superior head) and at the condylar process (inferior head). The medial pterygoid muscle passes inferior to the lateral pterygoid muscle on is posterolateral course toward the mandible. Depending on the course of the maxillary artery in relation to the inferior head of the lateral pterygoid muscle, there is a lateral/superficial variant and a medial/deep variant; the latter being less common. (6) perpendicular plate of the palatine bone. (**d**) (extreme lateral view) The masseter muscle (7) is located lateral to the temporalis muscle (2); its fibers oriented in a more oblique direction. (**e, f**) The medial pterygoid muscle (not shown) is recognized by fibers coursing in the vertical plane, complete drilling of the perpendicular plate of the palatine bone and the lateral pterygoid plate is required for its exposure from the endonasal perspective. Its smaller superficial head originates from the lateral aspect of the palatine pyramidal process and the maxillary tuberosity, whereas its bigger deep head originates from the medial surface of the lateral pterygoid plate and the pterygoid fossa. The medial pterygoid muscle (8) inserts at the medial surface of the ramus and angle of the mandible (9). The mandibular nerve (10) represents the largest of the three trigeminal divisions; it consists of a sensory root and a smaller motor root. Inferior to the foramen ovale (11), the mandibular nerve courses between the tensor veli palatini muscle and the Eustachian tube (12) posteromedially and the lateral pterygoid muscle anterolaterally; it provides meningeal and muscular branches and then divides into a smaller anterior trunk (13) and a larger posterior trunk (14). The anterior trunk courses laterally just below the roof of the infratemporal fossa; its provides various motor branches (deep temporal, masseteric, pterygoid) and the sensory buccal nerve. The otic ganglion is a peripheral ganglion formed by preganglionic parasympathetic fibers of the lesser petrosal nerve and sympathetic fibers from the plexus on the middle meningeal artery (5); the ganglion is located extracranially just inferior to the foramen ovale (11). The stylopharyngeal fascia originates on the styloid process and the base of the spina sphenoidalis, anterolateral to the external opening of the carotid canal. It blends into the sphenopharyngeal fascia (15) anteromedially to insert at the lateral pterygoid plate. It extends along the anterior aspect of the Eustachian tube and the tensor veli palatini muscle to separate the infratemporal fossa anteriorly from the poststyloid compartment of the parapharyngeal space posteriorly. From the endonasal endoscopic perspective, the Eustachian tube traverses the parapharyngeal space always anterior to the petrous segment of the internal carotid artery. (**g, h**) Detail of the region around the foramen ovale. The posterior trunk (14) provides the auriculotemporal nerve (16), as well as the lingual, mylohyoid, and inferior alveolar nerves (not identified in ambiguity). The middle meningeal artery (5) ascends medial to the lateral pterygoid muscle to enter the middle cranial fossa via the foramen spinosum (17). Due to the anteromedial to posterolateral line of sight of the endoscopic approach, the middle meningeal artery is usually found posterior to the mandibular nerve and the foramen ovale. The accessory meningeal artery reaches the middle cranial fossa either via the foramen ovale or the foramen venosum Vesalii

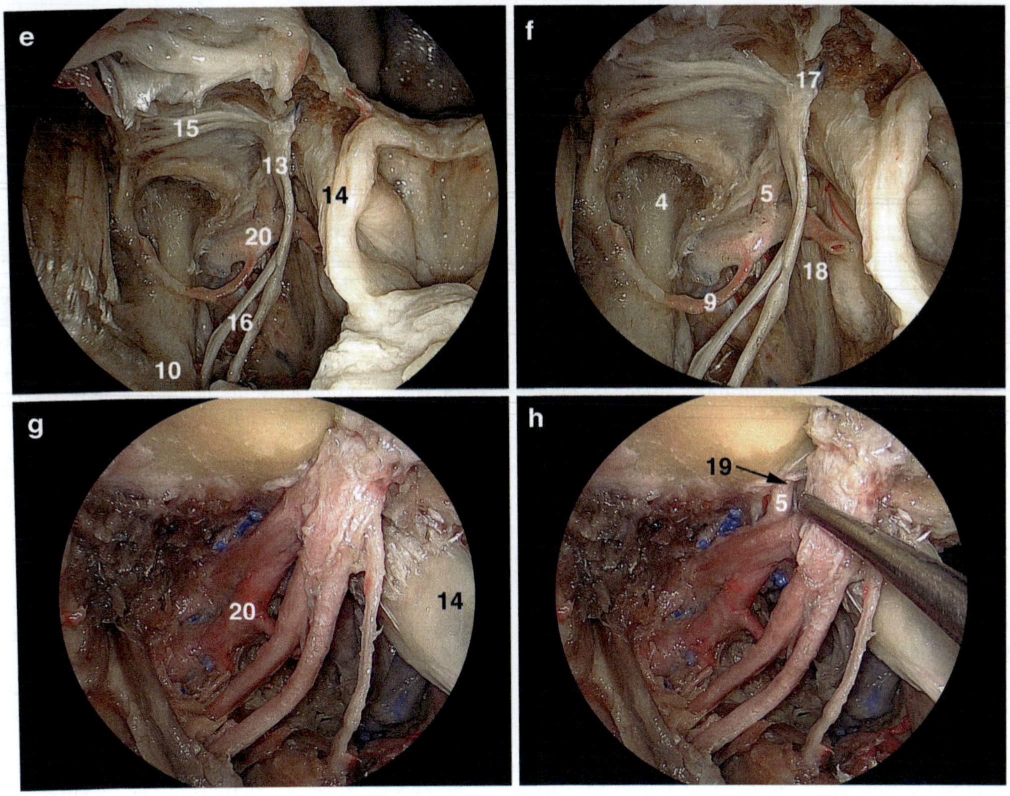

Fig. 22.4 (continued)

foramen ovale and the mandibular branch of the trigeminal nerve, when drilled flush to the cranial base the foramen ovale is found just posterolateral to it. The foramen spinosum is situated immediately posterolaterally to the foramen ovale, however, due to the anteromedial to posterolateral line of sight of the endoscopic approach, the foramen spinosum is encountered just behind the mandibular nerve as the middle meningeal artery traversing it enters the middle cranial fossa. Alternatively the inferior alveolar nerve can be followed as its courses under the lateral pterygoid muscle toward the foramen ovale [45]. The medial pterygoid plate also serves as the attachment of the superior constrictor muscle of the pharynx and the fibrous raphe to form the lateral layers of the wall of the nasopharynx; its medial plate therefore represents the lateral wall of the nasopharynx [46].

References

1. Hosseini SMS, Razfar A, Carrau RL, Prevedello DM, Fernandez-Miranda J, Zanation A, Kassam AB. Endonasal transpterygoid approach to the infratemporal fossa: correlation of endoscopic and multiplanar CT anatomy. Head Neck. 2012;34:313–20.
2. Fortes FSG, Sennes LU, Carrau RL, Brito R, Ribas GC, Yasuda A, Rodrigues AJ, Snyderman CH, Kassam AB. Endoscopic anatomy of the pterygopalatine fossa and the transpterygoid approach: development of a surgical instruction model. Laryngoscope. 2008;118:44–9.
3. Theodosopoulos PV, Guthikonda B, Brescia A, Keller JT, Zimmer LA. Endoscopic approach to the infratemporal fossa: anatomic study. Neurosurgery. 2010;66:196–203.
4. Alfieri A, Jho H-D, Schettino R, Tschabitscher M. Endoscopic endonasal approach to the pterygopalatine fossa: anatomic study. Neurosurgery. 2003;52:374–80.
5. Falcon RT, Rivera-Serrano CM, Miranda JF, Prevedello DM, Snyderman CH, Kassam AB, Carrau RL. Endoscopic endonasal dissection of the infratemporal fossa: anatomic relationships and importance of eustachian tube in the endoscopic skull base surgery. Laryngoscope. 2011;121:31–41.
6. Cavallo LM, Messina A, Gardner P, Esposito F, Kassam AB, Cappabianca P, de Divitiis E, Tschabitscher M. Extended endoscopic endonasal approach to the pterygopalatine fossa: anatomical study and clinical considerations. Neurosurg Focus. 2005;19:1–7.
7. Joo W, Funaki T, Yoshioka F, Rhoton AL. Microsurgical anatomy of the infratemporal fossa. Clin Anat. 2013;26:455–69.
8. Daniels DL, Mark LP, Ulmer JL, Mafee MF, McDaniel J, Shah NC, Erickson S, Sether LA, Jaradeh SS. Osseous anatomy of the pterygopalatine fossa. AJNR Am J Neuroradiol. 1998;19:1423–32.
9. Li L, London NR, Prevedello DM, Carrau RL. Anatomy based corridors to the infratemporal fossa: implications for endoscopic approaches. Head Neck. 2020;42:846–53.
10. Elhadi A, Almefty K, Mendes G, Kalani M, Nakaji P, Dru A, Preul M, Little A. Comparison of surgical freedom and area of exposure in three endoscopic transmaxillary approaches to the anterolateral cranial base. J Neurol Surg B Skull Base. 2014;75:346–53.
11. de Lara D, Filho LFSD, Prevedello DM, Carrau RL, Kasemsiri P, Otto BA, Kassam AB. Endonasal endoscopic approaches to the paramedian skull base. World Neurosurg. 2014;82:S121–9.

12. Li L, London NR, Prevedello DM, Carrau RL. Endonasal endoscopic transpterygoid approach to the upper parapharyngeal space. Head Neck. 2020;42:2734–40.
13. DelGaudio JM. Endoscopic transnasal approach to the pterygopalatine fossa. Arch Otolaryngol Head Neck Surg. 2003;129:441–6.
14. Al-Nashar IS, Carrau RL, Herrera A, Snyderman CH. Endoscopic transnasal transpterygopalatine fossa approach to the lateral recess of the sphenoid sinus. Laryngoscope. 2004;114:528–32.
15. Elhadi AM, Zaidi HA, Yagmurlu K, Ahmed S, Rhoton AL, Nakaji P, Preul MC, Little AS. Infraorbital nerve: a surgically relevant landmark for the pterygopalatine fossa, cavernous sinus, and anterolateral skull base in endoscopic transmaxillary approaches. J Neurosurg. 2016;125:1460–8.
16. Labib MA, Belykh E, Cavallo C, et al. The endoscopic endonasal eustachian tube anterolateral mobilization strategy: minimizing the cost of the extreme-medial approach. J Neurosurg. 2021;134:831–42.
17. Hofstetter CP, Singh A, Anand VK, Kacker A, Schwartz TH. The endoscopic, endonasal, transmaxillary transpterygoid approach to the pterygopalatine fossa, infratemporal fossa, petrous apex, and the Meckel cave: clinical article. J Neurosurg. 2010;113:967–74.
18. Oakley GM, Harvey RJ. Endoscopic resection of pterygopalatine fossa and infratemporal fossa malignancies. Otolaryngol Clin North Am. 2017;50:301–13.
19. Snyderman CH, Carrau RL, Kassam AB, Zanation A, Prevedello D, Gardner P, Mintz A. Endoscopic skull base surgery: principles of endonasal oncological surgery. J Surg Oncol. 2008;97:658–64.
20. Tiwari R, Quak J, Egeler S, Smeele L, Waal IV, Valk PV, Leemans R. Tumors of the infratemporal fossa. Skull Base Surg. 2000;10:1–9.
21. Hanakita S, Chang W-C, Watanabe K, Ronconi D, Labidi M, Park H-H, Oyama K, Bernat A-L, Froelich S. Endoscopic endonasal approach to the anteromedial temporal fossa and mobilization of the lateral wall of the cavernous sinus through the inferior orbital fissure and V1-V2 corridor: an anatomic study and clinical considerations. World Neurosurg. 2018;116:e169–78.
22. Shin M, Shojima M, Kondo K, Hasegawa H, Hanakita S, Ito A, Kin T, Saito N. Endoscopic endonasal craniofacial surgery for recurrent skull base meningiomas involving the pterygopalatine fossa, the infratemporal fossa, the orbit, and the paranasal sinus. World Neurosurg. 2018;112:e302–12.
23. Gerges MM, Godil SS, Younus I, Rezk M, Schwartz TH. Endoscopic transorbital approach to the infratemporal fossa and parapharyngeal space: a cadaveric study. J Neurosurg. 2020;133:1948–59.
24. Youssef A, Carrau R, Tantawy A, Ibraheim A, Solares A, Otto B, Prevedello D, Filho L. Endoscopic versus open approach to the infratemporal fossa: a cadaver study. J Neurol Surg B Skull Base. 2015;76:358–64.
25. Alves-Belo JT, Mangussi-Gomes J, Truong HQ, Cohen S, Gardner PA, Snyderman CH, Stefko ST, Wang EW, Fernandez-Miranda JC. Lateral transorbital versus endonasal transpterygoid approach to the lateral recess of the sphenoid sinus—a comparative anatomic study. Oper Neurosurg. 2018;16:600–6.
26. Yan R, Fang X. The endoscopic prelacrimal recess approach to the paramedian middle cranial base: an anatomical study. J Clin Neurosci. 2021;88:251–8.
27. Oyama K, Watanabe K, Hanakita S, Champagne P-O, Passeri T, Voormolen EH, Bernat AL, Penet N, Fukushima T, Froelich S. The orbitopterygoid corridor as a deep keyhole for endoscopic access to the paranasal sinuses and clivus. J Neurosurg. 2020;134(5):1480–9.
28. Watanabe K, Zomorodi AR, Labidi M, Satoh S, Froelich S, Fukushima T. Visualization of dark side of skull base with surgical navigation and endoscopic assistance: extended petrous rhomboid and rhomboid with maxillary nerve–mandibular nerve Vidian corridor. World Neurosurg. 2019;129:e134–45.
29. Rhoton A. Cranial anatomy and surgical approaches. Philadelphia: Lippincott Williams & Wilkins; 2003.
30. Hadad G, Bassagasteguy L, Carrau RL, Mataza JC, Kassam A, Snyderman CH, Mintz A. A novel reconstructive technique after endoscopic expanded endonasal approaches: vascular pedicle nasoseptal flap. Laryngoscope. 2006;116:1882–6.
31. Pinheiro-Neto CD, Paluzzi A, Fernandez-Miranda JC, Scopel TF, Wang EW, Gardner PA, Snyderman CH. Extended dissection of the septal flap pedicle for ipsilateral endoscopic transpterygoid approaches. Laryngoscope. 2014;124:391–6.
32. Fortes FSG, Carrau RL, Snyderman CH, Kassam A, Prevedello D, Vescan A, Mintz A, Gardner P. Transpterygoid transposition of a temporoparietal fascia flap: a new method for skull base reconstruction after endoscopic expanded endonasal approaches. Laryngoscope. 2007;117:970–6.
33. Kim JK, Cho JH, Lee Y-J, Kim C-H, Bae JH, Lee J-G, Yoon J-H. Anatomical variability of the maxillary artery: findings from 100 Asian cadaveric dissections. Arch Otolaryngol Head Neck Surg. 2010;136:813–8.
34. Zhang X, Wang EW, Wei H, Shi J, Snyderman CH, Gardner PA, Fernandez-Miranda JC. Anatomy of the posterior septal artery with surgical implications on the vascularized pedicled nasoseptal flap. Head Neck. 2015;37:1470–6.
35. Tanoue S, Kiyosue H, Mori H, Hori Y, Okahara M, Sagara Y. Maxillary artery: functional and imaging anatomy for safe and effective transcatheter treatment. Radiographics. 2013;33:e209–24.
36. Alvernia JE, Hidalgo J, Sindou MP, Washington C, Luzardo G, Perkins E, Nader R, Mertens P. The maxillary artery and its variants: an anatomical study with neurosurgical applications. Acta Neurochir. 2017;159:655–64.
37. Lieber S, Fernandez-Miranda J. Anatomy of the orbit. J Neurol Surg B Skull Base. 2020;81:319–32.
38. Battista JCD, Zimmer LA, Rodríguez-Vázquez JF, Froelich SC, Theodosopoulos PV, DePowell JJ, Keller JT. Muller's muscle, no longer vestigial in endoscopic surgery. World Neurosurg. 2011;76:342–6.
39. Battista JD, Zimmer L, Theodosopoulos P, Froelich S, Keller J. Anatomy of the inferior orbital fissure: implications for endoscopic cranial base surgery. J Neurol Surg B Skull Base. 2012;73:132–8.
40. Lasjaunias P, ter Brugge KT, Berenstein A. Surgical neuroangiography. 2nd ed. New York: Springer; 2001.
41. Pinheiro-Neto CD, Fernandez-Miranda JC, Rivera-Serrano CM, Paluzzi A, Snyderman CH, Gardner PA, Sennes LU. Endoscopic anatomy of the palatovaginal canal (palatosphenoidal canal). Laryngoscope. 2012;122:6–12.
42. Kassam AB, Vescan AD, Carrau RL, Prevedello DM, Gardner P, Mintz AH, Snyderman CH, Rhoton AL. Expanded endonasal approach: vidian canal as a landmark to the petrous internal carotid artery: technical note. J Neurosurg. 2008;108:177–83.
43. Wang W-H, Lieber S, Mathias RN, Sun X, Gardner PA, Snyderman CH, Wang EW, Fernandez-Miranda JC. The foramen lacerum: surgical anatomy and relevance for endoscopic endonasal approaches. J Neurosurg. 2019;131:1571–82.
44. Lang J. Skull base and related structures. 2nd ed. New York: Schattauer; 2001.
45. Leblanc A. The cranial nerves. 2nd ed. Berlin: Springer.
46. Pinheiro-Neto CD, Fernandez-Miranda JC, Wang EW, Gardner PA, Snyderman CH. Anatomical correlates of endonasal surgery for sinonasal malignancies. Clin Anat. 2012;25:129–34.

Endoscopic Transorbital Approach to the Optic Canal and Orbital Apex

23

Ben Ng, Hun Ho Park, and Calvin MAK

Abstract

Endoscopic transorbital approach (ETOA) to the skull base has gained popularity among skull base surgeons over the last decade to access orbital and intracranial lesions. Given its minimal morbidity, better cosmetic results, and minimal brain retraction, it provided an alternative minimally invasive approach to resecting orbital and intracranial lesions. Kris Moe et al. first described and published in 2010 (Moe KS et al. Oper Neurosurg 67:ons16–ons28, 2010). It serves to provide a distinct corridor for more laterally placed anterior skull base lesions or those which cross neurovascular structures that cannot be effectively addressed with endonasal approaches. The surgery can be performed with or without orbitotomy to increase surgical freedom for the deeply seated intracranial lesions.

Keywords

Endoscope · Transorbital · Orbital apex · Optic canal · Cavernous hemangioma · Indocyanine green

23.1 Introduction

With the development of microscopic and endoscopic instruments for use in neurosurgery, neurosurgeons are attempting to reduce morbidity and invasiveness during skull base procedures. Endoscopic transorbital approach (ETOA) provides a direct anterior surgical option through, which a corridor can be utilized laterally to the cavernous segment of the internal carotid artery (ICA) and cavernous sinus. This technique represents a minimally invasive and versatile means of addressing deep-seated skull base lesions. Kris Moe et al. initially introduced this method in June 2007 at the Pacific Coast Otolaryngology-Ophthalmology Society Annual Meeting, with his first case series being published 3 years later [1]. The aim is to give an additional path for tackling anterior skull base lesions or those that extend across neurovascular structures, which cannot be reached by endonasal surgeries alone. It is estimated that the central portion of the ventral anterior cranial fossa bounded laterally by orbits occupies around 20% of the anterior skull base, which is accessible via the endonasal route without crossing critical neurovascular structures [1]. With its minimal bone removal techniques and cosmetic advantages ETOA with the application of modern-day illumination and magnification capabilities via microscopic and endoscopic tools prove advantageous.

23.2 Surgical Methods

23.2.1 Step 1: Skin Incision

The skin incision is designed and created jointly with oculoplastic surgeons for optimal planning and minimizing wound complications. The orbit can be using superior, inferior, lateral, and medial approaches; an example of a superior lid crease incision is illustrated in Fig. 23.1a. Upon completion of this step, division of the orbicularis oculi muscle and stripping of the periosteum (Fig. 23.1b) ensue. Lateral orbital rim can be removed to increase the working angles and surgical freedom up to sixfold from our investigational studies (Fig. 23.1c).

B. Ng · C. MAK (✉)
Department of Neurosurgery, Queen Elizabeth Hospital, Hong Kong SAR, China
e-mail: calvin.mak@ha.org.hk

H. H. Park
Department of Neurosurgery, Gangnam Severance Hospital, Yonsei University Health System, Seoul, Korea

T. L. POON et al. (eds.), *Orbital Apex and Periorbital Skull Base Diseases*, https://doi.org/10.1007/978-981-99-2989-4_23

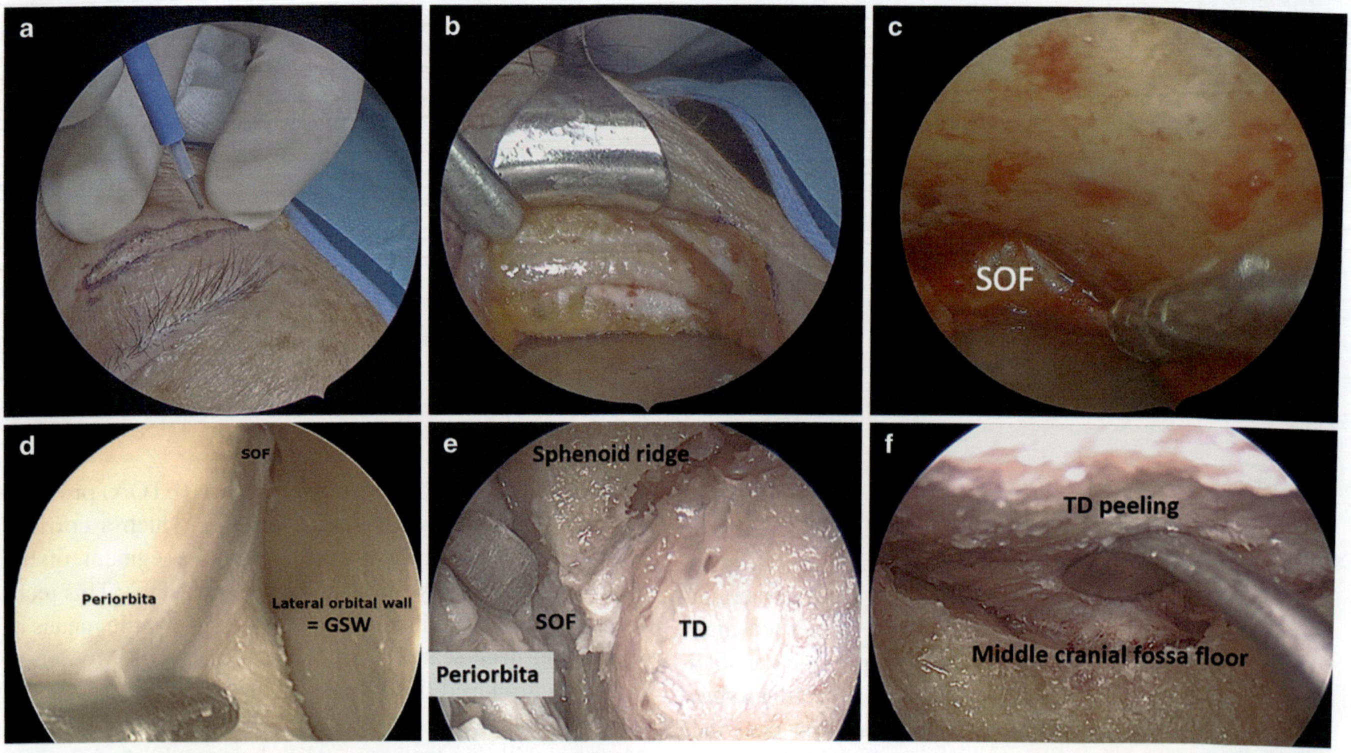

Fig. 23.1 (**a–f**) *(reprinted with permission, original from the last author)*: (**a**) Left lid crease incision. (**b**) Periosteum stripped and exposure of superolateral orbital rim. (**c**) Periorbita stripped to reach superior orbital fissure (SOF). (**d**) View after stripping of periobita from greater sphenoid wing (GSW) with exposure of superior orbital fissure (SOF). (**e**) Drilling of GSW to expose temporal dura (TD). (**f**) Temporal dura was elevated from middle cranial fossa floor. (reprinted with permission)

23.2.2 Step 2: Drilling of Greater Sphenoid Wing

The high-speed drill with a self-irrigation system was utilized to remove the greater sphenoid wing following the introduction of the endoscope. Maintaining copious irrigation throughout this process is vital in order to avoid thermal injuries to the orbital contents. It was shown that orbital compression of more than 1.5 cm was associated with a dramatic increase in intraocular pressure [2]. After the sphenoid wing has been removed, the meningo-orbital band is exposed and divided, thus establishing access to both the anterior and middle cranial fossa to unlock the anterior and middle cranial fossa (Fig. 23.1d–f).

23.2.3 Step 3: Extradural Dissection-Peeling of the Cavernous Sinus

The dura mater of the anterior and middle cranial fossa were separated, and the lateral wall of the cavernous sinus is then exposed via an extradural approach (Fig. 23.1f). This technique is analogous to extradural peeling of the cavernous sinus wall during craniotomy. The anteromedial triangle, created between the ophthalmic division (V1) and maxillary division (V2) of the trigeminal nerve, and anterolateral triangle formed between V2 and mandibular division (V3), can be identified (Fig. 23.2b). These two triangles are vital in guiding entrance into adjacent anatomical spaces such as petrous apex, infratemporal fossa, and cavernous sinus (Fig. 23.2a–d). Figure 23.2 shows the dissection via the left endoscopic transorbital approach.

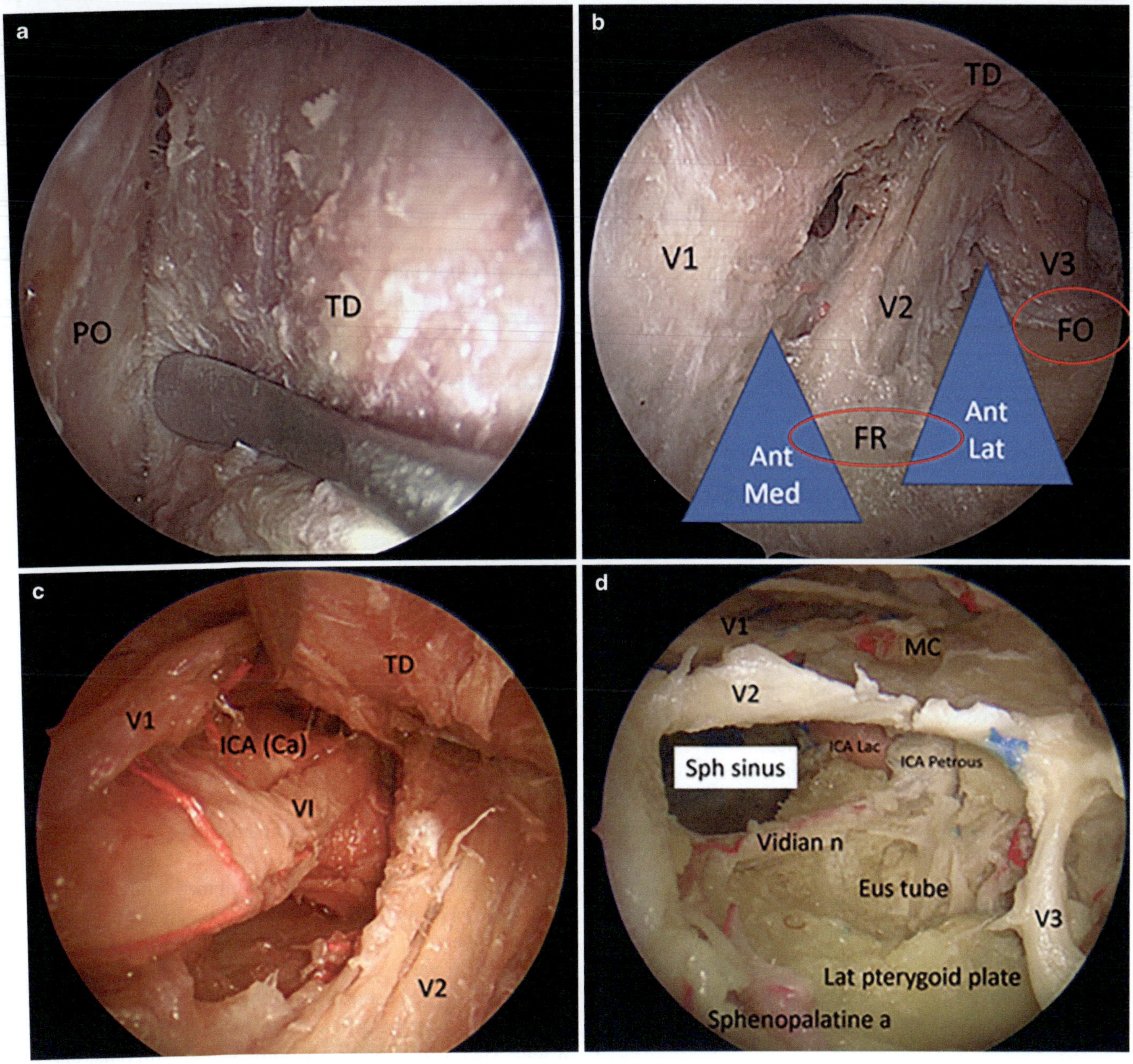

Fig. 23.2 (**a**–**d**) *(reprinted with permission, original from the last author)*: Left endoscopic transorbital view, with 30-degree endoscope. (**a**) Periorbita (PO) and temporal dura (TD) were split with dissector to expose the anterior cavernous sinus wall. (**b**) Anteromedial (Ant Med) and anterolateral (Ant Lat) triangles, which were bounded by ophthalmic (V1), maxillary (V2) and mandibular (V3) divisions of the trigeminal nerves were exposed. V2 exited via the foramen rotundum (FR) and V3 exited via the foramen ovale (FO). (**c**) Exposure of cavernous sinus content between V1 and V2, with temporal dura (TD) elevated. Abducens nerve (V1) travelled lateral to the cavernous segment of internal carotid artery (ICA(Ca)). (**d**) Exposure of infratemporal fossa between V2 and V3, the anterolateral triangle. Temporal dura was further elevated till Meckel's cave (MC) was seen. A pneumatized lateral recess of sphenoid sinus (Sph sinus) can be identified. Vidian nerve (Vidian n.) travelled superolaterally and served as a landmark to identify the petrous ICA and laceral segment of ICA (ICA Lac). Pterygoid muscles were removed to expose the Eustachian tube (Eus tube), sphenopalatine artery (sphenopalatine a), and lateral pterygoid plate (lat pterygoid plate)

23.3 Indications

The two most commonly described indications include repairing of cerebrospinal fluid (CSF) leaks and excision of skull base tumors.

The occurrence of iatrogenic and traumatic cerebrospinal fluid (CSF) leaks is a common cause for repair via a transorbital route. In most cases, the leak site was determined to be in the anterior cranial fossa, successfully addressed endoscopically from a transorbital approach [3].

For tumor excision, the most common indications are excision of spheno-orbital meningiomas and middle fossa schwannomas. The majority of the surgeries utilized only a transorbital approach while combined transorbital and endonasal approaches were used in some of the cases. The typical amount of time spent in the hospital afterward was approximately 3 days. Other indications described include cavernous hemangioma, intracranial abscesses, fibrous dysplasia, frontal mucocele, and fibroxanthoma [3, 4].

In our experience of over 30 cases, ETOA was used, either alone or in adjunct to other routes, to excise orbital tumor or vascular malformation, spheno-orbital meningiomata, trigeminal schwannomas, and infratemporal fossa tumors. Dura defects were repaired using artificial dura substitute and tissue glue. Abdominal fat graft was also used to repair large dura defects. We so far have not encountered any cases of CSF leakage nor pseudomeningocele.

Kong et al. recently conducted a case series to compare the efficacy of endoscopic transorbital approach (ETOA) and endoscopic transorbital approach combined with lateral orbitotomy in spheno-orbital meningioma resections. The results showed that ETOA with lateral orbitotomy had a higher gross total excision rate than ETOA alone. Our experience also suggests that this improved rate could be attributed to the improved surgical freedom from lateral orbitotomy, which can increase the surgical freedom from threefold to sixfold depending on the level of removal.

23.4 Complications

A systematic review of (ETOA) conducted by the Barrow Neurological Institute reported a complication rate of 13%, with permanent proptosis in one case [3]. CSF leaks were the most frequent complication, with most being transient. Other reported complications included diplopia, facial numbness, ptosis, levator muscle dysfunction, meningitis, periorbital hematoma, epiphora, superficial surgical site infection, and orbital pseudomeningocele [5].

23.5 Surgical Outcomes

Endoscopic transorbital approach (ETOA) has been demonstrated to be quite successful in treating cerebrospinal fluid leaks, ranging in success rate from 83 to 100%, with a recurrence rate of 7%. On the other hand, the rate of gross total excision of tumors surgically managed by this method is approximately 70%. Generally, patients presented with neurological deficits such as impaired visual acuity, ptosis, and reduced extraocular eye movement (EOM); most of these deficits were ameliorated postoperatively [3].

23.6 Discussion

Since its first description, the transorbital approach for endoscopic transorbital cranial surgery (ETOA) has been limitedly evaluated in contrast to traditional approaches such as craniotomies. Most existing studies are composed primarily of anatomical studies and case series. In 2020, our center initiated the utilization of this method; close collaborations between neurosurgeons and oculoplastic surgeons enabled a better aesthetic outcome through a minimal incision along natural creases of the skin. Satisfactory proptosis correction also provides good cosmetic outcome. Compared to craniotomies, there is no risk of temporalis muscle atrophy or injury to the facial nerve's frontal branch, and lower rates of cerebrospinal fluid leak than reported via the endonasal route. Moreover, less blood loss and quicker postoperative recovery is possible due to the minimal amount of brain retraction during surgery.

ETOA has the capability to be combined with other operative pathways, including endonasal and transoral routes. Through operating along multiple passages, ETOA provides an excellent view of important neurovascular structures using multi-angled endoscopes. Important cranial nerves and great vessels can be protected to facilitate the removal of lesions via ETOA alone, or in combination with other endoscopic corridors [6, 7].

Cadaveric dissection and the formation of a multidisciplinary surgical team are important components for the successful development of endoscopic transorbital approaches. While this surgical method may be unfamiliar to neurosurgeons and skull base, cadaveric dissection and anatomical studies facilitate a solid understanding of operative anatomy. Furthermore, oculoplastic surgeons and otolaryngologists contribute to mitigating morbidities and enhancing safety when treating complex head and neck tumors, to provide the best care and outcome to the patients.

Case 1

A 64-year-old Chinese woman exhibited decreased vision in her right eye (visual acuity of 0.6) with a relative afferent pupillary defect (RAPD) [8]. Fundoscopic examination indicated no swelling of the right optic disc, and automated visual field testing showed a deficit affecting the superior and infratemporal regions. Imaging with optical coherence tomography revealed subtle thinning of the retinal nerve fiber layer on the right side. Magnetic resonance imaging uncovered an oval mass that was hypointense on T1-weighted images and hyperintense on T2-weighted images with gradual enhancement, which was compatible with cavernous hemangioma.

Endoscopic transorbital excision of the tumor was performed with an indocyanine green (ICG) -assisted endoscope, through a lateral skin crease incision. A crescent-shaped superolateral orbital rim was removed to gain more surgical freedom. Periorbita was stripped to locate the superior orbital fissure. The meningo-orbital band was divided, and the greater wing of sphenoid bone was removed using a 3 mm high-speed diamond burr under irrigation. Lateral rectus muscle showed a rapid enhancement at 30 s after venous injection of ICG, while the lesion demonstrated delayed enhancement at 90 s. The tumor was then dissected away from the lateral rectus and the superior division of the oculomotor nerve, after which it was removed in an en bloc fashion. The supraorbital rim was replaced using two mini plates. Postoperatively, the patient enjoyed a good recovery, with right eye visual acuity of 0.8 and resolution of relative afferent pupillary defect (Fig. 23.3a–f).

Case 2

A 55-year-old man presented with progressive right eye proptosis. There is no diplopia with full extraocular muscle movement. Preoperative visual acuity of the right eye was 20/30. Serial MRI of the orbit showed an enlarging right intraconal lesion. Endoscopic transorbital surgery was performed to remove the lesion. Lateral canthotomy was performed, followed by a superomedial forniceal incision. Orbital fat was dissected away to expose the lesion. ICG was used, showing delayed enhancement at around 1 min 30 s of the lesion. The lesion was removed en bloc with a cryoprobe assisting the dissection. The advantages of using a cryoprobe are shrinking the lesion and attaching to the lesion firmly to facilitate dissection. The wound was closed by oculoplastic surgeons. Postoperative visual acuity was 1.0, with a resolution of proptosis (Fig. 23.4a–h).

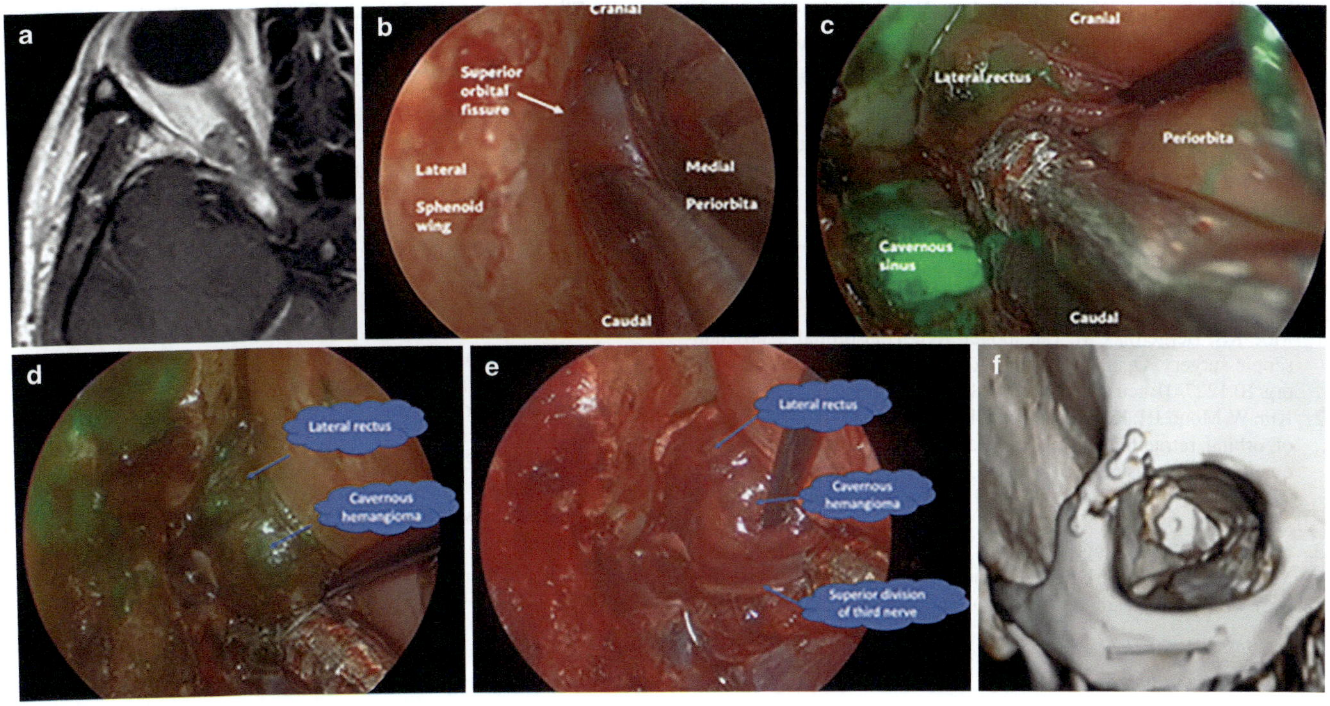

Fig. 23.3 (**a**): Contrast enhanced T1-weighted axial scan of right orbit showed a right orbital apex lesion with heterogenous enhancement, (**b**): Endoscopic view of meningio-orbital band at superior orbital fissure after stripping the periorbita from the sphenoid wing. (**c**): Indocyanine green (ICG) was injected showing early enhancement of the lateral rectus muscle at around 30 s. (**d**) Delayed ICG enhancement of cavernous hemangioma at around 1 min 30 s help to differentiate the cavernous hemangioma from the lateral rectus muscle. (**e**) The cavernous hemangioma was dissected from superior division of third nerve. (**f**) Lateral orbitotomy was reconstructed with miniplates

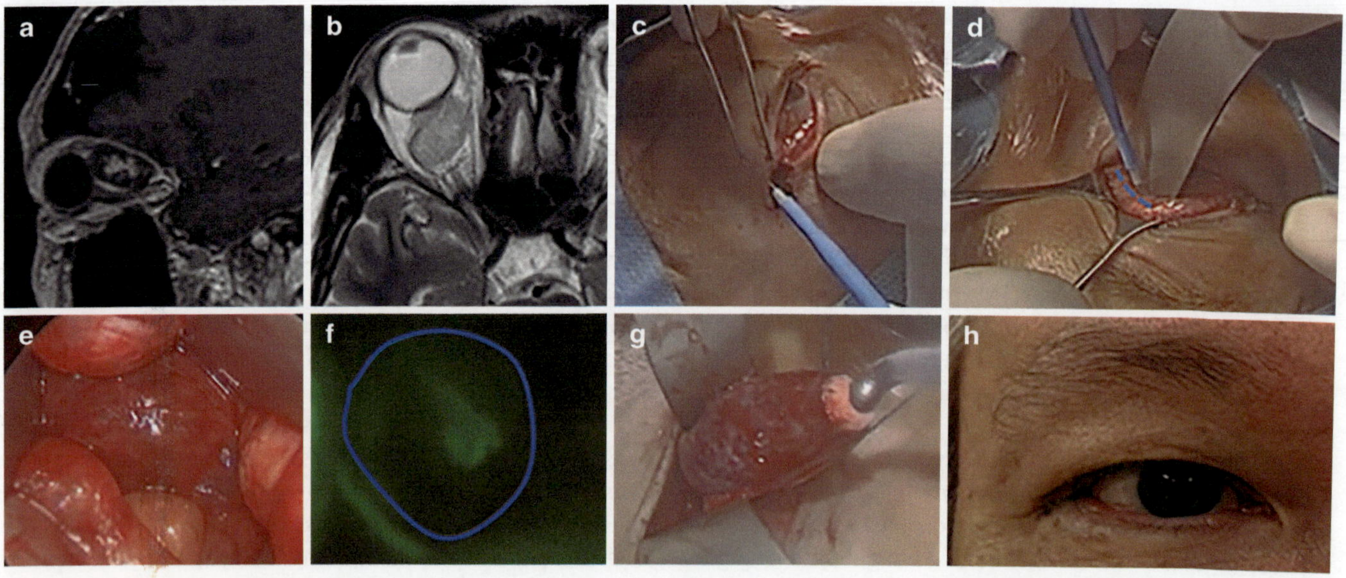

Fig. 23.4 (**a**) Coronal T1-weighted MRI showed a right intraconal lesion superior to optic nerve. (**b**) Axial T2-weighted MRI of the lesion. (**c**) Lateral canthotomy. (**d**) Superomedial forniceal incision(dotted line). (**e**) Exposure of the cavernous hemangioma after division of fat. (**f**) Delayed enhancement of the lesion (outline by the blue circle) helped to differentiate it from the surrounding. (**g**) Cryoprobe-assisted removal of the cavernous hemangioma (**h**) Excellent cosmetic outcome of the patient with resolution of proptosis

23.7 Conclusion

ETOA offered a direct anterior approach to the orbital apex and skull base pathologies lateral to the cavernous sinus and at the infratemporal fossa. Clinical outcomes with tumor excision and CSF leak repair are satisfactory, with acceptable transient morbidities. This minimally invasive approach also opens up potential for biportal or multiportal endoscopic skull base surgeries.

References

1. Moe KS, Bergeron CM, Ellenbogen RG. Transorbital neuroendoscopic surgery. Oper Neurosurg. 2010;67(3):ons16–28. https://doi.org/10.1227/01.neu.0000373431.08464.43.
2. Kim W, Moon JH, Kim EH, Hong CK, Han J, Hong JB. Optimization of orbital retraction during endoscopic transorbital approach via quantitative measurement of the intraocular pressure—[SevEN 006]. BMC Ophthalmol. 2021;21(1):76. https://doi.org/10.1186/s12886-021-01834-5.
3. Houlihan LM, Staudinger Knoll AJ, Kakodkar P, Zhao X, O'Sullivan MG, Lawton MT, Preul MC. Transorbital neuroendoscopic surgery as a mainstream neurosurgical corridor: a systematic review. World Neurosurg. 2021;152:167–179.e4. https://doi.org/10.1016/j.wneu.2021.04.104.
4. Ramakrishna R, Kim LJ, Bly RA, Moe K, Ferreira M. Transorbital neuroendoscopic surgery for the treatment of skull base lesions. J Clin Neurosci. 2016;24:99–104. https://doi.org/10.1016/j.jocn.2015.07.021.
5. Chen HI, Bohman LE, Emery L, Martinez-Lage M, Richardson AG, Davis KA, Pollard JR, Litt B, Gausas RE, Lucas TH. Lateral transorbital endoscopic access to the hippocampus, amygdala, and entorhinal cortex: initial clinical experience. ORL J Otorhinolaryngol Relat Spec. 2015;77(6):321–32. https://doi.org/10.1159/000438762.
6. Dallan I, Castelnuovo P, Locatelli D, Turri-Zanoni M, AlQahtani A, Battaglia P, Hirt B, Sellari-Franceschini S. Multiportal combined transorbital transnasal endoscopic approach for the management of selected skull base lesions: preliminary experience. World Neurosurg. 2015;84(1):97–107. https://doi.org/10.1016/j.wneu.2015.02.034.
7. di Somma A, Langdon C, de Notaris M, Reyes L, Ortiz-Perez S, Alobid I, Enseñat J. Combined and simultaneous endoscopic endonasal and transorbital surgery for a Meckel's cave schwannoma: technical nuances of a mini-invasive, multiportal approach. J Neurosurg. 2021;134(6):1836–45. https://doi.org/10.3171/2020.4.jns20707.
8. Fong Ng BC, Kwan Mak CH, Chan NL, Lam CW, Yuen HK, Poon TL. Indocyanine green–assisted endoscopic transorbital excision of lateral orbital apex cavernous hemangioma. World Neurosurg. 2022;158:167. https://doi.org/10.1016/j.wneu.2021.11.060.

Endoscopic Transorbital Approach for Orbital Apex Lesions

24

Chiman Jeon and Doo-Sik Kong

Abstract

In the era of neuroendoscopic surgery, an endoscopic transorbital approach via the superior eyelid crease has been proposed as a viable way to access the orbital apex and anterior and middle cranial fossa. In addition to the visualization of cranio-orbital tumors, a surgical corridor through this approach allows excellent visualization of the lateral cavernous sinus while avoiding the need for brain retraction. In addition, this approach allows a more direct and shorter anteromedial surgical access to Meckel's cave without violation of the temporalis muscle. This surgical technique could facilitate minimally invasive surgery for skull base tumors involving the orbital apex. In this chapter, we describe the step by step endoscopic transorbital approach to the orbital apex.

Keywords

Endoscopic · Transorbital · Orbital apex · Four-zone model

C. Jeon
Department of Neurosurgery, Korea University Ansan Hospital, Korea University College of Medicine, Ansan, South Korea
e-mail: caudate@korea.ac.kr

D.-S. Kong (✉)
Department of Neurosurgery, Samsung Medical Center, Sungkyunkwan University School of Medicine, Seoul, South Korea
e-mail: kds026@skku.edu

24.1 Introduction

The classic approaches to the orbital apex have involved a requirement for lateral or medial orbitotomy according to the circumferential extension of the lesion around the optic nerve or craniotomy, eventually combined with zygomatic osteotomy for larger lesions [1, 2]. However, transcranial approaches to the orbital apex are laborious and time-consuming with a high risk of temporalis muscle atrophy and operative morbidity associated with brain retraction and damage of critical neurovascular structures en route to the target lesion [3]. In the past few years, alternative approaches, including endoscopic approaches, have been suggested for the treatment of orbital apex lesions with the goal of decreasing the overall invasiveness of the procedure, tailoring the corridor, and, ultimately, achieving better visual and cosmetic outcomes [2]. In the era of neuroendoscopic surgery, an endoscopic transorbital approach (ETOA) has emerged as a recent technique of skull base surgery, enabling a superolateral corridor to the orbit as well as anterior and middle cranial fossae, although the idea itself is no longer novel.

Orbital apex lesions, including orbital tumors, remain a surgical challenge, because they often require an extensive fronto-temporo-orbital zygomatic approach and a multidisciplinary team approach to provide the best outcomes [3]. They mainly include cavernous hemangioma, meningioma, schwannoma, neurofibroma, and fibrous tumors, which have different characteristics and different imaging findings on CT or MRI [4]. The main goal of surgery for orbital apex lesions is to preserve or restore the vision by maximum safe resection of the lesions, with minimal morbidity. In this regard, selection of the optimal approach tailored to each orbital apex lesion is of utmost importance in order to obtain the best possible functional and cosmetic outcomes. For orbital apex lesions, various techniques have been described,

T. L. POON et al. (eds.), *Orbital Apex and Periorbital Skull Base Diseases*, https://doi.org/10.1007/978-981-99-2989-4_24

including transcranial approaches (such as pterional and supraorbital), lateral orbitotomies, transconjuctival, transantral, and transnasal transethmoidal approaches [2].

We have recently proposed a neuro-topographic four-zone model with the epicenter around the optic nerve on the coronal plane using endoscopic transorbital and endoscopic endonasal approaches, which successfully provided minimally invasive 360° circumferential access to the entire orbit with acceptable morbidity (Fig. 24.1) [5]. Although open transcranial approaches have classically been performed for access to the lesions located in zones I and II, our study demonstrated that ETOA resulted in clinical outcomes comparable to those achieved with conventional transcranial approaches with less morbidity. It provides a more direct and shorter operative corridor to the lesions located superiorly and laterally to the optic nerve via the superior eyelid crease incision. This access-related advantage is clinically associated with a shorter operation time, excellent cosmesis, reduced postoperative pain, a shorter hospital stay, a faster return to normal activities, and lower risks of CSF leak and wound infection [5–7].

We have previously demonstrated the feasibility of ETOA for paramedian skull base tumors, such as trigeminal schwannomas, spheno-orbital meningiomas, and other cranio-orbital tumors [5–9]. In this chapter, we will review the ETOA via the superior eyelid approach for the orbital apex lesions (Fig. 24.2).

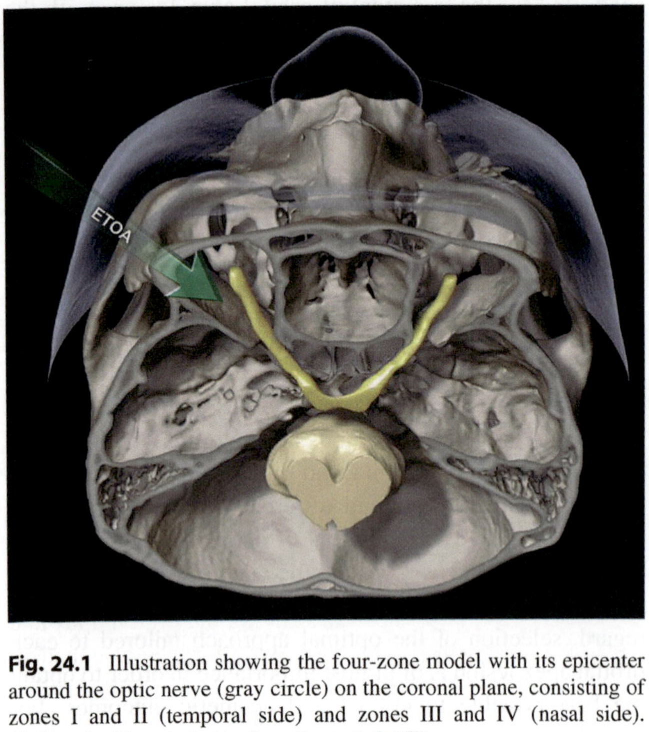

Fig. 24.1 Illustration showing the four-zone model with its epicenter around the optic nerve (gray circle) on the coronal plane, consisting of zones I and II (temporal side) and zones III and IV (nasal side). (Adapted with permission from Jeon et al. [5])

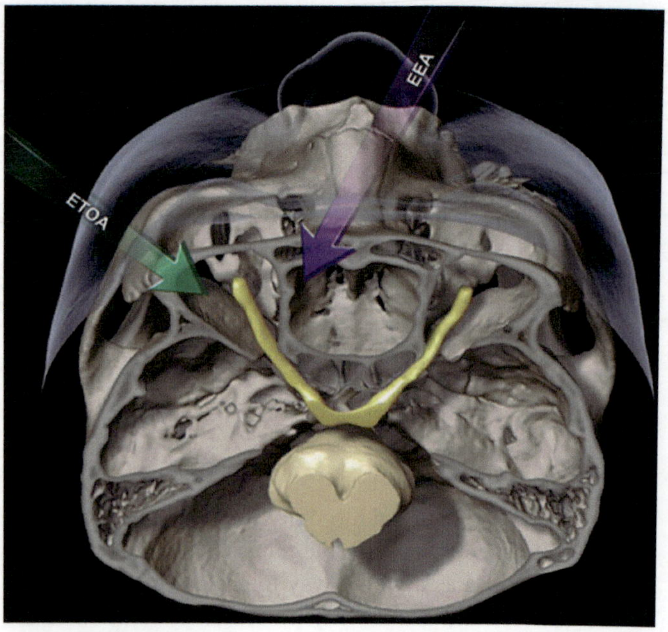

Fig. 24.2 3D reconstruction showing the surgical corridor to the orbital apex using ETOA. (Adapted with permission from Jeon et al. [5])

24.2 Procedure

24.2.1 Patient Position

All patients have preoperative imaging for intraoperative image guidance with computed tomography and magnetic resonance imaging. ETOA is performed by a multidisciplinary team, consisting of a neurosurgeon and oculoplastic surgeon. After induction of general anesthesia with endotracheal intubation, the patient is placed in a supine position with the head in a neutral or slightly flexed position in a Mayfield three-point fixation, and intraoperative multiplanar MRI–CT fusion neuronavigation is registered. Standard surgical preparation is then performed with 5% povidone-iodine solution on the periocular skin and eyelid margins. One should keep in mind that chlorhexidine is contraindicated on the face due to the potential risk of corneal damage. When draping the patient, both eyes should be left exposed so that the symmetry of the globe positions can be assessed intraoperatively. A lubricated corneal protector is placed over the ipsilateral eye to avoid corneal damage.

24.2.2 Surgical Technique

After infiltration of a local anesthetic with a mixture of 2% lidocaine with 1:100,000 epinephrine and 0.5% bupivacaine, a skin marking is made with a No. 15 Bard-Parker scalpel blade at the lateral half of the eyelid crease line for patients with an eyelid crease and at the same length of supraciliary line for patients without an eyelid crease (Fig. 24.3a). The line is extended approximately 1 cm laterally over the lateral orbital rim. The skin and orbicularis muscle flap are raised and extended superolaterally until the lateral orbital rim is reached, with the utmost care taken to avoid encroaching on the levator muscle and aponeurosis. Lateral orbital rim is not usually removed for orbital tumors. The periosteum is cut. A hand-held malleable retractor is gently set in place in an infero-medial fashion, and a rigid 0° endoscope is then introduced into the operative field. A subperiosteal dissection is undertaken in a lateral-to-inferomedial direction until the margins of the superior and inferior orbital fissures are identified (Fig. 24.3b). The cranio-orbital foramen (also known as Hirtl's foramen), through which the recurrent meningeal artery or meningolacrimal branch of the middle meningeal artery traverses, is a good anatomical landmark during the subperiosteal dissection. Being located 1–2 cm anterior to the superior orbital fissure, it is present in 50–60% of patients [10, 11]. After interrupting the recurrent meningeal branch with monopolar cauterization, further dissection to the edges of superior and inferior orbital fissures is made (Fig. 24.3c).

The superior orbital fissure is the next important landmark to identify prior to drilling the greater sphenoid wing and orbital roof (Fig. 24.3d). When dealing with exposing the margin of the IOF, it is essential to keep the subperiosteal dissection toward the inferomedial side. High-speed drilling of the sphenoid bone using a coarse diamond burr is carefully performed from lateral to medial, protecting the periorbita with a Silastic sheet (Fig. 24.3e). Minimal retraction force is applied with slight displacement of the orbital contents in an inferomedial direction while performing drilling as well as dissection. Given that the greater sphenoid wing has a wide triangular shape, drilling of the lateral orbital wall in the same direction also provides sufficient working space. Once the greater wing of the sphenoid bone is drilled until the dura mater covering the temporal pole comes into view, the hand-held malleable retractor is removed. Subsequently, natural retraction with the surgical instruments is intermittently carried out, resulting in minimal retraction force.

Above all, extreme care should be taken to minimize the retraction-induced pressure on the globe, which may induce

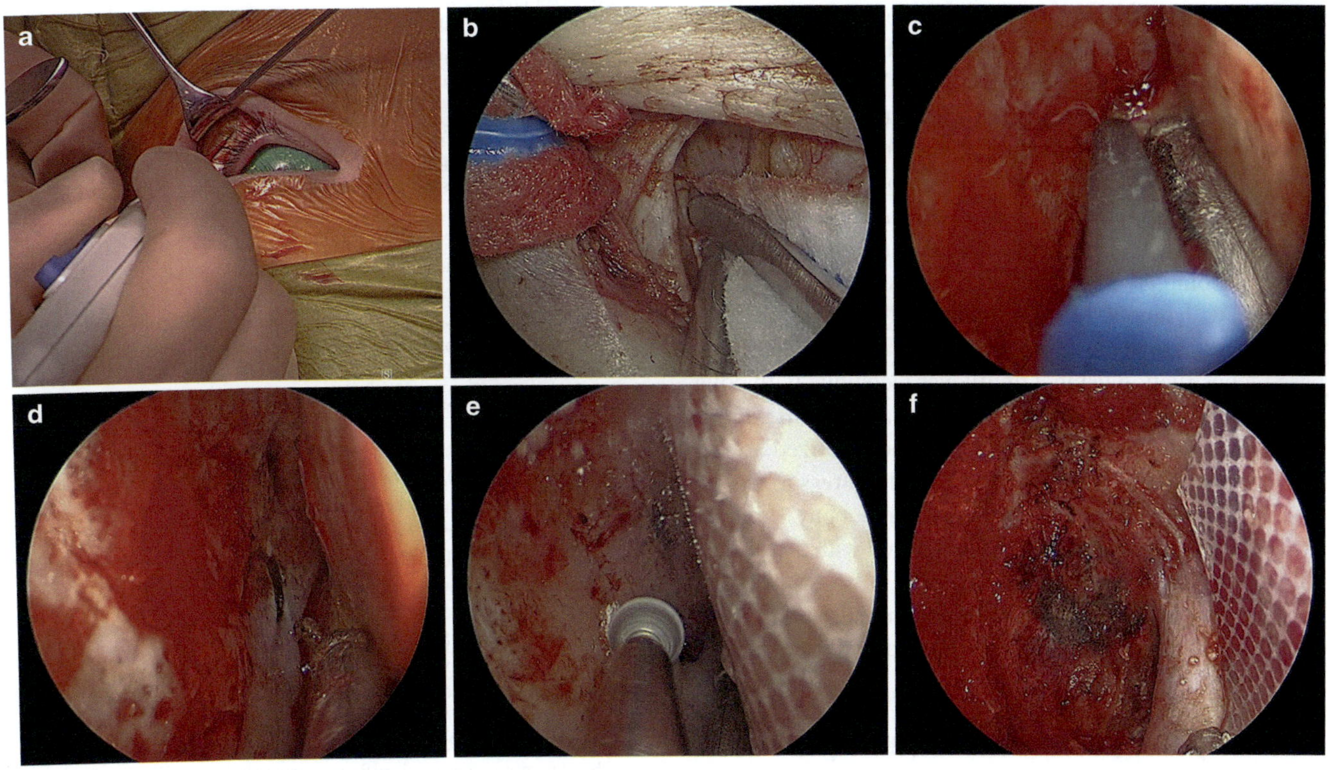

Fig. 24.3 Key steps approaching the orbital apex during endoscopic transorbital approach. (**a**) Superior eyelid crease incision after placement of a lubricated corneal protector over the ipsilateral eye. (**b**) Subperiosteal dissection on the superolateral orbital rim. (**c**) Coagulation of the recurrent meningeal artery at the cranio-orbital foramen. (**d**) Exposure of the superior orbital fissure. (**e**) Drilling of the greater sphenoid wing after placement of a silastic sheet along the periorbita. (**f**) Exposure of the orbital apex, meningo-orbital band, frontal dura, and temporal dura

the oculo-cardiac reflex, while dissecting the periorbita or drilling the greater sphenoid wing. In addition, an elevated intraocular pressure due to globe retraction during ETOA might lower the eye perfusion pressure, potentially leading to perioperative visual loss. We recommend the instruments be withdrawn from the operative corridor every 15 min while checking the pupils. If necessary, additional osteotomy of the lateral orbital rim using chiseling, so-called an extended ETOA, may be helpful in selected cases to avoid excessive retraction of the globe and to gain adequate working space.

Under guidance of neuronavigation, the periorbital overlying the lesion or the tumor capsule is appropriately opened, and the tumor is carefully removed. Microsurgical technique is used throughout tumor removal.

For the orbital apex lesions extending into Meckel's cave or cavernous sinus, an interdural dissection plane should be obtained. At this phase, the key anatomical landmark is the meningo-orbital band (MOB) (also known as the fronto-orbital-temporal polar dura), tethering the frontotemporal basal dura to the periorbita, which leads directly to the interdural space of the cavernous sinus without interrupting the intradural space (Fig. 24.3f). A slight incision at the MOB and a peel-off technique is used to gently dissect the interdural layers between the outer membrane of the cavernous sinus and the dura propria. This avascular dissection plane introduces the route to Meckel's cave and, most importantly, avoids profuse bleeding from the cavernous sinus. The intersection of the dura allows for entry into the cavernous sinus with direct visualization of the V1 and V2 space. Such an approach, through the anteromedial triangle, enables a Hakuba approach along the lateral border of the outer membrane of the cavernous sinus in an anteroposterior direction. The tumor is then removed by applying the same microsurgical techniques as for the conventional transcranial approach.

After complete resection of the lesion, hemostasis is achieved with bipolar forceps and Floseal®. In cases in which the dura mater is opened and/or CSF leakage is evident, skull base reconstruction using a multilayer technique with collagen matrix, autologous fascia, or acellular allogenic dermis is performed. A wedge-shaped piece of polymerized absorbable Medpor can be introduced as a rigid buttress to prevent postoperative enophthalmos when a large bony defect is expected. Finally, the periosteum is sutured with 5-0 absorbable suture, and the skin is closed with 6-0 fast-absorbing plain gut. No lumbar drainage is usually required postoperatively, unless the frontal sinus is breached during surgery.

24.3 Tips for ETOA to the Orbital Apex

- A multidisciplinary team with expertise in endoscopic techniques, consisting of a neurosurgeon, orbital surgeon, and otolaryngologist is essential in ETOA.
- When approaching the orbital apex via the ETOA, one should keep in mind key anatomical landmarks, such as recurrent meningeal artery, superior orbital fissure, and meningo-orbital band.
- Because long-standing globe retraction may often cause elevation of orbital pressure, resulting in cardiac arrhythmias, frequent monitoring of pupil size, heart rate, and blood pressure, along with electrocardiography, are required, and intermittent release from retraction of the eyeball is recommended. One should be cognizant and cautious of the potential risk of postoperative visual loss due to retraction of the ipsilateral globe during ETOA.
- As with any novel surgical technique, a concerning drawback is the long learning curve that is required for the maneuverability of the zero-degree and angled endoscopes in a narrow operative field via the transorbital corridor. It is thus important that practice in the cadaver laboratory be made mandatory to gain familiarity with this minimally invasive approach.

References

1. Paluzzi A, Gardner PA, Fernandez-Miranda JC, et al. "Round-the-Clock" surgical access to the orbit. J Neurol Surg B Skull Base. 2015;76(1):12–24.
2. Luzzi S, Zoia C, Rampini AD, et al. Lateral transorbital neuro-endoscopic approach for intraconal meningioma of the orbital apex: technical nuances and literature review. World Neurosurg. 2019;131:10–7.
3. Roth J, Fraser JF, Singh A, et al. Surgical approaches to the orbital apex: comparison of endoscopic endonasal and transcranial approaches using a novel 3D endoscope. Orbit. 2011;30(1):43–8.
4. Mendoza-Santiesteban E, Mendoza-Santiesteban CE, Berazain AR, et al. Diagnosis and surgical treatment of orbital tumors. Semin Ophthalmol. 2010;25(4):123–9.
5. Jeon C, Hong SD, Woo KI, et al. Use of endoscopic transorbital and endonasal approaches for 360 degrees circumferential access to orbital tumors. J Neurosurg. 2020:1–10.
6. Jeon C, Hong CK, Woo KI, et al. Endoscopic transorbital surgery for Meckel's cave and middle cranial fossa tumors: surgical technique and early results. J Neurosurg. 2018:1–10.
7. Kong DS, Young SM, Hong CK, et al. Clinical and ophthalmological outcome of endoscopic transorbital surgery for cranioorbital tumors. J Neurosurg. 2018;131(3):667–75.
8. Kong DS, Kim YH, Hong CK. Optimal indications and limitations of endoscopic transorbital superior eyelid surgery for spheno-orbital meningiomas. J Neurosurg. 2020;134(5):1472–9.
9. Park HH, Hong SD, Kim YH, et al. Endoscopic transorbital and endonasal approach for trigeminal schwannomas: a retrospective multicenter analysis (KOSEN-005). J Neurosurg. 2020;133(2):467–76.
10. Abed SF, Shams P, Shen S, et al. A cadaveric study of the cranio-orbital foramen and its significance in orbital surgery. Plast Reconstr Surg. 2012;129(2):307e–11e.
11. Erturk M, Kayalioglu G, Govsa F, et al. The cranio-orbital foramen, the groove on the lateral wall of the human orbit, and the orbital branch of the middle meningeal artery. Clin Anat. 2005;18(1):10–4.

Endoscopic Transorbital Approach to Infratemporal Fossa

25

Calvin MAK and Ben Ng

Abstract

The infratemporal fossa is a space that communicates with the orbit and pterygopalatine fossa. This chapter describes the endoscopic transorbital approach in a step-by-step fashion to the infratemporal fossa and displays key endoscopic images to delineate the anatomical details. Different approaches to the infratemporal fossa are compared and discussed. An illustrated case of parapharyngeal space carcinoma was described by using a triportal endoscopic technique.

Keywords

Infratemporal fossa · Transorbital · Endoscope · Mandibular nerve · Pterygopalatine fissure · Triportal

25.1 Introduction

The infratemporal fossa (ITF) is an important space for skull base surgeons to be familiar with. It houses multiple neural and vascular structures and provides a corridor to different compartments of the inferolateral skull base. Superiorly, it is bounded by the inferior surface of the greater wing of the sphenoid. Inferiorly, it is bounded by the attachment of the medial pterygoid muscles to the mandible. The anterior border is defined by the posterior aspect of the maxilla, and the posterior border is defined by the mastoid and styloid processes of the temporal bone. The lateral pterygoid plate forms the medial border, and the ramus of the mandible forms the lateral border of the ITF.

There are a few important structures and surgical compartments adjacent to the ITF. The foramen ovale and foramen spinosum opens to the roof of the ITF. The medial border communicates with the pterygopalatine fossa through the pterygomaxillary fissure at the anteroposterior aspect of the medial border. The cartilaginous eustachian tube is at the posteromedial aspect of the ITF, covering the horizontal portion of the petrous internal carotid artery (ICA). The orbit communicates with the superolateral corner of the ITF via the inferior orbital fissure (IOF) [1].

The content of ITF includes the following:

- The inferior part of the temporalis muscle, the lateral and medial pterygoid muscles
- Mandibular nerve (V3) and the branches
- Chorda tympani branch of facial nerve
- Otic ganglion
- Maxillary artery [2]
- Accessory meningeal artery
- Venous plexuses

Both benign and malignant tumors can occur at the infratemporal fossa (Table 25.1) [3]. Due to the deeply seated location and wide range of possible pathologies, the histological proof is often required, followed by surgical excision. Conventional surgical approaches include different craniofacial approaches, which can involve extensive soft tissue dissection, craniotomy, and facial bone incisions. Endoscopic

Table 25.1 Examples of tumors of the infratemporal fossa

Benign tumors	Malignant tumors
Schwannoma	Adenoid cystic carcinoma
Meningioma	Nasopharyngeal carcinoma
Nasopharyngeal fibroma	Squamous cell carcinoma
Hemangioma	Adenocarcinoma
Lipoma	Sarcoma (including post-irradiation)
	Osteosarcoma
	Lymphoma

C. MAK (✉) · B. Ng
Department of Neurosurgery, Queen Elizabeth Hospital, Hong Kong SAR, China
e-mail: calvin.mak@ha.org.hk

T. L. POON et al. (eds.), *Orbital Apex and Periorbital Skull Base Diseases*, https://doi.org/10.1007/978-981-99-2989-4_25

transorbital approach provides a new surgical approach to the ITF that is minimally invasive. It also allows superior visualization and dissection for deep structures, owing to direct visualization with high-resolution endoscope.

25.2 Approach to ITF by ETOA

The approach to the ITF is via a standard endoscopic transorbital approach (ETOA) in the previous chapter. If the lesion at the ITF has a low inferior extent, the supraorbital rim can be removed by high-speed drill and plated upon wound closure, in order to gain a wider surgical corridor.

After exposing the middle fossa dura, maxillary nerve (V2) and mandibular nerve (V3), the foramen ovale was unroofed with a high-speed diamond drill. The lateral aspect of the anterolateral triangle was also drilled along V3. The lateral pterygoid muscle was slightly retracted inferiorly to allow access to the lateral pterygoid plate. After opening the periosteum along V3, the anterior trunk of V3 can be identified, namely, the buccal nerve, deep temporal nerve, and masseteric nerve (Fig. 25.1).

The posterior trunk of V3 and the rest of the content of the infratemporal fossa can be identified after the removal of the lateral pterygoid muscle. These would also be visualized in presence of lesions occupying the fossa, with the lateral pterygoid muscle displaced or invaded. The posterior trunk of V3 consisted of three branches, including the auriculotemporal nerve, inferior alveolar nerve, and lingual nerve, which was joined by the chorda tympani (Fig. 25.2).

The middle meningeal artery arises from the internal maxillary artery, travels superiorly, and enters the foramen spinosum. The auriculotemporal nerve crossed anteriorly to the middle meningeal artery among all the studied specimens. The accessory meningeal artery lies posterior to the inferior alveolar nerve in the majority. It may cross the inferior alveolar nerve through fenestration within the nerve as an anatomical variation, according to our dissected cadaveric specimens. The artery continued to supply the lateral pterygoid muscle and ascended to form the artery to foramen ovale (Fig. 25.3). The Eustachian tube descended from the middle ear to the nasopharynx, lying just posterior to the foramen ovale. The Eustachian tube marks the location of the petrous segment of the internal carotid artery, which can be identified just posterior to the Eustachian tube.

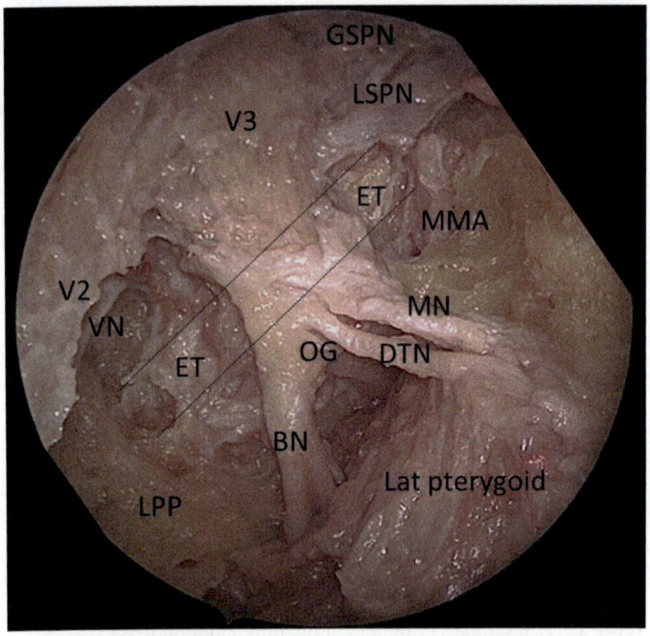

Fig. 25.1 ETOA view of anterior trunk of mandibular nerve. Dotted lines showed the course of Eustachian tube (ET) running posteriorly. *V2* maxillary nerve, *V3* mandibular nerve, *LSPN* lesser superficial petrosal nerve, *VN* vidian nerve, *MMA* middle meningeal artery, *LPP* lateral pterygoid plate, *Lat pterygoid* lateral pterygoid, *MN* masseteric nerve, *DTN* deep temporal nerve, *OG* otic ganglion, *BN* buccal nerve

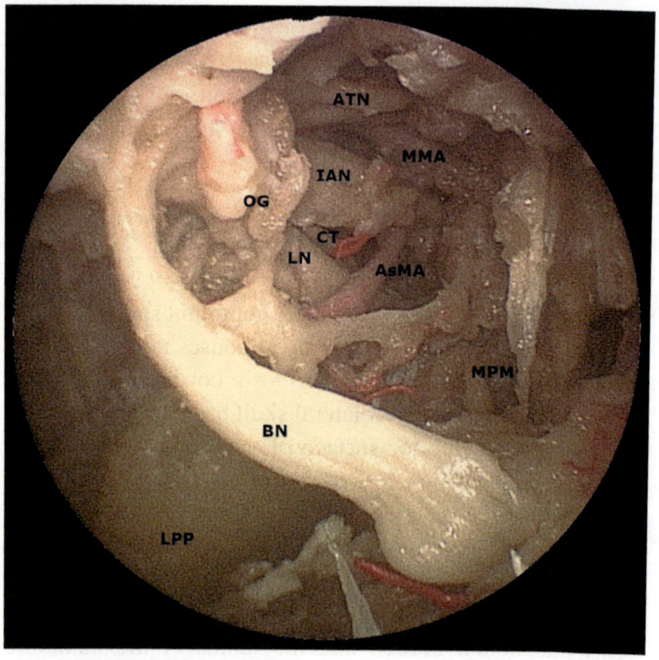

Fig. 25.2 ETOA view of posterior trunk of mandibular nerve (with lateral pterygoid muscle removed) and its branches. *ATN* auriculotemporal nerve, *IAN* inferior alveolar nerve, *LN* lingual nerve, *CT* chorda tympani, *BN* buccal nerve, *OG* otic ganglion, *MMA* middle meningeal artery, *AsMA* accessory meningeal artery, *MPM* middle pterygoid muscle, *LPP* lateral pterygoid plate

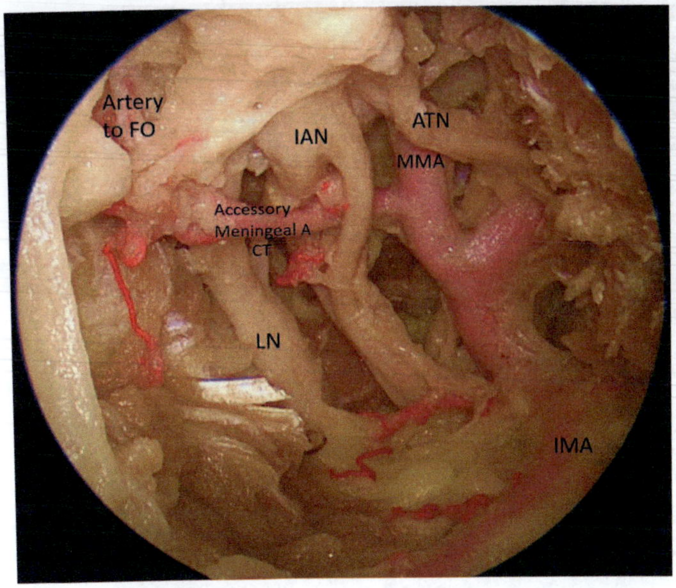

Fig. 25.3 Magnified ETOA view of posterior trunk of mandibular nerve. Anatomical variation showing fenestration of inferior alveolar nerve (IAN), which the accessory meningeal artery passed through. *ATN* auriculotemporal nerve, *LN* lingual nerve, *CT* chorda tympani, *IMA* internal maxillary artery, *MMA* middle meningeal artery, *FO* foramen ovale

Table 25.2 Comparison of approaches to ITF

	Craniotomy	Endoscopic endonasal	Endoscopic transorbital
	Preauricular subtemporal	Transpterygoid	Anterolateral triangle
Exposure of ITF	Superficial & lateral compartment	Medial compartment	Superior & deep compartment
Skin incision	Large	No	Minimal
Access to structures			
Maxillary nerve	++	++	++
Petrous ICA	+++	+	++
Maxillary Artery	+++	++	+
Complications			
Temporalis atrophy	+++	–	–
Pterygoid muscle weakness	+	+++	–
Frontalis weakness	++	–	–
CSF leak	–	+	–

25.3 Comparison of Different Approaches

Table 25.2 highlights the difference among different approaches to the ITF, including preauricular subtemporal, endoscopic endonasal transpterygoid, and endoscopic transorbital approaches. ETOA requires minimal skin incision in the superior lid crease or subbrow region and is cosmetically more pleasant than the open approach with minimal risk of temporalis atrophy and frontalis weakness. ETOA offers access to the maxillary nerve and mandibular nerve through the anterolateral triangle between these two nerves. In particular, the petrous portion of the carotid artery can be controlled after gaining access to the cartilaginous portion of the Eustachian tube. This is useful for biportal endoscopic surgery (transorbital and endonasal) to achieve en bloc resection of malignant tumors, where the carotid artery can be safeguarded directly under endoscopic vision. There is also a low chance of leakage of cerebrospinal fluid for this pure extradural approach.

25.4 Case Illustration

The patient is a 57-year-old gentleman with good past health who presented with recurrent right otorrhea for a few years. On physical examination, the right tympanic membrane was moist and perforated. The facial nerve function was intact. There was no head and neck swelling or mass. Magnetic resonance imaging (MRI) of the head and neck showed a 4 cm lipomatous lesion at the right parapharyngeal space (Fig. 25.4a–c). Nasoendoscopy showed a whitish firm mass obliterating the right Eustachian tube (Fig. 25.5a, b). Biopsy yielded a well-differentiated liposarcoma. The tumor was resected via a triportal approach. The first portal was robotic transoral approach in which a palatal flap was created to provide access to the tumor . The infero-medial aspect of the tumor was dissected up to the level of the nasopharynx using robotic system (Da Vinci Xi) (Fig. 25.5d, e). The second portal was the transorbital approach in which the superior orbital fissure was opened by drilling the greater wing of the sphenoid. V2 and V3 were identified. The tumor was situated postero-medial to V2 and V3. The superior pole of the tumor

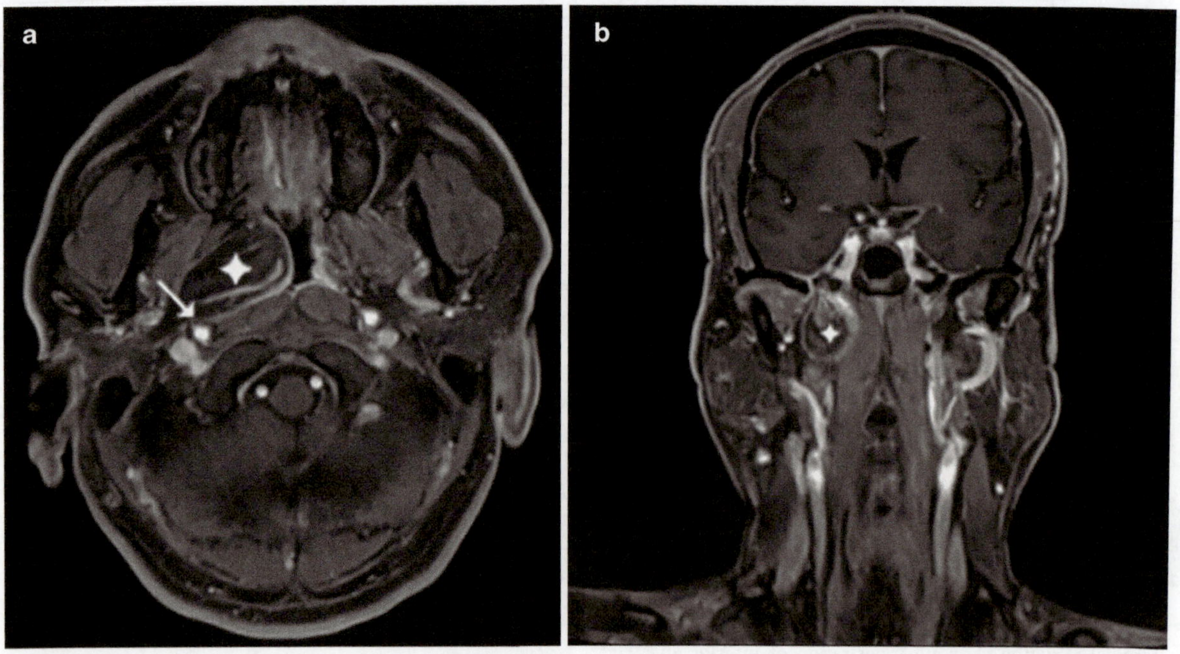

Fig. 25.4 Anatomy and characteristics of the tumor on contrast MRI. (**a**) Axial T1-weighted post-contrast MRI showed a 4 cm lipomatous lesion (♦) with internal enhancing septations, at the right parapharyngeal space (PPS). The lesion abutted the right ICA posteriorly (arrow), and bulged into the lateral wall of the nasopharyngeal mucosa medially. (**b**) Coronal T1-weighted post-contrast MRI showed the lesion extended down to the inferior aspect of the right petrous bone

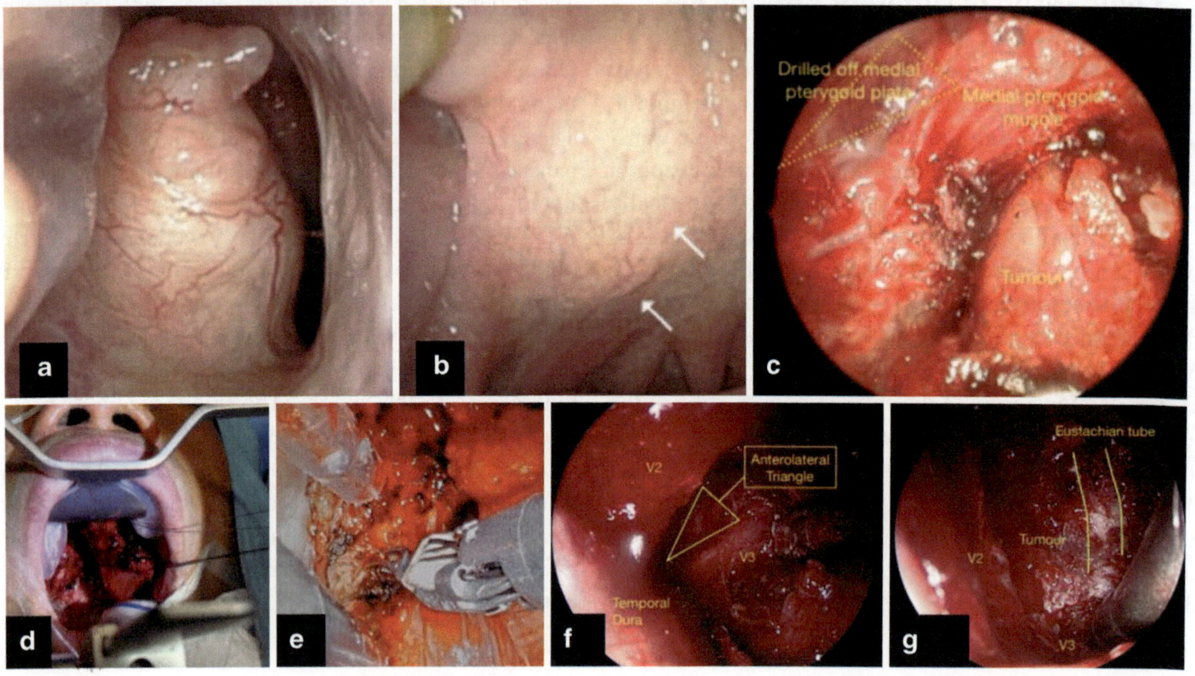

Fig. 25.5 (**a**–**g**) Surgical steps of the right parapharyngeal space tumor using triportal endoscopic approach, including ETOA. (**a**–**c**) Endoscopic endonasal view. (**a**) The tumor bulged out and obliterated the right Eustachian tube. (**b**) Smooth swelling over the right side of the soft palate. (**c**) The posterior aspect of the medial pterygoid plate was drilled to expose the anteromedial aspect of the tumor. The dissection continued with the identification of ICA, which was protected at the posterolateral aspect of the tumor via the transorbital port. (**d**, **e**) Transoral view. (**d**) A palatal flap was raised to provide access to the tumor. (**e**) The inferomedial aspect of the tumor was dissected to the level of the nasopharynx using the Da Vinci Xi robotic system. (**f**, **g**) Endoscopic transorbital view. (**f**) The inferior orbital fissure was opened by drilling the greater wing of the sphenoid. V2 and V3 were identified. The tumor was located posteromedial to V2 and V3. (**g**) The superior pole of the tumor was dissected away from the Eustachian tube

was dissected away from the Eustachian tube (Fig. 25.5f, g). The third portal was endo-nasal approach in which the posterior end of the medial pterygoid plate was drilled to expose the antero-medial aspect of the tumor (Fig. 25.5c). The dissection continued with the ICA identified and protected at the posterolateral aspect of the tumor by the trans-orbital port.

Surgical management of parapharyngeal space tumor is often challenging owing to the anatomical complexity of this area and adjacent critical neurovascular structure. The triportal minimally invasive surgery described above is a novel technique. Transcervical, cervical-parotid and mandibulotomy are the commonly reported approaches to resect parapharyngeal space tumors. However, they are bounded by either exposure limitations or high surgical morbidities. The use of endonasal and/or transoral routes with endoscope has been attempted to improve visualization and reduce surgical morbidities, yet their application is limited in tackling lesions situated in upper and lateral infratemporal fossa/parapharyngeal space. ETOA to the infratemporal fossa illustrates its advantage to overcome such shortcomings and provide an additional operative corridor.

References

1. Isolan GR, Rowe R, Al-Mefty O. Microanatomy and surgical approaches to the infratemporal fossa: an anaglyphic three-dimensional stereoscopic printing study. Skull Base. 2007;17(5):285–302. https://doi.org/10.1055/s-2007-985193.
2. Alvernia JE, Hidalgo J, Sindou MP, et al. The maxillary artery and its variants: an anatomical study with neurosurgical applications. Acta Neurochir (Wien). 2017;159(4):655–64. https://doi.org/10.1007/s00701-017-3092-5.
3. Tiwari R, Quak J, Egeler S, et al. Tumors of the infratemporal fossa. Skull Base Surg. 2000;10(1):1–9. https://doi.org/10.1055/s-2000-6789.

Surgical Treatment for Traumatic Optic Neuropathy

26

Yi Kui Zhang, Hunter Kwok Lai YUEN, and Wencan Wu

Abstract

Traumatic optic neuropathy (TON) is a severe and potentially blinding condition. Even though the role of surgical decompression is still debatable, many surgeons think that surgical decompression will be beneficial to selected cases. In this chapter, we will discuss how to perform endoscopic trans-ethmoid optic canal decompression (ETOCD) in TON.

Keywords

Traumatic optic neuropathy · Surgical decompression · Transnasal · Endoscopic · Optic canal decompression

26.1 Epidemiology

Traumatic optic neuropathy (TON) is an uncommon cause of visual loss after head injury, the incidence is around 2% in all head and/or facial injuries [1–3], and the degree of damage may range from simple contusion to complete avulsion of the optic nerve. Direct TON (DTON) refers to direct optic nerve injury with significant anatomical disruption to the optic nerve, for example, from a projectile penetrating the orbit at high velocity or optic nerve avulsion, or those with optic canal fracture with bony impingement onto the optic nerve. Indirect TON (ITON) is caused by the transmission of forces to the optic nerve from a distant site, without any overt damage to the surrounding tissue structures. Sometimes, occult optic canal fracture may be missed, both direct and indirect mechanisms can contribute to optic nerve damage, and a clear distinction between DTON and ITON is not always possible.

For those cases with complete optic nerve transection or avulsion, there is no proven treatment. In this chapter, we are focusing on those TON with radiologically intact optic nerve after closed head trauma, and we will simply refer these as ITON. In ITON, the damage mostly occurs at the intracanalicular segment of the optic nerve. Some of the ITON may turn up to have DTON component due to occult optic canal fracture with or without bony impingement onto the optic nerve that were noted during surgical intervention [4]. The vast majority of ITON patients are young males [5, 6], and nearly 80% ITON patients presented with visual acuity worse than 20/200 soon after trauma [6]. Spontaneous visual recovery occurs in around 50% of ITON patients at 3-month follow-up [6, 7].

26.2 Pathophysiology of TON

In DTON, the damage is caused by the direct injury itself, such as optic nerve transection. For ITON, the exact underlying mechanism of optic nerve damage is unknown. It is hypothesized that the force causing frontal head injury transmits along the bony orbital wall to the optic canal causing damage to the intracanalicular portion of optic nerve and its vasculature. In some cases, optic canal fracture could be revealed by high-resolution skull CT scan or as an intraoperative finding during trans-nasal endoscopic surgical decompression surgery [8]. In addition, both holographic finding and virtual biomechanical analysis discovered that forces from the frontal head can cause skeletal distortion of the optic canal via stress propagation [9–12]. Furthermore, some special anatomical features of the optic canal render

Y. K. Zhang · W. Wu
Department of Orbital and Oculoplastic Surgery, Eye Hospital of Wenzhou Medical University, Wenzhou, Zhejiang, China

H. K. L. YUEN (✉)
Hong Kong Eye Hospital, Hong Kong SAR, China

Department of Ophthalmology and Visual Sciences, The Chinese University of Hong Kong, Hong Kong SAR, China
e-mail: yuenkl1@ha.org.hk

T. L. POON et al. (eds.), *Orbital Apex and Periorbital Skull Base Diseases*, https://doi.org/10.1007/978-981-99-2989-4_26

the intracanalicular optic nerve more vulnerable to mechanical stress, these include the following: (1) firm adhesion between the dura around the intracanalicular optic nerve and the optic canal periosteum [4, 9, 10] and (2) the small subarachnoid space surrounding the intracanalicular optic nerve with minimal cerebrospinal fluid [13]. Following the aforementioned primary mechanical injury, secondary damage will occur because of ischemia and neuroinflammation [1, 7, 10]. Consequential compartment syndrome (optic nerve swelling within the confined optic nerve canal) may also contribute to visual loss and progressive optic nerve damage.

26.3 Management of TON and Proposed Indication for Surgical Decompression

Currently, no consensus exists from studies published to date on a preferred treatment for TON including ITON. Possible treatment options include high dose or "mega" dose corticosteroid treatment and/or optic canal decompression. The role of these treatments is debatable, and these treatments didn't yield better visual outcome compared with observation alone according to the nonrandomized International Optic Nerve Trauma Study and others [6, 7, 14]. As such, surgical intervention should be cautious and decided on a case-by-case basis with informed consent from patients.

Although there is no consensus on indication of optic canal decompression, we will consider the possibility of surgical intervention when TON patients meet the follow criteria: (1) the patient suffer from substantial visual loss (usually worse than 20/200) with poor response to corticosteroid treatment, (2) absence of intraocular injury or apparent skull base fracture (except for the canal fracture), and (3) the patient is completely conscious who can consent to the surgical treatment, after being informed of the unproven benefit and the potential complications of the surgery.

26.4 Surgical Approaches

The rational of surgical optic canal decompression is to relieve the presumably elevated intracanalicular pressures resulted from the secondary inflammatory response after the primary injury. It also aims to remove any bony impingement onto the optic nerve, sometimes such bony impingement may not be identified by CT scan. According to our previous study of 1275 cases, TON patients with optic canal fracture had better visual improvement after endoscopic trans-ethmoid optic canal decompression (ETOCD) surgery than those without optic canal fracture [8].

There are many surgical approaches to decompress the optic canal, including trans-cranial, trans-orbital, and trans-ethmoid pathways, via neurosurgical operative microscope or transnasal endoscopic appraoch [15]. Trans-nasal endoscopic approach can provide excellent assess to the optic canal and its neighboring structures with minimal surgical trauma. This also provides magnified view under bright illumination, which enables delicate surgical manipulation of the optic canal under direct visual guidance. As such, in properly performed cases, the surgical morbidity is minimal. Furthermore, there is no cutaneous incision or facial scar. In this chapter, we will discuss this minimally invasive ETOCD surgery.

26.5 Basic Setup of ETOCD

The basic components of a ETOCD setup are as follows (Fig. 26.1):

1. Trans-nasal endoscopy system, including illumination system (light source, optic fiber) and camera system (Fig. 26.1).
2. Endoscopic powers system (Fig. 26.1), including microdebrider, tricut blade, and microdrill.

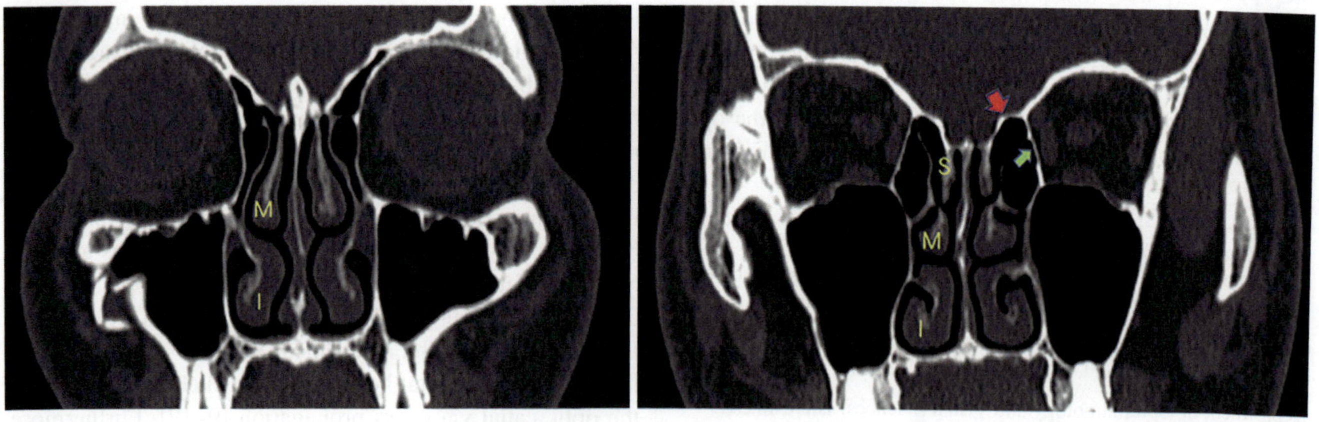

Fig. 26.1 CT scan images of nasal turbinates. *S* superior turbinate, *M* middle turbinate, *I* inferior turbinate. Thin medial orbital wall (green arrow) and skull base (red arrow) are shown as well on the right panel

3. Essential surgical instruments:
   (a) Periosteal elevator
   (b) Vacuum aspirators with different sizes
   (c) Bone cutter (remove bony tissue in the nasal cavity)
   (d) Endoscopic grasping forceps (grasp tissue debris or cottonoid)
   (e) MVR knife (dural incision)

26.6 Surgical Procedures of ETOCD

Precise identification of the anatomical landmarks during the surgery is essential for a safe and effective ETOCD surgery. The surgeon should be familiar with the patient's CT scan before surgery. Intraoperatively, the following anatomical landmarks should be identified and tackled in a stepwise fashion via trans-nasal endoscopic approach: inferior turbinate, middle turbinate, uncinate process, ethmoid bulla, superior turbinate, sphenoid ostium, sphenoid sinus, and optic canal. A key principle during a ETOCD surgery is that the surgeon should not remove or excise tissue superiorly or temporally without certainty, as this may enter into the cranium or orbital cavity accidentally through the thin skull base or medial orbital wall, which may be fractured and displaced after head trauma. The detailed procedures of ETOCD are listed as follows (Fig. 26.1).

1. **Surgical positioning**
   The patient is in supine position with their head slightly elevated (about 10°) to prevent fluid accumulation in the nasal cavity or sphenoid sinus. The surgeon can stand or sit to the right side of the patients according to their preference. Sitting posture with elbow supported allows the surgeon to hold the endoscope with good stability with minimal lower limb muscular fatigue. The patient's face should be turned slightly toward the surgeon to facilitate endoscopic manipulation.
2. **Skin and nasal cavity preparation**
   The patient's entire facial skin is prepared by 5% povidone iodine and then draped with sterile drapes to expose the peri-nostril area. One percent povidone iodine (1:5 diluted with saline water) is applied to irrigate the patient's nasal cavity and then aspirated. To achieve local vasoconstriction and reduce tissue swelling, cottonoids containing 1:1000 adrenaline are inserted into the nasal cavity and maintained for around 20 s. Care should be taken not to injure the nasal mucosa or the middle turbinate during insertion and removal of these packing material. Iatrogenic damage to middle turbinate will cause swelling and hemorrhage, which will impede the access to the deeper structures especially the sphenoid sinus.
3. **Uncinate process exposure and removal**
   Exposure and removal of the uncinate process provides an entrance to the ethmoid bulla and ethmoid sinus (Fig. 26.2). The middle turbinate should be medialized gently toward the nasal septum to enhance the visualization of the uncinate process and part of the ethmoid bulla (Fig. 26.3).
4. **Ethmoid bulla exposure**
   Place cottonoids onto the exposed uncinate process to gain more surgical space and then remove the uncinate process by an endonasal scissor and periosteal elevator to expose the ethmoid bulla (Fig. 26.4). Alternatively, uncinectomy can be performed by backbiter forceps. It is better to cut the inferior end of the uncinate process first and then cut its superior end following a vertical incision into the uncinate process (Fig. 26.4).

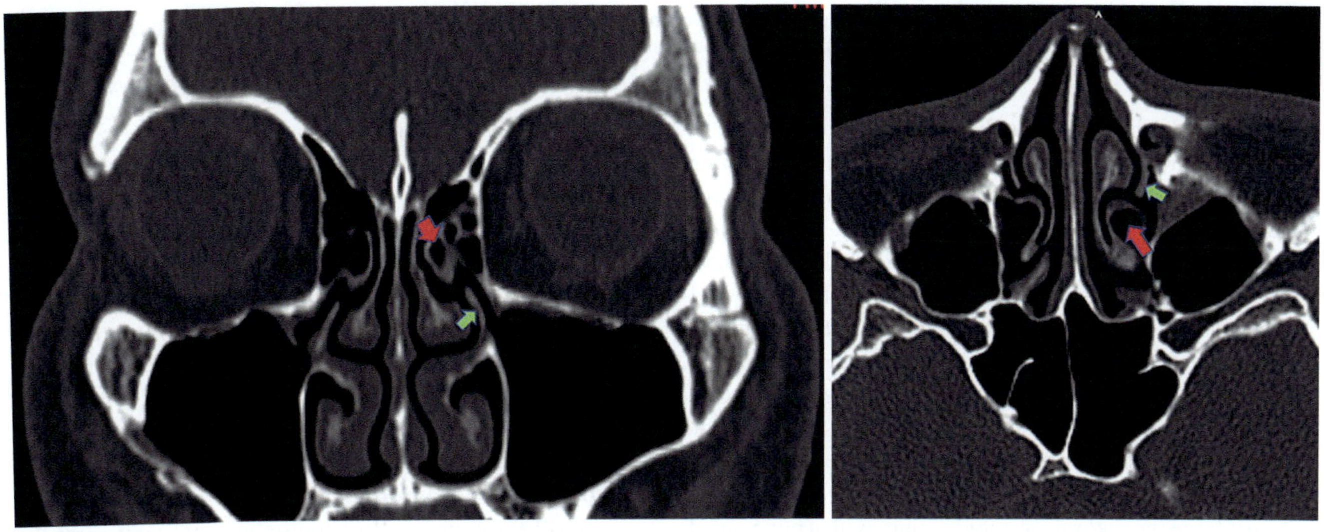

Fig. 26.2 CT scan images of uncinate process (green arrow) and ethmoid bulla (red arrow) on the coronal (left panel) and horizontal (right panel) planes

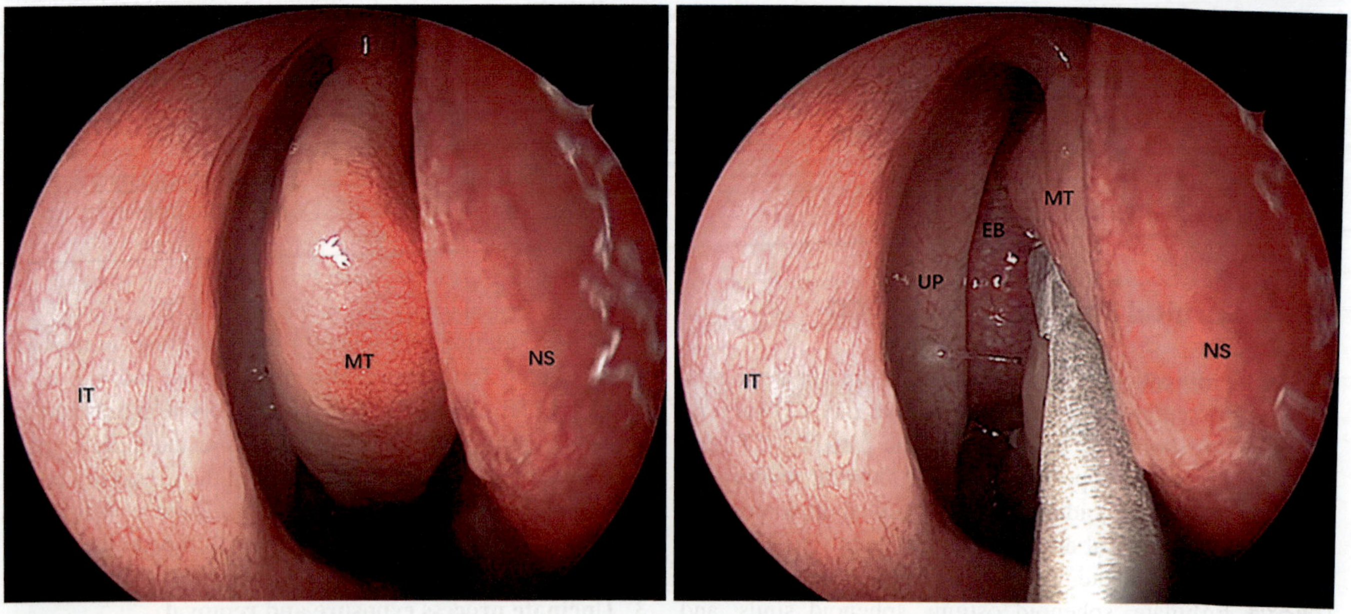

Fig. 26.3 Endoscopic images of inferior turbinate (IT), middle turbinate (MT), nasal septum (NS) on the left panel, and uncinate process (UP) with ethmoid bulla (EB) on the right panel

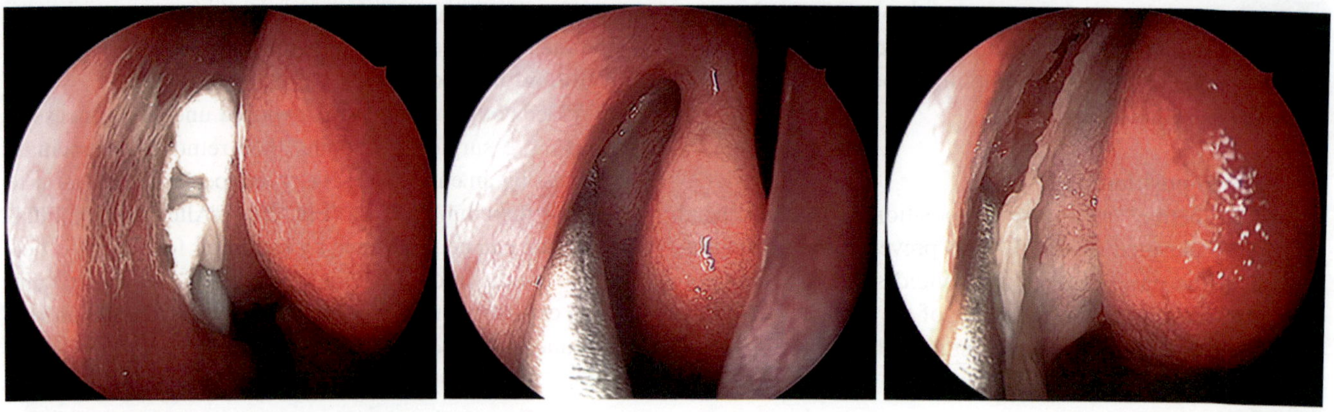

Fig. 26.4 Endoscopic images showing uncinate process removal. Left panel: the cottonoid are inserted onto the exposed uncinate process for vasoconstriction; mid and right panels: vertical incision is made into the uncinate process

5. **Superior turbinate and sphenoid ostium exposure**

   The sphenoid ostium, which usually sit posteriorly and inferiorly to the superior turbinate, provides a natural portal to access the sphenoid sinus (Fig. 26.5). There are two ways to expose the superior turbinate, either by partial ethmoidectomy performed temporally to the mid-turbinate or lifting the mid-turbinate to locate the superior turbinate between the mid-turbinate and nasal septum. After the removal of the superior turbinate, the surgeon can use a periosteal elevator with vacuum aspirator on the tip to identify the sphenoid ostium.

6. **Sphenoid sinus exposure**

   Enlarge the natural sphenoid ostium with a bone punch or a microdebrider to fully expose the sphenoid sinus. Be careful not to injure the sphenopalatine artery, which usually sits beneath the sphenoid ostium.

7. **Optic canal exposure**

   The optic canal protrusion is usually located temporally and superiorly on the posterior wall of the sphenoid sinus, and the carotid artery protrusion lies beneath the optic canal. Between these two protusion is the opticocarotid recess. Surgical navigation system is helpful to provide intraoperative guidance. In case of optic canal fracture with associated hematoma, make sure that the hematoma is not pulsating as it could be a traumatic pseudo-aneurysm from the carotid or ophthalmic arteries, or cavernous sinus (Fig. 26.6).

8. **Optic canal decompression**

   Drill the bony wall of the optic canal very carefully with diamond bur after peeling off the overlying sinus mucosa. When the optic canal bony wall became thin and semi-transparent after diamond bur drilling, remove it

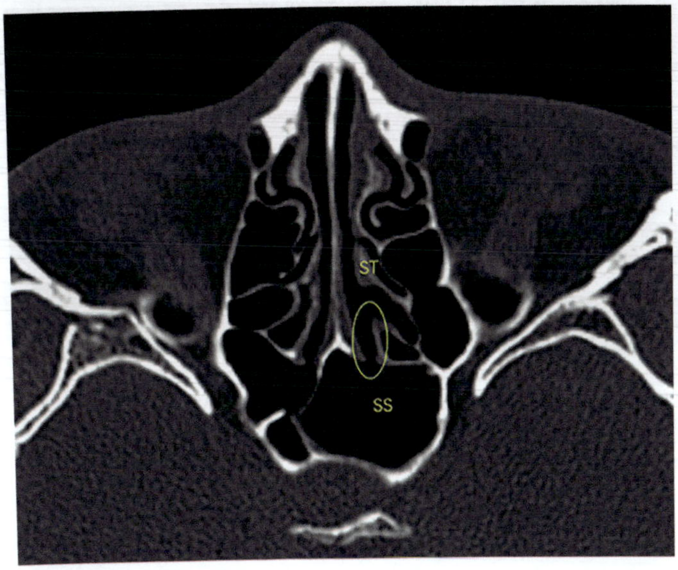

Fig. 26.5 CT scan images of superior turbinate (ST), sphenoid ostium (yellow circle) and sphenoid sinus (SS)

with a periosteal elevator. In case of bony impingement onto the optic nerve, we recommend to drill its neighboring bony wall first and then carefully remove the bony piece away. There is no consensus on the required extent of the optic canal decompression. To reduce the chance of iatrogenic injuries to skull base or cavernous sinus, we usually remove the bony wall along the full length of the optic canal, including its orbital and cranial ends, with 50% of its circumstance. Then we perform small and multiple dural incisions on the entire intra-canalicular optic nerve and the common tendinous ring for further decompression (Fig. 26.7). Subsequently, we gently placed several pieces of merogel filled with corticosteroid over the exposed optic nerve, to reduce post operative inflammation and to provide partial insulation of the exposed optic nerve from the nasal cavity.

9. **Postoperative management**

Intravenous methyl-prednisolone and broad-spectrum antibiotics are administrated for 3 days after the ETOCD

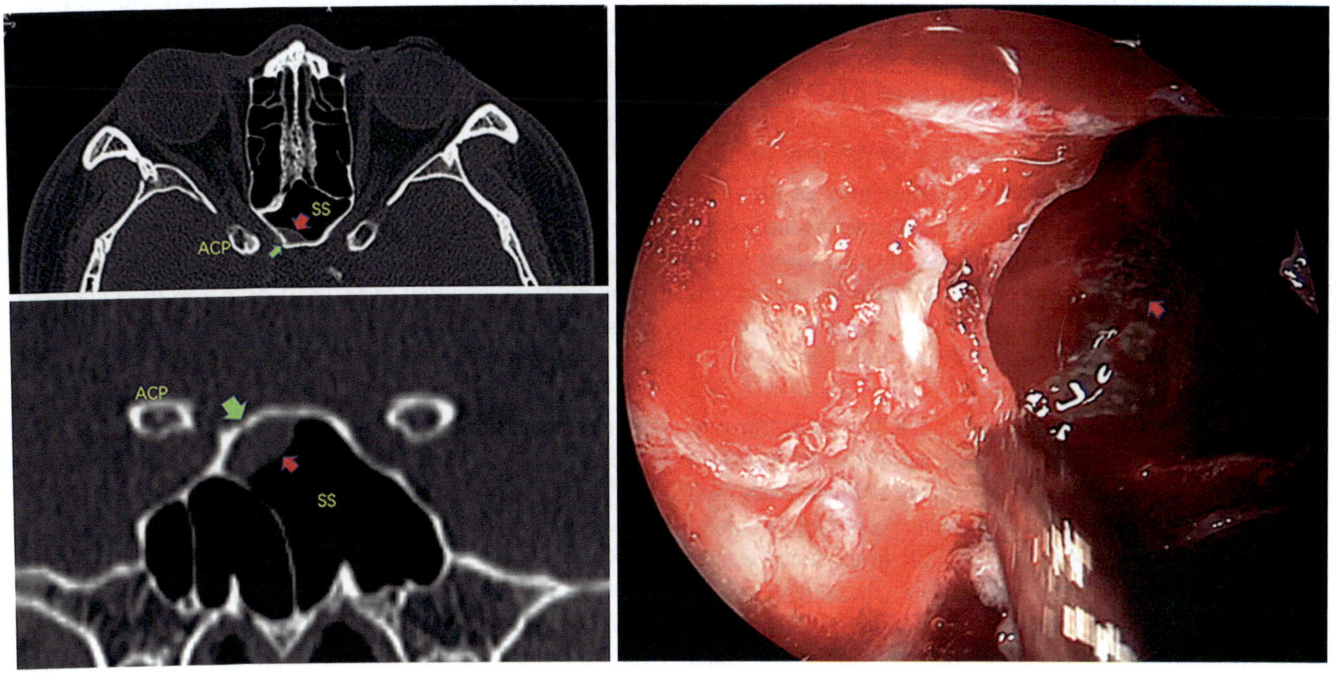

Fig. 26.6 Hematoma on the optic canal with optic canal fracture. Left panel: CT scan images of hematoma (red arrow), optic canal fracture (green arrow), sphenoid sinus (SS) and anterior clinoid process (ACP). The majority of the optic canal is located between the SS and the ACP. Right panel: endoscopic view of the hematoma with dark purple color without pulsation

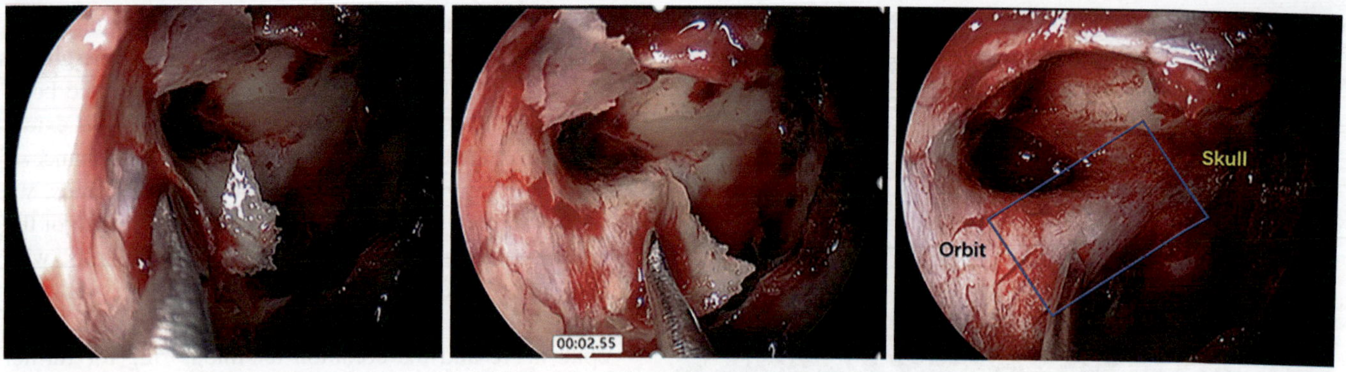

Fig. 26.7 Endoscopic images showing optic canal decompression. Left and mid panels: a periosteal elevator is used to chisel the remaining thin canal wall after drilling; right panel: dural incision is made by an MVR knife

surgery. Nasal corticosteroid and decongestants are used for 1–3 months. Patients are instructed to avoid nose-blowing or intensive physical activity for 2 weeks postoperatively. Routine trans-nasal endoscopic examination of the ethmoid sinus is taken at 1 week after the surgery. Follow-ups are carried out at 2 weeks, 1, 3, 6, and 12 months postoperatively.

26.7 Potential Complications of ETOCD

In properly performed cases, the risk of ETOCD is small with minimal morbidity. Due to the proximity of the optic canal to the ipsilateral carotid artery, cavernous sinus, skull base, and medial orbital wall, caution must be taken to not injure these neighboring structures, especially for the patients with possible skull base instability after trauma. CT angiography (CTA) should be considered in case of suspected carotid artery pseudoaneurysm.

Common but mild complications ETOCD include transient postoperative nasal pain and mild epistaxis. Patients are instructed not to swallow nasal discharge because swallowed blood may irritate their stomach and cause vomiting. In case of a postoperative cerebrospinal fluid leak (transparent watery nasal discharge with or without headache), the patients should be on strict bed rest for a few days and receive systemic antibiotics to prevent potential infectious meningitis and intra-cranial infection. Most of the postoperative CSF rhinorrhea will cease spontaneously following strict bed rest for days. Surgical intervention may be considered for a persistent cerebrospinal fluid leak (up to 2 weeks of conservative treatment).

26.8 The Future of ETOCD Surgery

Both the optic nerve and the spinal cord belong to the central nervous system. In 2021, a study published in the Lancet Neurology found that surgical decompression within 24 h of acute spinal cord injury (SCI) was associated with better sensorimotor recovery. The earlier the decompression was performed, the better the recovery would be 1 year after the injury. If the surgery was done later than 36 h after the injury, the beneficial effect plateaued with time [16]. It might also be true for the optic canal decompression surgery for TON. Future studies can explore the effect of time of ETOCD on the visual outcome of the TON patients. However, challenges exist for such clinical studies due to the following reasons: (1) the incidence of TON (around 1 in 1 million [17]) is much lower than that of SCI (10–50 per million [18]); (2) considerable variation exists in TON patients, such as age, severity of TON, time to surgery, medication received; (3) few patients with TON following head trauma can receive optic canal decompression surgery within 24 h. Therefore, preclinical studies with large animal model of TON, which allows ETOCD surgery as in TON patients, is of great importance.

Furthermore, ETOCD surgery provides a minimally invasive approach to access the injured intracanalicular optic nerve. The exposed sphenoid sinus could be employed as a reservoir for local delivery of neuroprotective drugs/stem cells/biomaterials to repair the intracanalicular optic nerve. With large animal model of TON, therapeutic strategies succeeded in the SCI model or TON rodent model can be tested and selected preclinically.

References

1. Guy WM, et al. Traumatic optic neuropathy and second optic nerve injuries. JAMA Ophthalmol. 2014;132:567–71.
2. Pirouzmand F. Epidemiological trends of traumatic optic nerve injuries in the largest Canadian adult trauma center. J Craniofac Surg. 2012;23:516–20.
3. al-Qurainy IA, Stassen LF, Dutton GN, Moos KF, el-Attar A. The characteristics of midfacial fractures and the association with ocular injury: a prospective study. Br J Oral Maxillofac Surg. 1991;29:291–301.
4. Thale A, Jungmann K, Paulsen F. Morphological studies of the optic canal. Orbit. 2002;21:131–7.
5. Lee KF, Muhd Nor NI, Yaakub A, Wan Hitam WH. Traumatic optic neuropathy: a review of 24 patients. Int J Ophthalmol. 2010;3:175–8.
6. Levin LA, Beck RW, Joseph MP, Seiff S, Kraker R. The treatment of traumatic optic neuropathy: the international optic nerve trauma study. Ophthalmology. 1999;106:1268–77.
7. Yu-Wai-Man P, Griffiths PG. Steroids for traumatic optic neuropathy. Cochrane Database Syst Rev. 2013;2013(6):CD006032.
8. Yan W, et al. Incidence of optic canal fracture in the traumatic optic neuropathy and its effect on the visual outcome. Br J Ophthalmol. 2017;101:261–7.
9. Gross CE, DeKock JR, Panje WR, Hershkowitz N, Newman J. Evidence for orbital deformation that may contribute to monocular blindness following minor frontal head trauma. J Neurosurg. 1981;55:963–6.
10. Anderson RL, Panje WR, Gross CE. Optic nerve blindness following blunt forehead trauma. Ophthalmology. 1982;89:445–55.
11. Nagasao T, et al. Biomechanical analysis of likelihood of optic canal damage in peri-orbital fracture. Comput Assist Surg (Abingdon). 2018;23:1–7.
12. Huempfner-Hierl H, Bohne A, Wollny G, Sterker I, Hierl T. Blunt forehead trauma and optic canal involvement: finite element analysis of anterior skull base and orbit on causes of vision impairment. Br J Ophthalmol. 2015;99:1430–4.
13. Liugan M, Xu Z, Zhang M. Reduced free communication of the subarachnoid space within the optic canal in the human. Am J Ophthalmol. 2017;179:25–31.
14. Yu-Wai-Man P. Traumatic optic neuropathy-clinical features and management issues. Taiwan J Ophthalmol. 2015;5:3–8.
15. Oh H-J, Yeo D-G, Hwang S-C. Surgical treatment for traumatic optic neuropathy. Korean J Neurotrauma. 2018;14:55–60.
16. Maas AIR, Peul W, Thomé C. Surgical decompression in acute spinal cord injury: earlier is better. Lancet Neurol. 2021;20:84–6.
17. Singman EL, et al. Indirect traumatic optic neuropathy. Mil Med Res. 2016;3:2–2.
18. Singh A, Tetreault L, Kalsi-Ryan S, Nouri A, Fehlings MG. Global prevalence and incidence of traumatic spinal cord injury. Clin Epidemiol. 2014;6:309–31.

Part V

Radiotherapy for Neoplasm

External Radiotherapy for Orbital Apex Lesions: Principles and Practice

27

Jeannie Chik, K. M. Cheung, Chi Ching Law, James Chow, Gavin Cheung, K. H. Au, C. W. Y. Kong, and K. H. Wong

Abstract

Tumors arising from the orbital apex represents a therapeutic challenge due to the proximity to vast amount of neurovascular bundles. Neoplasms located in this anatomically confined region usually cause significant symptoms even for small sizes. A small change in size of the lesions will make significant improvement in function and quick symptom relief. Therefore, timely treatment for symptomatic cases is pivotal to avoid debilitating neurological symptoms and maintain quality of life. Management is dictated by the causative pathology, and tissue biopsy is often difficult. Comprehensive clinical evaluation with neuro-imaging studies with or without histological diagnosis is needed to determine the nature of the lesion and formulate treatment plan. This chapter will introduce common tumors found in the orbital apex, different aspects of radiotherapy including radiotherapy techniques, target volume delineation, and toxicities of radiotherapy.

Keywords

Orbital apex neoplasm · Three-dimensional conformal radiotherapy · Intensity-modulated radiation therapy · Volumetric modulated arc radiation therapy · Stereotactic radiosurgery · Fractionated stereotactic radiotherapy

J. Chik (✉) · K. M. Cheung · C. C. Law · J. Chow · G. Cheung
K. H. Au · C. W. Y. Kong · K. H. Wong
Department of Clinical Oncology, Queen Elizabeth Hospital, Hong Kong SAR, China
e-mail: cyk632@ha.org.hk; ckm792@ha.org.hk; lccz01@ha.org.hk; cch932@ha.org.hk; CTC069@ha.org.hk; akhz01@ha.org.hk; kwy803@ha.org.hk; wongkh@ha.org.hk

27.1 Introduction

Orbital apex has crowded anatomic structures with neurovascular bundles passing through it. Lesions located in this anatomically confined region usually cause significant symptoms, and neoplasms are the common pathologies. They include those originating from the orbital apex tissues, direct extension, or perineural spread of the neoplastic lesions arising from adjacent structures or metastases from other primary sites (Table 27.1).

Symptoms mainly arise from the mass effects of the lesions, infiltration of the neovascular bundles by the lesions, and the impaired function of the intraocular muscles. A slight tumor

Table 27.1 Orbital apex neoplasms

Primary lesions originating from tissues at orbital apex	
Malignant	Benign
• Non-Hodgkin lymphoma – MALToma (mucosa-associated lymphoid tissue lymphoma) – Diffuse large B cell lymphoma – Peripheral T cell lymphoma – Follicular lymphoma • Adenoid cystic carcinoma • Others: – Squamous cell carcinoma – Soft tissue sarcoma such as rhabdomyosarcoma	• Cavernous venous malformations (hemangioma) • Neural tumors – Optic nerve glioma – Schwannoma • Meningioma – Optic nerve sheath meningioma • Others: – Hemangiopericytoma
Direct extension or perineural spread of neoplastic lesions from • Anteriorly: anterior orbital structures, eye, lacrimal appendage, eyelids, and conjunctiva • Laterally: paranasal sinuses • Posteriorly: cavernous sinus, pituitary gland, and middle cranial fossa • Inferiorly: head and neck squamous cell carcinoma and adenoid cystic carcinoma, and nasopharyngeal carcinoma	
Metastatic lesions [1] • **Frequent primary sites:** breast cancer (42%), lung cancer (11%), prostate cancer (8.3%), melanoma (5.2%), gastrointestinal tract cancer (4.4%) and kidney cancer (3.2%)	

T. L. POON et al. (eds.), *Orbital Apex and Periorbital Skull Base Diseases*, https://doi.org/10.1007/978-981-99-2989-4_27

growth at that area will threaten vision and warrants early intervention. A small regression of the lesions will make significant improvement in function and quick symptom relief [2]. Therefore, timely treatment for symptomatic cases is pivotal to avoid debilitating neurological symptoms and maintain quality of life. Even management of orbital apex lesions is dictated by the causative pathology and needs thorough assessment. Comprehensive clinical evaluation should be conducted to confirm diagnosis, assess the impacts of the lesion on the patient, and estimate the prognosis of the disease. Neuro-imaging studies including MRI and contrast CT scan of the brain and orbits can delineate the nature and extent of the lesion, guide histological diagnosis, formulate the treatment plan, and define the target volumes of radiotherapy. Staging work-up is indicated when malignancy is diagnosed or suspected.

Although histological diagnosis of the lesions at the orbital apex is challenging and risky, it needs to be considered in certain clinical scenarios. Clinical presentations of most cases regardless of histology are quite similar, while imaging studies have limitations in differentiating chronic invasive fungal sinusitis from inflammatory pseudotumor [3]. When a malignant disease is suspected or infectious causes should be excluded, biopsy is necessary for prompt diagnosis and early treatment. Multidisciplinary team approach is advocated to define the most appropriate way for histological diagnosis.

Surgical resection is commonly the treatment of choice for lesions confined to the orbit to achieve rapid symptom relief by acute decompression. However, it is technically difficult and risky due to the dense network of critical neurovascular structures within the orbit [4]. For orbital apex lesions, surgical treatment will lead to significant complications and may be infeasible. Radiotherapy can be an alternative treatment not only for neoplastic but also some inflammatory orbital apex lesions.

27.2 Radiotherapy

Radiotherapy is the use of ionizing radiation to treat patients with malignant neoplasm and occasionally benign diseases by delivering a precisely measured dose of irradiation to a defined tumor volume with as minimal damage as possible to the surrounding healthy tissues. The main aims include the following: to eradicate the tumor, arrest tumor progression, relieve symptoms, achieve better quality of life, and prolong survival [5]. Radiotherapy can be of curative intent when adopted as a primary treatment, in postoperative cases when there is residual disease or high risk of relapse, or of palliative intent when the disease is beyond cure. The practice of radiotherapy is guided by the treatment purposes, the nature and extent of the lesion, proximity of the lesion to critical organs at risk, and patient factors such as general condition, comorbidities, and symptoms.

Radiotherapy for orbital apex lesions is very challenging. It should be effective to lead to shrinkage of the lesions for symptom relief even though total eradication of the tumors may not always be possible. With advanced radiotherapy technology, a high tumor control rate of nearly 90% with preservation of the eye can be achieved in orbital tumors [6].

27.2.1 Planning

Considering the intimate relationship of the lesions with the optic nerve and limitation of the radiation doses to the optic apparatus, radiotherapy planning for orbital apex lesions is sophisticated and individualized. High conformality of radiation to cover the lesions with appropriate treatment margin and accurate delivery of radiation doses are the core components of radiotherapy to achieve the treatment aims.

Radiotherapy planning for lesions in this complicated area requires accurate delineation of the lesions and their relationship with adjacent critical tissues. MRI adds details about proximity and involvement of the vital soft tissue structures around the lesions and evaluates the status of surgical margins if any. Joint assessment of the patients and review of the imaging studies by neurosurgeons, ophthalmologists, radiologists, and radiation oncologists will ensure accurate delineation of the lesions.

Regardless of radiotherapy techniques, stringent immobilization of the patient during treatment is crucial. The patient should be treated in a comfortable and reproducible position, which is suitable for acquisition of diagnostic staging imaging. It is commonly achieved by customized thermoplastic cast with the patient supine and the neck in a comfortable position as showed in Fig. 27.1.

27.2.2 Target Volumes [7, 8]

Radiotherapy target volumes are determined by the nature of the irradiated lesions. For benign orbital apex lesions with well-defined borders, such as cavernous venous malformation (hemangioma) and optic nerve sheath meningioma (ONSM), their gross tumor volumes (GTV) can be accurately defined by imaging studies. The planning target volume (PTV) can then be directly generated by adding a quantitative margin to the GTV, taking into consideration the repositioning uncertainties and alignment of treatment beams between fractions. Such lesions are amenable to highly conformal radiotherapy with a tight margin, allowing higher radiation dose delivered to the lesions while minimizing the radiation dose to adjacent normal tissues (Fig. 27.2).

Malignant lesions involving the orbital apex will have infiltrating borders, and MRI should be taken as reference when contouring the GTV. The clinical target volume (CTV)

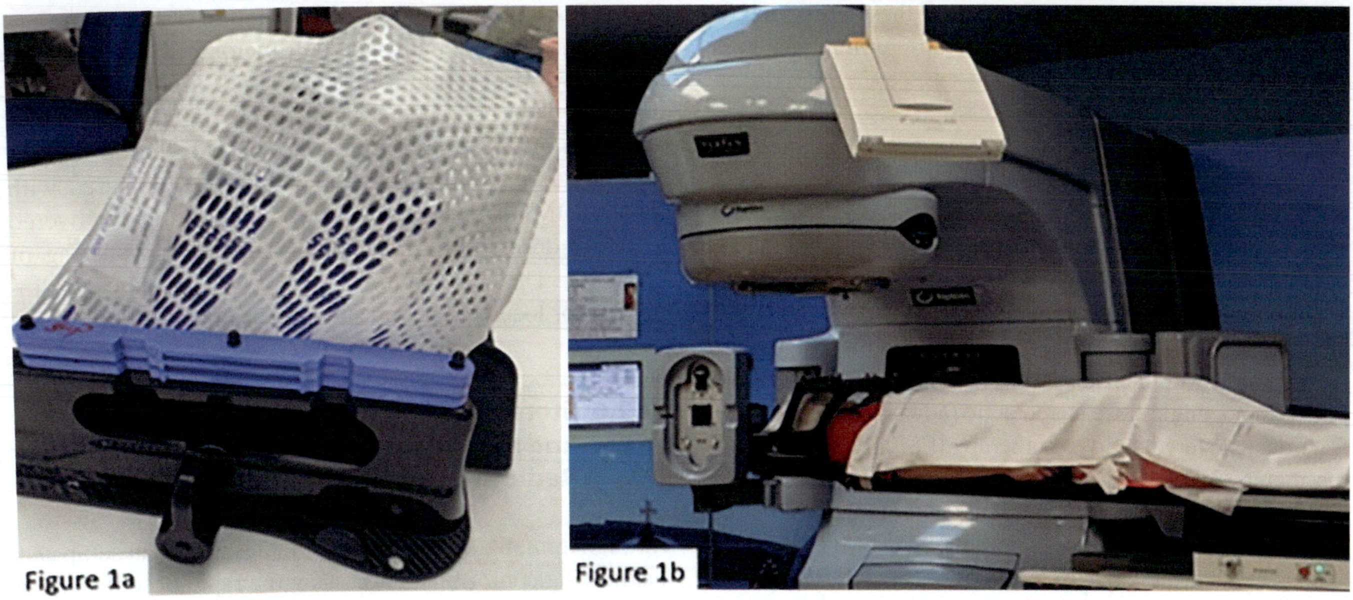

Fig. 27.1 (**a**) A customized thermoplastic cast used for stringent patient immobilization during radiation. (**b**) A patient who is immobilized by a customized thermoplastic cast mounted with a removable frame to the treatment coach is receiving stereotactic radiotherapy

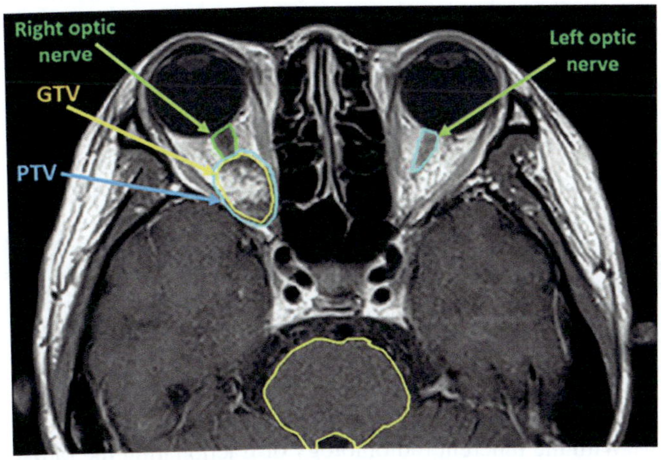

Fig. 27.2 A patient with cavernous venous malformation (hemangioma) treated by fractionated stereotactic radiotherapy. Yellow line is the gross tumor volume (GTV), which is contoured according to the well-defined lesion on the MRI. Blue line is the planning target volume which is generated directly by adding 1 mm margin to the GTV

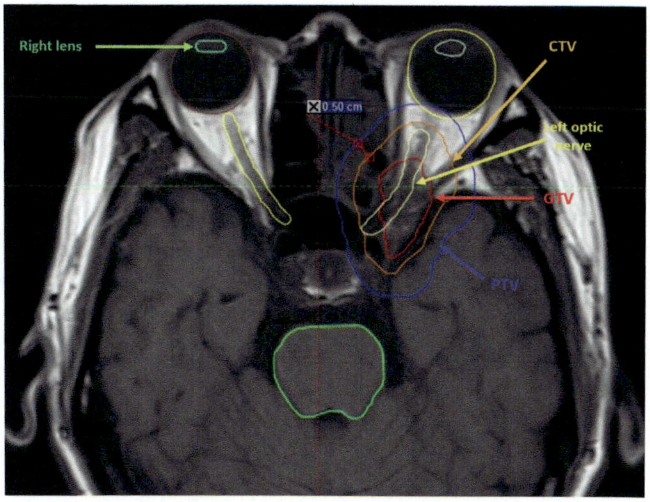

Fig. 27.3 Radical IMRT for primary adenoid cystic carcinoma involving the left orbital apex (70 Gy at 100% I.L. in 35 fractions over 6.5 weeks). Red line is the gross tumor volume (GTV), which is contoured on the planning CT scan with reference to the MRI scan; organ line is the clinical target volume (CTV), which is generated by adding 1 cm margin to the GTV to cover the subclinical disease around the primary with normal brain tissue trimmed out; blue line is the planning target volume (PTV), which is generated by adding 5 mm margin to the CTV

is then defined by a margin to the GTV to encompass any subclinical diseases, which depends on the anatomy of the affected areas and the nature history of the lesion. In adjuvant radiotherapy setting, where the lesion has been totally or partially removed by surgery, the GTV is defined by the gross residual disease if any, while the surgical bed as one of the potential areas of subclinical disease should be covered in the CTV. The planning target volume (PTV) is then generated by adding a margin to the CTV, to account for uncertainties of beam alignment, intra- and inter-fraction motions (Fig. 27.3).

Since there is no lymphatic drainage inside the orbit, prophylactic irradiation of regional lymph nodes is generally not indicated for those neoplasms confined in the orbit. However, some malignant and benign tumors can extend from the posterior orbit or the orbital apex to the middle cranial fossa through the superior orbital fissure and the optic canal, or into the pterygopalatine fossa and the masticator space via the inferior orbital fissure. Coverage of these areas may be necessary when planning of radiotherapy for malignant diseases located at the orbital apex.

27.2.3 Radiotherapy Techniques

With technology advancement, radiotherapy techniques have been extensively evolving, developing from two-dimensional technique, through three-dimensional conformal radiotherapy (3D -CRT), intensity-modulated radiation therapy (IMRT) and volumetric modulated arc radiation therapy (VMAT), to single-dose stereotactic radiosurgery (SRS) and fractionated stereotactic radiotherapy (FSRT), and even proton therapy. These advanced radiotherapy techniques allow high radiation doses delivered to smaller volumes with minimal visual and neurological complications when treating lesions at the orbital apex.

27.2.4 Three-Dimensional Conformal Radiotherapy (3D-CRT)

3D-CRT will be employed when a relatively large area is to be irradiated, while the total dose of radiotherapy can be kept well below the thresholds of critical organs at risk (OARs) or when the OARs can be shielded from radiation. Employing a few fixed treatment fields to achieve target coverage, the planning process is relatively simple. Because of its relatively spatial inaccuracies in patient setup and difficulty of achieving sharp dose fall off in neighboring organs, the drawback of 3D-CRT is inclusion of large area of normal tissues within radiation fields, and this may cause significant long-term complications even though acute side effects may be minimal. Therefore, standard dose fractionation at daily fraction of 1.8–2 Gy is commonly applied for radical radiotherapy using 3D-CRT, allowing sufficient time for sensitive normal structures to repair and regenerate during the interval between fractions. One example is primary radiotherapy for orbital MALToma, in which the whole orbit is irradiated and the therapeutic dose is lower than OARs.

27.2.5 Intensity-Modulated Radiation Therapy (IMRT) and Volumetric Modulated Arc Radiation Therapy (VMAT)

IMRT and VMAT are both advanced radiotherapy technologies, which generate treatment plans with high conformality to target. IMRT modulates the intensity of the radiation beam as well as its geometric shape to deliver complex dose distributions, using forward or inverse treatment planning. VMAT is similar IMRT, except that it generates highly conformal dose distribution with a single rotation of the LINAC gantry. During each rotation, the radiation beam is continuously shaped by the multi-leaf collimator with the dose rate and gantry speed optimized to generate highly conformal dose distributions. Comparing with IMRT, VMAT has the advantage of shorter treatment time, but the conformality is lower for highly irregular-shaped lesions. Compared with 3D-CRT, IMRT and VMAT allow radiation to be delivered at higher doses with greater conformality and sparing of OARs [9]. They are commonly employed in radical radiotherapy for localized neoplastic lesions at the orbital apex.

27.2.6 Stereotactic Radiosurgery (SRS) and Fractionated Stereotactic Radiotherapy (FSRT)

Through minimizing spatial inaccuracies in patient setup and maximizing conformity, harnessing the rapid dose fall-off at radiation beam edges, stereotactic radiosurgery (SRS) and fractionated stereotactic radiotherapy (FSRT) allow higher dose per fraction, which results in a higher biologically equivalent dose to the target without increasing the risk of complications in surrounding tissues. The margin for PTV from GTV/CTV can be as tight as 0.5–1 mm. They can be delivered by Gamma Knife, Cyberknife, or Linear Accelerator. Traditionally, it was reluctant to use SRS in the posterior orbit as the visual pathway is sensitive to a large single dose of radiation [10], and it is also technically difficult to avoid irradiation to the optic nerve. A single dose of 8–12 Gy is considered threshold for development of optic neuropathy [10, 11]. Nevertheless, a few series have reported the use of SRS in various types of intra-orbital lesions with good outcomes, including metastatic tumors [12], cavernous venous malformations [13–15], and optic nerve sheath meningiomas [16] (Table 27.2).

With the inherent radiobiology of fractionating the radiation dose, there is less risk of toxicity to normal structures with FSRT than SRS. Therefore, FRST is safer for lesions in proximity to the optic nerve by keeping the nerve dose below the dose constraint [19]. A Korean series reported favorable treatment outcomes of FSRT for benign orbital apex lesions [17, 20] and suggested it might be considered as the initial treatment of choice for cavernous venous malformations [17]. Klink also reported the results of a case with optic sheath meningioma treated by FSRT with 36 Gy given in six fractions, in which the patient's visual acuity and field remained stable while the appearance of the tumor did not change [18] (Table 27.2).

Other series have reported the results of using stereotactic radiotherapy system with standard daily fraction size of 1.8–2 Gy to treat benign lesions at the orbit and orbital apex. This approach enables a higher total dose delivered to the lesion while keeping the dose to the optic tract within the safety threshold [2, 21–24] (Table 27.3).

Table 27.2 Outcomes of stereotactic radiosurgery (SRS) and fractionated stereotactic radiotherapy (FSRT) for orbit/orbital apex lesions

Series	Subjects	Dose and machine type	Outcomes
Stereotactic radiosurgery (SRS) for orbit/orbital apex lesions			
Klingenstein 2012 [12]	16 patients with orbital metastases	16.5–21 Gy (median: 18 Gy) by CyberKnife	13 (87%) had stable disease
Liu 2012 [13]	23 patients with orbital cavernous venous haemangioma	12–20 Gy (median dose: 15 Gy) by Gamma Knife	20 (87%) out of 23 patients had a decrease in tumor size 11 (79%) out of 14 patients had visual improvement
Thompson 2000 [14]	1 patient with intra-orbital hemangioma after partial resection two times	16 Gy by Gamma Knife	46% reduction in size with no change in vision
Kim 2008 [15]	8 patients with orbital tumors: 5 whose optic apparatus at least 2 mm from the lesion and 3 being blind	13–20 Gy (median dose: 14 Gy) by Gamma Knife	6 (75%) out of 8 achieved tumor control at a median follow-up of 20.9 months
Kwon 2005 [16]	2 patients with optic nerve glioma and 1 patient with optic sheath meningioma	15 Gy to patient with optic sheath meningioma 8 Gy and 12 Gy to two patients with optic nerve glioma, respectively, by Gamma Knife	Patient with optic sheath meningioma had tumor shrinkage with resolving exophthalmos Both patients with optic nerve glioma had tumor size reduction and visual improvement
Fractionated stereotactic radiotherapy (FSRT) for orbital apex lesions			
Kim 2015 [17]	23 patients with orbital apex tumors: 8 cavernous hemangioma, 8 meningioma and 7 schwannoma	18–22 Gy in 4 fractions at 50% isodose line (range: 50–55%) by Gamma Knife	17 (74%) had tumor shrinkage (mean volume reduction of 53.9%), and 16 (70%) achieved visual improvement All cavernous hemangiomas had tumor control (mean volume reduction of 68.3%)
Klink 1998 [18]	1 patient with optic sheath meningioma	36 Gy in 6 fractions	Patient's visual acuity and field remained stable while the appearance of the tumor was not changed

Table 27.3 Outcomes of radiotherapy using stereotactic radiotherapy system with standard dose-fractionation for orbit/orbital apex lesions

Series	Subjects	Dose and machine type	Outcomes
Ratnayake 2019 [21]	6 patients with orbital cavernous venous malformation	45–50.5 Gy at 85–95% isodose line at 1.8–2 Gy per fraction, by 6 MV LINAC	All had tumor shrinkage (average volume reduction by 63%) and symptom improvement without complications
Rootman 2012 [2]	5 patients with orbital cavernous venous malformation with 2 extending to cavernous sinus and 1 extending through superior orbital fissure	40–49.59 Gy at 90% isodose line at 1.62–2 Gy per fraction, by 6MV LINAC	All achieved visual improvement and shrinkage of the lesions (average volume reduction by 60%) without complications
Maaijwee 2012 [22]	3 patients with radiologically cavernous venous malformation at orbital apex	50.4 Gy in 28 daily fractions	All achieved tumor shrinkage and two had improvement of visual acuity, without any adverse effects
Pacelli 2011 [23]	5 patients with orbital ONSM with 4 contained intra-orbitally and 1 having intracranial extension through the optic nerve canal	50.4 Gy in 28 daily fractions	All experienced subjective improvement in vision and had no radiological progression. No late side effects reported
Paulsen 2012 [24]	109 patients (113 eyes) with primary* (*n* = 37) or secondary* (*n* = 76) ONSM	50.4 Gy in 28 daily fractions with a safety margin of 5 mm and then boost with 3.6 Gy in two fractions with a safety margin of 2 mm, by 6MV LINAC (median dose: 54 Gy)	Regression of the tumor (5 eyes): 4% Progression of the tumor (4 eyes): 3.6% Stable (104): 92% Visual acuity was preserved in 94.8% after 3 years and 90.9% after 5 years

ONSM orbital optic nerve sheath meningioma, *primary ONSM* ONSM arising from the sheath of the intraorbital or the intracanalicular portions of the optic nerve, *secondary ONSM* ONSM originating from intracranial meningeal structures with subsequent invasion of the optic canal and orbit

Table 27.4 Radiation dose tolerance of organs at risk (OARs) in radiotherapy for orbit

	Single institute (Queen Elizabeth Hospital, HK)			Quantec [29]		UK consensus [30]				EPTN consensus [31]
	Stereotactic RT			SRS		Stereotactic RT				
						1 Fr (Gy)		5 Fr (Gy)		
	1 Fr (Gy)	5 Fr (Gy)	EQD2 (Gy)	1 Fr (Gy)	EQD2 (Gy)	Optimal	Mandatory	Optimal	Mandatory	EQD2 (Gy)
Brainstem (D_{max})	$D_{0.1cc} < 12.5$	$D_{0.1cc} < 30$	54	<12.5	54	<10	<15	<23	<31	$D_{0.03cc} < 54$
Chiasm	$V_{8Gy} < 0.2$ cc	$V_{23Gy} < 0.2$ cc	–	–	–					
Chiasm (D_{max})	$D_{0.035cc} < 10$	$D_{0.035cc} < 25$	54	<12	55	<8		<22.5		$D_{0.03cc} < 55$
Optic nerve	$V_{8Gy} < 0.2$ cc	$V_{23Gy} < 0.2$ cc	–	–	–					
Optic nerve (D_{max})	$D_{0.035cc} < 10$	$D_{0.035cc} < 25$	54	<12	55	<8		<22.5		$D_{0.03cc} < 55$
Eye (D_{max})	–	–	50	–	–	<8		–		$D_{0.03cc} < 50$
Lens (D_{max})	–	–	6–10	–	–	<1.5		–		$D_{0.03cc} < 10$
Lacrimal gland										$D_{mean} < 25$
Pituitary gland										$D_{mean} < 45$ $D_{mean} < 20$
Whole brain minus GTV	$D_{10cc} < 12$ $D_{50\%} < 5$	–		V_{12Gy} < 5–10 cc		$D_{10cc} < 12$ $D_{50\%} < 5$		–		$V_{60Gy} < 3$ cc

EQD2 equivalent dose in 2 Gy per fraction, D_{max} is defined as the maximum dose to 0.1 cc, 0.03 cc or 0.035 cc of the OAR volume ($D_{0.1\ cc}$, $D_{0.03\ cc}$ or $D_{0.035\ cc}$, respectively), D_{mean} mean dose, $D_{50\%}$ mean dose to 50% of the OAR volume, $V_{8\ Gy}$ volume of OAR with dose >8 Gy

27.2.7 Side Effects of Radiotherapy

The normal ocular tissues have a spectrum of radiation tolerance. Orbital bones, muscle, and fat can tolerate high radiation doses, whereas the lens, eyelashes, retina, and lacrimal system are more radiosensitive [25]. In the posterior orbit, where any lesions will lie in proximity to the optic nerve, there will bear a significant risk of optic neuropathy if a large dose of radiation given to this area. Under the standard dose fraction size of 1.8–2 Gy, the risk of damage with 50 Gy in 25 daily fractions is around 1% [26]. Based on studies on optic nerve tolerance to SRS, radiation optic neuropathy rates are low when a dose of 10–12 Gy applied to a functioning optic nerve [10, 27, 28]. In contrast, a higher overall dose of radiation to the same region can be delivered in multiple fractionated doses. In daily fractionated RT, the optic nerve is more sensitive to the dose per fraction rather than the total dose [29].

Other long-term risks include non-optic cranial neuropathy, retinopathy, pituitary dysfunction, and secondary malignancy. Although tumor control is the primary goal, treatment plans should be shaped to avoid the radiosensitive normal tissue at the anterior part of the orbit, including retina, lacrimal system, and lens. A total dose of higher than 45 Gy and a daily fraction greater than 1.9 Gy significantly increases the risk of retinopathy [29]. Radiation necrosis is another significant potential complication of radiotherapy and has a higher chance to occur in patients who are hereditarily sensitive to radiation, receive re-irradiation, or treated with high dose SRT/FSRT. Table 27.4 summarizes recommended radiation dose tolerance of the key organs at risk for radiotherapy to the orbital apex lesions.

References

1. Goldberg RA, Rootman J, Clin RA. Tumors metastatic to the orbit: a changing picture. Surv Ophthalmol. 1990;35(1):1–24.
2. Rootman BD, Rootman J, Gregory S, et al. Stereotactic fractionated radiotherapy for cavernous venous malformations (haemangioma) of the orbit. Ophthal Plast Reconstr Surg. 2012;28(2):96–102.
3. Cho SW, Lee WW, Ma DJ, et al. Orbital apex lesions: a diagnostic and therapeutic challenge. J Neurol Surg B Skull Base. 2018;79:386–93.
4. Mendoza-Santiesteban E, Mendoza-Santiesteban EC, Berazain AR, et al. Diagnosis and surgical treatment of orbital tumours. Semin Ophthalmol. 2010;25:123–9.
5. Halperin EC. The discipline of radiation oncology. In: Halperin EC, Wazer DE, Perez AC, Brady LW, editors. Perez and Brachy's principles and practice of radiotherapy. 7th ed. Philadelphia: Lippincott Williams & Wilkins; 2019. p. 2–70.
6. Kuhnt T, Müller AC, Werschnik C, et al. Radiotherapy of eye and orbit tumors. Klin Monbl Augenheikld. 2004;221(12):1033–45.
7. International Commission on Radiation Units and Measurements. ICRU report no. 50: prescribing, recording, and reporting photon beam therapy. Bethesda: ICRU, 1993.
8. International Commission on Radiation Units and Measurements. ICRU report no. 50: prescribing, recording, and reporting photon beam therapy (Supplement to ICRU report 50). Bethesda: ICRU, 1999.
9. Finger PT. Radiation therapy for orbital tumors: concepts, current use, and ophthamic radiation side effects. Surv Opthhalmol. 2009;54(5):545–68.
10. Leber KA, Berglöff J, Pendl G. Dose-response tolerance of the visual pathways and cranial nerves of the cavernous sinus to stereotactic radiosurgery. J Neurosurg. 1998;88(1):43–50.
11. Tishler RB, Loeffler JS, Lunsford LD, et al. Tolerance of cranial nerves of the cavernous sinus to radiosurgery. Int J Radiat Oncol Biol Phys. 1993;27(2):215–21.
12. Klingenstesin A, Kufeld M, Wowra B, et al. CyberKnife radiosurgery for the treatment of orbital metastases. Technol Cancer Res Treat. 2012;11(5):433–9.

13. Liu X, Xu D, Zhang Y, et al. Gama knife surgery in patients harboring orbital cavernous haemangiomas that were diagnosed on the basis of imaging findings. J Neurosurg. 2010;113 Suppl:39–43.
14. Khan AA, Niranjan A, Kano H, et al. Stereotactic radiosurgery for cavernous sinus or orbital haemangiomas. Neurosurgery. 2009;65(5):914–8; discussion 918.
15. Kim MS, Park K, Kim JH, et al. Gamma knife radiosurgery for orbital tumors. Clin Neurol Neurosurg. 2008;110(10):1003–7.
16. Kwon Y, et al. Visual changes after gamma knife surgery for optic nerve tumors. Report of three cases. J Neurosurg. 2005;102 suppl:143–6.
17. Kim BS, Im YS, Woo KI, et al. Multisession gamma knife radiosurgery for orbital apex tumours. World Neurosurg. 2015;84(4):1005–13.
18. Klink DF, Miller NR, Williams J. Preservation of residual vision 2 years after stereotactic radiosurgery for a presumed optic nerve sheath meningioma. J Neuroophthalmol. 1998;18:117–20.
19. Giaccia AJ, Hall EJ. Radiobiology for the radiologist. 7th ed. Alphen aan den Rijn: Wolters Kluwer; 2011.
20. Goh AS, Kim YD, Woo KI, et al. Benign orbital apex tumors treated by multisession gamma knife radiosurgery. Ophthalmology. 2013;120(3):635–41.
21. Ratnayake GS, McNab AA, Dally MJ, et al. Fractionated stereotactic radiotherapy for cavernous venous malformations of the orbital apex. Ophthalmic Plast Reconstr Surg. 2019;35(4):322–5.
22. Maaijwee K, Nowak PJ, van den Bosch WA, et al. Fractionated stereotactic radiotherapy for cavernous haemangioma of the orbital apex. Acta Ophthalmol. 2012;90:e655–7.
23. Pacelli R, Cella L, Conson M, et al. Fractionated stereotactic radiation therapy for orbital optic nerve sheath meningioma—a single institution experience and a short review of the literature. J Radiat Res. 2011;52:82–7.
24. Paulsen F, Doerr S, Wilhelm H, et al. Fractionated stereotactic radiotherapy in patients with optic nerve sheath meningioma. Int J Radiat Oncol Biol Phys. 2012;82(2):773–338.
25. Mayo C, Martel MK, Marks LB, et al. Radiation dose-volume effects of optic nerves and chiasm. Int J Radiat Oncol Biol Phys. 2010;76(3 Suppl):S28–35.
26. Morita A, Coffey RJ, Foote RL, et al. Risk of injury to cranial nerves after gamma knife radiosurgery for skull base meningiomas: experience in 88 patients. J Neurosurg. 1999;90(1):42–9.
27. Stafford SL, Pollock BE, Leavitt JA, et al. A study on the radiation tolerance of the optic nerves and chiasm after stereotactic radiosurgery. Int J Radiat Oncol Biol Phys. 2003;55(5):1177–81.
28. Parsons JT, Bova FJ, Fitzgerald CR, et al. Radiation optic neuropathy after megavoltage external-beam irradiation: analysis of time-dose factors. Int J Radiat Oncol Biol Phys. 1994;30(4):755–63.
29. Marks LB, Yorke ED, Jackson A, et al. The use of normal tissue complication probability (NTCP) models in the clinic. Int J Radiat Oncol Biol Phys. 2010;76(3 supp):S10–9.
30. Hanna GG, Murray L, Patel R, et al. UK consensus on Normal tissue dose constraints for stereotactic radiotherapy. Clin Oncol. 2018;30(1):5–14.
31. Lambrecht M, Eekers DB, Alapetite C, et al. Radiation dose constraints for organs at risk in neuro-oncology; the European Particle Therapy Network consensus. Radiat Oncol. 2018;128:26–36.

External Photon Radiotherapy for Benign Orbital Apex Lesions

28

K. M. Cheung, Jeannie Chik, Christine Kong, and K. H. Wong

Abstract

Management of benign orbital apex lesion is challenging as biopsy and surgical resection are often difficult due to proximity of critical neurovascular structures. Experienced multidisciplinary team is important to identify the diagnosis and decide on optimal treatment plan. Radiotherapy is indicated for symptomatic cases or those with increasing size threatening vision. Treatment aim is to preserve vision, to relieve symptoms, and to arrest growth of tumor. This chapter focuses on treatment approach and radiotherapy techniques for benign orbital apex lesions including cavernous venous malformation, hemangiopericytoma, Schwannoma, meningioma, and Graves ophthalmopathy.

Keywords

Vision preservation · Optic nerve · Cavernous venous malformation · Hemangiopericytoma · Schwannoma · Meningioma · Graves ophthalmopathy · Intensity-modulated radiation therapy · Stereotactic radiotherapy

The management of benign lesions at the orbital apex is complicated due to the tight space packed with critical nervous and vascular structures. Diagnosis of a lesion in this area is always a challenge and mainly relies on imaging studies as biopsy and surgery are inherently risky in this tight space. Attempts at complete resection of tumors in this critical location may result in direct injury to or vascular impairment of the optic apparatus followed by vision loss [1] and damage of other cranial nerves. Surgery should be reserved for selected cases in whom there is a sufficient space to handle the optic apparatus [2] or immediate decompression is indicated for rapidly progressing lesions. Close surveillance with serial imaging and visual field testing can be one of the treatment options for asymptomatic cases.

Radiotherapy is indicated for symptomatic cases and those benign yet potentially vision-threatening lesions at the orbital apex. The primary aims are to arrest the disease progression and achieve tumor shrinkage to relieve the symptoms while maintaining visual acuity. The therapeutic ratio (cost/benefit) of the radiation treatment should be carefully weighted, and the treatment margins should be as tight as possible for discrete lesions. Standard fractionation at 1.8 Gy per day up to a total dose of 50.4–54 Gy will be the choice of treatment for preservation of visual function. In selected cases, FSRT can be considered.

When being used for treatment of benign conditions, one of the most serious side effects of radiotherapy would be the risk of radiation carcinogenesis. Current observation is reassuring. In a US series including 276 patients who received SRS for benign conditions with 3216 patient-years follow-up, no radiation-associated cancer was observed [3].

28.1 Cavernous Venous Malformation (Hemangioma)

Background. Cavernous venous malformation (hemangioma) is the most common orbital benign lesion in adults. It mainly affects middle aged individuals with female predominance. It is a congenital vascular malformation in which growth is triggered by localized low grade vascular changes followed by subsequent development of vascular network and expansion in size. Patients usually present with insidious onset of diplopia or decreased vision over months to years.

Management. Diagnosis is by orbital imaging studies, usually MRI. Management is mainly surgical and is reserved to those having symptoms secondary to mass effects [4]. For

K. M. Cheung · J. Chik (✉) · C. Kong · K. H. Wong
Department of Clinical Oncology, Queen Elizabeth Hospital, Hong Kong SAR, China
e-mail: cyk632@ha.org.hk

T. L. POON et al. (eds.), *Orbital Apex and Periorbital Skull Base Diseases*, https://doi.org/10.1007/978-981-99-2989-4_28

lesions located close to the orbital apex and the optic nerve, surgery is deemed technically difficult and of high risk. Radiotherapy is therefore a feasible option with great potential in achieving tumor shrinkage and symptom control.

External beam radiotherapy using standard dose fractionation is safe and widely accessible. It can be performed on standard LINAC. Rootman et al. have reported his experience on five patients, delivering radiation dose ranging from 40 Gy in 20 fractions to 49.59 Gy in 29 fractions. Resolution of visual field defects and tumor shrinkage was observed in all cases, and the magnitude of tumor shrinkage was on average 60% (32–79%). In the cohort, no complication was noted [5]. The risk of radiation-induced optic nerve injury is low, as the dose used was lower than dose constraints for optic pathway (maximum point dose, Dmax = 54 Gy).

Stereotactic radiotherapy is another feasible approach but requires specialized LINAC or radiotherapy equipment, for example, Gamma Knife. The main advantage will be fewer treatment fractions due to the capability of delivering a higher dose-per-fraction with stringent immobilization techniques. The higher precision of immobilization and the special radiotherapy planning technique employed in stereotactic radiotherapy allow dose escalation within treatment target and rapid dose falloff in neighboring tissues, which would potentially improve clinical outcomes without increasing toxicity. Young and colleagues have described their experience in treating 12 patients with Gamma Knife technique, delivering a dose of 16–24 Gy in four fractions at tumor margins (prescription isodose 50%) with the maximal dose of 33.3–48 Gy within the treatment target. The maximal dose to the optic apparatus was limited to the same dose level at the tumor margin by extra caution of placing small collimator shots to achieve a stiff and fast dose falloff. Results were encouraging, with over 80% of patients experiencing improvement of visual field and all cases showing tumor shrinkage from a mean of 3104mm^3 (range 221–8500 mm^3) to 658 mm^3 (range 120–3350 mm^3). Moreover, no radiotherapy-related morbidity was noted during the follow-up period of 2 years [6].

Case 1 Cavernous Hemangioma at Right Orbital Apex (Fig. 28.1a–d)

A 32-year-old lady presented with visual blurring of right eye. MRI shows T1 isointense, T2 FS hyperintense, contrast enhancing lesion with gradual filling pattern, suggestive of cavernous hemangioma. She refused surgery and opted for stereotactic radiotherapy. Stereotactic radiosurgery at 20 Gy in five fractions over 1 week was prescribed.

Case 2 Right Cavernous Sinus Hemangioma (Fig. 28.2a–d)

A 57-year-old lady presented with left facial and tongue burning sensation persistent, mild headache. She experienced no visual disturbance all along. MRI baseline showed a T2 hyperintense homogeneously contrast enhancing mass is seen in right sellar/parasellar region with encasement of the right internal carotid artery and displaces the pituitary gland and stalk to the left. Features compatible with cavernous sinus hemangioma. Stereotactic radiotherapy 27.5 Gy in 5 Fr was given. Facial dysasethesia decreased after radiotherapy. Post treatment MRI 18 months after radiotherapy showed decrease in size of lesion.

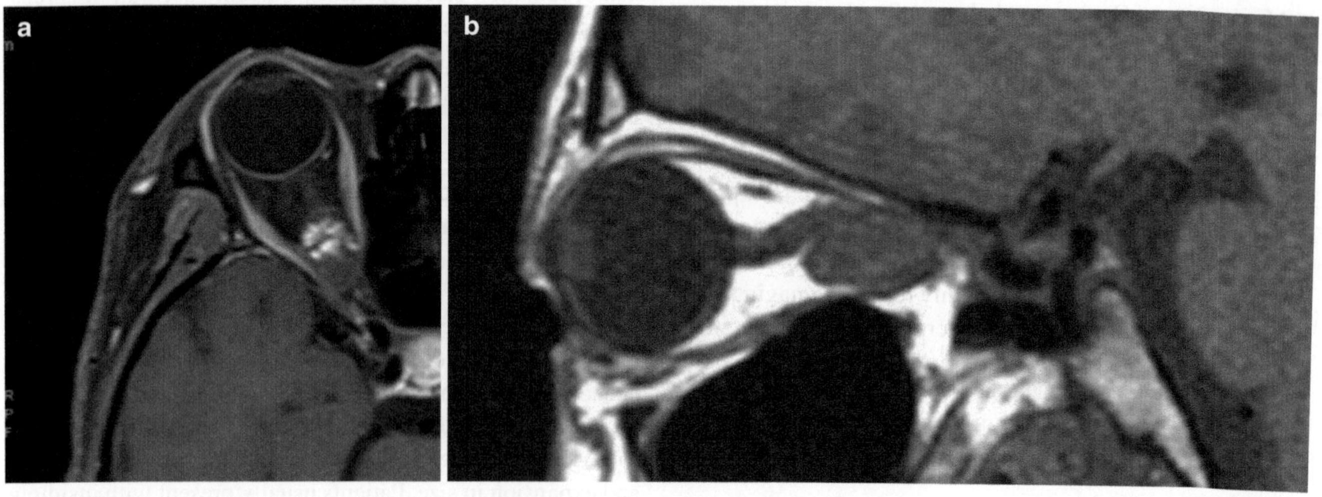

Fig. 28.1 (**a** and **b**) Pre-treatment MRI T1 images shows a contrast-enhancing hemangioma at orbital apex (left). The close anatomical relationship between the lesion and neighboring organs is evident. The tumor is compressing the right optic nerve and is close to optic chiasm, frontal lobe, and retina (right). (**c** and **d**) Radiotherapy treatment of orbital apex hemangioma. (above) GTV is delineated in yellow. A tight PTV of 1 mm is applied. 20 Gy in five fractions (4 Gy per fraction) was prescribed and 100% isodose line was prescribed in red, which shows good conformality to PTV. (below) The diagram shows radiation dose to each target per fraction. The sharp dose falloff is shown by the negligible dose in right lens and optic chiasm (<0.5 Gy)

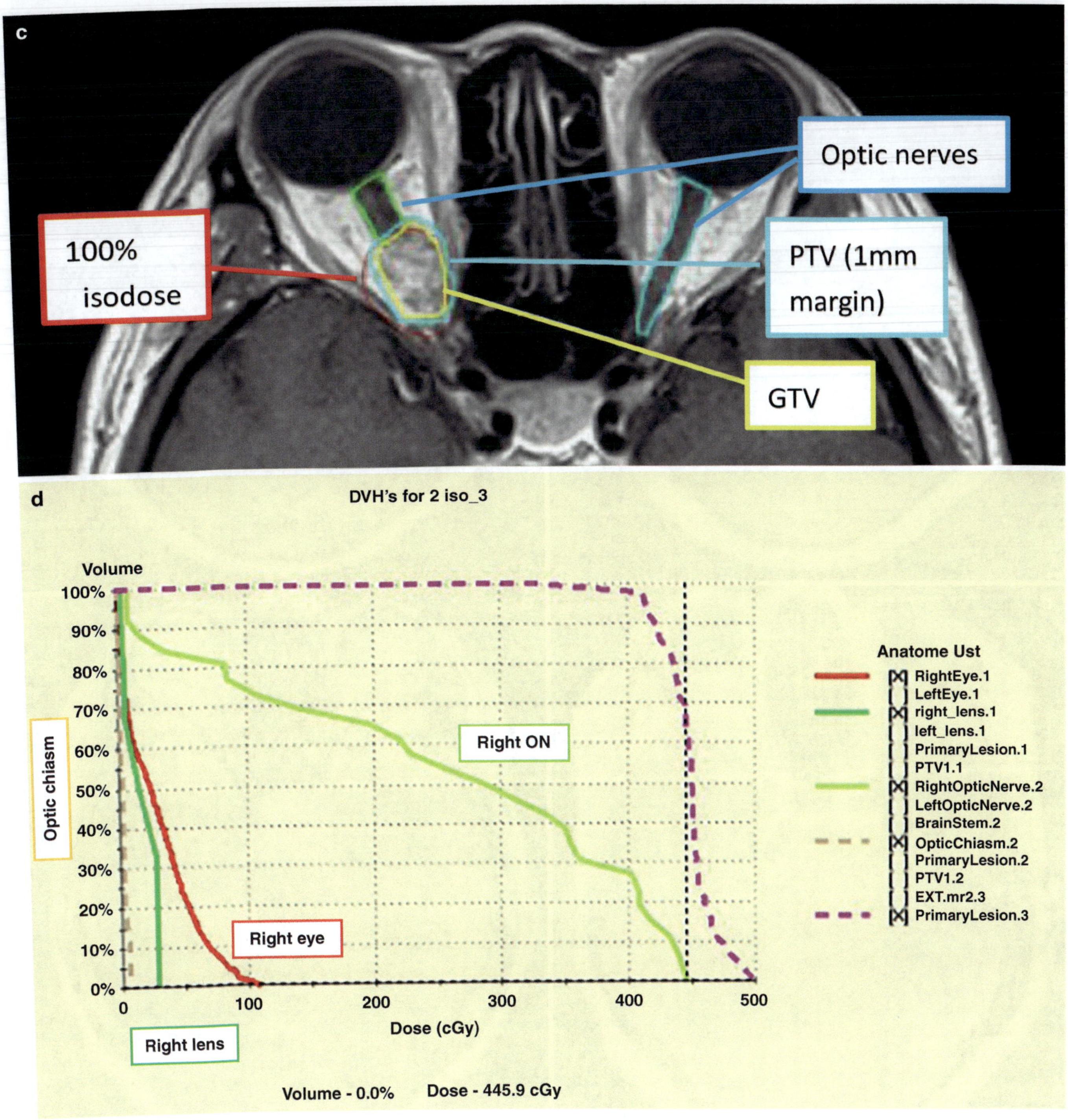

Fig. 28.1 (continued)

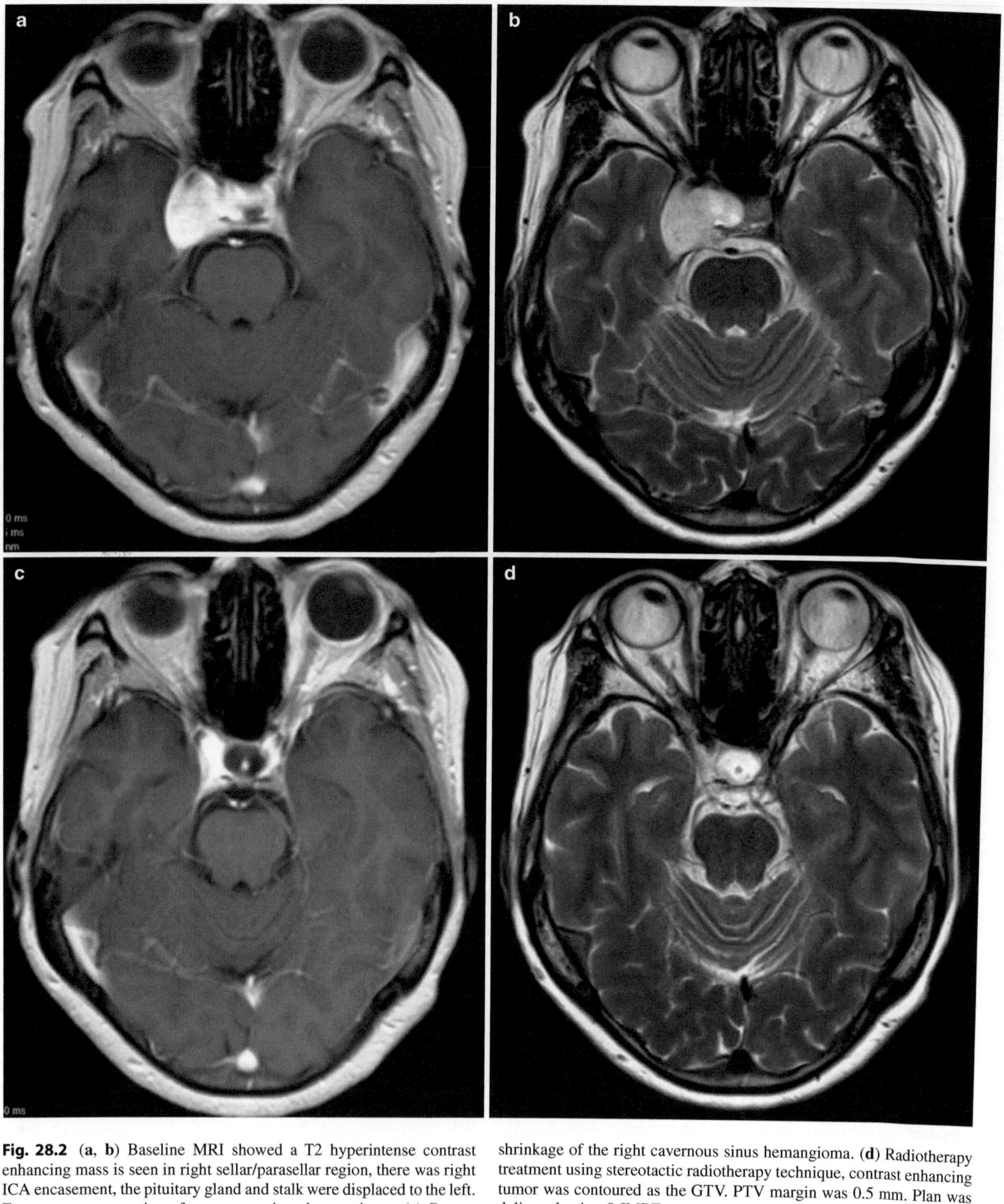

Fig. 28.2 (**a**, **b**) Baseline MRI showed a T2 hyperintense contrast enhancing mass is seen in right sellar/parasellar region, there was right ICA encasement, the pituitary gland and stalk were displaced to the left. Features are suggestive of cavernous sinus hemangioma. (**c**) Repeat MRI 18 months after SRT showed that there was significant interval shrinkage of the right cavernous sinus hemangioma. (**d**) Radiotherapy treatment using stereotactic radiotherapy technique, contrast enhancing tumor was contoured as the GTV. PTV margin was 0.5 mm. Plan was delivered using 9 IMRT noncoplanar beams. Dose received by targets and OAR as shown in the Table 28.1

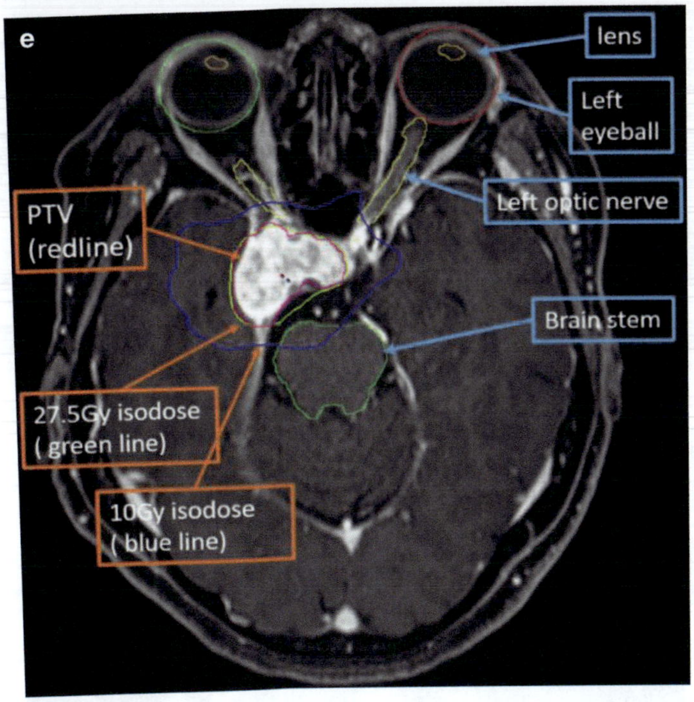

Fig. 28.2 (continued)

Table 28.1 Dose received by targets and organs-at-risk for SRT plan of Case 2

Dose fractionation	% IL of max	Target volume (cc)	Treatment volume (cc)	Min. dose (Gy)	Max. dose (Gy)	% coverage	Brainstem Dmax (Gy)	Brainstem D1cc (Gy)	OC Dmax (Gy)	Lt ON Dmax (Gy)	Rt ON Dmax (Gy)
27.5 in 5 Fr	80	8.378	10.64	20.78	34.67	99.2	26.01	12.69	24.29	15.88	24.64

28.2 Hemangiopericytoma

Background. Hemangiopericytoma belongs to a combined entity of soft tissue tumors called solitary fibrous tumor/hemangiopericytoma (SFT/HPC) according to the WHO 2016 classification. It is an uncommon ocular neoplasm and accounts for only 1–3% of ocular tumors [7, 8]. It mainly affects middle-aged individuals with no sex predilection [9]. It is generally a slow growing tumor arising from pericytes, of which 30% are malignant with a very long interval of up to 2–3 decades between initial diagnosis and metastases [10]. This condition is reported to affect conjunctiva, lacrimal gland, and optic nerve. Symptoms are mainly proptosis, pressure, pain, and visual loss, which are usually difficult to distinguish from other benign intra-orbital pathologies [11].

Management. Considering its locally aggressive nature, surgical excision is required but frequently challenging because they are commonly vascular, friable, and ill-defined due to the lack of true capsule in some cases [12]. With a recurrence risk up to 30%, adjuvant radiotherapy is generally advised, mainly based on the favorable experience extrapolated from other intracranial SFT as data are scarce for orbital haemangiopericytoma [13]. There were reports showing the successful use of radiotherapy either before or after surgery. Radiotherapy fractionation ranged from 40 Gy in 20 daily fractions to 59.8 Gy in 33 daily fractions [12–14]. Intensity-modulated radiotherapy (IMRT) is the current standard owing to its capability of high dose conformality to target and sparing of nearby organs-at-risk (OARs) with its swift dose fall-off, especially when the presence of optic apparatus nearby, which are radiation sensitive. There is no consensus on target delineation in radiotherapy contouring. Both pre-op and post-op images would be taken into consideration. Gross tumor volume (GTV) will encompass gross residual tumor and will be expanded into high-dose planning target volume (PTV) with 60 Gy prescribed (PTV60). Clinical target volume (CTV) will cover areas with subclinical disease and is generated by expanding the GTV by 2 cm circumferentially, trimming along anatomical borders. CTV will be expanded into the prophylactic dose PTV (PTV54) with 54 Gy prescribed. Treatment will be given in 30 daily fractions over 6 weeks using simultaneous integrated boost (SIB) technique.

Stereotactic radiotherapy (SRS) is also reported to be feasible in a number of cases using gamma knife [14, 15]. Tata et al. reported a successful salvage of recurrent lesion adhering to the optic nerve by a single session SRS of 16 Gy at 50% IL. Significant shrinkage of the tumor was noted with no neurological complication at 18 months [15]. Brzozowska et al. reported a case of posterior orbit tumor receiving partial excision and adjuvant SRS. Single fraction radiosurgery was delivered by linear accelerator with Brainlab, using a single dose of 20 Gy at 100% IL. The treated lesion and neurological function remained stable at 3 years, yet a metastatic focus was subsequently developed at the frontal lobe [14].

Case Illustration Hemangiopericytoma of Right Eye (Fig. 28.3a–d)

Case of a 43-year-old lady who suffered from hemangiopericytoma causing proptosis and visual blurring. MRI shows 2.5 cm right orbital mass with nonspecific pattern of T1 and T2 isointensity and avid enhancement. She received maximal tumor debulking followed by adjuvant IMRT with conventional fractionation of 60 Gy in 30 fractions over 6 weeks. The tumor volume and her vision both remained stable after radiotherapy over a follow-up period of 5 years.

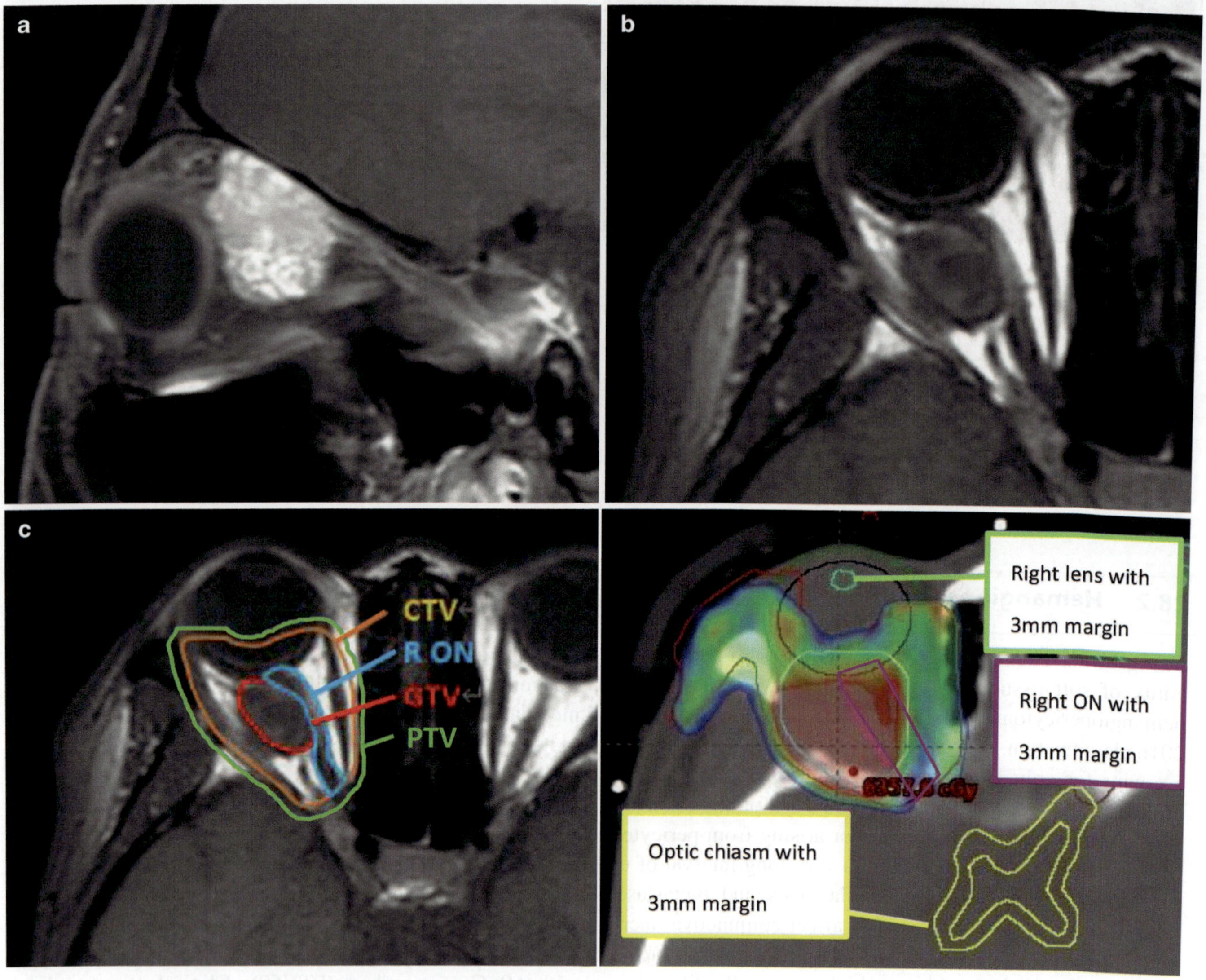

Fig. 28.3 (**a** and **b**) MRI reveals an avidly enhancing superior orbital mass with close relationship with right optic nerve causing inferior and medial displacement. It is also close to eyeball and frontal lobe. (**c** and **d**) On upper left, GTV was defined by the residual tumor, CTV was created by expansion of GTV by 2 cm and trimming along anatomical confines. PTV was 3 mm. Upper right shows the organs-at-risk (OAR), which included bilateral optic nerves (Dmax <54 Gy), eyeball (Dmax <54 Gy), lens (Dmax <6 Gy), and brain (V60 < 30%). The rest shows dose distribution represented by color wash, with green area denoting 54 Gy and red area 60 Gy. While the optic nerve fell into target volume, planners tried to avoid hotspot and keep the dose as cold as possible over the optic nerve area (lower left). XR beam from various angles and planes are used to produce a radiotherapy plan with high conformality. (lower right) The tumor volume and her vision both remained stable after radiotherapy over a follow-up period of 5 years

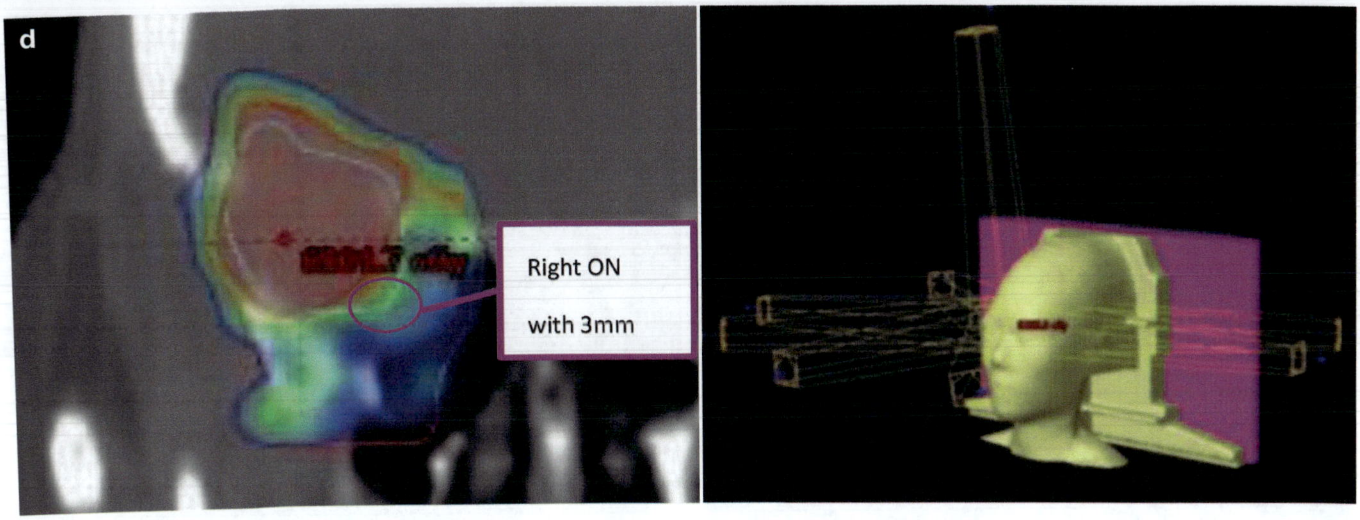

Fig. 28.3 (continued)

28.3 Schwannoma

Background. Schwannoma is a benign neoplasm of myelin-producing Schwann cells. These tumors can affect all peripheral nerves and most of the intracranial nerves. Uncommonly, Schwannomas can arise from any intracranial nerves traversing the orbit. Theoretically, Schwannoma cannot develop in optic nerve due to its embryonic origin of oligodendrocytes, but optic nerve Schwannoma still rarely occurs and is thought to originate from autonomic fibers innervating optic nerve vessels [16]. It mainly occurs in middle-aged individuals [17]. It is associated with neurofibromatosis both types 1 and 2, with respective dysregulation of RAS and Merlin proteins, leading to Schwann cells hyperplasia and tumorigenesis. Common presentations include proptosis and visual change which develop over many years [17]. While malignant transformation to malignant peripheral nerve sheath tumor is rare, symptoms tend to evolve quicker than expected (over a few months or 1–2 years) [17].

Investigations. Imaging study using magnetic resonance imaging (MRI) allows assessment of the nature of the lesion and involvement of surrounding soft tissues. The specific MRI features of Antoni B regions of schwannoma, which appears non-enhancing, T1 hypointense and T2 hyperintense, will help differentiate it from other tumors. Computed tomography (CT) enables reliable assessment of bony structures. Schwannoma commonly molds surrounding bony structures and fissures without erosion. Common differentials include neurofibroma, hemangioma, and lymphoma [18].

Management. Basically, surgery is the mainstay of treatment. Tumor is ideally excised with capsule preserved intact. When the tumor is unreachable or unresectable, or recurs after surgery, radiotherapy is commonly used to secure local control. Fractionated stereotactic radiosurgery (FSRT) has been used for treatment of orbital benign tumors, especially those located close to the optic apparatus. Jo et al. have reported their experience of fractionated gamma knife radiosurgery to mainly orbital apex lesions, which included schwannoma. Using rigid immobilization and a fractionation scheme of 20 Gy in four fractions prescribed at 50% isodose, 12 h apart, the treatment was well tolerated and devoid of long-term side effects. All subjects experienced durable disease control and volume reduction ranged from 14 to 92% [19]. Goh et al. also described favorable experience using same technique, with all patients experienced improvement of visual acuity and an average tumor volume reduction of 76% (range = 70–87%) [20].

Case Illustration (Fig. 28.4a–d)

A 62 year-old gentleman had right orbital schwannoma presented with painless proptosis. He received surgical debulking but had recurrence after 3 years. FSRT was offered.

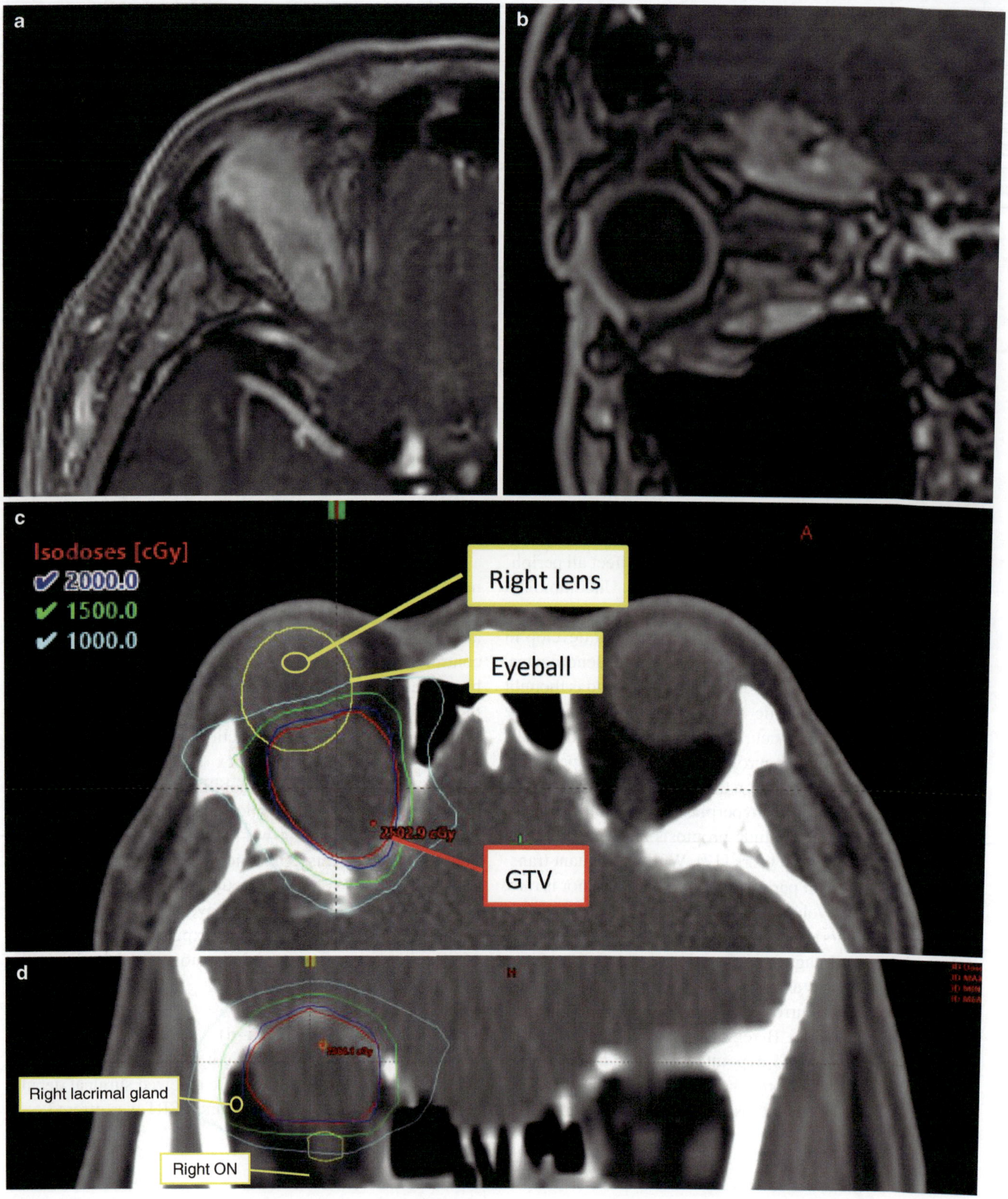

Fig. 28.4 (**a**, **b**) MRI shows a superior orbital lesion inseparable from superior rectus muscle, having intermediate T1 and T2 signal and patchy enhancement pattern. (**c**, **d**) GTV was contoured in red color. The radiation dose was 20 Gy in five fractions, prescribed at 78% IL. The isodose curves of 10 Gy, 15 Gy, and20 Gy were as shown, illustrating rapid dose falloff and high dose conformity. The maximum dose of right optic nerve was 21.2 Gy (mainly the upper part close to GTV as shown in the lower image), optic chiasm 2.38 Gy, right lens 1.3 Gy. Mean dose of right lacrimal gland 13.1 Gy

28.4 Optic Nerve Sheath Meningioma

Background. Meningioma that occurs in the orbital apex can be classified into two types. Primary optic nerve sheath meningioma (ONSM) arises from the intra-orbital portion of the optic nerve. Secondary ONSM is invasion from intracranial meningioma into the optic canal and orbit [21]. Primary ONSM is rare, more prevalent in young women and patients with neurofibromatosis 2 [22]. Patients commonly present with symptoms caused by optic nerve damage leading to decreased visual acuity and visual field deficits. Tumor mass effect may also cause headache, proptosis, and diplopia [22–24]. Diagnosis is made based on ophthalmological examination and MRI [22, 24]. Treatment aims to preserve vision while avoid local progression. Asymptomatic patients can be observed. Surgery carries a significant risk of blindness and is usually reserved as debulking surgery for patients with proptosis or when diagnosis is uncertain that warrants histology confirmation [22]. Radiotherapy is the treatment of choice for patients with visual impairment, which is effective for tumor control while giving high chance of preservation of vision. Stereotactic radiotherapy greatly improves precision and gives promising treatment result [22–24].

Radiotherapy. Indication of radiotherapy includes visual impairment and asymptomatic patients with radiological progression. Studies treating ONSM with radiotherapy reported favorable radiologically local control rate of 90–100% [24]. The rate of preservation of vision was reported to be 77–100% [23, 25–28]. Concerning treatment toxicities, with radiotherapy dose of up to 54 Gy, the risk of optic nerve injury is less than 5% [22], patients with surgery and diabetes mellitus have higher risk of optic nerve injury [24]. Radiation retinopathy can occur when the dose is over 50 Gy with a latency period of 6 months to 3 years [22]. Pituitary function deterioration has been reported in up to 19% when the dose to pituitary gland was above 45 Gy [22, 24].

Radiotherapy can be delivered using IMRT technique. Stereotactic radiotherapy using standard dose fractionation gives high precision and can minimize radiation doses to surrounding normal tissues. During delivery of radiotherapy, patient is immobilized with thermoplastic cast with eyes closed and should be instructed to keep eyes still to avoid movement of the target. GTV includes the gross tumor and care should be taken to include the portion of optic nerve in the optic canal. No CTV margin is required for WHO G1 meningioma. PTV margin is 3–5 mm for thermoplastic cast without image guidance, and 1–2 mm for stereotactic radiotherapy. Radiation beams should be avoided from entry or exit through the contralateral eye. Organs at risks include eyeballs, optic nerve, optic chiasm, pituitary gland, lens, and brain stem. Dose of 50.4–54 Gy in 1.8 Gy per fraction is recommended.

28.4.1 Case Illustration

Case 1 (Fig. 28.5a–d) Optic Nerve Sheath Meningioma in a 10-Year-Old Boy with Known Neurofibromatosis Type 2

Surveillance MRI brain showed an enhancing mass encasing most of the right optic nerve, involving the orbital apex and extending across the optic canal, with perineural enhancement along right intracranial optic nerve and a 6 mm enhancing nodule lateral to the prechiasmatic optic nerve. Optic chiasm and ipsilateral optic tract were not involved. Right eye vision was normal. Features were compatible with optic nerve sheath meningioma (ONSM). Interval MRI in one year showed progressive enlargement of optic nerve mass. External beam radiotherapy with 50.4 Gy in 1.8 Gy per fraction size was given. Post treatment MRI at 10 months showed the right ONSM was static. Right eye vision was normal all along.

Case 2 (Fig. 28.6a–e) Grade 1 Petroclival Meningioma

A 37-year-old lady was diagnosed large Grade 1 right petroclival meningioma with invasion to right orbital apex, right temporal lobe, abutting on right cavernous sinus and brain stem. Partial excision was performed three times on July 8, 2014; June 30, 2015; and July 24, 2015. The second operation was complicated with right sixth cranial nerve palsy. Ventriculoperitoneal shunt was performed for hydrocephalus on July 31, 2015. MRI in September 2016 showed slightly progression of the retroclival part of the tumor, indenting onto the pons. External radiotherapy with 54 Gy given in 30 daily fractions completed on December 14, 2016. MRI brain in January 2018 showed mild reduction in size of the retroclival part of the tumor. Clinically, the patient had static right sixth cranial nerve palsy and partial right seventh cranial nerve palsy since radiotherapy.

Case 3 (Fig. 28.7a–c) Left Cavernous Sinus Meningioma

A 64-year-old lady presented with facial dysesthesia and left sided headache. MRI brain showed left lateral cavernous sinus meningioma with suspected thickening of left trigeminal nerve. It was decided to treat with stereotactic radiotherapy in view of worsening symptoms. SRT using a dose 27.5 Gy in 5 Fr over 2 weeks was given. Left headache and facial dysesthesia decreased after radiotherapy and post-radiotherapy reassessment MRI is pending.

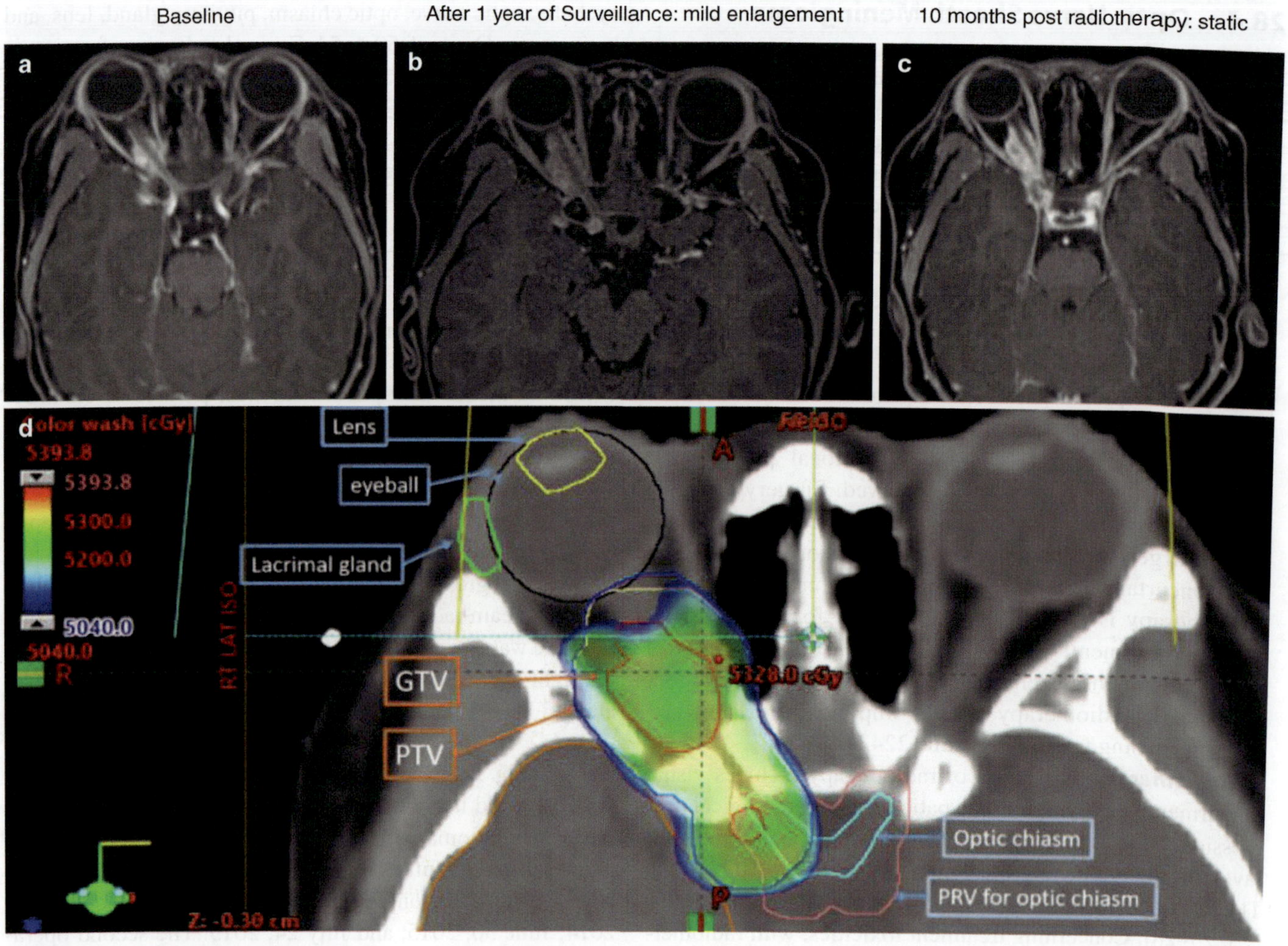

Fig. 28.5 (**a**–**c**) A 10-year-old boy with known Neurofibromatosis type 2 was detected to have an ONSM involving right optic nerve by surveillance MRI. Interval MRI in one year showed progressive enlargement of optic nerve mass. External beam radiotherapy with 50.4 Gy in 1.8 Gy per fraction size was given. Post treatment MRI at 10 months showed the right ONSM was static. Right eye vision was normal all along. (**d**) Radiotherapy treatment using IMRT technique with 50.4 Gy given in 28 daily fractions. Immobilization by means of thermoplastic cast was used and simulation was done with 1 mm fine cut CT. Gross tumor was contoured as GTV (red line) and no CTV margin was required for Grade 1 meningioma. Margin for PTV (blue line) was 5 mm to account for setup error and optic nerve movement. No Gazing target was adopted. Treatment was delivered with eyes closed

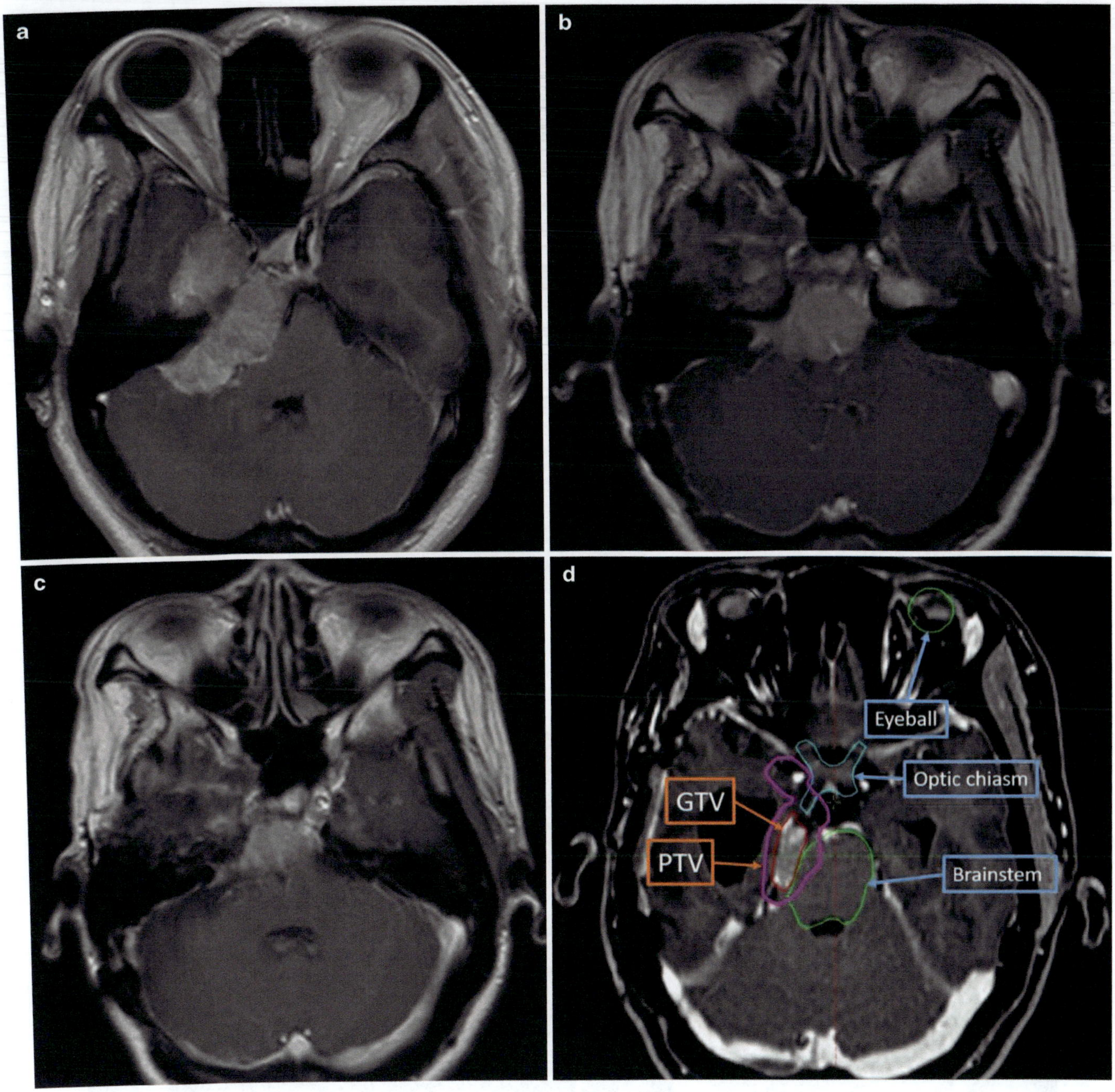

Fig. 28.6 (**a**) Baseline. (**b**) Recurrence after three partial excisions. (**c**) One year after external radiation. (**d**) Target volumes and organs at risk. (**e**) Radiotherapy treatment using IMRT technique with 54 Gy given in 30 daily fractions. Immobilisation by means of thermoplastic cast was used. Gross tumor was contoured as GTV. No CTV margin is required for Grade 1 meningioma and PTV margin was 3 mm

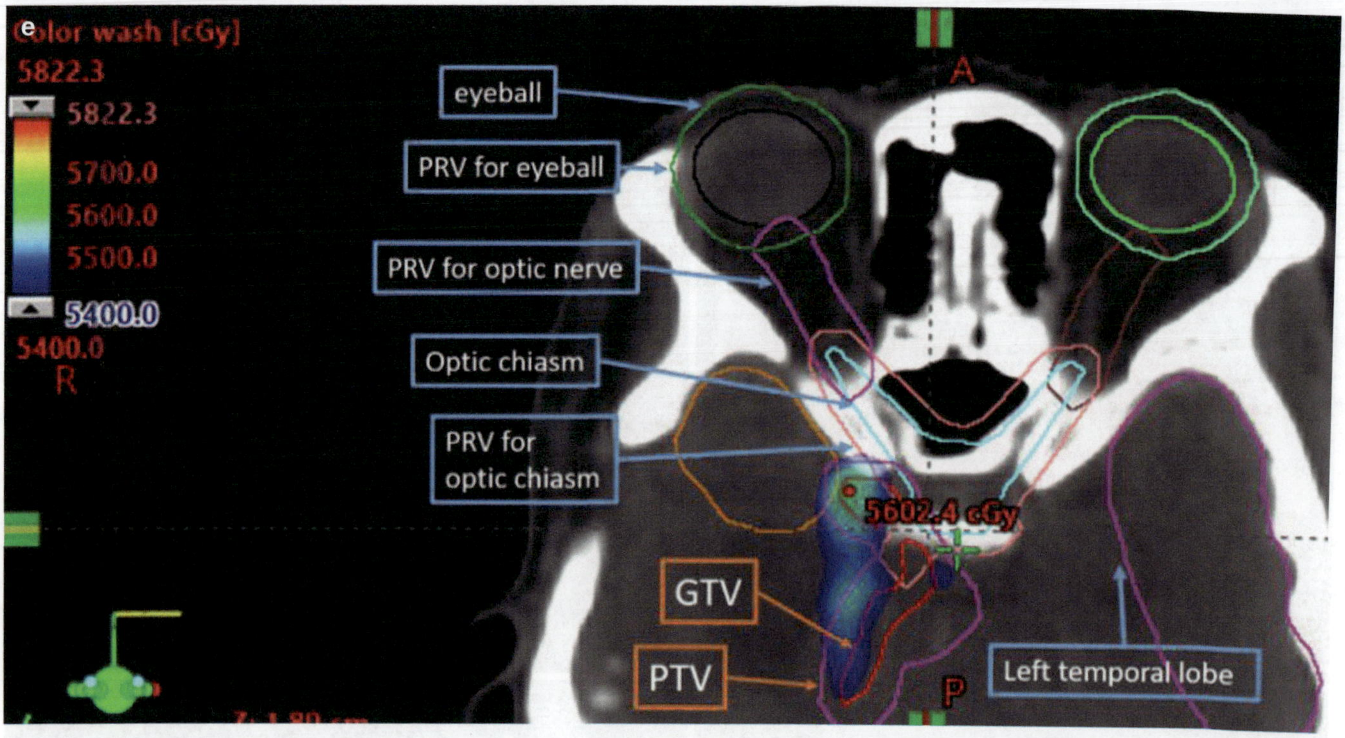

Fig. 28.6 (continued)

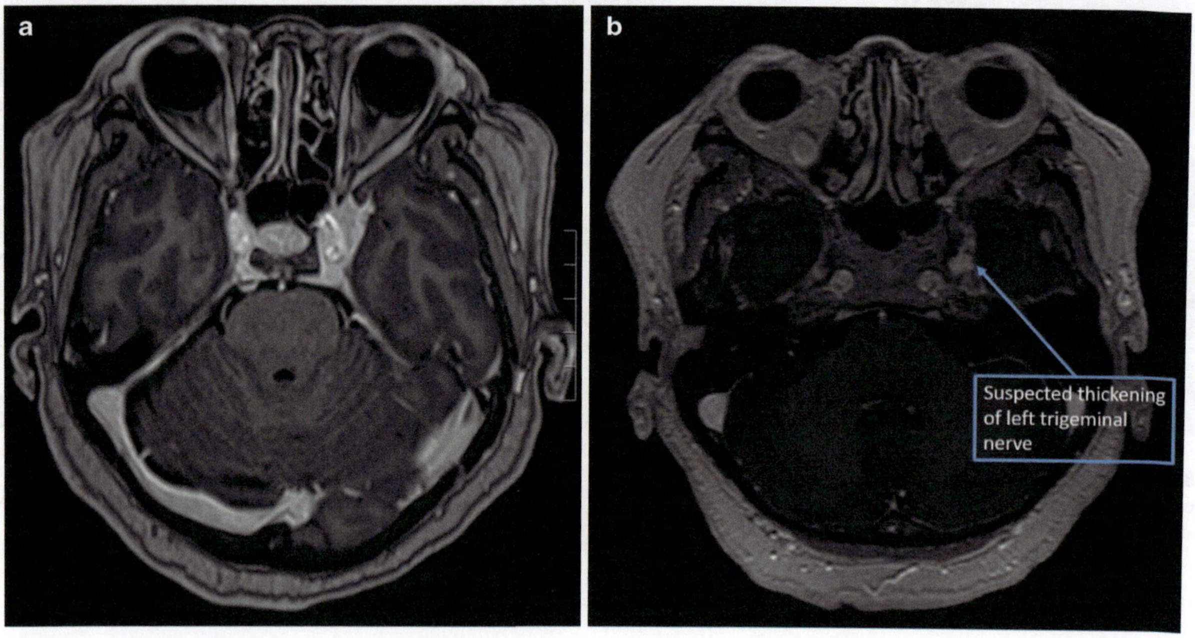

Fig. 28.7 (**a**, **b**) Baseline MRI showed a left lateral cavernous sinus meningioma with suspected thickening of left trigeminal nerve. (**c**) Radiotherapy treatment using stereotactic radiotherapy technique, contrast enhancing tumor was contoured as the GTV. PTV margin was 0.5 mm. SRT was delivered using 10 IMRT noncoplanar beams. Dose received by targets and OAR as shown in the Table 28.2 below

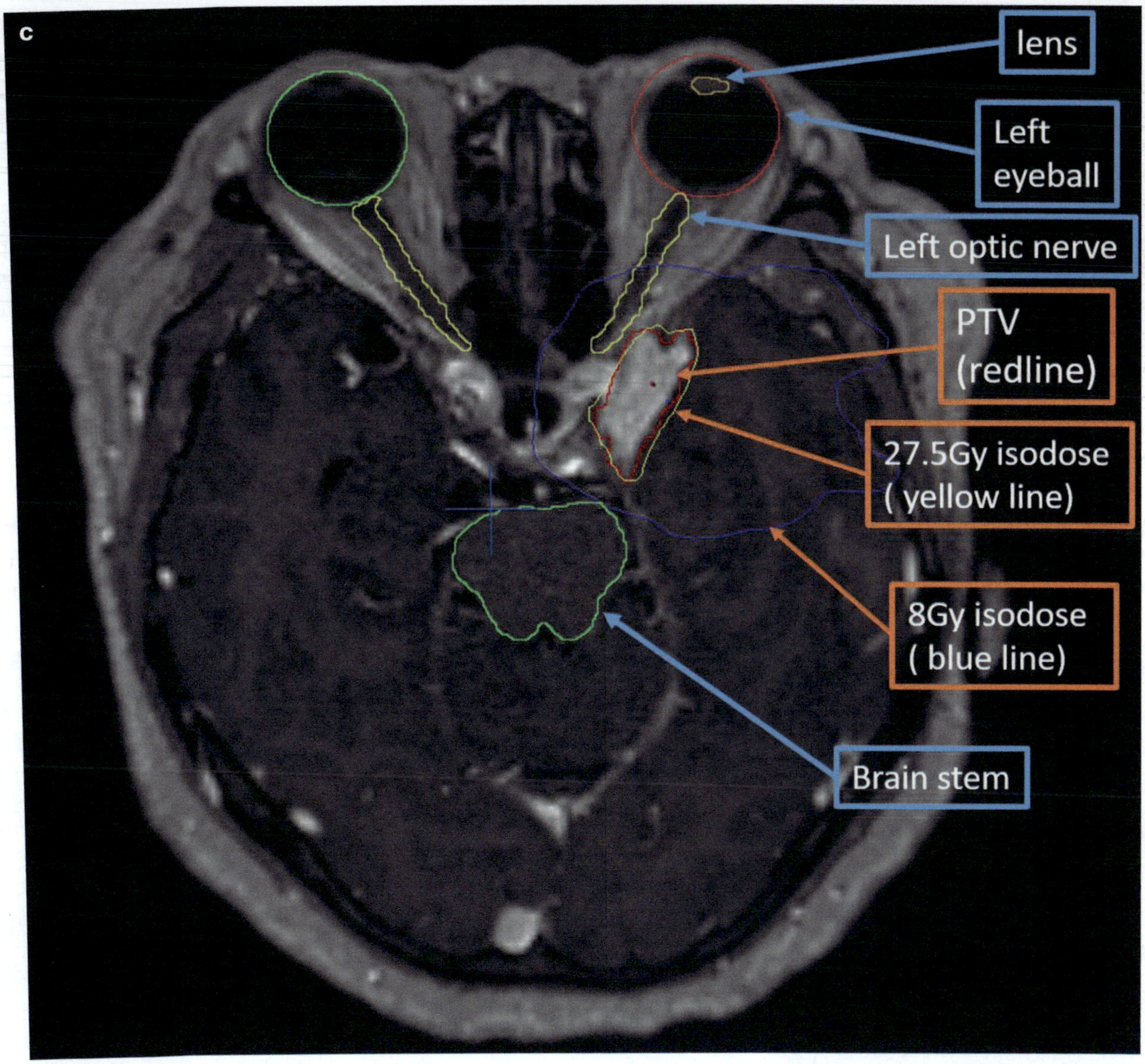

Fig. 28.7 (continued)

Table 28.2 Dose received by targets and organs-at-risk for SRT plan of Case 3

Dose fractionation	% IL of max	Target volume (cc)	Treatment volume (cc)	Min. dose (Gy)	Max. dose (Gy)	% coverage	Brainstem Dmax (Gy)	Brainstem D1cc (Gy)	OC Dmax (Gy)	Lt ON Dmax (Gy)	Rt ON Dmax (Gy)
27.5 Gy in 5 Fr	80	4.685	7.825	24.28	34.11	99.4	11.48	6.51	18.46	24.84	3.66

28.5 Graves Ophthalmopathy

Background. Graves' ophthalmopathy (GO) is a clinically significant disease entity, which affects retro orbital tissues. It affects around 25% of patients with thyrotoxicosis [29]. While the disease course of mild GO is benign, with over 50% experiencing clinical remission of symptoms after treatment of thyrotoxicosis, those with clinically significant or visual-threatening GO seldom resolve on its own. The condition may last for years, and a few of them (~3%) will worsen and require more aggressive intervention [29].

Management. Removal of exacerbating factors is essential in management of GO. Smoking cessation is the key. Treatment with selenium is also shown to decrease severity of GO. While for active and clinically significant GO defined as clinical activity score (CAS) ≥3, corticosteroid treatment is shown to effectively improve the severity of GO. In case of sight threatening condition, timely decompression surgery will help salvage vision.

External orbital radiation is mainly used for moderate to severe GO in combination with steroids or only when intravenous glucocorticoids are contraindicated or ineffective. Radiotherapy aims to reduce retro-orbital infiltration of lymphoid cells and active inflammation. Trials have revealed that combination of radiotherapy with systemic steroid is superior to steroid alone in improving disease activity of GO [30]. Outcomes of radiotherapy alone is conflicting; some studies comparing steroid and radiotherapy observed comparable results, but radiotherapy was more tolerable [31], yet some reported no major benefit but only improvement in diplopia [32].

Despite the advances in intensity-modulated radiotherapy techniques, the most common radiotherapy is still lateral opposing radiation fields delivered by 4–10 MV LINAC and 3D planning (Fig. 28.8). Clinical target volume (CTV) will include retro-orbital tissues and muscles. Planning target volume (PTV), which accounts for daily setup error of radiotherapy treatment, is usually 3–5 mm with the patient immobilized by thermoplastic cast. A half-beam block technique

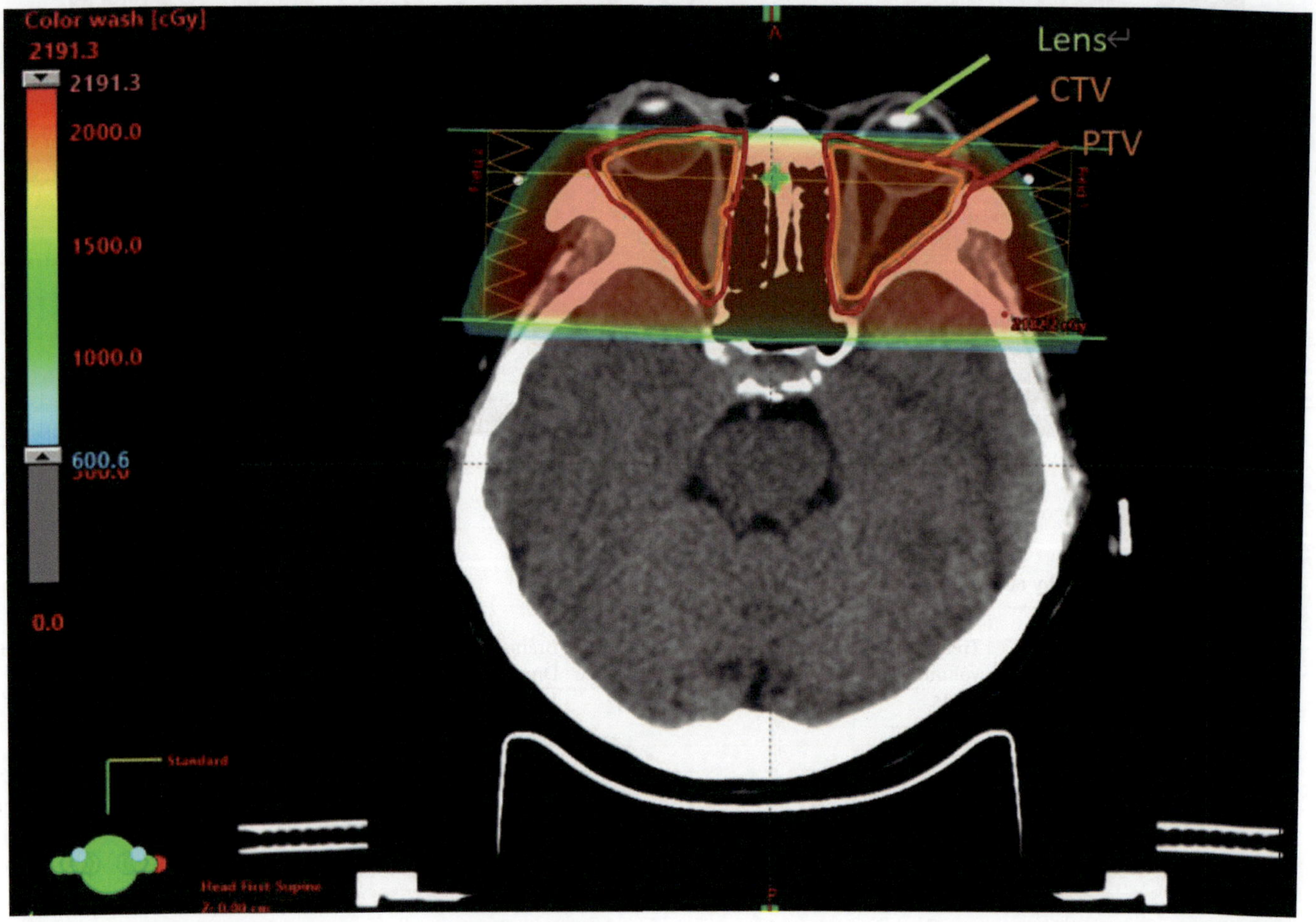

Fig. 28.8 Case of active Graves' orbitopathy presenting with diplopia. CT images shows bilateral thickened rectus muscle. Treatment included systemic steroids and concurrent radiotherapy to both orbits. CTV encompassed the whole retro-orbital area and was shown in orange. It was then expanded by 3 mm to form the PTV. Total radiation dose of 20 Gy was given in 10 daily fractions over 2 weeks. Area irradiated by over 6 Gy of radiation was represented in color wash. Both lenses, with maximum dose tolerance of 6 Gy, was safely excluded from the radiation field. Patient reported improvement in diplopia in 3 months' time with no ocular side-effects after a follow-up period of 2 years

at the anterior field border ensures minimal divergence of beam edge and minimize scattering to lens, which is an organ at risk (OAR) sensitive to radiation. Lens dose is documented during radiotherapy limited to as low as possible, as while conventional dose constraint of lens is 6 Gy, radiation dose as low as 0.5 Gy can predispose to increased risk of cataract [33]. Acute and chronic side effects are generally mild. Elevated risk of cataract was only observed in group of patients using older cobalt units but not in contemporary LINAC.

References

1. Zabramski JM, Kiris T, Sankhla SK, et al. Orbitozygomatic craniotomy. Technical note. J Neurosurg. 1998;89(2):336–41.
2. Baumert BG, Villà SG, et al. Early improvements in vision after fractionated stereotactic radiotherapy for primary optic nerve sheath meningioma. Radiother Oncol. 2004;72(2):169–74.
3. Sherry AD, Bingham B, Kim E, et al. Secondary malignancy following stereotactic radiosurgery for benign neurologic disease: a cohort study and review of the literature. J Radiosurg SBRT. 2020;6(4):287–94.
4. Pargament J, Nerad J, Burkat CN, Yen MT, Goel S. Orbital cavernous venous malformation (cavernous hemangioma). Website of American Academy of Ophthalmology https://eyewiki.aao.org/Orbital_Cavernous_Venous_Malformation_(Cavernous_Hemangioma. Accessed 31 Jan 2021.
5. Rootman DB, Rootman J, Gregory S, Feldman KA, Ma R. Stereotactic fractionated radiotherapy for cavernous venous malformations (hemangioma) of the orbit. Ophthalmic Plast Reconstr Surg. 2012;28(2):96–102.
6. Young SM, Kim KH, Kim Y, et al. Orbital apex venous cavernous malformation with optic neuropathy: treatment with multisession gamma knife radiosurgery. Br J Ophthalmol. 2019;103:1453–9.
7. Karcioglu ZA, Nasr AM, Haik BG. Orbital hemangiopericytoma: clinical and morphologic features. Am J Ophthalmol. 1997;124:661–72.
8. Furusato E, Valenzuela I, Fanburg-Smith J, et al. Orbital solitary fibrous tumor: encompassing terminology for hemangiopericytoma, giant cell angiofibroma and fibrous histiocytoma of the orbit: reappraisal of 41 cases. Hum Pathol. 2011;42(1):120–8.
9. Sujatha S, Sampath R, Bonshek RE, Tublo AB. Conjunctival haemangiopericytoma. Br J Ophthalmol. 1994;78:497–9.
10. Croxatto JO, Font RL. Hemangiopericytoma of the orbit: a clinicopathologic study of 30 cases. Hum Pathol. 1982;13(3):210–8.
11. Burkat CN, Lee NG, Yen MT. Haemangiopericytoma. Eye Wiki, American Academy of Ophthalmologists. https://eyewiki.aao.org/Hemangiopericytoma#cite_note-croxtto5-6. Accessed 10 Mar 2021.
12. Shinder R, Jackson TL, Araujo D, et al. Preoperative radiation therapy in the management of recurrent orbital hemangiopericytoma. Ophthalmic Plastic Reconstr Surg. 2011;27(5):e126–8.
13. Ciliberti MP, D'Agostino R, Gabrieli L, Nikolaou A, Sardaro A. The radiation therapy options of intracranial hemangiopericytoma: an overview and update on a rare vascular mesenchymal tumor. Oncol Rev. 2018;12(2):354.
14. Brzozowska A, Juszczynska J, Jarosz B, et al. Radiotherapy in patients with solitary fibrous tumour of the orbit—a case report and literature review. Oncol Radiother. 2017;1(39):19–27.
15. Tata A, Cohen-Inbar O, Sheehan JP. Treatment of orbital solitary fibrous tumour with gamma knife radiosurgery and systematic review of literature. BMJ Case Rep. 2016;2016:bcr2016217114.
16. Kim DS, Choi JU, Yang KH, et al. Optic sheath schwannomas: report of two cases. Childs Nerv Syst. 2002;18:684–9.
17. Rose GE, Wright JE. Isolated peripheral nerve sheath tumours of the orbit. Eye (Lond). 1991;5(Pt 6):668–73.
18. Khan SN, Sepahdari AR. Orbital masses: CT and MRI of common vascular lesions, benign tumors, and malignancies. Saudi J Ophthalmol. 2012;26(4):373–83.
19. Jo KI, Im YS, Kong DS, Seol HJ, Nam DH, Kim YD, Lee JI. Multisession gamma knife surgery for benign orbital tumors. J Neurosurg. 2012;117(Suppl):102–7.
20. Goh ASC, Kim YD, Woo KI, Lee JI. Benign orbital apex tumors treated with multisession gamma knife radiosurgery. Ophthalmology. 2013;120(3):635–41.
21. Jeremic B, Pitz S. Primary optic nerve sheath meningioma: stereotactic fractionated radiation therapy as an emerging treatment of choice. Cancer. 2007;110(4):714–22.
22. Soldà F, Wharram B, De Ieso PB, Bonner J, Ashley S, Brada M. Long-term efficacy of fractionated radiotherapy for benign meningiomas. Radiother Oncol. 2013;109(2):330–4.
23. Ratnayake G, Oh T, Mehta R, et al. Long-term treatment outcomes of patients with primary optic nerve sheath meningioma treated with stereotactic radiotherapy. J Clin Neurosci. 2019;68:162–7.
24. Paulsen F, Doerr S, Wilhelm H, Becker G, Bamberg M, Classen J. Fractionated stereotactic radiotherapy in patients with optic nerve sheath meningioma. Int J Radiat Oncol Biol Phys. 2012;82(2):773–8.
25. Andrews DW, Faroozan R, Yang BP, et al. Fractionated stereotactic radiotherapy for the treatment of optic nerve sheath meningiomas: preliminary observations of 33 optic nerves in 30 patients with historical comparison to observation with or without prior surgery. Neurosurgery. 2002;51(4):890–904.
26. Baumert BG, Villà S, Studer G, et al. Early improvements in vision after fractionated stereotactic radiotherapy for primary optic nerve sheath meningioma. Radiother Oncol. 2004;72(2):169–74.
27. Narayan S, Cornblath WT, Sandler HM, Elner V, Hayman JA. Preliminary visual outcomes after three-dimensional conformal radiation therapy for optic nerve sheath meningioma. Int J Radiat Oncol Biol Phys. 2013;56(2):537–43.
28. Lesser RL, Knisely JPS, Wang SL, Yu JB, Kupersmith MJ. Long-term response to fractionated radiotherapy of presumed optic nerve sheath meningioma. Br J Ophthalmol. 2010;94(5):559–63.
29. Cawood T, Moriarty P, O'Shea D. Recent developments in thyroid eye disease. BMJ. 2004;329(7462):385–90.
30. Bartalena L, Marcocci C, Chiovato L, et al. Orbital cobalt irradiation combined with systemic corticosteroids for Graves' ophthalmopathy: comparison with systemic corticosteroids alone. J Clin Endocrinol Metab. 1983;56(6):1139–44.
31. Prummel MF, Mourits MP, Blank L, et al. Randomized double-blind trial of prednisone versus radiotherapy in Graves' ophthalmopathy. Lancet. 1993;342(8877):949–54.
32. Mourits MP, van Kempen-Harteveld ML, García MB, et al. Radiotherapy for Graves' orbitopathy: randomised placebo-controlled study. Lancet. 2000;355(9214):1505–9.
33. Ainsbury EA, Bouffler SD, Dorr W, et al. Radiation cataractogenesis: a review of recent studies. Radiat Res. 2009;172:1–9.

External Photon Radiotherapy for Malignant Orbital Apex Lesions

29

Jeannie Chik, K. M. Cheung, James Chow, Gavin Cheung, C. W. Y. Kong, and K. H. Wong

Abstract

Orbital apex malignancies are rare. This diagnosis must be considered whenever there is a rapidly enlarging orbital mass. Histological diagnosis is mandatory to guide treatment. Multimodality treatment is often required. Radical radiotherapy should be delivered with acceptance of higher radiation toxicities to achieve cure. For advanced or metastatic disease, treatment aim is to control symptom and maintain quality of life and to minimize toxicities. This chapter focuses on treatment approach and radiotherapy techniques for malignant orbital apex tumors including lymphoma, adenoid cystic carcinoma, direct invasion, or metastases from other primary malignancies.

Keywords

Orbital apex malignancies · Lymphoma · Adenoid cystic carcinoma · Nasopharyngeal carcinoma · Orbital apex metastases · Intensity-modulated radiation therapy · Stereotactic radiotherapy

Primary and secondary orbital malignancies are rare, and they must be considered whenever there is a rapidly or relentlessly progressive disease [1]. All significantly enlarging mass in the orbit should be biopsied to establish histological diagnosis for guiding definitive treatment. For localized malignant lesion without distant metastasis or extensive involvement of adjacent structure, the intent of treatment is mainly curative. The key purpose of radiotherapy is for eradication of all the malignant cells if technically feasible. The treatment margins should be adequate to cover subclinical diseases, while the total radiation dose should be high enough to achieve the curative purpose according to the radiosensitivity of the lesions. A higher risk of radiation side effects is acceptable.

However, for those with locally extensive malignant lesions beyond cure or when distant metastases existing, the intent of radiotherapy is mainly palliative. The treatment becomes focus on symptom control and quality of life. Significant acute radiotherapy complications should be avoided.

29.1 Lymphoma

Background. Lymphoma accounts for over 50% of orbital malignancies [2]. It can be either localized or part of an advanced stage disease. Systemic therapy (with chemotherapy and/or targeted therapy) is the main treatment modality of the latter with use of radiotherapy as palliation or consolidation treatment. This section focuses on primary orbital lymphoma.

Primary orbital lymphoma accounts for around 1% of all non-Hodgkin's lymphoma [3]. Majority of orbital lymphoma is due to Mucosa-Associated Lymphoid Tissue lymphoma (MALT lymphoma or MALToma) [4]; less frequent histology includes diffuse large B cell lymphoma or NK/T cell lymphoma. Risk factors for orbital MALToma include advanced age (median age at around 60 years old), immunosuppression and chlamydia psittaci infection [5]. Common presentations include salmon-red patch for conjunctival involvement, mass, exophthalmos, ophthalmoplegia, and visual disturbances. If there is presence of systemic involvement, patients may have palpable lymph nodes, B symptoms (e.g., fever, night sweats, weight loss), and hepatosplenomegaly.

Approach. Before formulating the treatment, complete workup should be conducted for diagnosis, staging, and fitness for various treatments. These include blood tests

J. Chik (✉) · K. M. Cheung · J. Chow · G. Cheung · C. W. Y. Kong
K. H. Wong
Department of Clinical Oncology, Queen Elizabeth Hospital, Hong Kong SAR, China
e-mail: cyk632@ha.org.hk

T. L. POON et al. (eds.), *Orbital Apex and Periorbital Skull Base Diseases*, https://doi.org/10.1007/978-981-99-2989-4_29

(complete blood count, biochemistry, hepatitis, and HIV status), bone marrow examination, and imaging of the orbital region (CT or MRI orbit) and the trunk (CT neck, thorax, abdomen, and pelvis). Figure 29.1 shows an example of MRI appearance of a patient diagnosed with right orbital MALToma involving the orbital apex. Although gaining popularity, PET/CT does not have a high sensitivity to MALToma [6] and other low-grade lymphomas due to slow-growing nature of these lesions; it should be done when high grade or advanced stage lymphoma is suspected.

Biopsy is crucial to identify the histology of the disease, which may have an impact on treatment. Fine needle aspiration is not preferred, as it lacks information of cellular architecture and adequate tissue for flow cytometry or additional immunohistochemistry [7]. On the other hand, complete excision is not required, as it is difficult to achieve adequate margins without causing significant morbidity. Ophthalmologist should be engaged in monitoring disease-related vision impairment and treatment-induced morbidity.

Management. Radiotherapy using three-dimensional technique with conventional fractionation is the primary treatment of choice for primary localized low-grade orbital lymphoma. Patient will be treated in supine position with the head immobilized with a thermoplastic cast. CT simulation will be done in treatment position, and registration of the planning CT images with previous diagnostic imaging studies should be done to ensure accurate delineation of the gross tumor. A wax may be placed in front of the eye as a bolus to allow building up of adequate radiation dose to the target. The gross tumor volume (GTV) includes the disease identified radiologically and clinically; yet invariably, the clinical target volume (CTV) would cover the whole orbit constrained to the bone [8], as multifocal microscopic disease is not uncommon for MALToma. An exception would be conjunctival MALToma, in which good disease control can be achieved even with radiotherapy to the disease site alone with adequate margin [9]. A further expansion of 3–5 mm is adopted to generate the planning target volume (PTV), accounting for setup errors. A total dose of 24 Gy in 12 daily fractions would be given for MALToma and other low-grade lymphomas [10]. High-grade lymphomas involving the orbitare usually treated with combined modality treatment using chemotherapy and radiotherapy. Radiation dose for high-grade lymphomas ranges from 30 to 40 Gy in 2 Gy per fraction, and dosage also takes into account the aggressiveness of disease and their response to chemotherapy [11].

The main principle of radiotherapy beam arrangement is to deliver radiotherapy dose conformally while minimizing doses to neighboring structures. Conformal 3-D radiotherapy or intensity-modulated radiotherapy (IMRT) should be the state-of-the-art treatment [11]. Common beam arrangements for conformal radiation technique would include anterior oblique and lateral oblique wedged pairs as illustrated in Fig. 29.2, or non-coplanar superior-inferior oblique beam pairs.

Outcomes of radiotherapy for primary orbital MALToma is excellent, with the local control rate over 90% [12]. Side effects of radiotherapy include conjunctivitis, dry eyes, and cataract; otherwise, the radiotherapy dose is within tolerance of many neighboring critical structures such as retina, optic nerve and chiasm, brain stem, and temporal lobe.

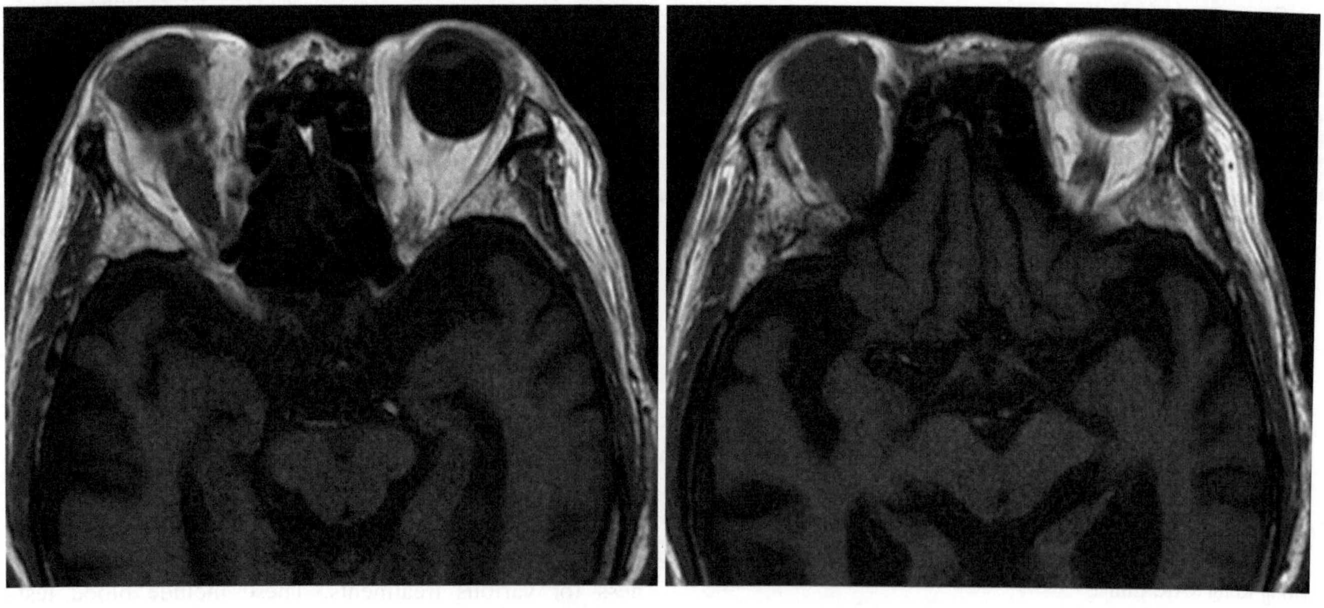

Fig. 29.1 MRI axial cuts of a patient having right orbital MALToma involving the orbital apex

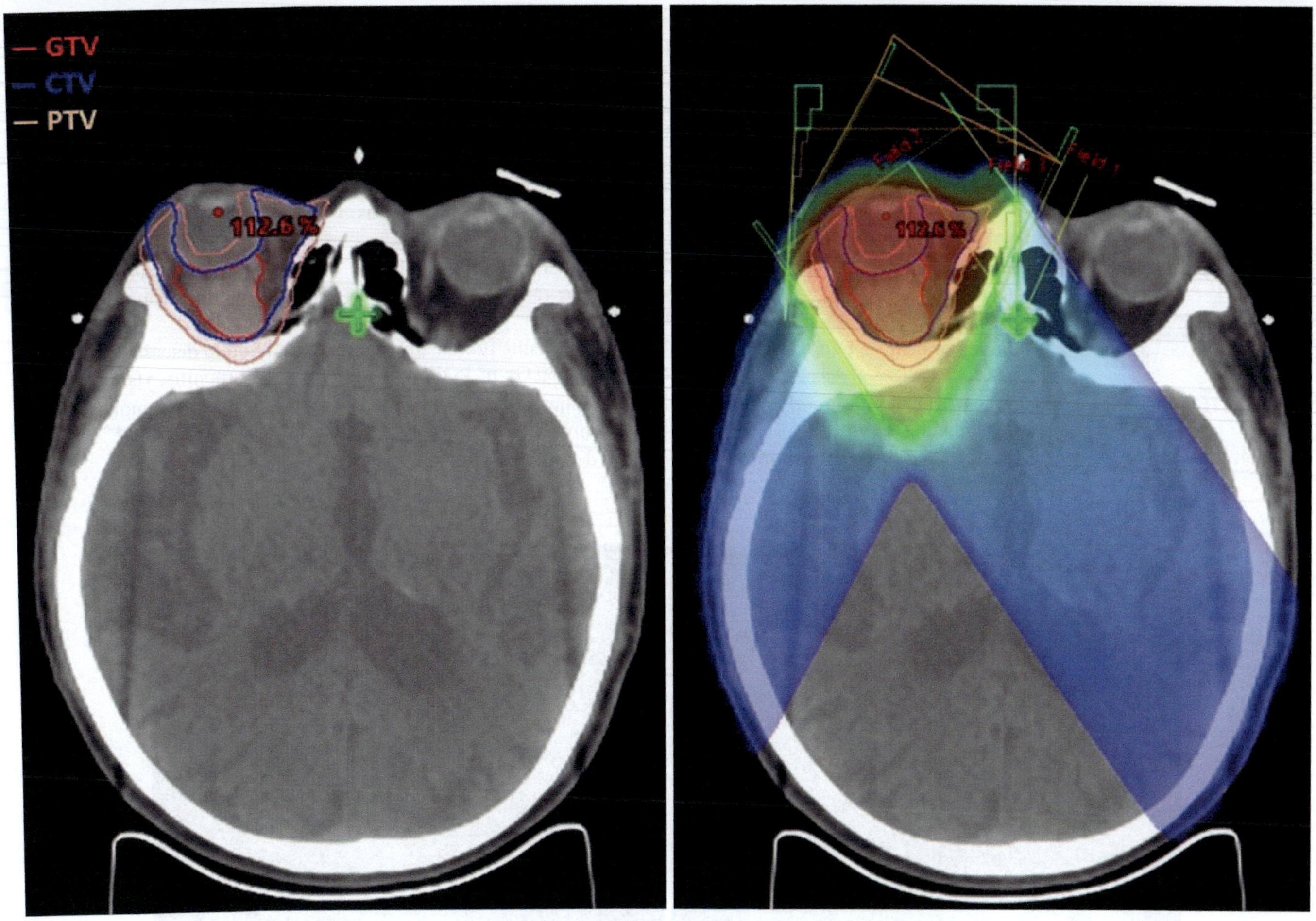

Fig. 29.2 Target volumes (left) and beam arrangement (right) of radiotherapy for the same patient in Fig. 29.1 with right orbital MALToma

29.2 Primary Orbital Apex Malignant Tumors

29.2.1 Adenoid Cystic Carcinoma

Orbital adenoid cystic carcinoma (ACC) accounts for approximately 1–4% of orbital tumors and usually arises from the lacrimal gland [13, 14]. Orbital ACC without lacrimal gland involvement is rare and assumed to arise from the ectopic lacrimal gland tissue within the medial orbit [15, 16]. Only six cases have been reported in the literature (Table 29.1). Patients usually presents with decreased visual acuity and proptosis (Table 29.1). MRI often shows an orbital apex mass mimicking optic nerve sheath meningioma [13, 19]. Diagnosis should be confirmed with a biopsy. The disease course tends to be aggressive with propensity of bony erosion and perineural spread to skull base and intracranial region [20, 21]. Although this entity is rare, one should have a high index of suspicion when approaching an orbital apex mass, given the aggressive nature of disease needing multimodality treatment.

Multimodality treatment approach is required in most cases, with surgical removal followed by adjuvant radiotherapy or chemotherapy [13–15]. In inoperable cases such as those with intracranial extension, radical radiotherapy up to 70 Gy with or without concurrent chemotherapy is recommended. Postoperative radiotherapy has been shown to reduce local recurrence [22]. Given the scant number of reported cases in the literature, we have the opportunity of encountering an ACC of the orbital apex, which was treated using primary radical radiotherapy, as illustrated in Figs. 29.3 and 29.4.

Table 29.1 Six reported cases of orbital ACC without lacrimal gland involvement

Case report	Age, sex	Presenting symptoms	Location of tumor	Treatment given	Outcome
Shields 1997 [17]	26, M	Orbital mass	Nasal aspect of the left orbit	Orbital exenteration followed by postoperative radiotherapy (64.8 Gy, number of fractions not reported)	Remained well at 6 months post treatment, no recurrence
Lin 2008 [15]	60, F	Headache, orbital fullness	Inferior orbit	Orbital exenteration followed by adjuvant radiotherapy (dose not reported) and chemotherapy using paclitaxel plus cisplatin for 2 cycles	Not reported
Venkitaraman 2008 [14]	51, M	Vision impairment, proptosis, headache	Left orbital apex	Orbital exenteration followed by postoperative radiotherapy (50 Gy in 25 daily fractions)	Alive and stable after treatment (duration not reported)
Walsh 2013 [13]	53, F	Vision impairment	Left orbital apex	Radiotherapy using proton and photon to a total dose of 70 Gy in 35 daily fractions	Stable disease at 13 months, vision static
Li 2016 [16]	70, F	Vision impairment, left facial numbness	Left orbital apex	Orbital exenteration, followed by radiotherapy (60 Gy in 30 daily fractions)	Stable at 18 months
Muttagi 2017 [18]	38, F	Headache, proptosis, diplopia	Right retro-orbit	Surgical decompression	Not reported

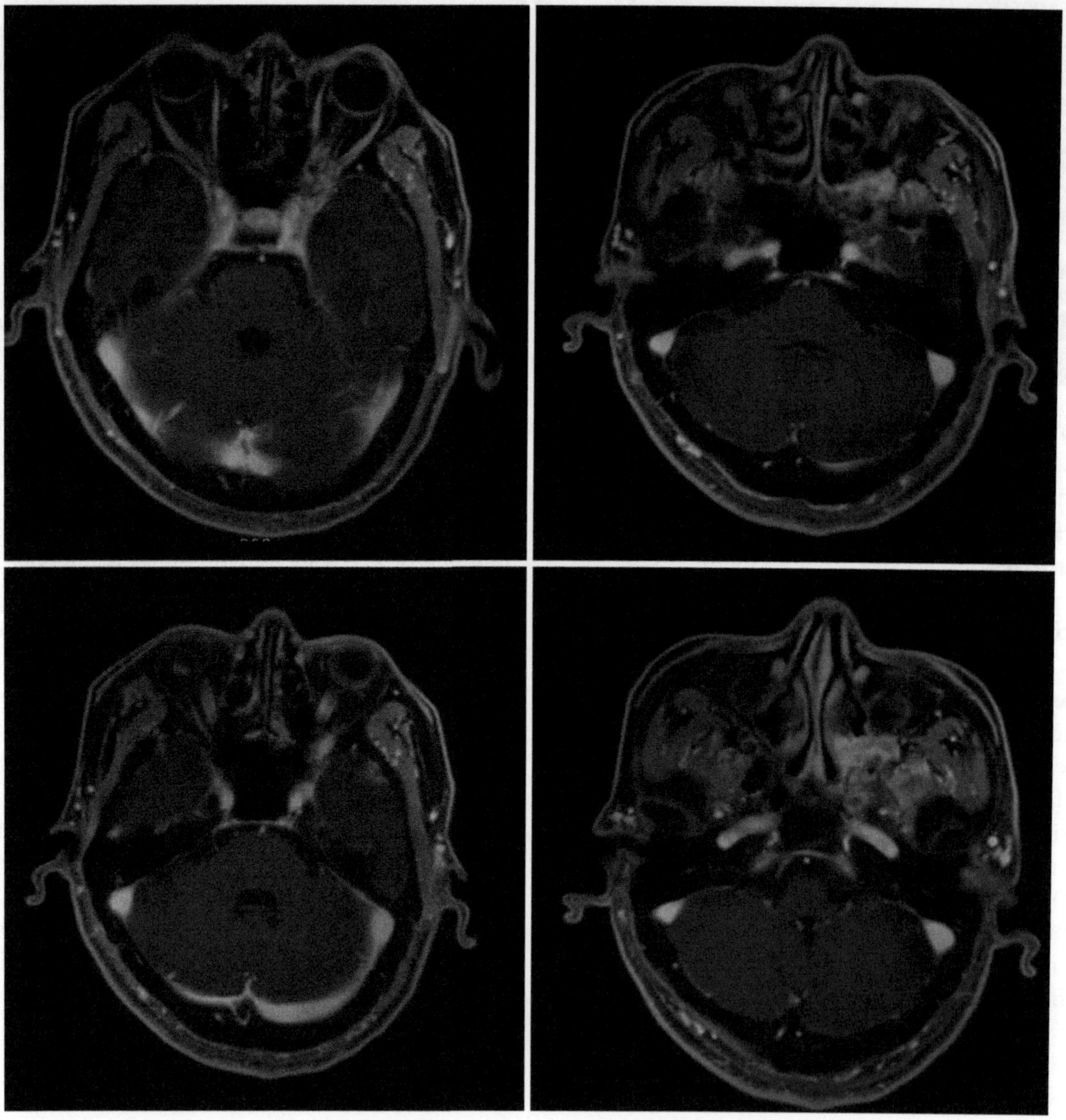

Fig. 29.3 A 55-year-old gentleman presented with progressive left visual loss. CT brain and orbit showed an abnormal mass at the left orbital apex with compression onto the left optic nerve and left extra-ocular muscles. Left optic canal decompression was performed and biopsy of the mass showed adenoid cystic carcinoma. MRI showed an infiltrative mass at the left orbital apex. Superiorly, it was distorting the left optic canal and compressing the left optic nerve. Posteriorly, it showed intracranial extension to the left cavernous sinus. Inferiorly, it extended to the left pterygomaxillary fissure. Medially, it invaded the left nasal cavity

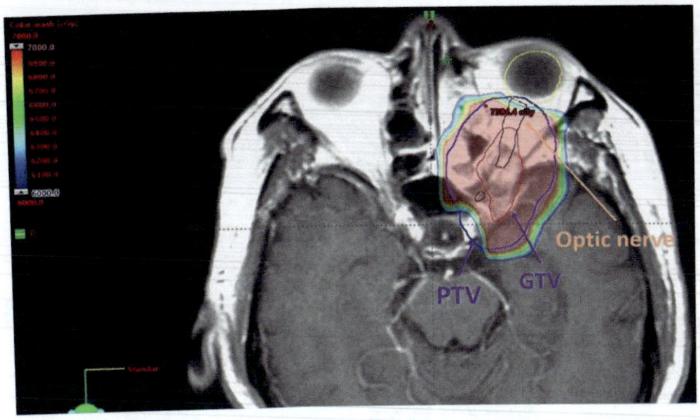

Fig. 29.4 The patient with primary ACC of the orbital apex, mentioned in Fig. 29.3 received a course of radical radiotherapy using IMRT with a total dose of 70 Gy given in 35 daily fractions to PTV and intended for a sacrifice left eye treatment

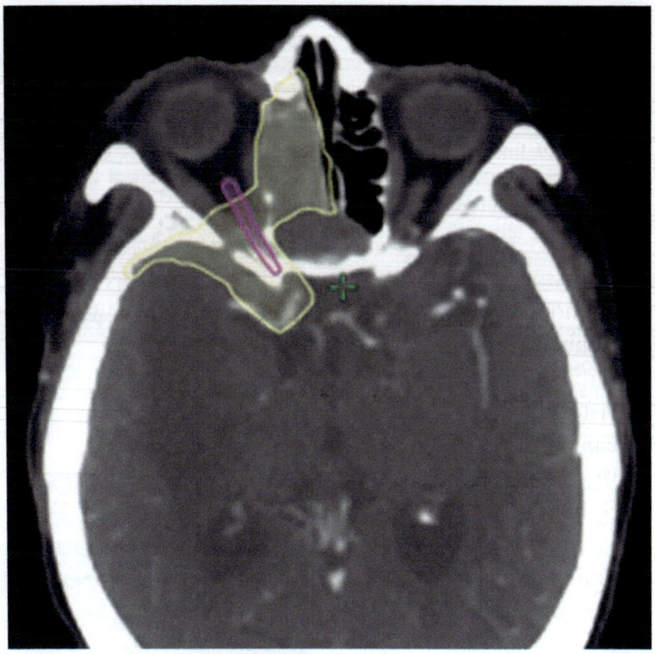

Fig. 29.5 Case of locally advanced NPC with direct extension to right orbital apex. This patient presented with right visual loss and ophthalmologic assessment confirmed right optic neuropathy. The right optic nerve (purple) transverses within the gross tumor volume (GTV) of the nasopharyngeal tumor (yellow)

29.3 Malignant Lesions Extended from Adjacent Tissue: Nasopharyngeal Carcinoma

Background. Nasopharyngeal carcinoma (NPC) is an endemic cancer in East and Southeast Asia. Chemoradiotherapy is the standard of care for loco-regionally advanced disease [23]. Given the central location of the primary nasopharyngeal tumor and its proximity to the base of skull, direct extension to the orbital apex is possible in advanced diseases. Anatomically, the route of local infiltration for NPC often takes a step-wise path of low tissue resistance: starting from the nasopharyngeal mucosa at the fossa of Rossenmuller, extends to the pterygopalatine fossa through sphenopalatine foramen, and then spreads superiorly via inferior orbital fissure and further reaches orbital apex [24]. Spread pattern analyses from large NPC cohorts have reported a 3.9% incidence of orbital involvement, whereas 1.1% of tumors were found to invade the orbital apex at diagnosis [25, 26]. Consequent to the infiltration of optic nerve, approximately 1% of all NPC patients present with optic neuropathy, which often co-manifest with other cranial neuropathies—typically the III, V, VI, and XII nerves [27]. Despite the generally radio- and chemo-sensitive nature of NPC, prognosis of NPC patients who have orbital involvement is worse than other less advanced counterparts. In a territory-wide cohort from Hong Kong, which included patients exclusively treated with intensity-modulated radiotherapy, the estimated 5-year local failure-free survival and 5-year progression-free survival for patients with T4 tumors were 76% and 52%, respectively, in stark contrast to 90% and 70% in patients with T3 tumors [28].

Management. Management of non-metastatic NPC with orbital apex involvement is challenging. Current international guidelines recommend treating gross nasopharyngeal tumor to a dose of 70 Gy equivalent [29], and radiation dose lower than 66.5 Gy have been shown to compromise local control [30]. This tumoricidal radiation dose is significantly higher than the typical safety constraints for optic nerve, and optic chiasm (e.g., maximum dose of 54 Gy) hence represents a treatment dilemma for radiation oncologists and dosimetrists (Fig. 29.5). In order to maximize the chance of tumor control, optic constraints on the involved side may be loosened at treatment planning (Fig. 29.6). Such an approach represents a trade-off between the risk of mono-ocular visual impairment versus disease control and should be adopted after detailed discussion with patients weighing in their individual views and preferences. Importantly, it should be emphasized that the dose-toxicity relationship for radiation optic neuropathy holds a sigmoidal function; therefore, extra effort should be made at radiotherapy planning to minimize hotspots within the traversing optic nerve, especially in cases where it is embedded within high-dose target volume.

Another widely adopted treatment strategy for advanced NPC is induction chemotherapy. In recent years, multiple randomized trials have confirmed the dosimetric and survival advantage of giving additional chemotherapy before definitive chemoradiotherapy [31–33]. Given the highly promising response rates of 80–90%, induction chemotherapy can induce early tumor shrinkage within the crowded

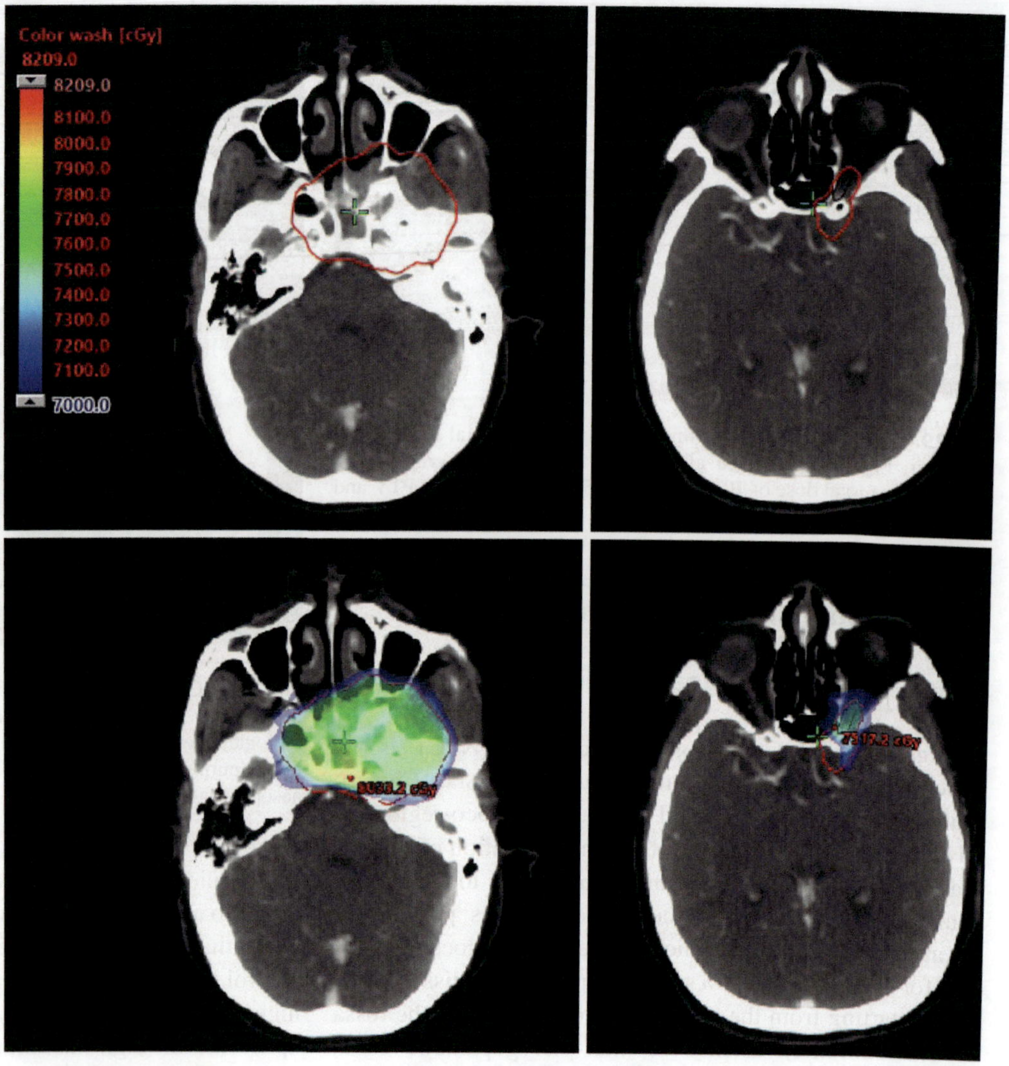

Fig. 29.6 Case of locally advanced NPC with direct extension to left orbital apex. Red line indicates high-dose planning target volume (PTV) 70 Gy. Black line highlighted the left optic nerve. This patient consented for loosening the left optic nerve radiation dose constraint in exchange for optimal target coverage. The left optic nerve, which situated within high-dose PTV, received a maximal point-dose of 73.2 Gy. He remained disease-free with normal vision for 6 years after induction chemotherapy followed by concurrent chemo-radiotherapy

orbital apex, thereby hastening the recovery of optic neuropathy [34]. Following tumor shrinkage after induction chemotherapy, recent randomized evidence also supported de-escalation of radiotherapy volumes based on post-chemotherapy disease extents [35]. When carefully executed, this approach may help reduce the risk of radiation optic neuropathy without affecting treatment effect. Long-term efficacy and safety data are eagerly awaited.

29.4 Orbital Apex Metastases

Background. Among intraocular tumors, metastases account for 1–13% of all orbital tumors [36]. Choroidal metastases are more common due to the rich vascular supply [37, 38]. Extraocular orbit metastases are rare and occur less frequently [39]. The prevalence of extraocular orbital metastases in cancer patients is 2–4.7% [36]. Breast and lung cancers are the common malignancies which causes orbital metastases [37, 38].

Management. Common presenting symptoms include periorbital mass, proptosis, diplopia, decreased vision, and pain [36]. Studies have shown that early treatment could give higher chance of preservation of vision [40]. Hence, when there is a high index of suspicion, timely recognition and delivery of treatment is warranted. In cases where a solitary metastasis to the orbit with no other primary sites identified, biopsy may be necessary [41]. CT or MRI of orbit should be performed and often shows a retro-orbital mass. Treatment is aimed both at preserving vision and improving symptom control for the remainder of the patient's life. External beam radiotherapy (EBRT) has been shown to be effective with minimal toxicity [42–47]. With the advancement of new and effective systemic therapies, radiotherapy should be delivered in conjunction with appropriate systemic treatment to achieve maximal response.

Radiotherapy Technique. Typically, radiotherapy is given by conformal technique with CT simulation with registration of the contrast planning CT with diagnostic MRI images. The gross tumor would be contoured as GTV. CTV is generated by adding 1–1.5 cm margin to GTV, cropping away from anatomical barriers. PTV margin ranges from 3 to 5 mm. Dose fractionation of 30–40 Gy in daily fractions of 2 Gy gives effective symptom palliation of 57–90% [43, 46]. In patient with poor general condition or with limited life expectancy, shorter fractionations including 20 Gy in five fractions, 30 Gy in ten fractions should be considered with comparable response achieved [40].

It has been controversial whether to irradiate bilateral orbits for unilateral orbital metastases. Rosset et al. showed that three out of 26 patients (11%) with unilateral disease developed contralateral metastases when only the involved eye was irradiated [42]. In a prospective study by the German Cancer Society (ARO 95-08), unilateral disease was treated by unilateral irradiation using a lateral field to deliver a dose of 40 Gy in 20 fractions, with the posterior contralateral choroid receiving 50–70% of the total dose (20–28 Gy) for suspected micrometastases. None of these patients developed contralateral choroidal metastasis during the median follow up time of 11.5 months [48]. The risk of retinopathy was reported in up to 5% when doses between 30 Gy in 10 fractions and 40 Gy in 20 fractions were given [46, 49]. We advocate the approach of giving radiotherapy to the affected eye only using conformal technique, which allows radiotherapy to the contralateral eye to be feasible if metastases arise in the future. Organs at risk should include the lens, optic nerve, chiasm, eyeball, and brain stem. Potential side effects include skin irritation and conjunctivitis, and patient should be treated with eyes opened to avoid permanent corneal and conjunctival damage. Figure 29.7a, b shows a conformal RT plan for a patient with breast cancer with orbital apex metastases.

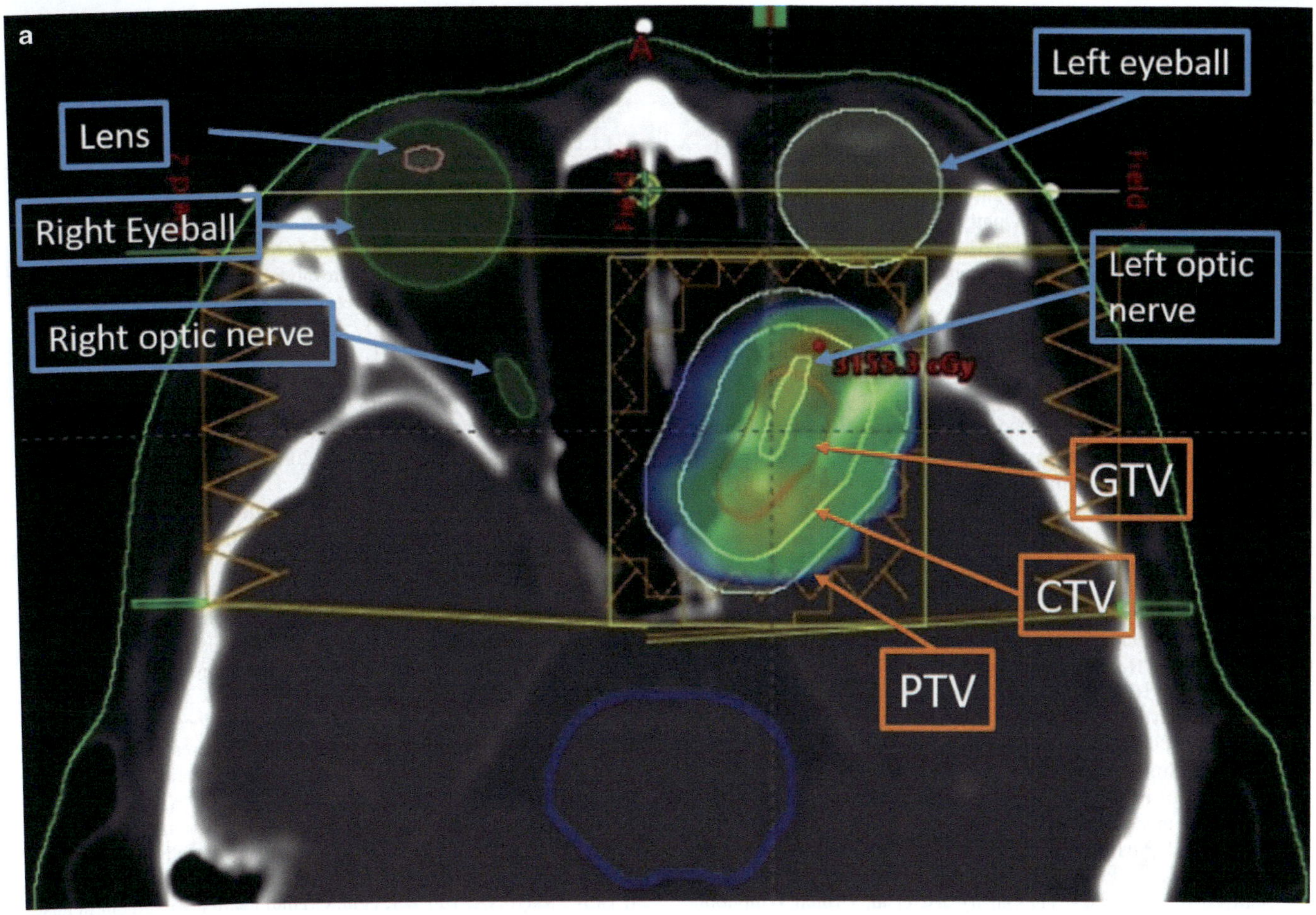

Fig. 29.7 (**a**, **b**) Case of radiotherapy to the orbital apex metastasis from breast cancer. Patient was diagnosed to have metastatic breast cancer. She presented with gradual left vision loss over 2 months. PETCT showed soft tissue density at left orbital apex with increased FDG uptake (SUVmax 5.0). The tumor adhered to the left optic nerve. Palliative radiotherapy with a total dose of 30 Gy in ten fractions over 2 weeks was prescribed. A noncoplanar beam configuration with vertical and lateral opposing field was adopted to spare radiotherapy dose to the contralateral eyeball and retina. Patients left eye visual acuity was light perception only. After radiotherapy, her vision remained static but succumbed to breast cancer 12 months later.

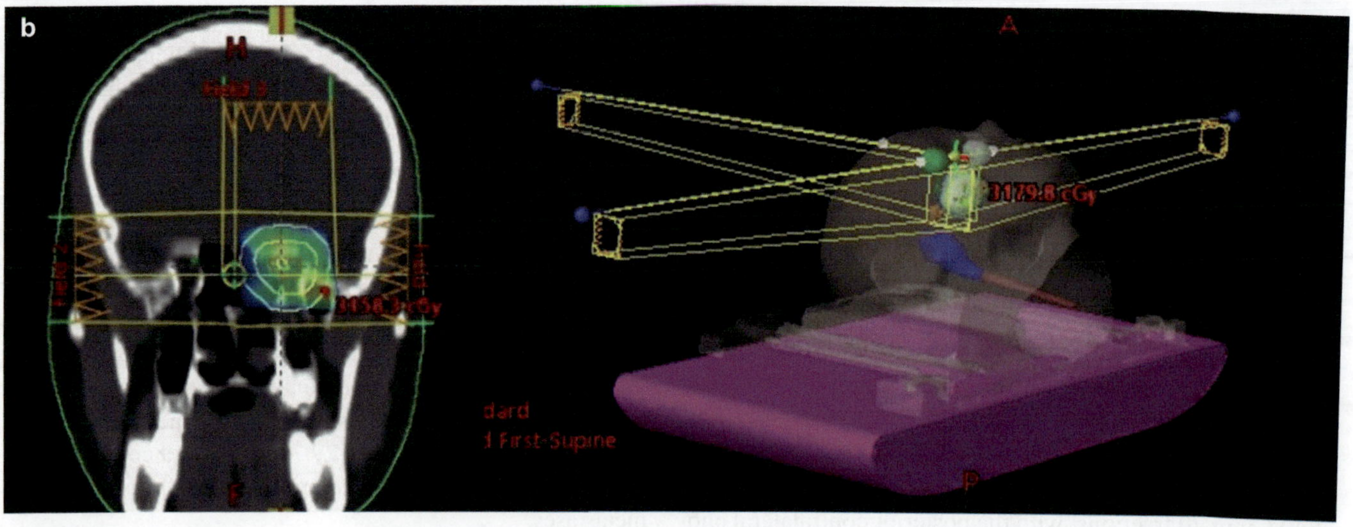

Fig29.7 (continued)

References

1. Verity HD, RE. Benign and malignant diseases of the orbit—a review. J Biomed Clin Res. 2011;4:3–16.
2. Margo CE, Mulla ZD. Malignant tumors of the orbit. Analysis of the Florida Cancer Registry. Ophthalmology. 1998;105:185–90.
3. Eckardt AM, Lemound J, Rana M, et al. Orbital lymphoma: diagnostic approach and treatment outcome. World J Surg Oncol. 2013;11:73.
4. Fung CY, Tarbell NJ, Lucarelli MJ, et al. Ocular adnexal lymphoma: clinical behavior of distinct World Health Organization classification subtypes. Int J Radiat Oncol Biol Phys. 2003;57:1382–91.
5. Stefanovic A, Lossos IS. Extranodal marginal zone lymphoma of the ocular adnexa. Blood. 2009;114:501–10.
6. Perry C, Herishanu Y, Metzer U, et al. Diagnostic accuracy of PET/CT in patients with extranodal marginal zone MALT lymphoma. Eur J Haematol. 2007;79:205–9.
7. Hehn ST, Grogan TM, Miller TP. Utility of fine-needle aspiration as a diagnostic technique in lymphoma. J Clin Oncol. 2004;22:3046–52.
8. Hoskin PJ, Diez P, Gallop-Evans E, et al. Recommendations for radiotherapy technique and dose in extra-nodal lymphoma. Clin Oncol (R Coll Radiol). 2016;28:62–8.
9. Binkley MS, Hiniker SM, Donaldson SS, et al. Partial orbit irradiation achieves excellent outcomes for primary orbital lymphoma. Pract Radiat Oncol. 2016;6:255–61.
10. Lowry L, Smith P, Qian W, et al. Reduced dose radiotherapy for local control in non-Hodgkin lymphoma: a randomised phase III trial. Radiother Oncol. 2011;100:86–92.
11. Yadav B, Sharma S. Orbital lymphoma: role of radiation. Indian J Ophthalmol. 2009;57:91–7.
12. Stafford SL, Kozelsky TF, Garrity JA, et al. Orbital lymphoma: radiotherapy outcome and complications. Radiother Oncol. 2001;59:139–44.
13. Walsh RD, Vagefi MR, McClelland CM, et al. Primary adenoid cystic carcinoma of the orbital apex. Ophthalmic Plast Reconstr Surg. 2013;29:e33–5.
14. Venkitaraman R, Madhavan J, Ramachandran K, et al. Primary adenoid cystic carcinoma presenting as an orbital apex tumor. Neuroophthalmology. 2008;32:27–32.
15. Lin SC, Kau HC, Yang CF, et al. Adenoid cystic carcinoma arising in the inferior orbit without evidence of lacrimal gland involvement. Ophthalmic Plast Reconstr Surg. 2008;24:74–6.
16. Li B, Iordanous Y, Wang Y, et al. Adenoid cystic carcinoma presenting as an orbital apex mass with intracranial extension. Can J Ophthalmol. 2016;51:e65–7.
17. Shields JA, Shields CL, Eagle RC, et al. Adenoid cystic carcinoma developing in the nasal orbit. Am J Ophthalmol. 1997;123:398–9.
18. Muttagi VK, Gairola M, Ahlawat P, et al. Rare presentation of adenoid cystic carcinoma presenting as retro-orbital mass: a case report. Ophthalmology. 2017;1:28–31.
19. Morioka T, Matsushima T, Ikezaki K, et al. Intracranial adenoid cystic carcinoma mimicking meningioma: report of two cases. Neuroradiology. 1993;35:462–5.
20. Kostick DA, LJ. Lacrimal gland tumors. In: Tasman W, JE, editor. Duane's clinical ophthalmology. 20th ed. Philadelphia: Lippincott Williams and Wilkins.
21. McDonald HR, Char DH. Adenoid cystic carcinoma presenting as an orbital apex syndrome. Ann Ophthalmol. 1985;17:757–9.
22. Brada M, Henk JM. Radiotherapy for lacrimal gland tumours. Radiother Oncol. 1987;9:175–83.
23. Chen YP, Chan ATC, Le QT, et al. Nasopharyngeal carcinoma. Lancet. 2019;394:64–80.
24. Dubrulle F, Souillard R, Hermans R. Extension patterns of nasopharyngeal carcinoma. Eur Radiol. 2007;17:2622–30.
25. Liang SB, Sun Y, Liu LZ, et al. Extension of local disease in nasopharyngeal carcinoma detected by magnetic resonance imaging: improvement of clinical target volume delineation. Int J Radiat Oncol Biol Phys. 2009;75:742–50.
26. Li WF, Sun Y, Chen M, et al. Locoregional extension patterns of nasopharyngeal carcinoma and suggestions for clinical target volume delineation. Chin J Cancer. 2012;31:579–87.
27. Li JC, Mayr NA, Yuh WT, et al. Cranial nerve involvement in nasopharyngeal carcinoma: response to radiotherapy and its clinical impact. Ann Otol Rhinol Laryngol. 2006;115:340–5.
28. Au KH, Ngan RKC, Ng AWY, et al. Treatment outcomes of nasopharyngeal carcinoma in modern era after intensity modulated radiotherapy (IMRT) in Hong Kong: a report of 3328 patients (HKNPCSG 1301 study). Oral Oncol. 2018;77:16–21.

29. Lee AW, Ng WT, Pan JJ, et al. International guideline for the delineation of the clinical target volumes (CTV) for nasopharyngeal carcinoma. Radiother Oncol. 2018;126:25–36.
30. Ng WT, Lee MC, Chang AT, et al. The impact of dosimetric inadequacy on treatment outcome of nasopharyngeal carcinoma with IMRT. Oral Oncol. 2014;50:506–12.
31. Zhang Y, Chen L, Hu GQ, et al. Gemcitabine and cisplatin induction chemotherapy in nasopharyngeal carcinoma. N Engl J Med. 2019;381:1124–35.
32. Sun Y, Li WF, Chen NY, et al. Induction chemotherapy plus concurrent chemoradiotherapy versus concurrent chemoradiotherapy alone in locoregionally advanced nasopharyngeal carcinoma: a phase 3, multicentre, randomised controlled trial. Lancet Oncol. 2016;17:1509–20.
33. Cao SM, Yang Q, Guo L, et al. Neoadjuvant chemotherapy followed by concurrent chemoradiotherapy versus concurrent chemoradiotherapy alone in locoregionally advanced nasopharyngeal carcinoma: a phase III multicentre randomised controlled trial. Eur J Cancer. 2017;75:14–23.
34. Luk YS, Shum JS, Sze HC, et al. Predictive factors and radiological features of radiation-induced cranial nerve palsy in patients with nasopharyngeal carcinoma following radical radiotherapy. Oral Oncol. 2013;49:49–54.
35. Yang H, Chen X, Lin S, et al. Treatment outcomes after reduction of the target volume of intensity-modulated radiotherapy following induction chemotherapy in patients with locoregionally advanced nasopharyngeal carcinoma: a prospective, multi-center, randomized clinical trial. Radiother Oncol. 2018;126:37–42.
36. Ahmad SM, Esmaeli B. Metastatic tumors of the orbit and ocular adnexa. Curr Opin Ophthalmol. 2007;18:405–13.
37. Fernandes BF, Fernandes LH, Burnier MN Jr. Choroidal mass as the presenting sign of small cell lung carcinoma. Can J Ophthalmol. 2006;41:605–8.
38. Kreusel KM, Wiegel T, Stange M, et al. Choroidal metastasis in disseminated lung cancer: frequency and risk factors. Am J Ophthalmol. 2002;134:445–7.
39. Shields CL, Shields JA, Gross NE, et al. Survey of 520 eyes with uveal metastases. Ophthalmology. 1997;104:1265–76.
40. Chik JYK, Leung CWL, Wong KH. Palliative radiation therapy for patients with orbital and ocular metastases. Ann Palliat Med. 2020;9:4458–66.
41. Allen R. Orbital metastases: when to suspect? When to biopsy? Middle East Afr J Ophthalmol. 2018;25:60–4.
42. Rosset A, Zografos L, Coucke P, et al. Radiotherapy of choroidal metastases. Radiother Oncol. 1998;46:263–8.
43. Wiegel T, Bottke D, Kreusel KM, et al. External beam radiotherapy of choroidal metastases—final results of a prospective study of the German Cancer Society (ARO 95-08). Radiother Oncol. 2002;64:13–8.
44. Roy S, Madan R, Gogia A, et al. Short course palliative radiotherapy in the management of choroidal metastasis: an effective technique since ages. J Egypt Natl Canc Inst. 2016;28:49–53.
45. Huh SH, Nisce LZ, Simpson LD, et al. Proceedings: value of radiation therapy in the treatment of orbital metastasis. Am J Roentgenol Radium Ther Nucl Med. 1974;120:589–94.
46. Rudoler SB, Corn BW, Shields CL, et al. External beam irradiation for choroid metastases: identification of factors predisposing to long-term sequelae. Int J Radiat Oncol Biol Phys. 1997;38:251–6.
47. Hahn E, Laperriere N, Krema H, et al. Clinical outcomes of hypofractionated radiation therapy for choroidal metastases: symptom palliation, tumor control, and survival. Pract Radiat Oncol. 2017;7:388–95.
48. Wiegel T, Kreusel KM, Schmidt S, et al. Radiotherapy of unilateral choroidal metastasis: unilateral irradiation or bilateral irradiation for sterilization of suspected contralateral disease? Radiother Oncol. 1999;53:139–41.
49. Wiegel T, Kleineidam M, Schilling A. [Choroid metastasis in a patient with adenocarcinoma of the cervix. A case report]. Strahlenther Onkol. 1995;171:539–542.

Proton Therapy for Malignant Orbital Apex Lesions

30

Chi Ching Law

Abstract

Radiotherapy for malignant orbital apex lesions is challenging because of the close proximity of organs at risk that are vulnerable to radiation damage at low- and medium-dose range. By virtue of its unique characteristic of Bragg peak, proton beam has the advantage of delivering conformal radiation dose to the tumor target and minimizing dose to the surrounding normal tissues. This chapter will review the dosimetric difference between proton and conventional photon therapies, as well as clinical studies of proton therapy for malignant tumors of the orbital apex.

Keywords

Lacrimal gland adenoid cystic carcinoma · Orbital apex · Optic pathway gliomas · Orbital rhabdomyosarcoma · Photon therapy · Proton therapy · Radiotherapy

30.1 Introduction to Proton Beam

Proton beam has distinct physical characteristic from megavoltage photon beam in conventional radiotherapy (Fig. 30.1) [1]. After a short build-up region, megavoltage photon beam exhibits an exponential attenuation of energy deposition with increasing depth in tissue. In contrast, proton beam has the unique dose deposition profile known as Bragg peak, characterized by a sharp fall-off of dose deposition at a specific depth with virtually no exit dose beyond the tumor target.

A single Bragg peak is too narrow to treat most tumors in clinical practice. By stacking multiple Bragg peaks of variable energies, a uniform dose region can be created at the depth of target volume (spread-out Bragg peak) (Fig. 30.1) [1]. Although this modulation increases the entrance dose, the spread-out Bragg peak still delivers lower doses to the normal tissue proximal to the target and no exit dose distal to the target compared with photon beam [2].

Protons are accelerated to therapeutic energies (70–250 MeV) using cyclotrons or synchrotrons [2]. An accelerated proton beam is too thin for the treatment of three-dimensional tumor targets. The thin proton beam is broadened laterally and sculpted to conform to the target volumes by two main strategies: (1) passively scattered proton technique and (2) pencil beam scanning technique.

In passively scattered proton technique, the thin proton beam is broadened laterally and longitudinally using rotating modulation wheel and one or two scatterers [2, 3]. Custom-made beam

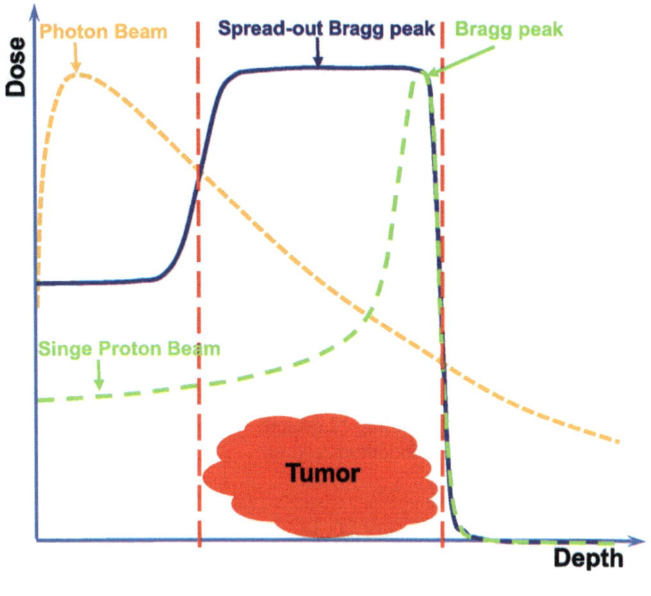

Fig. 30.1 Comparison of depth dose distribution of proton beam versus photon beam: megavoltage photon beam (dashed yellow line), single proton beam (dashed green line), and spread-out Bragg peak (solid blue line). (Adapted from Hu, M., Jiang, L., Cui, X. et al. *Proton beam therapy for cancer in the era of precision medicine. J Hematol Oncol* ***11**, 136 (2018).* https://doi.org/10.1186/s13045-018-0683-4)

C. C. Law (✉)
Department of Clinical Oncology, Queen Elizabeth Hospital, Hong Kong SAR, China
e-mail: lccz01@ha.org.hk

T. L. POON et al. (eds.), *Orbital Apex and Periorbital Skull Base Diseases*, https://doi.org/10.1007/978-981-99-2989-4_30

shaping devices (Lucite compensator and brass aperture) are required to model the beam to the shape of the target volumes.

In pencil beam scanning technique, individual proton beams are magnetically scanned across the tumor in the required location and depth [2, 3]. This technology can deliver highly conformal radiation dose to complex target without the use of patient-specific beam shaping devices. Importantly, it allows the delivery of intensity-modulated proton therapy which is a sophisticated technique of proton therapy analogous to intensity-modulated photon radiotherapy [2, 4].

30.2 Dosimetric Comparison Between Proton and Photon Radiotherapy for Malignant Orbital Apex Lesions

Dosimetric comparison examines the relative target volume coverage and radiation doses to organs at risk in different radiotherapy treatment plans. Owing to the rarity of malignant orbital apex lesions, only a handful of dosimetric studies are available in the literature comparing head-to-head between proton therapy with various photon therapy techniques (intensity-modulated, 3-dimensional conformal and lateral photon therapies) (Table 30.1). Compared with photon therapies, proton therapies achieve comparable tumor target coverage and lower radiation doses to organs at risk in the ipsilateral orbit, the contralateral orbit, and the adjacent brain.

Miralbell et al. provided an illustrative example comparing intensity-modulated proton therapy with intensity-modulated photon therapy in an optic nerve meningioma (Fig. 30.2) [8]. While achieving similar tumor target coverage, proton therapy produced relatively lower doses to organs at risk in the low- and medium-dose region.

This is of particular relevance in orbital apex because most of its organs at risk are susceptible to radiation damage even in the low- and medium-dose range. Importantly, the degree of reduction in the radiation dose to the organs at risk is clinically significant with respect to their dose constraints, potentially mitigating the risk of growth hormone deficiency, cognitive impairment, dry eye syndrome, and cataract (Table 30.2) [7]. Take lens as an example, the dose constraint for the end point of cataract is maximum radiation dose of less than 6 Gy [9]. Ladra et al. demonstrated that passively scattered proton therapy was associated with a lower percentage of patients having lens dose >6 Gy when compared with intensity-modulated photon therapy for orbital rhabdomyosarcoma (21% versus 45%) [7].

Another important finding in the dosimetric comparison study is the lower integral dose achieved by proton therapy as compared with photon therapy [7]. This advantage of proton therapy could potentially mitigate the relative risk of second malignant neoplasm (SMN) [1, 10]. Miralbell et al. estimated that the expected incidence of radiation-induced SMN could be reduced by a factor of >2 with proton therapy compared

Table 30.1 Dosimetric studies comparing proton and photon radiotherapy for malignant neoplasms of orbital apex

Study	Neoplasm (number of patients)	Comparators	Results of dosimetric comparison	
			TTC	Sparing of organs at risk
Yock et al. [5]	Pediatric orbital rhabdomyosarcoma (*n* = 7)	Passively scattered prT vs. 3D conformal phT	Comparable	Lower doses achieved with prT to: – Ipsilateral orbital structures (retina, optic nerve, orbital bone & lens) – Contralateral orbital structures (retina, optic nerve, orbital bone & lens) – Brain structures (hypothalamus, pituitary, temporal lobes & chiasm)
Fuss et al. [6]	Pediatric optic pathway glioma (*n* = 7)	Passively scattered prT vs. 3D conformal phT vs. lateral phT	Better tumor conformity with prT	Lower doses achieved with prT to: – Contralateral optic nerve – Brain structures (chiasm, pituitary gland, both temporal lobes and frontal lobes)
Ladra et al. [7]	Pediatric rhabdomyosarcoma including 12 orbital rhabdomyosarcoma	Passively scattered prT vs. intensity-modulated phT	Comparable	Lower doses achieved with prT to: – Ipsilateral & contralateral orbital structures (lens, retina, optic nerve & lacrimal gland) – Brain structures (hypothalamus, pituitary & temporal lobes) – Integral non-target dose
Miralbell et al. [8]	Orbital and paraorbital tumors (*n* = 4) including 1 optic nerve meningioma	Intensity-modulated prT vs. intensity-modulated phT	Comparable	Lower doses achieved with prT to: – Ipsilateral orbital structures (lens, lacrimal gland, retina) – Contralateral orbital structures (lens, lacrimal gland, retina & optic nerve) – Brain structures (optic chiasm, pituitary gland & brain stem) – Integral non-target dose

phT photon therapy, *prT* proton therapy, *TTC* tumor target coverage

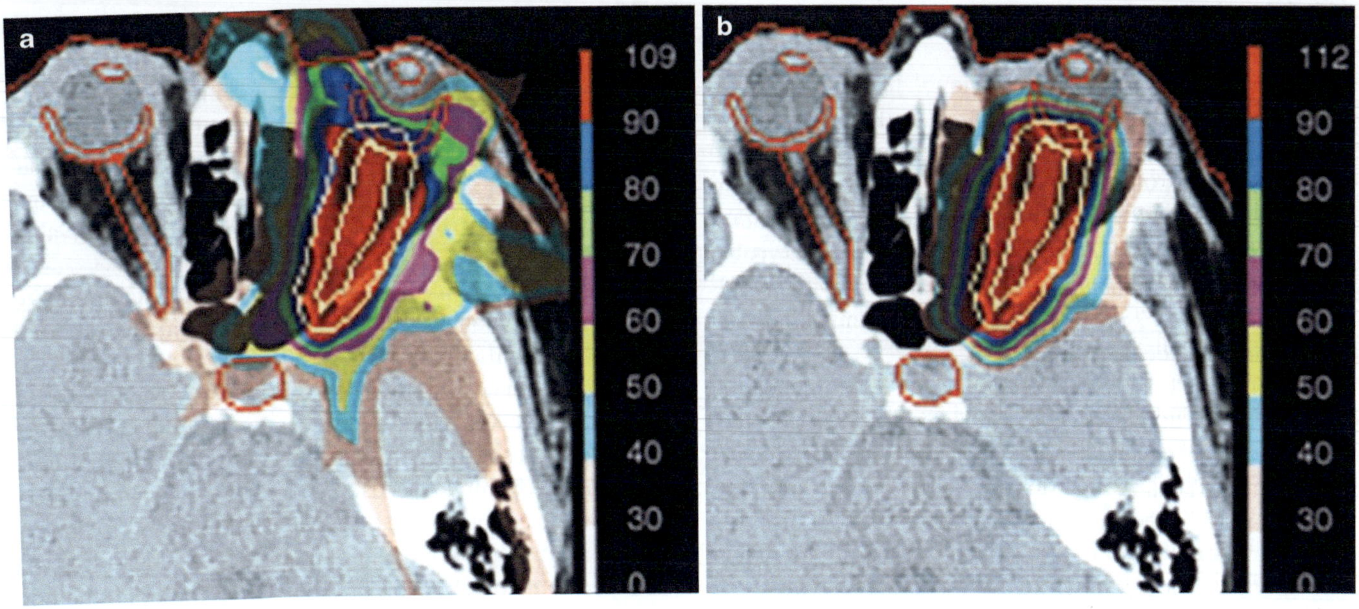

Fig. 30.2 Comparison of dose distribution in an optic nerve meningioma between (**a**) intensity-modulated photon therapy and (**b**) intensity-modulated proton therapy. (Adapted from *Miralbell R, Cella L, Weber D*, et al. *Optimizing radiotherapy of orbital and paraorbital tumors: intensity-modulated X-ray beams* vs. *intensity-modulated proton beams. Int J Radiat Oncol Biol Phys. 2000;47(4):1111-9*)

Table 30.2 Comparison of organs at risk sparing between passively scattered proton therapy and intensity-modulated photon therapy in orbital rhabdomyosarcoma

Late effects of radiotherapy	Organs at risk	Radiation dose constraints [9]	Comparison of radiation dose to organs at risk [7]		
			Dose parameters	Passively scattered prT	Intensity-modulated phT
Growth hormone deficiency	Pituitary gland	D_{mean} <25 or 30 Gy	Mean pituitary dose	4 Gy	15 Gy
Cognitive impairment	Temporal lobe	D_{mean} < 30 Gy	Mean temporal lobe V30	1.7 times higher with IMRT	
Dry eye syndrome	Lacrimal gland	D_{max} < 40 Gy	Dose >35 Gy	4% patients	15% patients
Cataract	Lens	D_{max} < 6 Gy	Dose >6 Gy	21% patients	45% patients

D_{mean} mean radiation dose, D_{max} maximum radiation dose, *prT* proton therapy, *phT* photon therapy, *V30* volume of the organ at risk receiving at least 30 Gy

with photon therapy in the scenario of para-meningeal rhabdomyosarcoma infiltrating left orbit [11]. In the study by Chung et al. including over 1000 pediatric and adult patients, a lower incidence of second cancers was found among patients treated with proton therapy compared with photon therapy [12]. This finding is echoed by another analysis, including 450,373 patients identified in the National Cancer Database, showing an overall lower risk of second cancer with proton therapy compared with intensity-modulated photon therapy [13].

30.3 Clinical Studies of Proton Therapy for Neoplasms in Orbital Apex

Based on its dosimetric superiority over conventional photon techniques, proton therapy has great potential to improve the therapeutic ratio of radiotherapy for tumors of the orbital apex. However, clinical data on the treatment outcomes and complications of proton therapy for such tumors is scarce in the literature, owing to the rarity of such tumors and the limited access to proton therapy.

30.4 Orbital Rhabdomyosarcoma

30.4.1 Background

Orbital rhabdomyosarcoma (ORM) constitutes around 10% of all pediatric rhabdomyosarcoma [14]. It mostly presents with localized disease without regional or distant spread. The commonest histology is embryonal rhabdomyosarcoma, which carries more favorable prognosis than alveolar subtype. The standard of care consists of systemic chemotherapy and local radiotherapy, with the remarkable event-free and overall survival rates at 10 years of 77% and 85%, respectively [15, 16].

30.4.2 Radiotherapy Target Volumes and Dose Fractionation

Gross target volume (GTV) 1 is defined as the visible tumor volume at diagnosis prior to any chemotherapy or surgical resection [17]. GTV1 plus a 0.5–1 cm margin gives the clinical target volume (CTV) 1 to account for potential microscopic disease. Gross target volume (GTV) 2 is the visible tumor volume after chemotherapy and/or surgery. CTV2 is defined as the GTV2 plus a 0.5–1 cm margin and all areas at risk of harboring occult spread.

The current Children's Oncology Group recommendation is to give a total dose of 45 Gy or 50.4 Gy in 1.8 Gy per fraction, depending on the tumor response to the neoadjuvant chemotherapy [18]. A total dose of 45 Gy is used for complete remission, whereas a total dose of 50.4 Gy for partial response. In case of total dose of 50.4 Gy, a volume reduction can be considered after 36 Gy for tumors having good response to chemotherapy, with the CTV2 receiving the remainder of the prescription dose.

30.4.3 Clinical Study of Proton Therapy in Orbital Rhabdomyosarcoma

In the prospective phase II study by Ladra et al. on 57 children with rhabdomyosarcoma (including 13 patients with primary ORM), all patients received chemotherapy and proton therapy [7]. The local control rate at 5-year was 92%. The 5-year event-free survival and overall survival rates were 92% and 100%, respectively. Regarding radiotherapy-induced adverse events, facial hypoplasia was noted in 8%, dry eye in 17%, cataracts in 8% patients, while no patient had endocrine abnormalities.

30.5 Optic Pathway Gliomas

30.5.1 Background

Representing 5% of pediatric central nervous system tumors, optic pathway gliomas (OPGs) occur predominately in children in their first decade of life [19, 20]. Most OPGs are low-grade, with juvenile pilocytic astrocytoma being the commonest pathology [21]. OPGs have a strong association with the tumor predisposition syndrome neurofibromatosis type 1 (NF1), with at least 30% of OPG patients having NF-1 [19]. NF-1 associated OPGs have earlier onset, more indolent clinical course and may even regress spontaneously. In contrast, sporadic OPGs are more aggressive in behavior.

The management approach for OPGs should take into consideration patient' age, symptom, NF-1 status, and the tumor extent [22]. The treatment options include observation, surgery, chemotherapy, and radiotherapy. Observation is appropriate in children who are asymptomatic or with NF-1 associated OPGs. Treatment should be initiated when there is visual deterioration. OPGs are generally not amenable to complete resection. Chemotherapy is the mainstay initial treatment, achieving 10-year progression-free survival of 44% [23].

Radiotherapy represents an effective local treatment for OPGs. Improvement or stabilization in vision was reported in 81% of patients treated by radiotherapy [24]. Good long-term overall survival rates of over 90% have been reported [25, 26]. However, radiotherapy carries significant risks of late toxicities especially in younger children, including vasculopathy (Moyamoya disease), endocrine dysfunction, neurocognitive effects, and second malignancy. Hence, radiotherapy is generally recommended in older children (>10 year old) or upon progression after multiple chemotherapy regimens [27].

30.5.2 Radiotherapy Target Volumes and Dose Fractionation

GTV is defined as the macroscopic disease [28, 29]. CTV encompasses the GTV plus 0.5–1 cm margin to cover regions at risk of microscopic tumor infiltration. The recommended prescription dose is 50.4–54 Gy.

30.5.3 Clinical Studies of Proton Therapy in Optic Pathway Gliomas

Prospective study on proton therapy by Indelicato et al. included 174 children with low-grade glioma, (diencephalon/optic pathway in 52% of cases) [30]. Chemotherapy was given before radiotherapy in 42% of patients. The therapeutic outcomes were remarkable, with 5-year local control rate of 85%. The 5-year progression-free and overall survival rates were 84% and 92%, respectively. Regarding radiotherapy-induced adverse events, grade 2 endocrine deficiency occurred in 39 patients (22%). Only 4% patients developed serious toxicities, such as brainstem necrosis, symptomatic vasculopathy, retinopathy, and second malignancy.

Hug et al. reviewed 27 pediatric patients with low-grade gliomas treated with proton therapy at Loma Linda University Medical Centre [31]. Of 7 patients with OPGs, the visual function improved in 2 patients and remained stable in 4 patients (one patient was blind prior to radiotherapy). Moyamoya disease occurred in one NF-1 associated OPG patient.

30.6 Adenoid Cystic Carcinoma of the Lacrimal Gland

30.6.1 Background

Adenoid cystic carcinoma (ACC) is the commonest malignant epithelial neoplasm of the lacrimal gland, accounting for 66% of cases [32]. The recommended treatment strategy is combined surgery and postoperative radiotherapy [33]. Advancement in imaging and radiotherapy technologies allows globe sparing approach in selected cases [34].

30.6.2 Radiotherapy Target Volumes and Dose Fractionation

In the study by Lesueur et al., the target volumes included the postoperative residual tumor, tumor bed, and the potential sites of microscopic spread [35]. Three risk level CTVs were defined as:

1. CTV1: In case of biopsy only or presence of gross residual tumor, CTV1 was defined as GTV plus 3 mm anatomical margin. In case of clear or microscopically positive resection margin, it was defined as the operative bed plus 3 mm anatomical margin. The globe and the optic nerve were trimmed from CTV1.
2. CTV2 covered the optic canal, the external wall of orbit, and the ipsilateral half of the orbit.
3. CTV3 encompassed the ipsilateral cavernous sinus.

The corresponding PTV1, PTV2, and PTV3 were formed by adding isotropic margins of 1, 2, and 3 mm to these CTVs, respectively. The prescription doses were 73.8 Gy RBE to PTV1, 63 Gy RBE to PTV2, and 54 Gy RBE to PTV3 in 1.8 Gy RBE daily fraction.

30.6.3 Clinical Studies on Proton Therapy for Lacrimal Gland Adenoid Cystic Carcinoma

Three single-institution retrospective studies reported the outcomes of lacrimal gland ACC treated with surgery and high-dose adjuvant proton therapy (Table 30.3). Majority of cases received globe-preserving surgery. Using either passively scattered or pencil beam scanning technique, proton therapy was given at a median dose of 60–73.8 Gy RBE. The local control and survival rates were promising. With the median follow-up duration of 67.4 months, Lesueur et al. reported the therapeutic outcomes of 3-year overall survival of 78% and 3-year progression-free survival of 58%. Apart from low-grade ocular and endocrinal complications, high grade skull bone osteitis and brain radiation necrosis were reported.

Table 30.3 Clinical studies on the combined surgery and proton therapy for lacrimal gland adenoid cystic carcinoma

Study	Lacrimal gland tumors (number of patients)	Treatments	Therapeutic outcomes	Toxicities
Wolkow et al. [36]	ACC (n = 18)	OT: Globe-preserving surgery RT: Passively scattered prT ± combined phT Median RT dose: 72 CGE (range 66–76 CGE)	Median FU duration of 13 years LR: 4/18 DR: 3/18	Brain damage (n = 3), retinopathy (n = 10), optic neuropathy (n = 5), cataract (n = 10), dry eye requiring artificial tears (n = 18), severe keratopathy (n = 10)
Lesueur et al. [35]	ACC (n = 15)	OT: Globe-preserving surgery (60%) or exenteration (40%). RT: Passively scattered prT in 12 patients, pencil beam scanning prT in 3 patients Median RT dose: 73.8 Gy RBE (range 64–75.6 Gy RBE)	Median FU duration of 67.4 months LR: 6/15 3-year OS: 78% 3-year local PFS: 70% 3-year PFS: 58%	Grade I-II dry eye (n = 4), grade I cataract (n = 1), grade I hyperprolactinemia (n = 6), grade I pan-hypopituitarism (n = 1), grade IV osteitis of the skull bone (n = 1), brain radio-necrosis (n = 4)
Holliday et al. [37]	Malignant epithelial tumors of orbit & ocular adnexa (n = 20) [ACC in 7 patients]	OT: Orbit-sparing surgery RT: Passively scattered prT in 4 patients, intensity-modulated prT in 6 patients Median RT dose: 60GyRBE (range 50–70 Gy RBE)	Median FU duration of 27.1 months LR: 0/12 RNR: 1/12 DR: 1/12	Grade III epiphora (n = 3), grade III exposure keratopathy (n = 3)

ACC adenoid cystic carcinoma, *CGE* cobalt gray equivalent, *DR* distant relapse, *DFS* disease-free survival, *FU* follow-up, *LR* local relapse, *OT* operation, *OS* overall survival, *prT* proton therapy, *phT* photon therapy, *PFS* progression-free survival, *RBE* relative biological effectiveness, *RT* radiotherapy, *RNR* regional nodal relapse

30.7 Summary

Owing to the unique Bragg peak characteristic with zero exit dose beyond tumor target and lower entrance dose proximal to target, proton beam can achieve superior sparing of organs at risk compared with conventional photon therapy. Orbital apex is the optimal anatomical site to explore the benefit of proton therapy, in view of the close proximity of organs at risk to tumor target. Dosimetric studies have consistently demonstrated that proton therapy can produce comparable target coverage and better sparing of critical normal structures, especially in low- and medium-dose regions. Due to the rarity of neoplasms in orbital apex and the limited access to proton therapy, published clinical data on proton therapy in treating such tumors are limited but promising.

References

1. Hu M, Jiang L, Cui X, et al. Proton beam therapy for cancer in the era of precision medicine. J Hematol Oncol. 2018;11:136. https://doi.org/10.1186/s13045-018-0683-4.
2. Mohan R, Grosshans D. Proton therapy—present and future. Adv Drug Deliv Rev. 2017;109:26–44.
3. Mohan R, Mahajan A, Minsky BD. New strategies in radiation therapy: exploiting the full potential of protons. Clin Cancer Res. 2013;19(23):6338–43.
4. Miller DW. A review of proton beam radiation therapy. Med Phys. 1995;22(11 Pt 2):1943–54.
5. Yock T, Schneider R, Friedmann A, et al. Proton radiotherapy for orbital rhabdomyosarcoma: clinical outcome and a dosimetric comparison with photons. Int J Radiat Oncol Biol Phys. 2005;63(4):1161–8.
6. Fuss M, Hug EB, Schaefer RA, et al. Proton radiation therapy (PRT) for pediatric optic pathway gliomas: comparison with 3D planned conventional photons and a standard photon technique. Int J Radiat Oncol Biol Phys. 1999;45(5):1117–26.
7. Ladra MM, Szymonifka JD, Mahajan A, et al. Preliminary results of a phase II trial of proton radiotherapy for pediatric rhabdomyosarcoma. J Clin Oncol. 2014;32(33):3762–70.
8. Miralbell R, Cella L, Weber D, et al. Optimizing radiotherapy of orbital and paraorbital tumors: intensity-modulated X-ray beams vs. intensity-modulated proton beams. Int J Radiat Oncol Biol Phys. 2000;47(4):1111–9.
9. Scoccianti S, Detti B, Gadda D, et al. Organs at risk in the brain and their dose-constraints in adults and in children: a radiation oncologist's guide for delineation in everyday practice. Radiother Oncol. 2015;114(2):230–8.
10. Hall EJ. Intensity-modulated radiation therapy, protons, and the risk of second cancers. Int J Radiat Oncol Biol Phys. 2006;65(1):1–7.
11. Miralbell R, Lomax A, Cella L, et al. Potential reduction of the incidence of radiation-induced second cancers by using proton beams in the treatment of pediatric tumors. Int J Radiat Oncol Biol Phys. 2002;54(3):824–9.
12. Chung CS, Yock TI, Nelson K, et al. Incidence of second malignancies among patients treated with proton versus photon radiation. Int J Radiat Oncol Biol Phys. 2013;87:46–52.
13. Xiang M, Chang DT, Pollom EL, et al. Second cancer risk after primary cancer treatment with three-dimensional conformal, intensity-modulated, or proton beam radiation therapy. Cancer. 2020;126(15):3560–8.
14. Shields JA, Shields CL. Rhabdomyosarcoma: review for the ophthalmologist. Surv Ophthalmol. 2003;48(1):39–57.
15. Oberlin O, Rey A, Anderson J, et al. Treatment of orbital rhabdomyosarcoma: survival and late effects of treatment results of an international workshop. J Clin Oncol. 2001;19:197–204.
16. Raney RB, Walterhouse DO, Meza JL, et al. Results of the intergroup rhabdomyosarcoma study group D9602 protocol, using vincristine and dactinomycin with or without cyclophosphamide and radiation therapy, for newly diagnosed patients with low-risk embryonal rhabdomyosarcoma: a report from the Soft Tissue Sarcoma Committee of the Children's Oncology Group. J Clin Oncol. 2011;29(10):1312–8.
17. Terezakis S, Ladra M. Pediatric rhabdomyosarcoma. In: Merchant TE, Kortmann RD, editors. Pediatric radiation oncology. Cham: Springer International Publishing Switzerland; 2018.
18. Ermoian RP, Breneman J, Walterhouse DO, et al. 45 Gy is not sufficient radiotherapy dose for group III orbital embryonal rhabdomyosarcoma after less than complete response to 12 weeks of ARST0331 chemotherapy: a report from the Soft Tissue Sarcoma Committee of the Children's Oncology Group. Pediatr Blood Cancer. 2017;64(9):10.1002/pbc.26540.
19. Dutton JJ. Gliomas of the anterior visual pathway. Surv Ophthalmol. 1994;38(5):427–52.
20. Miller NR. Primary tumours of the optic nerve and its sheath. Eye (Lond). 2004;18(11):1026–37.
21. Binning MJ, Liu JK, Kestle JR, et al. Optic pathway gliomas: a review. Neurosurg Focus. 2007;23(5):E2. https://doi.org/10.3171/FOC-07/11/E2.
22. Fried I, Tabori U, Tihan T, et al. Optic pathway gliomas: a review. CNS Oncol. 2013;2(2):143–59.
23. Gnekow AK, Falkenstein F, von Hornstein S, et al. Long-term follow-up of the multicenter, multidisciplinary treatment study HIT-LGG-1996 for low-grade glioma in children and adolescents of the German Speaking Society of Pediatric Oncology and Hematology. Neuro Oncol. 2012;14(10):1265–84.
24. Tao ML, Barnes PD, Billett AL, et al. Childhood optic chiasm gliomas: radiographic response following radiotherapy and long-term clinical outcome. Int J Radiat Oncol Biol Phys. 1997;39(3):579–87.
25. Tsang DS, Murphy ES, Merchant TE. Radiation therapy for optic pathway and hypothalamic low-grade gliomas in children. Int J Radiat Oncol Biol Phys. 2017;99(3):642–51.
26. Erkal HS, Serin M, Cakmak A. Management of optic pathway and chiasmatic-hypothalamic gliomas in children with radiation therapy. Radiother Oncol. 1997;45(1):11–5.
27. Loakeim-Ioannidou M, MacDonald SM. Evolution of care of orbital tumors with radiation therapy. J Neurol Surg B Skull Base. 2020;81(4):480–96.
28. Merchant TE, Kun LE, Wu S, et al. Phase II trial of conformal radiation therapy for pediatric low-grade glioma. J Clin Oncol. 2009;27(22):3598–604.
29. Cherlow JM, Shaw DWW, Margraf LR, et al. Conformal radiation therapy for pediatric patients with low-grade glioma: results from the Children's Oncology Group Phase 2 Study ACNS0221. Int J Radiat Oncol Biol Phys. 2019;103(4):861–8.
30. Indelicato DJ, Rotondo RL, Uezono H, et al. Outcomes following proton therapy for pediatric low-grade glioma. Int J Radiat Oncol Biol Phys. 2019;104(1):149–56.
31. Hug EB, Muenter MW, Archambeau JO, et al. Conformal proton radiation therapy for pediatric low-grade astrocytomas. Strahlenther Onkol. 2002;178(1):10–7.
32. Bernardini FP, Devoto MH, Croxatto JO. Epithelial tumors of the lacrimal gland: an update. Curr Opin Ophthalmol. 2008;19:409–13.
33. Mendenhall WM, Morris CG, Amdur RJ, et al. Radiotherapy alone or combined with surgery for adenoid cystic carcinoma of the head and neck. Head Neck. 2004;26:154–62.

34. Woo KI, Yeom A, Esmaeli B. Management of lacrimal gland carcinoma: lessons from the literature in the past 40 years. Ophthalmic Plast Reconstr Surg. 2016;32(1):1–10.
35. Lesueur P, Rapeaud E, De Marzi L, et al. Adenoid cystic carcinoma of the lacrimal gland: high dose adjuvant proton therapy to improve patients outcomes. Front Oncol. 2020;10:135.
36. Wolkow N, Jakobiec FA, Lee H, et al. Long-term outcomes of globe-preserving surgery with proton beam radiation for adenoid cystic carcinoma of the lacrimal gland. Am J Ophthalmol. 2018;195:43–62.
37. Holliday EB, Esmaeli B, Pinckard J, et al. A multidisciplinary orbit-sparing treatment approach that includes proton therapy for epithelial tumors of the orbit and ocular adnexa. Int J Radiat Oncol Biol Phys. 2016;95(1):344–52.

GPSR Compliance

The European Union's (EU) General Product Safety Regulation (GPSR) is a set of rules that requires consumer products to be safe and our obligations to ensure this.

If you have any concerns about our products, you can contact us on ProductSafety@springernature.com

In case Publisher is established outside the EU, the EU authorized representative is:

Springer Nature Customer Service Center GmbH
Europaplatz 3
69115 Heidelberg, Germany

Batch number: 10705953

Printed by Printforce, the Netherlands